Over 4,000 products reviewed, plus the latest hair care information

Don't Go Shopping
for
Hair Care Products
Without Me

Completely revised
and updated **2nd** *Edition*

*One-of-a-kind guide
to manageable, gorgeous hair
on any budget!*

PAULA BEGOUN

Best-Selling Author of
Don't Go to the Cosmetics Counter Without Me

Subscribe today to 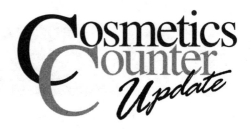 Cosmetics Counter Update

Dear Reader,

Why should you subscribe to my bimonthly newsletter? Because the cosmetics industry is always changing, and as much as I would like to tell you that **Don't Go to the Cosmetics Counter Without Me** provides ALL the product reviews you'll ever need, that simply wouldn't be the truth. There are new products and new cosmetic lines created practically every day, which is the exact reason I created *Cosmetics Counter Update*.

In each issue of *Cosmetics Counter Update* you'll find:

- **An endless array of the latest product reviews**
- **Full evaluations of new lines**
- **Answers to readers' "Dear Paula" questions**
- **Clear explanations of new research and studies**
- **Critiques of makeup techniques**
- **Hair-care product reviews**

I personally guarantee my newsletter. If you are not 100% satisfied, you will receive an immediate refund. Please give *Cosmetics Counter Update* a try. See if you, like many other readers, notice a money-saving difference in your beauty budget. I look forward to hearing from you!

Warmest regards,

Paula Begoun

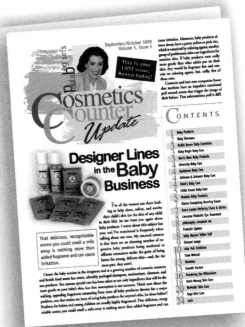

Cosmetics Counter Update:
Beauty and Brains

Finally, a newsletter for women like you!

❏ 1 Year **Cosmetics Counter Update** (US) $25.00 _____

❏ 1 Year **Cosmetics Counter Update** (Canada) $35.00 _____

❏ 1 Year **Cosmetics Counter Update** (All Other Countries) $45.00 _____

❏ E-mail Subscription to **Cosmetics Counter Update** $12.50

    E-mail address _____ _____

❏ One-Time Introductory copy of **Cosmetics Counter Update** $ 1.00 _____

❏ **The Beauty Bible** $16.95 _____

❏ **Don't Go to the Cosmetics Counter Without Me**, 4th Edition $19.95 _____

❏ **Don't Go Shopping for Hair Care Products Without Me**, 2nd Edition $14.95 _____

❏ Paula's Choice Skin Care brochure   **FREE**

	If your order totals	Add	
	$00.00–$20.00	$5.00	All Prices Are Listed in US Funds
Shipping	$20.01–$40.00	$6.00	
Charges	$40.01–$60.00	$7.00	**Subtotal** _____
	$60.01–$80.00	$8.00	**WA State Residents Add 8.6% Sales Tax** _____
	$80.01–$100.00	$9.00	**Shipping (for book orders only)** _____
	$100.01 and up	$10.00	**TOTAL** _____
	No shipping charges for newsletter		

❏ My check or money order is enclosed (make payable to Beginning Press and send your order to:

    Beginning Press, 13075 Gateway Drive, Suite 160, Seattle, WA 98168)

❏ Please charge my credit card (account number listed below)

Printed Name _____

Address _____

_____

Phone # _____

Signature _____

Credit Card # _____ Expiration Date _____

(Visa, MasterCard, American Express, and Discover Accepted)

Call (800) 831-4088 to order now
www.cosmeticscop.com   DG4AD

Editors: Sigrid Asmus, Kris Fulsaas
Art Direction, Cover Design, and Typography: Studio Pacific, Inc.
Printing: Publishers Press
Research Assistants: María Brown, Susan Hinkle, Elizabeth Janda, Laura Peterson, Melissa Roeder, Kathy Siegler, and Nicole Turgeon
Special Acknowledgments: Michelle Criminale of *Salon Criminale*
Special Thanks: Marco Hair Salon for Cover Photo Styling

Copyright © 1995, 2000 Paula Begoun

Publisher: Beginning Press
             13075 Gateway Drive, Suite 160
             Seattle, Washington 98168

First printing for this edition: January 2000

ISBN   1-877988-26-X
        1 2 3 4 5 6 7 8 9 10

This book is distributed to the United States book trade by:
        Publishers Group West
        1700 Fourth Street
        Berkeley, CA 94710
        (800) 788-3123

and to the Canadian book trade by:
        Raincoast Books
        8680 Cambie Street
        Vancouver, B.C. V6P 6M9
        (800) 663-5714

Publisher's Note

The intent of this book is to present the author's ideas and perceptions about the marketing, selling, and use of hair-care products. The author's sole purpose is to present consumer information and advice regarding the purchase of hair-care products. Nowhere herein does the publisher endorse the use of one product over another. The information and recommendations presented strictly reflect the author's opinions, perceptions, and knowledge of the subject and products mentioned. You may find success with a particular product that is not recommended or even mentioned herein, or you might be partial to a $50 hair-care routine. It is your inalienable right to judge products by your own criteria and standards and to disagree with the author.

More important, because skin often reacts to external stimuli, any product could cause a negative reaction at one time or another. If you develop a skin sensitivity to a hair-care product, stop using it immediately and consult your physician. If you need medical advice about your skin, scalp, or hair, it is best to consult a dermatologist or your personal physician.

Table of Contents

Contents

Contents

Contents

About the Author

I am the author and publisher of several best-selling books on the cosmetics industry. My first was *Blue Eyeshadow Should Be Illegal* (the first edition was published in 1985 and was revised four times and reprinted dozens more). In 1992 I wrote and published the first edition of *Don't Go to the Cosmetics Counter Without Me* (which is now in its fourth edition). In 1994, I wrote and published the first edition of *Don't Go Shopping for Hair Care Products Without Me*. In 1996 I wrote and published *The Beauty Bible*, which updated all of the information in my book *Blue Eyeshadow Should Be Illegal*. Altogether, I have sold over 2 million books.

I am also a syndicated columnist with Knight Ridder News Tribune Service and I have a regular column in the *New York Daily News*. Over the years, my writing has been strictly based on my earnest desire to get beyond the hype and chicanery of the cosmetics industry and to provide straightforward information that a consumer can really use to look and feel more beautiful.

Though I have studied many aspects of the cosmetics and hair-care industry over the past 20 years, I am not a cosmetics chemist, a doctor, or a scientist of any kind. My expertise is, like that of any other consumer reporter who covers such topics as food, cars, or toys, based on extensive research in the area about which I am writing. What makes my situation unique is that I also have years of personal experience from working as a professional makeup artist and aesthetician, and from selling makeup and skin-care products at department stores, salons, and my own stores. I have also worked extensively with hairstylists and hair-care formulators over the years.

I have used my reporting background to continually and extensively research the cosmetics and hair-care industry over the past 14 years. I base all my comments on comprehensive interviews with dermatologists, oncologists, chemists, and cosmetic and hair-care ingredient manufacturers, and on information I've gleaned from industry magazines and medical journals. I am constantly reviewing scientific abstracts and studies. I do not capriciously or abruptly make any conclusions. Everything I report is supported by studies and information from experts in the field. Naturally, there are many who disagree with my assertions, and I do the best I can to present other points of view whenever I can. However, I assure you that a great number of people in the industry agree with my conclusions, even if they can't do so publicly.

In many ways, I am surprised that reviewing, researching, investigating, and questioning the beauty industry is what I do for a living. But a direct course of action and purpose has led me since 1978, when I started working in the beauty industry, as I've tried to uncover the truth inside the bottles and behind the sales pitches of the skin-care, makeup, and hair-care industries.

The demand to know what works and what doesn't has grown since I wrote my first book back in 1985, mostly because the industry has grown by monstrous proportions. The number of new product lines emerging every day is sheer madness. Between infomercials, multilevel direct-marketing lines, home shopping network lines, new lines at the department stores and drugstores, and the endless parade of new product launches from existing lines, it turns out the first edition of this book was only a beginning.

The hair-care industry has gone through many changes over the years. In many ways, it has gotten more complicated as the research into hair care has increased and become more exciting. But then again, in many ways, it has stayed the same. There are only so many ingredients that can clean hair, only so many that can cling to hair and condition it, and there are even fewer options for ingredients that can keep it in place during and after styling. When it comes to skin-care formulations, a cosmetics chemist has literally thousands of ingredients to choose from that can have a positive impact on the skin. By comparison, there are only a handful of ingredients available to a hair-care chemist. In some ways that makes my job of analyzing hair-care products far easier than analyzing skin care or makeup. On the other hand, because hair styling is such a core beauty issue for most women and the variables around hair styles and preferences are so vast, it makes it that much more difficult to separate the hype and hyperbole from the honesty. We all want to have perfect hair and it must be that *next* product that will give us what we want.

My goal with this edition of *Don't Go Shopping for Hair Care Products Without Me* is to examine, evaluate, and clarify all the new hair-care data and research out there in order to help each person choose the best products possible for his or her specific needs.

The amazing number of letters I receive from women asking me to continue doing what I'm doing and the wonderful thank-you letters I receive daily are gratifying and encouraging. Sometimes I absolutely need the encouragement. The beauty industry, as you can well imagine, is not often a friendly place for me. Perhaps the most difficult part for me is keeping a straight face when I hear the crazy things said about hair-care products. Combating this endless parade of useless and bizarre information can be maddening. But it's my job and, thankfully, it has been far more rewarding than I ever expected.

How I Do My Reviews

If you've ever felt uncertain about a hair-care product, or didn't have the time, energy, or ingredient knowledge to figure out which shampoos wouldn't build up on your hair, which conditioners would really make coarse, dry hair feel silky and soft, which hairsprays didn't create helmet hair, which gels didn't flake or leave a sticky residue, or whether or not any of the claims on the labels were true, I hope this book will answer all those questions for you. I've also included a summary chapter of best finds and buys to create the best look for your hair type—but try not to jump to that section first. It is important to read the chapters about formulation and hair facts so you have a better understanding about what is genuinely possible for your hair and what are marketing fictions and lies. It is also important for you to read the individual product reviews so you understand *exactly* what you are buying. I might recommend 20 good shampoos for thin or fine hair, but each one might be good for a different reason.

In the product review section of this book, each product is described in terms of its reliability, value, performance, effect, and feel. Within every category of product—shampoos, conditioners, treatments, dandruff shampoos, hair serums, pomades, gels, mousses, hairspray, perms, and dyes—I have established specific criteria (I explain those criteria at length in Chapter Nine, *Product Reviews*), and I evaluate products using those strict standards. For example, a shampoo for someone with an oily scalp, according to my criteria, should be gentle but effective, contain no conditioning agents, minimal detangling agents (which can also build up on hair), and no irritants (which can cause an itchy, dry scalp). Conditioners for coarse, dry hair should leave a soft, smooth feel on the hair with no heavy or greasy after-feel. Hairsprays that claim they provide a firm hold should do just that, but not feel sticky, flake, or be hard to brush through. I relied on my 15 years of researching the hair-care industry, myriad interviews with hair-care chemists, and discussions with hundreds of hair-care professionals to help establish guidelines for the quality of every product type.

Many elements of what a product would do for hair care were evaluated by analyzing its ingredient list and comparing it to the claims made about the product. If a shampoo claims it won't strip hair color or that it is good for sensitive skin, but it contains ingredients that break down the hair shaft or irritate the scalp, it would be rated poorly and not be recommended. If a conditioner claims it can hydrate hair, then it should contain ingredients that can keep water in the hair and not dry it out with drying ingredients. If a conditioner claims it can make hair feel silky, it should contain ingredients that create that effect. If a gel or mousse claims it can hold hair in place without feeling sticky it shouldn't contain sticky ingredients. Moreover, I have made a point of challenging the inflated claims made about such ingredients as yeast, herbal extracts, botanicals, seaweed extracts, placenta extracts, vitamins, minerals, and other overly hyped ingredients. Until a company provides substantiated or peer-reviewed research conducted in vivo (meaning on a live person and not in vitro—in a petrie dish, or on animal studies alone), you should treat their claims as nothing more than snake oil and marketing artifice. I used this standard of substantiation for all product types.

While ingredient evaluations played a large part in my assessments, I also purchased over $25,000 worth of hair-care products (all of the styling products) selected from each of the 120 lines reviewed in this book. Each product was applied to hair and examined for texture and performance. If a product said it could make hair feel thicker and fuller but it didn't, then it was not recommended for that purpose. If a product said it wouldn't leave a film or sticky residue, but it did, then it was not recommended, and so on.

Hair-Care Chemists

Although I complain profusely about the way hair-care companies can invent or twist the truth about their products and about the way some cosmetics companies won't grant me interviews, I want to give my heartfelt thanks to the companies that actually do provide me with information and interviews. I know this might seem like a strange departure, given that I don't always agree with the information that I'm sent or told, but these resources are always welcomed and appreciated more than I can say. It is my intent to provide the best information possible, and whenever I can see the cosmetics industry's point of view, my reporting is that much more accurate. Granted, it often fans the flames of my ire about false claims and misleading information, but it also helps me tell consumers when and where there are wonderful products to be found.

And there are wonderful, exquisite products out there. I know I tend to emphasize the negative when it comes to crazy claims, exorbitant prices, and poor quality, but I also extol the boundless parade of superlative products. I am hardly anti-hair care! Far from it. I am in awe of how well hair-care products work. Where would we be without the brilliant work of the hair-care chemists who make the exquisite products we use? It is because of their astonishing skill that we have shampoos that effortlessly clean hair, conditioners that make hair easy to comb and silky to touch, dyes that can change hair color in a matter of minutes, perms that can alter the very structure of hair, changing curly manes to straight tresses and vice versa—and of course, glorious styling products that keep hair exactly where you want it.

I want to sincerely thank all the companies who have provided so much of their time and information to me for this book, as well as for my newsletter and my other books. We often don't see eye to eye, but despite our differences, more companies than ever have been generous and forthcoming with information and products.

I also want to thank all the hair-care chemists everywhere who strive to produce better and better products that continue to make the beauty industry so incredibly beautiful. I also want to ask those same chemists to do the best they can, whenever they can, to combat the insane marketing departments they have to work with. I know most of you don't believe even a fraction of what the advertisements, salespeople, infomercial hucksters, or editorials in fashion magazines say about the products you create. Your work is rooted in science, not hyperbole. I know this is risky business. After all, creating products that no one buys is not going to get anyone a promotion, and the marketing department knows all too well what women love to hear, no matter how ridiculous. But try anyway, just to put a bit of fresh air into an otherwise very cloudy business.

Industry Statistics

Collectively, we spend billions of dollars a year on hair. In 1998 we spent over $42 billion at the salon. According to the cosmetics industry magazine *Drug and Cosmetic Industry,* "the hottest categories are hair volumizing, thickening, and growth stimulating. Nioxin [a company known for its advertisements about increased hair growth] sold an estimated $50 million in products." For hair-care products at both the salon and the drugstore, we spent over $5 billion in the United States to help groom our tresses. How does it add up? Well, we're laying out $2 billion on shampoo; $1.4 billion on conditioners; $700 million on hairsprays; $600 million on gels and mousses; $2 billion on hair-coloring products; $150 million on men's hair products; and $400 million on permanents and hair straighteners. Add to that the money we spend getting our hair professionally cut and colored (no accurate industry figures are available, but it is estimated to be in the millions) and it's obvious we have a lot invested in trying to make our hair look good.

An estimated 50 percent of American women over the age of 25 color their hair. At least 80 percent of the technical work being done in salons concerns changing hair color or concealing gray, while only 20 percent is in the realm of permanent waves. A mere decade ago, those numbers were reversed. (I should note that salons that cater to an African-American clientele consistently perform permanent waves—for straightening hair—for approximately 85 percent of their customers, with a growing number having braiding done.) Why the radical change from permanent waves to hair coloring? In part it reflects the aging of the population. Baby boomers are turning gray, and just as they spend money fighting wrinkles, they spend money battling gray hair.

Statistics may not have much to do with your own personal hair-care needs, but they often tell companies how to approach their marketing campaigns, and that affects how you spend money. It can cost millions of dollars to introduce a new product to consumers. How a product is presented determines its success or failure. Because we are coloring our hair more and more frequently, those of us who never had damaged hair are now battling frizzies, split ends, and "growout." Those, in turn, require new products and new guarantees. Many current product innovations are aimed directly at the needs of the newly graying consumer. Aging baby boomers (I'm in this category too) need to believe that the products they are buying will protect their hair, prevent fading, slow growout, and repair the damage the chemical assault has forged.

To say that statistics drive product marketing is an understatement. Another clear example is the fact that approximately 40 percent of women in the United States complain that their hair is too fine, too limp, or too flat. Full, thick hair is the order of the day, and women feel it acutely when their hair won't behave accordingly. Cosmetics companies are very aware of this huge number because it represents such a vast segment of the hair-care buying population. The result? Scads of lines and product types promising thicker, fuller hair. Do any of these work? I'll get to that later.

CHAPTER ONE

Don't Go Shopping for Hair Care Products Without Me

Detangling an Industry

Because there are many who will take issue with the information in this book, let me state from the very beginning: I have nothing against hairstylists. In fact, just the opposite is true. I unconditionally encourage women to put their trust, tresses, and money in the hands of a talented and skilled hairstylist. In comparison to buying hair-care products, it is almost impossible to waste money on a stylist whose work you admire. Because I believe in the irrefutable value of finding a good stylist, I want to make it abundantly clear that this book does not in any way, shape, or form try to replace the expert service performed by an accomplished hairstylist.

I also want to state up front how wonderful I think many hair-care products really are. While I frequently find skin-care and makeup products that are harmful to skin, I can't often say the same for hair-care products. There are more great hair-care products than there are bad ones. It is actually difficult to find really bad or harmful hair-care products (though there are definitely those that can cause an itchy scalp; dry, flyaway hair; or allergic reactions and skin irritation). More often than not, hair-care products perform well and live up to at least some small aspect of the claim on the label (but just one small aspect can be exceedingly disappointing to the consumer).

By the same token, when it comes to the chemists formulating hair-care products, I am quite frequently in awe of what they do. Their innovations and creativity have given us a plethora of products that are nothing less than modern-day sensations. Shampoos efficiently clean hair, conditioners make it feel silky, dyes change color in an instant, perms alter its structure, and styling products allow you to keep just about any shape you can coerce out of your clean, conditioned, dyed, and styled locks. Amazing! Simply amazing!

After all this praise, you may now be wondering, if I have such deep respect for hairstylists and hair-care formulations, why would I then write a book suggesting women should only go shopping for hair-care products with me instead of trusting the recommendations of their hairstylist or the companies making hair-care products? The answer is simple: **You can't rely on the information you receive from your hairstylist or from the hair-care company that makes the products you are thinking of buying.**

The fundamental fact is that most hair-care companies don't tell you the truth about their products! Most all hair-care companies make bogus or misleading claims about what their products can and can't do, and that can hurt your hair as well as your pocketbook. Because of this industrywide deceit, it is essential for every consumer to have more objective information so we don't have to waste money or damage our hair.

What about hairstylists? After conducting hundreds of interviews, I found that most hairstylists were not intentionally trying to be misleading or purposely giving out wrong information about hair-care products. Quite the contrary; they seemed to earnestly believe what they were saying regarding what they knew about hair. Yet, more often than not, their information was wrong or ambiguous (I untangle some of these myths at length throughout this book). Unfortunately, most hairstylists are exclusively trained to cut and style hair; they are not trained to understand physiology or hair-care formulations. In fact, the only knowledge most hairstylists have about hair-care products comes directly from the hair-care companies whose products they are selling. Therein lies the problem—and I mean a really big problem. **Hairstylists are being trained by the very companies that make false or misleading claims about their hair-care products.** In place of complicated chemical analysis, hair stylists echo the very falsehoods they've been taught by the companies who provide their training, namely, the designers or salon lines that come up with a wide variety of specious justifications to warrant their overinflated prices.

Between advertising and hairstylists, there isn't much accurate information available to the consumer, and fashion magazines only make things worse. Consumers need to be very skeptical about what they read in fashion magazines. When you think about it, how often do you see an article in a fashion magazine that doesn't have something nice to say about any hair-care product, or about any cosmetics line that happens to be one of its advertisers? About as often as you see an overweight model. If an article doesn't cast a critical eye on a particular company's claims or product selection or if it buries the cautionary words in the middle of the report, be suspicious. I always love it when fashion magazines offer their lists of the "Top 100 Products Our Readers Like Best." As long as the magazine was taking the time to find out what products their readers liked best, what about the products they didn't like? There isn't a woman anywhere in the world who hasn't purchased a hair-care product she hated! Why not provide that information as well? Because fashion magazines can't do that!

The majority of fashion reporters have their journalistic hands tied by the demands of the companies that advertise in the publications for which they write. And there is little impetus to change things. If a magazine depends on advertisers, it is simply prohibitive to tick off that vital source of revenue. When cosmetics companies spend thousands or millions of dollars a year advertising in a magazine, a writer for that magazine cannot be expected to criticize that company's products and stay employed. **This commingling of editorial and advertising control results in gushing "news" stories that are little more than company publicity pieces and biased product recommendations. All the news that's fit to print—as long as it's what the cosmetics industry wants the consumer to know.**

Inasmuch as I find the technical or editorial information in fashion magazines to be prejudiced by the power of the magazines' advertisers (and therefore completely unreliable), their pictorial essays regarding the latest hairstyles or hair-color trends are nothing less than brilliant. Fashion magazines are the quintessential source for fashion news and lore, and should be consulted whenever the need arises for a fashion update. I can't imagine making a change in my hair without checking first to see what the model or celebrity I admire is wearing these days. It is when we go beyond the pictures to the product *advertorials* (not editorials, because they are hardly independent or autonomous) that the issue gets lost. By the time you are finished reading this book, you will have a better understanding of just how crazy much of the hair-care information you are receiving—from many different sources—really is.

Why Hair Is So Important

Feeling and looking beautiful is a wonderful, satisfying, joyous process as well as a state of mind in which women can revel with much pleasure and reward. Yet all the delightful and beautiful possibilities can get zapped by frustration caused by poor information and broken promises. Is there anything quite as irksome as spending $20 on a lavishly hyped conditioner or $50 on a whole new range of hair-care products, or spending anywhere between $5 (for a drugstore product) to $200 (at a high-end salon) for a new hair color or perm, only to end up with more problems than you started with and none of the changes you were hoping for? (Ironically, studies indicate that just as many women are disappointed by the hair color they receive from a stylist as they are from the products they buy at the drugstore.)

The truth is, hair care isn't easy (I wish it were effortless, but we all know better) because hair care and contemporary definitions of beauty are complicated topics.

Hair-care problems from both external and internal sources can be exceedingly technical and difficult to understand. There are over 100,000 hairs on your head. That's a lot of hair to take care of. **Also, hair isn't stagnant: it can change from day to day, depending on the weather (particularly the moisture content in the air), month to month (depending on hormonal activity), season to season (drier versus wetter months), and year to year (because hair changes radically as we get older).** And then there's the scalp's complex structure and function, which are dependent on numerous factors from hormones, health, and the environment to the products you use. All this makes it an understatement to say that hair care is a complex and multifaceted issue.

Hair biology and physiology are indeed fundamental issues, but how they affect our appearance is of vital concern. The hair on our head is one of the first things people notice about us and, whether we like it or not, it reveals to the world where we stand in terms of beauty, fashion, and age. In our culture, attentively coifed tresses are an obligatory component of beauty. For some, that means having smooth, silky, flowing tresses; for others, it can mean a precisely cut Mohawk dyed a rainbow of colors, a voluminous mane of tightly twisted curls, or perhaps a short, neatly trimmed haircut. Whatever way you go, it is the attention our hair receives that makes our product choices so important.

Two more aspects of our hair complicate matters even further. The first is that we often don't like the hair we are born with. It is either too thick, too thin, too straight, too curly, too coarse, too dry, or too *something* we don't like. Altering the genetic structure of hair is a struggle for many. The second issue is that hair displays the effects of time by turning gray or becoming thinner well before any of us want to see that happen. Trying to prevent or hide the results of that occurrence is a preoccupation for many of us. Preventing loss, hiding gray, or making hair go against its predisposed nature is technically more complicated than all the other needs of hair care combined.

True or False

There are ways to make sense of all this, but the initial step is to acquire a clear understanding of how the hair-care industry works, and then of how your hair works. The best place to start is with some basic facts so you can better differentiate between fact and fiction when it comes to your hair. If you can understand these before you go shopping for hair-care products, see another infomercial promising flawless results, have a friend introduce you to a new multilevel company selling hair-care products, or read another fashion magazine, you will have a better perspective on what you are really buying, what these products can and can't do, whether what you are using is worth the money, and, most important, whether any of them can be damaging to your hair.

Here are some of the major myths I hope you will let go of as you read this book:

Expensive hair-care products are better than inexpensive ones. (VERY FALSE)

Inexpensive hair-care products are watered down, while expensive hair-care products are more concentrated. (FALSE)

Salon products are better than drugstore products. (FALSE)

Natural ingredients are better than synthetic ones. (COMPLETELY FALSE)

Silicone is bad for hair. (1,000 percent FALSE)

You can repair damaged hair. (not humanly possible)

You can protect hair from heat damage. (not humanly possible)

You can perm and color hair without causing more damage if you wait a few weeks between treatments. (FALSE)

Hair-care products can protect your hair from damage caused by blow-dryers or styling tools. (FALSE)

Dyeing hair is dangerous and can cause cancer. (controversial, but not substantiated)

Inexpensive hair-care products can strip hair color. (FALSE)

There are hair-care products that can protect from sun damage. (FALSE)

Sodium lauryl sulfate and other hair-care ingredients can cause cancer. (FALSE)

Cosmetic hair-care products can grow hair. (ALMOST FALSE—cosmetic companies can't, but pharmaceutical companies with FDA-approved drugs can)

Here are the facts I will explain at length in the chapters that follow:

1. **According to the Food and Drug Administration (FDA) (www.FDA.gov), hair-care companies can legally lie to you.** Hair-care companies do not have to substantiate claims or prove efficacy of any kind. The only part of a hair-care product firmly regulated by the FDA is the ingredient labeling, and that is impossible for most consumers to decipher.

2. **Expensive hair-care products are not better than inexpensive cosmetics.** Women who spend more money on cosmetics do not have better hair than those with a tighter budget. (Of course, women who can afford great stylists can have great haircuts—though all women who overprocess their hair have hair like straw no matter who the stylist is.) Start reading ingredient listings, and you will notice there is little to no difference between inexpensive and expensive lines.

3.   **Believing in a hair-care line doesn't make sense.** Many expensive lines are produced by the same companies that make the inexpensive lines.

4.   **Hair-care chemists are not chained to one company, so there is no reason to believe that one company has secrets another one isn't privy to.** Plus, if the research is legitimate, it is published and accessible to everyone.

5.   **We have all bought products we disliked from expensive lines, so that should negate the belief that expensive automatically means better.** Regardless of what we empirically know to be true, the pressure from advertisements, hairstylists, and infomercials often overpowers our own knowledge. The bottom line: There are good and bad products in a wide variety of price ranges. Price is not an indicator of quality.

6.   **There is no such thing as an all-natural hair-care product.** Natural ingredients cannot clean hair, cling to hair, or perform any function of conditioning or styling. Most of the natural ingredients included in hair-care products are there for marketing purposes only and, more often than not, actually get in the way of a product's performance. There are plenty of natural ingredients that are problematic for the hair and scalp, and there are lots of synthetic ingredients you do not want to do without. It only takes a quick glance at an ingredient label to notice that names like cetrimonium bromide, methylparaben, or quaternium-16 are not natural, although they and thousands of other "unnatural" ingredients are the backbone of every hair-care product you will ever use, despite the claims you may read on the label.

     What is most insidious is the plethora of companies on the Internet making claims about "all-natural," extolling what their products don't contain, but then never providing a complete ingredient list. Do not buy a product unless you know every ingredient that's in it. A listing of only plants is always a lie!

7.   **There are no miracle ingredients that can cure your hair-care woes.** There are no patented marvels separating one product's performance from another.

8.   **When a model's hair looks beautiful in an ad or on television, it is never because of the products being used.** It is due to the hours of diligent work by a hairstylist, the photographer's talent, and lots of digital touch-ups before the picture is ever shown to the public.

9.   **What does make a great deal of difference to your hair is the kind of styling tools you use and how you use them.** Learning good styling techniques is far more worth your time than shopping for hair-care products.

10. **There are no hair-care products that can repair, fix, correct, restructure, reform, change, reconstruct, restore, rebuild, or alter damaged hair.** Hair is

dead; it cannot be repaired or permanently added on to in any way. You can no more mend a hair strand than you can mend a dead leaf or a rock.

11. **There are no hair-care products that can protect hair from heat damage.** Hairstyling tools get as hot as 350 degrees Fahrenheit, and you cannot prevent that kind of heat from harming hair. Could you imagine protecting skin from that kind of heat with a hair-care product? If you can't do it for skin, you can't do it for hair.

12. **Advertising is a one-sided game of beautiful photography and overblown claims.** It is very easy to be seduced by new advertising, new products, or a new product line that the hair-care industry produces, but "new" does not automatically mean better and the ads never make any product sound bad.

13. **Sun is damaging for hair.** There is no way around that. Sun breaks down the hair shaft, causes hair color to fade, and actually degrades the structure of hair.

14. **There are no products that can protect hair from sun damage.** The only sure-fire way to protect your hair from sun damage is to wear a hat! There are no hair-care products with an SPF rating. Until that changes, the claims about sun protection are fraudulent and completely bogus.

15. **There are no cosmetic hair-care products that can make hair grow.** None, period! However, this does not include Rogaine (minoxidil), which is not a cosmetic; it is a pharmaceutical with radically different FDA testing and substantiation requirements.

16. **Please think twice (or change channels) when buying products from an infomercial or from a home shopping network.** These are long, overextended ads, nothing more. No matter how wonderful they make their products sound, you are receiving a bizarrely one-sided point of view. Each "show" is more glorious and spectacular than the next, and what you choose to believe is based on how seduced you are by the claims and the enthusiastic responses of the participants. Clearly the producers of the infomercial are not going to include people who have a contradictory or dissenting point of view.

17. **Terms and phrases like "hypoallergenic," "dermatologist tested," "exclusive formula," "all natural," and all other unsupported generalizations about a product are simply untrue.** Remember the number-one fact! According to the FDA, hair-care companies do not have to prove their claims. There are no FDA guidelines or specifications for any of these marketing labels.

Does Expensive Mean Better?

The number-one myth you need to come to terms with is the notion that expensive or salon hair-care products are somehow superior to drugstore versions. Before I can convince you of what you probably already suspect I'm building up to, I want to explain how to separate perceptions, emotional reactions, and opinions from facts.

Many consumers feel that if they buy salon products, they will achieve a "salon look" for their hair. In many ways, that is a logical conclusion. Most of us know that we always look better after a salon appointment. A good hairstylist can make hair defy gravity, smooth out frizzies as if they never existed, coax previously flat, limp hair into abundant voluminous waves, and transform perfectly straight hair into winsome, natural-looking curls. We know their talent plays a large part in what they can do, but when we see those products being strategically applied, we assume there must be something special inside those bottles of conditioner, jars of gel, and cans of hairspray. Plus, most hairstylists wince every time a client confesses to using a drugstore product instead of a salon product. On top of all that, their suggestions of what to use and how important it is to use the best products for your hair are so convincing. Surely a stylist who can do magic with hair must know all there is to know about hair-care products! All this glamour, allure, and professionalism provide more than enough evidence to persuade us that there must be something exceptional about salon products. But the beguiling stumbling blocks don't stop there.

Another reason many women become enamored with salon products is because drugstores are just so overwhelming. At the drugstore, we get hit in the face with literally hundreds of product choices. In our bewilderment, the only differences we see are the colors of the bottles, the names we are most familiar with from advertisements, and, if we are bargain hunting, the price tags. There is no way to discern actual differences, and no one to tell us which product will do what we want and need.

At the hair salon, none of this confusion exists. Not only is the selection much smaller (most salons carry only a handful of lines, versus dozens and dozens at large drugstores or beauty supply houses), but eager stylists and the people behind the counter are there to gush over the effectiveness of each of the products they sell. It is important to recognize that your hairstylist's recommendations are most likely influenced by a commission for selling the products instead of whether or not he or she truly likes them. I have interviewed many hairstylists who confided that they prefer products purchased at the drugstore, but that they were required to sell the products the salon sold.

Ultimately, there is also the issue of prestige. A stylist who charges $60 for a haircut and $80 for a hair color, but recommends Citre Shine Shampoo at $5 for 12 ounces or L'Oreal's Colorvive conditioner at $3 for 10 ounces, seems to be doing something contradictory. Whether or not the drugstore product is better is irrelevant because it just doesn't carry the sophistication and distinction of the salon lines. Forget the fact that most all of the more expensive products are either made by the same companies that make the less expensive products, or that the same basic contract manufacturer is making many salon lines as well as many of the drugstore lines. What about the fact that L'Oreal owns Redken, Dial owns Nexxus, Wella owns Sebastian, and Bristol Meyers owns Matrix? How does that figure into the equation?

With all this status pressure and the stylists' image at stake, it's a wonder women ever deign or dare to buy hair-care products from the drugstore. How could drugstore products begin to compete with the salon setting and its influence on us? They often can't, despite their quality, and that's where our emotions get in the way of reality.

It is true that good products can help generate a change in your hair, but there are good products in all price ranges! Expensive has nothing to do with quality! Salon products aren't what make your hair look so wonderful after leaving your stylist. Rather, it is the skill of the hairstylist that creates the final results regardless of the products being used. The most wonderful products in the world can't make up for a lack of artistic ability or technique. A blow-dryer held at the proper angle and used with the right brush can yield miracles. The perception that the products are assisting in the effect is not realistic. They may be good products, but the assumption that those are the only products that work just isn't true.

You may be shocked to learn that drugstore lines or lines we perceive as being "cheap" or a bargain (and therefore not very good) are often the very lines that spend the most money on research and development of their products. Companies like Revlon, Clairol, and L'Oreal spend millions of dollars a year on product research. Smaller companies cannot even begin to afford that kind of expenditure. L'Oreal has some of the most stunning state-of-the-art laboratories you can imagine, and spends, on average, $360 million a year for product development that is performed by a veritable brigade of cosmetic scientists and researchers. Procter & Gamble, Clairol, and Revlon run a close second, third, and fourth, respectively. On the other hand, almost all salon lines are produced by contract manufacturers. Sebastian products may be coming from the same place as 25 to 50 other hair-care lines in all price ranges. A company that makes $4 shampoos is often making $20 shampoos too. The technology and the scientific capacity don't change, and the ingredients are the same and come from the same sources—only the color, shape, and design of the bottle are different. Let go of the illusion that salon lines spend more money on research and that the quality of their products is somehow superior; the facts tell us otherwise.

We have so many misconceptions and misunderstandings about salon versus drugstore products that the fallacies spiral around each other like a maze of propaganda. **I'm not suggesting that there aren't reasons to shop for hair-care products at salons, because there are, but those reasons should be based on fact, not advertising or media hype.**

Here are some of the myths we believe about buying salon products versus drugstore products:

• **Everyone needs pampering in a salon.** Absolutely, but buying products that might not be worth the money is not my idea of being pampered.

• **Drugstore lines are weak and full of alcohol. Salon lines are more concentrated.** That is not what my research discovered. "Watery" products can be found at both the salon and the drugstore, and the same goes for products containing alcohol. Besides, alcohol is not necessarily the only hair culprit; there are other ingredients, some sounding natural or exotic, that can also be damaging to the hair. All in all, there is nothing inherent in salon products that will make them last one hour longer or be any more effective than a drugstore product.

• **Salon products have fewer surfactants (cleansing agents) and wax-type ingredients than drugstore lines.** Nothing could be further from the truth. In fact, just the opposite can be true. It only takes a quick review of the ingredient listing to determine this. Surfactants are uniform throughout the industry. You will not find one shampoo ingredient in a salon line that can't also be found in a drugstore line. The same is true for conditioning and thickening agents. In the long run, it all depends on the individual product.

• **Salon products use better grades of cosmetics than drugstore ones do.** I have heard this one more times than I can count, although I have yet to ever find proof. I have called dozens and dozens of ingredient suppliers to ask if they sell different grades of ingredients, and the answer has always been a resounding "No." That's not to say that ingredient manufacturers don't have their selling angles to prove that their quality and service is better, but the claim doesn't hold up when it comes to the ingredients' actual specifications.

• **Drugstore products can damage hair or fade hair color.** Because the same shampoo and conditioning agents tend to be used in virtually all products, that statement is completely unfounded. There are ingredients that can cause hair problems, but they show up in both the inexpensive and expensive stuff.

• **Hairstylists can pick the right product for your needs.** That definitely can be true, but, as we all know, hairstylists can also be wrong. Many hairstylists are intimately familiar with the hair products they sell and with the results those products provide. For that reason, shopping at the hair salon with the advice of a stylist is certainly one way to go—if you remember that many hairstylists recommend what their salon sells simply because they have to or because they are paid a commission on their sales.

• **You can try hair-salon products first.** If you feel you can evaluate a product's performance from having your hairstylist use it on your head first, that is a good reason to buy hair-salon products. However, keep in mind that the way your hair feels and looks after you see your stylist might not have anything to do with the products used but, rather, with the way your hair was styled. Remember, similar products could be available for less (but unless you are able to interpret the ingredient list, there is no way for you to know).

• **I am overwhelmed by the selection of products at the drugstore. It is just too large for me to make a comfortable decision.** Boy, is that the truth! A sea of products and a dearth of reliable information. It's enough to make anyone crazy. But that's why you're reading this book! It takes a good deal of the guesswork and worry out of your choices.

• **I would never feel confident dyeing my hair with drugstore products.** I understand the feeling. Yet all the evidence indicates that the risk of using drugstore products is the same as having a hairstylist do it for you. This is particularly true if the goal is only to lighten or darken the hair a shade or two or to cover gray. There are horror stories from both the salon and the drugstore sides of the color world. Hairstylists can custom-blend a color for you, but it still doesn't mean your hair will end up being the color you want. Nevertheless, I strongly suggest that if you want to make a drastic change in hair color (going three or more shades lighter or radically changing your hair color), it is probably best to start at the hair salon before you venture to the drugstore.

• **Salon products contain fewer ingredients you may be allergic to.** Nothing could be further off the mark than this. Hair-care products in all price ranges from all types of companies have shockingly similar ingredients. Just read the labels: The evidence is plainly written in the ingredient list. From the preservatives to the conditioning agents and everything else in between, salon and drugstore products have more similarities than differences. There are times when the salon line is loaded with botanicals and fragrance, yet more often than not, those are the very plants and essential oils that cause allergic reactions and skin sensitivities.

• **Styling products available at the drugstore are just awful in comparison to those sold in hair salons.** My research just did not prove that. Regardless of price, the crux of the matter is that all hair-care companies have good and bad products. Even more to the point, all of us have bought products we didn't like from expensive lines. Does that mean all expensive lines are bad? No, not any more than buying an occasional inexpensive product you didn't like should represent the overall quality at the drugstore. At the drugstore, it is trickier to discover for yourself what works, but hopefully my research will help alert you to the mistakes that happen in all price ranges.

As you read through the chapters on product formulation and the specific product reviews, you will discover that hair-care products sold by hair salons are not intrinsically better, more sophisticated, more appropriate, or superior to drugstore lines. In many cases just the opposite is true, or, at the very least, there is no real differ-ence between the expensive versus the inexpensive. **What is 100 percent true is that the differences between any two products or product lines, both negative and positive, are not identifiable by price or by the celebrity name on the package.**

At this juncture some of you are probably saying to yourself, "I've used inexpen-sive products and expensive products, and, for the most part, I prefer the expensive products. They just work better." I can't argue with your personal experience, but you must realize how much your personal experience is influenced by the claims and the marketing image of the product. I've repeatedly heard from cosmetics chemists that it is difficult to rely on a consumer's opinion of a given product because the consumer tends to believe what she is told, especially by someone perceived to be an authority figure.

There are actually studies that reveal just how impressionable we are. One such study was conducted by giving 100 women two "different" hair conditioners. They were told that one was a very expensive salon conditioner and the other was an inexpensive drugstore conditioner. The women were then asked to rate how they liked each one. **More than 80 percent of those participating said they felt the "ex-pensive" version performed better than the less expensive version. After the study was over, the women discovered that the two products were virtually identical—the only difference was what they had been told about the product's relative price!**

The Salon Guarantee

Perhaps the final and most powerful draw for buying salon hair-care products is the "salon guarantee," which is, for the most part, nothing more than a gimmick. The labels on the back of products from companies such as Aveda, KMS, Paul Mitchell, Sebastian, Scruples, and dozens of other hair-care lines usually state something like this: "Retail sale of this product by anyone other than a professional is unauthorized by the manufacturer, and warranties do not apply." Aveda's disclaimer is probably the most elaborate of them all: "To protect consumers and insure product integrity, Aveda maintains contractual agreements with authorized distributors, salons, and licensed professionals (Aveda Certified Professionals) for the sale of its products. These agree-ments prohibit Aveda products from being sold by any drugstore, supermarket, or other unauthorized retailer. Aveda will take legal action against such unauthorized retailers for interfering with its contractual agreements." It almost sounds like it would be against the law if you borrowed it from a friend without permission from Aveda.

So, what do these "guarantees" actually guarantee, and how is the consumer protected if the products are sold only at a hair salon instead of anywhere else? Good questions, but the answers aren't clear.

For all the hoopla about product guarantees, none of the hairstylists I interviewed agreed about what was guaranteed, or were even sure what the guarantees referred to. Comments ranged from assurances that you would be certain to get an authentic salon-only product and not an imitation, to the belief that it was nothing more than a marketing ploy aimed at the salon owners to make them feel they were getting the rights to an "exclusive" line, or that it was merely a return policy. According to the companies, the guarantee indeed refers to accepting returns and is a warranty that you are getting the right stuff. It is also a distribution warning. If you buy a salon-only product (and they are increasingly available outside of salons) at a drugstore or discount store, the manufacturing company won't give you a refund if you're not happy with it. They will only refund your money if you purchased the product at a hair salon.

On the other hand, most of the drugstore companies I talked to said they would be glad to give customers a refund any time they were dissatisfied with anything they purchased. So the catch to these guarantees is that women rarely return hair-care products that don't work. Women collect hair-care products much the same way they collect makeup. When they don't like a product, they put it aside and buy another. The woman who asks for her money back is the exception.

So, how does a salon-only product end up at a drugstore in the first place? No one is exactly clear or forthcoming about this, but unless the hair-care company sues, and a couple have, people are not arrested for selling salon-only products in a drugstore. More often than not, it isn't a distribution problem at all. Some hair-care companies sell their products wherever they can to improve their cash flow. Many hair-care companies even have a professional line and a drugstore line with, not surprisingly, identical ingredient lists.

Some salon-only companies told me that the only way you can be sure you aren't getting a cheap imitation or a knockoff is to buy the product only at a hair salon. That is possibly a valid concern, but not a serious one, because even if you aren't getting an authentic product, the risk to the consumer is nonexistent. Other companies claim to reproduce popular formulas and these imitations are clearly marked as such, so most consumers are not in any doubt about what they are buying.

It is debatable whether or not knockoffs of this nature are an ethical direction for cosmetics companies. I happen to take offense to these kinds of products. First of all, the practice suggests that there is something superior about the products being imitated, and that isn't always the case. Paul Mitchell may indeed have some very good products, but there is nothing about awapuhi or The Conditioner that is necessarily worth knocking off. I also happen to agree with the position of the salon-only hair-care companies: These knockoff brands are capitalizing on another entrepreneur's efforts. I wouldn't want someone to do that to me. What if someone came out with a book called *Don't Go Shopping for Salon or Drugstore Hair Products Without This Book*? I would not be happy. Products should stand on their own, each with its own identity and marketing plan. While generics are probably a fine option for the consumer to try, putting the emphasis on one line's success and not on the value of an individual product is a misleading way to sell products.

What the professional or salon-only guarantee really turns out to be is a marketing device used to enhance value and add price points. Salons don't want to sell products that the consumer can get from any drugstore shelf; where is the exclusivity in that? Markup is an essential part of a hair salon's profits (given that they are selling far fewer products than the drugstore), and you can't make much profit selling $6 shampoos or $5 hairsprays. Plus, where would the status and prestige be if the prices were so reasonable? Most women need to believe that their hair will be more beautiful if they spend more money on it, and hairstylists are more than willing to encourage that attitude.

Naturally Absurd

"Natural," as a marketing hook, is the fastest-growing and largest segment of the hair-care industry. Consumers are more likely to be swayed if some aspect of a shampoo, conditioner, or styling product appears to be formulated from natural ingredients. Though most cosmetics chemists cringe when you bring up the concept of "natural," they recognize that their products would be ignored without it. Almost all natural-sounding ingredients are nothing more than a charade, but it is a game that the hair-care chemist, hair-care company, and consumer are all more than willing to play. Each product beckons to the consumer with a menulike list of ingredients that sound good enough to eat. The drop of aloe, dash of lavender, hint of rosemary or ginseng, or of any of dozens of other plant offerings is there almost solely for image and little else.

Most consumers are so enamored by the power of "natural" that there is no question in their minds whether any of this natural stuff is really good. **Sadly, while some natural ingredients can have helpful properties for skin, in hair care most all natural ingredients have little to no impact or influence on the health, cleanliness, strength, or smoothness of hair.** If only I had a dime for every woman who has said to me, "Well, the products I'm using must be good—they're all natural and pure." And if only I had the opportunity to say in response, "The products you are using cannot be remotely or even partly all natural. You have simply bought into one of the biggest and most successful marketing scams of all time because the functional ingredients in your products are not natural in the least."

In essence, you could take all of the natural-sounding ingredients out of a product and you would still have an effective shampoo, conditioner, or styling product that would leave hair clean, soft, and manageable. Take out all the so-called chemical-sounding ingredients and all you would have is tea (which is what plant extracts often are) and dirty, unconditioned, and unmanageable hair.

Consumers want to believe that natural ingredients such as plant extracts and vitamins can somehow nourish the hair and revitalize it, changing it into something better than it was before. Nothing could be further from the truth. All of the plants and vitamins in the world can't change a dead leaf or a rock, and they can't change the very dead hair on your head. There is no evidence that any of these ingredients provide any substantive benefit for hair. When you read the ingredient lists for these so-called natural products, you find that all the standard hair-care ingredients, used throughout the industry, are also there.

When pushed for evidence that natural ingredients make a difference, companies stoop to references to folklore or history for proof, but that proves nothing. Egyptians may have used certain plants for their hair but that doesn't mean it worked. Cleopatra might have used exotic plants to take care of her hair, but we have no proof she had great hair! Are we assuming she looked like Elizabeth Taylor in the movie *Cleopatra*? We don't know if hair treatments from the past worked; we know only that they were used. When it comes to hair, I would, without question, choose the standard, much less exotic-sounding ingredients—such as polyquaternium-16, dimethicone, cyclomethicone, or PVP (polyvinylpyrrolidone)—to get my hair to feel soft and stay in place, rather than lavender extract or vitamin D, and so would hair-care chemists. Paying for the illusion of benefit from natural ingredients does absolutely nothing for your hair, but it can surely hurt your pocketbook.

Too Good to Be True

Selling snake oil is a game that has been around for centuries upon centuries. Modern-day vendors have refined the art, and the Internet has taken it to new heights. But what exactly is "selling snake oil"? Any sales technique that tries to convince you that a product can live up to your wildest dreams without any negative side effects is the essence of snake-oil salesmanship. Scams like this are abundant in the world of hair care, but even more so in the world of hair-growth treatments and products promising to correct hair damage and make thin, fine hair feel thicker and fuller.

Consumers have heard for years that if it sounds too good to be true, it is—but we just don't want to believe it. Whatever the emotional or psychological reasons are that make us weak in the presence of such otherwise repetitive and blatant deceptions, it costs us a lot of money and wasted time. Perhaps what we need are a few reminders of how to identify a potential scam when we see one. If you can recognize fraudulent marketing contrivances, it will go a long way toward helping your hair and your budget.

If a company claims that its research or products are being suppressed by the government or by big pharmaceutical companies, it is guaranteed that you have encountered a hoax. This is a pathetic attempt to cash in on our fear that Big Brother or big capitalist interests are keeping you from something truly spectacular for your health. Legitimate, verifiable research can be carried out by any company of any size. It does take some amount of money but, then, any investment in a business that sells products takes capital outlay. How dare a company attempt to make money (and some companies are making millions) without doing the work to prove its claims are plausible and without risk?

A corollary to the Big-Brother-is-out-to-get-us ploy is the one that states "we are releasing our products without FDA approval because it would take too long for us to wait for their endorsement." Of course it takes a long time to prove something is safe and effective, and if a product really can do something significant (like play around with your hormones, in the case of hair-growth products) don't you want to know if there is a risk of cancer or other biochemical and systemic side effects? The FDA asks for serious proof, and we should demand no less if someone is asking us to spend our hard-earned money.

Another sure sign you and your hair are being taken for a ride is if the company claims the secret ingredient is from some faraway, exotic land. As nice as it would be if there were such miracles hiding in the rain forest of some remote region of the world, there just aren't. Regardless of locale, whether it comes from New Jersey or the Amazon, if an ingredient can perform, then the research and resulting patent wouldn't be a secret; it would be shared with the world just like all legitimate research is.

One of the most frustrating fraudulent schemes taking place in the world of cosmetics is the use of pseudoscience. Studies are quoted, scientific-sounding publications or journals are cited, well-known universities are mentioned, doctors in good standing are referred to, and serious-sounding awards are attributed to whatever product is being sold. Sadly, more often than not, the studies are taken out of context or misquoted, the study is done on a tiny population (86 percent of eight people is not proof of anything), the journal mentioned doesn't exist or is published by the same company making the product, or the study itself or the results are meaningless given the methodology they used—something very hard for the average person who isn't familiar with scientific protocol to understand. Even more ludicrous, though it happens often, is that the doctor or university mentioned has never heard of the ingredient or product or there is no such award given anywhere in the world.

How do you know when the science referred to isn't true? The clearest sign you're being scammed is when the results are sweeping and there is no downside. When the conclusions only point to the product being sold as being the absolute best, most wondrous thing ever created, with no negative reactions, you can be assured you're about to be taken in by a great marketing ruse.

An addendum to the scientific, proof-positive approach to snake-oil selling tactics is the all-embracing, absolutely-everyone-loves-our-products approach. Infomercials do this form of selling the best. Glowing enthusiasm, stunning befores and afters, and no downside or risks are extolled by seemingly impartial users. Yet the reason why hundreds of lines are being sold is that the previous ones weren't really the "best" after all (plus women are amazingly fickle about the products they like). Also, do you think these companies are ever going to air the voices of the women who aren't happy?

Medical expertise is the most seductive selling tactic of all. A neat white coat and stethoscope draped around the spokesperson or owner of a product line are all it takes to establish instant credibility with most consumers. Physicians are believed almost instinctively, and whether or not the product is related to their field, if they are doctors, we believe they must know. It just isn't true. Doctors and medical experts exaggerate their positions and lie about products to make sales just like the worst of them. Expensive products and overly hyped, ordinary formulations abound in physicians' offices. Again, if it seems all positive and wonderful and miraculous, it just isn't true. Besides, it is the rare dermatologist or physician who has any knowledge about cosmetic or hair-care formulations and research. If you look at dermatological or plastic surgery journals, those research papers have little or nothing to do with formulations like this.

It's ironic that American medical know-how can sell a horde of nonmedical products, while at the same time the notion that a product is anything but American-made or developed from Western science is a strong come-on for a large range of susceptible consumers. Companies love taking advantage of the belief that anything foreign-made, particularly if it's from the Far East, must be better for you and contain better, more effective ingredients. The selling points are distinctive: either the research has taken place in a far corner of the world such as India or China, or the ingredient has been hidden away in a remote forest or jungle somewhere. Hair-care or skin-care revelations from outside the purview of Western medicine are impossible to confirm or refute because there is rarely any hard data to analyze. A bigger mystery is why people are so quick to believe that American technology is not up to speed with these distant locales. Most of these areas have medical and health standards that are far below ours.

It's interesting to note that if you are in most any part of the world outside of the United States, the major selling point to consumers is that the product is made in the United States! Isn't that amazing! In China, products are sold with English words written on the label to give the impression they aren't made in China, while here in the United States, products are sold with Chinese- or Japanese-styled letters to impress consumers. I guess all you marketers really have to do is figure out a consumer's weakness and go after it.

The final potentially phony advertising inducement is a bit confusing. While I love money-back guarantees and consider them a primary, major motivation when finalizing a purchase, these guarantees are pointless in the world of hair-growth products (or for products claiming to make hair stop growing). Most money-back policies are good for a 30-day period, but it takes months to discover if a hair-related product is working because hair growth takes months to develop. Hair growth is also cyclical, so a product may seem to work and then a few months later the hair you thought grew back may actually fall out.

Hair History

Men and women alike spend a lot of time and money worrying about the condition of their hair, and for good reason. Hair makes a powerful social statement. It is the rare person who can go very long without paying attention to the state of affairs growing out of his or her head. What we've done to and with our hair over the centuries has illustrated not only social and financial status (from wigs for the 18th-century British and French elite, to no style at all for the working class in Eastern Europe), but political and religious leanings as well. During the 1960s there was no question what your politics were if you were a man and your hair hung below your ears. When it comes to religion, the Rastafarians are known for their distinctive dreadlocks, and religious Jewish men are distinguishable by their long, curled sideburns.

While we take great pains today to get our hair to look attractive and make a statement, it doesn't begin to compare to what our ancestors routinely underwent. French court women of the 15th century plucked their foreheads in order to push their hairline back an inch or two to give the effect of added height. Towering wigs were introduced by Louis XIV, who disliked being short and thought a large hairpiece would somehow fool people. The women at court picked up this absurd style and wore immense contraptions on their heads that were decorated with brocade, ribbons, jewelry, works of art, and even figurines. Because they washed their hair only once or twice a year, they were subject to chronic head lice infestations. The varmints even took up residence in those grandiose wigs.

Over millennia, hairstyles have ranged from intricate braids and plaits to large bananalike curls and ringlets to carefully pinned buns and chignons. Head coverings have included layers of veiling; colorful, intricately wrapped scarves and kerchiefs; and an array of hats, both practical and fanciful. To say we have it easier today is an understatement.

Even in this century, however, each decade has seen gyrations of fashion, and women have obediently followed the dictates of the pundits of chic and forced their hair into submission (except for the inevitable, lucky few who were blessed with the right hair at the right time). At the turn of the century, every Gibson girl was crowned by a pompadour, while Clara Bow bobs were all the rage in the Roaring '20s. In the 1930s and '40s, soft but structured permanent waves began by hugging the head and ended up brushing the shoulders. Women in the 1950s and early '60s went to the hair salon for their weekly appointment, got their dos lacquered in place, then diligently kept them fresh with clips, wrappings, and nets that they wore to bed. If you were young in the 1960s and early '70s, you probably were desperate for stick-straight hair. (I either slept on orange juice cans or laid my too-curly, waist-length hair on an ironing board for my older sister to iron—yes, *iron*, with my mother's Hamilton Beach—into a straight, well pressed line.) The late 1970s brought Farrah Fawcett and her carefully tousled mane with bangs bent back and up. Gels and sprays were absolutely necessary in order to keep those gravity-defying bangs in a neat, swept-up curve, along with the advent of the handheld blow-dryer and the world of haircare changed forever.

In the 1980s, curly, "natural"-looking hair arrived with a vengeance, replacing the lifeless, vertical hair of the previous two decades. Of course, women who wanted curly hair that supposedly required no care went in droves to hair salons to get a perm. What a joke! There was nothing about permanent waves that made hair easier to care for (more often than not, permed hair was fried hair and required persistent conditioning) or that made it look particularly natural (a perm usually looked like a perm).

Now, as we head into the 21st century, we have returned to the stick-straight hair I had to put up with in the '60s. Actresses like Nicole Kidman and Minnie Driver, well known for their tightly curled, abundant manes, are sporting ultrastick-straight hairdos that must take hours to create and maintain. Everyone from Calista Flockhart to Jennifer Aniston has a hairstyle that wouldn't dare to have a bend or curve.

Yet there is also an element of do-what-you-want with your hair. Curly, slicked back, wavy, full, flat, short, long, ringlets, and much more are all options (though straight is still by far the main fashion choice). With all these hairstyle options come the products to maintain the specific look—and, boy, do we have choices! The market is so crowded with so many different products, color options, and varieties of perms that it's hard to know what to do and what not to do. Hairstyles may not be as complicated as they once were, but finding the right products for your hair can be an awesome task. I want to help make it simpler.

CHAPTER TWO

To the Root of the Matter

Hair Basics 101

If you take no other information in this book to heart, the two following facts are the ones you must understand in order to take better care of your hair:

1. **Hair is dead (notice that when you cut hair, you don't say "ouch"), and once it has been damaged it cannot be repaired in any way, shape, or form.** Repeated blow-drying, brushing, styling, chemical processing, and sun exposure degrade hair and the damage cannot be mended or restored.

2. **Hair has a particular genetic or hormonally generated nature; you can work with it and spend time controlling it, and find products that simulate a different feel, but you cannot alter it permanently into something else.** Perms and hair straighteners, of course, can make a huge difference. The effect grows out and there are definite negative consequences to the process, but that's an entirely different story from thinking something can be altered for good.

The pursuit of products that will finally make your dream hair come true is an endless one. What most women desire and hope for is that they will find a product line (at any cost) that will be able to make thick, heavy hair lighter and fuller; thin hair thicker and fuller; curly, frizzy hair straighter and smoother; straight hair curlier; coarse hair silkier; frizzy hair smoother; and on and on and on. Whatever it is you want to hear, the hair-care industry is willing to tell you. To name just a handful of claims: Overprocessed, completely destroyed hair can somehow be brought back to life. Split ends can be mended into a harmonious whole. Frizzy manes can be miraculously transformed into flowing, silky waves. Thin hair can be made thick. Dandruff can be cured. Dyeing hair won't cause damage. Is any of this possible? I know you want me to say yes unequivocally, but the truth is that the answer is both yes and no.

Primarily, what you can expect depends less on the products you use and far more on the actual texture and structure of your hair, how adept you are at wielding styling tools, and how much time and trouble you are willing to go through to achieve the desired results. All that varies from hair type to hair type and from person to person.

For example, if you have thin, limp hair you can only do so much to change how thick it can really feel or how full it can really look. Most of the products that simulate (notice I said *simulate* and not *create*) a thick feel can also build up and make the hair appear limp and sticky. Likewise, products that help hold the hair aloft for an appearance of fullness can leave a film on the hair.

If your hair is coarse and naturally frizzy you cannot expect to eternally tame it. If your hair has been double-processed (both permed and colored, even if you wait between processes, or colored twice in a brief span of time), it can never be restored to its original texture until it grows out. Hair that has been abused by blow-dryers on a daily basis, overbrushed (brushing causes more damage than you could ever imagine), or backcombed for fullness (which can absolutely destroy hair) can never be revived or renewed.

Now that you know what you can't expect, here's what you can. There are wonderful products on the market that can temporarily, from washing to washing, do some fairly incredible things to hair. Several ingredients can produce amazing results, from filling in the holes and tears in damaged hair cuticles, to imparting a silky-smooth texture to the rough sections of the hair shaft. Many ingredients can to some extent be absorbed by the hair shaft to help make the hair feel soft and manageable. Conditioners and shampoos can deposit temporary color on the hair to extend the life of your hair dye between touchups. Advances in sprays, gels, and mousses allow deftly formed styles to be kept in place with a relative amount of softness and ease of brushing.

Does this have to be expensive? Absolutely not. In later chapters, which deal more with actual product formulations, you will be shocked by the repetitive nature of hair-care products. In the world of skin care, a cosmetics chemist has over 50,000 different ingredients at his or her disposal from which to create a vast array of products with an almost limitless range of textures and performance traits. Hair-care formulations by comparison have none of that scope. **While there are literally thousands of ingredients that can help skin feel moist and soft, there are only a mere handful of ingredients that can clean hair or condition it.** Hair is very specific about what will cling to it and what you can use to clean it. The truly insane disparity in price tags in no way reflects differences in the products. Again, the information is all there on the ingredient label.

Hair Is Dead!

First and foremost, you need to know and remember that the hair you see on the top of your head, every inch of it, is dead as a doornail. The only portion of your hair that isn't dead is the hair you can't see, growing inside the hair follicle under your scalp. Because hair is dead, your options as to what you can do to take care of it are limited.

Hair-care companies want to convince you that, much like Frankenstein's monster, dead hair can be changed into ostensibly alive hair. How many products have you bought that said they would repair and reconstruct damaged hair, only to have your hair return to its original state after the next washing or when the weather changed? Yes, we all know that hair products such as conditioners and gels, and hair implements such as blow-dryers and curlers, can temporarily reshape hair. The trouble begins when we are led to believe that it is possible to *permanently* alter or improve damaged hair structure with shampoos, conditioners, and treatments. The only way hair can truly be altered is with certain hair-coloring products and with perms. That's it—and even so, you are not necessarily guaranteed long-term positive re- sults. Everything else is a sort of Band-Aid remedy that is easily removed after washing.

Before you go shopping for hair-care products again, or before you venture into a hair salon to get your hair dyed or permed, you need to know some basic facts about your hair in order to be a discerning, clear-eyed consumer. This isn't the most fascinating aspect of hair, but it is one more crucial step that will let you sift the facts from the fiction.

How Does Hair Grow?

Depending on the individual, approximately 5 million hair follicles cover the surface of the body at any given time. Of that total, there are about 100,000 to 120,000 strands of hair growing on the head. All those millions of hairs are developed and in place before a baby is even born. Biologically, it is impossible to grow more hair after birth. All the hair you are ever going to have is already there when you arrive.

Surprisingly, blondes usually have more hair on their heads than those with red or darker hair colors. What is even more surprising is that even though a single hair has a thickness of only 0.02 to 0.04 millimeters, it is remarkably strong, with a tensile strength equivalent to that of a thin strand of wire. Why, then, does hair seem to be so fragile? According to a March 1988 article in *Cosmetic Dermatology* by Dr. Zoe Draelos, hair easily stretches (unlike wire) and can do just fine when extended to 30 percent of its length. However, once it exceeds 30 percent, damage is certain, and at much past 80 percent of its original length, the hair shaft fractures. (Hair becomes even more vulnerable to breakage when the hair shaft is damaged, but more about that later.) This explains why the tension placed on hair by pulling it down with a round brush during blow-drying—or by tying the hair up tightly in a ponytail—can be so damaging.

Inside the hair follicle, deep below the skin, hair is going through a life cycle all its own. At any given time, all the hair on your body is either growing, resting (or dormant), or shedding. Hair grows in three distinct stages. The first stage is the

anagen (growth) stage. At this point, the hair is very busy developing in the hair follicle, a pocketlike structure located deep in the skin that houses the bulb-shaped root of the hair. At the very base of this root is an intricate network of capillaries and nerves that feed the embryonic hair. During the growth stage, each individual hair is formed by rapidly dividing cells that push forward and up through the follicle. As

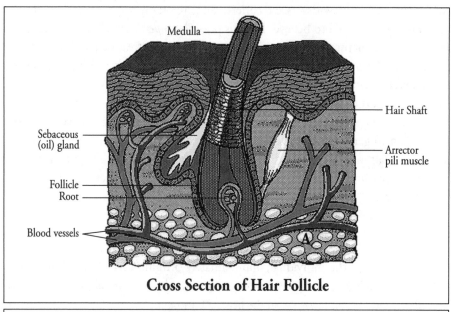

Cross Section of Hair Follicle

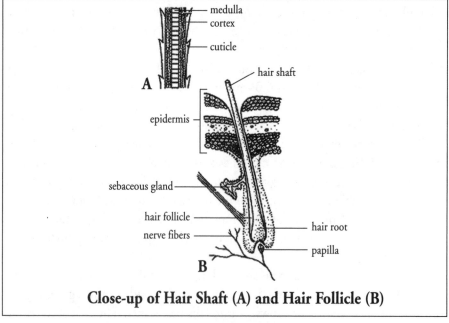

Close-up of Hair Shaft (A) and Hair Follicle (B)

they multiply and expand, the cells reach the surface, where they die and harden into what we know as hair. This growth stage can last anywhere from two to six years. During this phase, hair grows an average of about half an inch per month, or six inches a year (but that is only an average and it can vary drastically from very active hair growth to very slow growth for different people).

Over the entire period of growth, the hair can reach a length of approximately three feet, about the middle of the back for most women. Naturally, there are variations in length potential, and women with tresses six feet long have been reported, but there are also women who can't grow hair much past their shoulders. The reason for this is that length of hair is genetically predetermined, and that explains why some women feel they can never get their hair to grow past a certain point while other women can't get to a hairdresser often enough to keep up with the growout.

The next stage of hair life is the **catagen (transition) stage.** After two to six years of growth, the hair cells stop reproducing and the growth process is just about over. For about three to six weeks, the hair just lies around taking it easy while the root slowly moves up to the skin's surface.

Entering its last phase of life, the hair is ready to literally jump ship and shed. The **telogen (final) stage** is short-lived. At this point the hair root has moved almost to the surface (near the opening of the oil gland), where it is completely separated from the base of the follicle. In a matter of weeks the anagen (growth) stage begins again at the base of the hair follicle. Hair cells again start dividing and multiplying, generating a new shaft. This new hair sprouts to the surface, pushing the old hair out of its way. **So all that hair collecting on your brush, in the bottom of your drain, or on your clothing, about 25 to 100 hairs a day, is usually hair that has passed from the growth phase through the transition plateau and then, sadly, into the final period of shedding.**

At any given time, approximately 88 percent of scalp hair is in the anagen phase, 1 percent in the catagen phase, and 11 percent in the telogen phase. Thankfully, hair is predominantly in the growing phase (at least, if male pattern baldness has not started to take place), which explains why we end up having more hair than less, despite the ones we lose on a daily basis.

Although everyone's hair goes through the same life cycle, not all hair is the same. Hair has very clear, inherited differences. African hair mostly grows in an alternating curved/flat sequence that imparts a coiled, corkscrewlike shape to the hair and produces weak spots at every turn. Asian, Native American, and Hispanic hair is straight to slightly wavy, coarse, thick, and almost always black. European and Hindu hair textures vary greatly, from straight to curly, and thick to thin to coarse, and have a wide range of colors. Generally, what distinguishes African hair from European or Asian hair is the tight, spiral growth pattern. The fragile nature of this corkscrew structure causes endless problems for African-American hair. (For information about African-American hair problems and solutions, see Chapter Seven, *For African-American Women*.)

Why Does Hair Stop Growing?

Alopecia is the technical name for hair loss. There are several forms of alopecia, but the kind affecting most men (over 75 percent) and some women (about 40 percent), or 99 percent of everyone if you include the process of hair thinning that takes place as we age, is called **androgenetic alopecia.** Another more popular name for this type of hair loss is "male pattern baldness." It is even called male pattern baldness for women due to the condition's relationship to male sex hormones. Commonly, male pattern baldness takes place in a horseshoe pattern, with the hair receding from the forehead back toward the neck. Male pattern baldness can also take place from the center of the scalp out. For women, male pattern baldness is more diffuse, taking place all over the scalp.

Despite the claims that hair-care companies are making, not much is actually understood about androgenetic alopecia, but a few aspects of what causes the problem are known. Principally, hair growth has a lot to do with hormonal activity, especially related to the male sex hormone group called androgens. Testosterone and dihydrotestosterone (DHT, a hormonal by-product of testosterone) are types of androgens produced in large quantities by the testes (and in women in smaller concentrations by the ovaries) that are responsible for the development of secondary male sex characteristics for both genders.

What makes testosterone and DHT so significant to hair loss is their fundamental role in the growth of facial and pubic hair. Some type of balance between the two hormones appears to create normal hair growth as well as other male attributes. Then, as we age, an increase of DHT in the blood takes place. Remember that the hair follicle has a rich supply of blood vessels at the root. This excess concentration of DHT in the blood is therefore concentrated at the hair follicle. Theoretically, this concentration of DHT is thought to inhibit hair growth and to eventually shrivel the actual size of the hair follicle. But this is only a hypothesis. It is not proven, because there are conflicting studies showing that increased levels of DHT are not the cause of balding.

One major conflicting piece of evidence disproving the theory that excess amounts of DHT in the blood reduce hair growth on the head is that this excess doesn't affect hair growth on the body. Quite the contrary; as we age, hair on the body increases and actually becomes thicker. Continuing research on balding still focuses on DHT and the notion that there are other concomitant factors implicated in the condition.

For women, it appears that their increased levels of estrogen (the primary female sex hormone) combat the effects of male androgens on hair growth. When estrogen levels decrease as women approach menopause, the consequences of androgen-related balding can begin to appear. Estrogen Replacement Therapy (ERT) raises estrogen levels and can stop the hair loss.

This issue of a reduction in estrogen triggering the influence of androgen-affected hair loss is significant for women who overexercise or exercise excessively and reduce their body fat content to below 15 percent. Female athletes who have diminished estrogen levels (often indicated by extremely light or nonexistent periods) tend to have increased levels of testosterone. This increase in male hormones and reduced estrogen can stimulate hair loss.

While research concerning hair loss has focused primarily on hormonal development, there is a good deal of discussion surrounding the issue of blood supply to the hair follicle. This one is another favorite of companies selling hair-care productsthat they claim help hair growth.

One of the side effects (or causes, depending on your marketing point of view) of hair loss is that the hair follicle shrinks and the blood vessels feeding the hair follicle wither and terminate. As the hair follicle becomes less vital, the hair it yields becomes finer and thinner (thereby needing less blood supply, which causes the deterioration of the blood vessels). Along with this thinner hair growth, the actual growth cycle (the anagen, catagen, and telogen phases) becomes shorter. Not only is the hair development diminished, but when the hair falls out during the telogen phase, there is a shorter anagen phase to re-create the hair growth.

This situation can then become more a marketing discussion, because hair-care companies want you to believe that the blood-flow issue is the primary factor affecting hair growth. Theoretically, if you can improve blood flow you should be able to improve hair growth. As logical as that sounds, it doesn't address the issue of what is causing the blood vessels to wither, and whether or not you can stop that from happening. We simply don't know the answer, and therein lies the puzzle. Lots of companies want you to believe they can increase blood flow or decrease the amount of DHT present, but no one has much proof that either of these is possible or even whether these factors are the real cause of hair loss.

The hype around DHT affecting hair growth is related to conflicting research studies. **Remember that not all hair follicles are negatively influenced by DHT, so it doesn't automatically follow that DHT must be eliminated.** Likewise, although efficient blood flow is needed for hair growth, if we don't know what culprit is causing the diminished capacity of the blood vessels, can we really affect any noticeable change in hair growth?

On the other hand, research concerning oral medications like Propecia (discussed in the next section, "Stopping Hair Loss") shows that blocking the formation of DHT can improve hair growth significantly. There are also studies showing that increased hair growth can be stimulated in mice using several different treatments, ranging from green tea to zinc. However, mice don't have the same hormones as humans, so very few researchers believe that those studies relate to the human condition.

There are a handful of other causes of hair loss, but they occur much less frequently than male pattern baldness. These causes of hair loss are alopecia areata, malnutrition, and thyroid problems. Of these, thyroid disorders can often be corrected with medication, and malnutrition can be completely reversed with a change in diet.

Alopecia areata is a frequent cause of hair loss, second only to male pattern baldness, but it is an extremely rare disorder. Alopecia areata is an autoimmune disease that can cause a general loss of body and scalp hair. (A complete, overall balding of this type is called alopecia universalis.) An autoimmune disease occurs when the body's immune system identifies a normal bodily function as if it were some problem bacteria, virus, or some other unwanted systemic presence. That triggers the immune system to attack an otherwise healthy human function. In other words, in this case the immune system attacks the hair follicle and causes hair loss. What causes this to take place is completely unknown and cannot be predicted or altered. However, in most cases, in time the hair will regenerate.

Stopping Hair Loss

I'm sure you've seen the ads: *Grow Hair in 12 Weeks! Stop Hair Loss Today! Stop Baldness Without Costly Drugs, Chemicals, or Surgery! Turn Fallout into Growout with Only One Hour of Your Time a Week!* Wouldn't that be nice? Then all you'd have to do is send in your three easy payments of $29.95 and receive a melange of vitamins, a special shampoo or conditioner, several scalp masks, a battery-run scalp massager, and who knows what else, and you too would look like the before-and-after pictures in the advertisements. Bald spot one day, waves of bushy hair a few weeks later. If any of this were possible, why would anyone be bald? There wouldn't be a naked scalp in the house.

Regrettably, most all of these concoctions are nothing more than snake-oil treatments, here today and gone tomorrow. Most of these products are only available via mail order, so the companies are hard to find, especially if you want to get your money back when the products fail, which they inevitably do. You would be better off throwing your money out the window. At least you wouldn't be funding these unscrupulous businesses that lure other hopeful but deceived consumers into wasting their money.

What makes all of this so difficult to sort through is that there are some ingredients with interesting studies showing some hopeful results. Such popular cosmetics ingredients as emu oil, zinc, polysorbate 80, superoxide dismutase, and green tea have shown promise—but is the possibility worth the trouble of rubbing this stuff all over your head? And which one do you choose? Then you have to get through all the companies selling products with not even a shred of evidence that they can do anything at all but clean your hair and make it easy to comb, just like any other shampoo and conditioner. None of these points has an easy answer, but throughout the Product Reviews, Chapter Nine, I attempt to point out the ones that hold out some hope, no matter how remote, and the others that will take your money and still leave you hairless.

Some hair loss is also caused by frequent and/or constant pressure on the hair follicle. Women who wear extremely tight ponytails or braids on a regular basis can experience bald spots, particularly around the hairline. African-American women who weave hair extensions into their own hair, plait heavy beadwork into cornrows, or wear tightly patterned braids can pull hair right out of the root. All of this is temporary and almost immediately rectified when the pressure is relieved. Winding rollers too tight, clipping them firmly to the head, and then sleeping on them can pull out hair and cause bald spots but, again, this is easily remedied by changing styling techniques. Searching for vitamins, shampoos, or special products to handle these predicaments only takes attention away from the real solution, which may be simply to change hairstyles.

Because a tiny percentage of hair loss is caused by an extreme condition where the hair follicle becomes blocked or clogged, a lot of hair-care companies claim that they can undo that blockage and thereby stimulate hair growth. While that may be true, there is nothing special about that process in the least. Any shampoo or product can do it. Shampooing more frequently, massaging the scalp gently with the fingertips and nails, and using less greasy (nonocclusive) conditioners and hair treatments usually cures the problem, at no extra cost, and it doesn't require special products.

Contributing to this problem of clogged pores or hair follicles, certain hair-care treatments and conditioners for dry scalp contain a large concentration of petrolatum, lanolin, cocoa butter, and/or heavy waxes that can build up on the scalp and clog the hair shaft. This is primarily true for African-Americans who are trying to treat dry scalp conditions caused by repeated hair straightening. Not only is African-American hair more fragile to begin with, but the very treatments used in styling the hair make it more susceptible to breakage and damage. Consequently, in an effort to prevent further damage, some African-American women wash their hair much less often than they should. Without regular shampooing, the heavy emollient conditioners can build up on the scalp, choking off the follicles' air supply and holding dead skin cells on the head. This in turn decreases circulation and prevents healthy hair growth. In worst-case scenarios, that can lead to hair falling out. Remember, the capillary network at the root of the hair feeds the hair cells as they divide and multiply. Without good circulation, the hair can't and won't grow to its full potential. (For more information on African-American hair problems and solutions, see Chapter Seven, *For African-American Women*.) But once again, it doesn't take special products to correct this. It's a matter of changing habits and styling products, not spending a fortune on products.

Other forms of hair loss can be caused by disorders of the immune system (such as alopecia areata, mentioned above), physical stress (expressed in repeated tugging and pulling on the hair, causing bald or thinning patches of scalp), and nutritional conditions caused by rapid weight loss or certain eating disorders. Baldness caused by diet or physical stress is easily reversed once the diet is corrected or the physical stress is stopped. Autoimmune disease such as alopecia areata (spontaneous hair loss) can occasionally be helped with oral medications such as steroids, but generally there is little, if anything, that can be done for that problem.

Pregnant women can suffer from hair loss or bask in greater hair growth. Pregnancy focuses all of the body's energy on taking care of the developing fetus. That means little attention is directed toward making new hair cells. When a hair falls out during the catagen (transition) stage of hair growth, generally there is no new hair preparing to emerge and take the old one's place. On the other hand, some pregnant women whose female hormones are flourishing have an extended anagen phase of hair growth and the transition stage never takes place. They just keep growing hair. At some point after the baby is born, the transition stage finally kicks in and the noticeable, sudden hair loss can be scary. Either way, don't be concerned: These are both temporary conditions that return to normal sometime during the first few months after the baby's birth or, in some cases, after the breast-feeding stage is over. Just be patient. Don't rush out and buy products to change what is happening; they won't work.

Hair Growing Possibilities

A good deal of this information was gleaned from Kevin J. McElwee's Web site, www.keratin.com. It has a wealth of information and should be reviewed by anyone looking further into the topic of hair loss and hair-loss treatments.

The only over-the-counter, topical pharmaceutical product that works (meaning it is approved by the FDA for claims regarding hair regrowth) is minoxidil. Minoxidil (once only available under the trade name Rogaine) is now available under different names from several different companies and can increase hair growth (it doesn't affect hormonal activity; rather, it appears to encourage increased growth patterns) in a statistically significant percentage of men and women. Extensive research and statistics released by the makers of minoxidil (again, approved and accepted by the FDA) suggest that this fairly inexpensive treatment (about $20 a month for life if you want the effects to continue) works for a percentage of people who use it according to instructions. According to the Mayo Clinic's *Women's Health Report* for May 1998, minoxidil is successful for 44 percent to 63 percent of women who try it. It is actually far less effective for men, working in only about 20 percent of men who use it. Dermatologist Arthur P. Bertolino, M.D., Ph.D., director of the hair consultation unit at New York University, in an article published in the December 1991 FDA *Consumer* magazine, said that minoxidil ". . . approximately 90 percent of the time at least slows down hair loss." The makers of Rogaine are even more cautious with their numbers, stating in their literature that "19 percent of women reported moderate hair regrowth, 40 percent had minimal regrowth, with men demonstrating less effectiveness."

No one is certain yet just how topical minoxidil works to promote hair growth. One theory is that it may convert tiny hair follicles that produce peach fuzz or invisible hair growth into large hair follicles that produce normal-size hairs. The most common side effects with this medication are itching and skin irritation, and once you stop using it, any hair that grew as a result will fall out.

Minoxidil works best in men who are balding at the crown instead of from the temples back. Also, for good results, it is essential to start treatment early. If you start showing signs of hair loss at age 30, that's when it should be started. Waiting even a few years after you've noticed the start of male pattern baldness can mean limited results from minoxidil.

Propecia, as I mentioned above, is the oral medication from Merck & Co. (technical name **finasteride**), and appears to be extremely effective in treating male pattern baldness. An article in the January 1998 issue of *Cosmetic Dermatology* stated, "The FDA's Dermatologic and Opthalmic Drugs Advisory Committee agreed in discussions that Propecia is efficacious in treating male pattern baldness." The article cited three studies "involving 1,879 men, ages 18 to 41, who had mild to moderate but not complete hair loss. . . . These studies, which lasted 24 months, demonstrated that treatment with Propecia prevented further hair thinning, and significantly increased hair growth in the majority of men (86 percent)." However, as an article in the November 17, 1997 issue of *Newsweek* pointed out, 42 percent of the men in the placebo group also showed improvement. Still, 86 percent is an impressive number. But don't get too excited—there are negatives to taking this drug. Propecia can cause birth defects for pregnant women and can decrease men's libido. However, as several doctors pointed out to me, the research showed the libido decrease was minor and that it was not significantly different from the placebo group. What the study warnings didn't point out was that finasteride in some people raised the levels of testosterone and increased the libido! For some that's a great side effect, and you get some of your hairline back at the same time!

By the way, Propecia works by inhibiting an enzyme called 5 alpha-reductase, which prevents testosterone from making DHT. It doesn't get rid of DHT, it prevents it from being produced. I'm pointing this out because there are hair-care companies that want you to believe they can alter or eliminate DHT from the outside in. They can't: It is a very specific enzyme, which can be controlled by Propecia, that affects testosterone, indirectly curbing production of DHT. Cosmetics can't perform the same action, though if they could, you would want the research to prove they aren't harmful, and there are no safety studies for any of these cosmetic hair-growth products.

Other than minoxidil, there are a handful of topical substances that show some evidence that they can reduce hair loss and stimulate hair growth. These hardly have abundant research, but studies do exist for them.

Tretinoin (trade name Retin-A or Renova) is a topical cream or gel that may influence improvement in cell development, which has benefit for many skin-care problems ranging from acne to wrinkles. Surprisingly, no one is actually sure why tretinoin can do that, but there are lots of studies indicating it does. Some dermatologists have begun formulating their own treatments for male pattern balding by mixing tretinoin with minoxidil for topical application. It is thought that tretinoin can increase the absorption of minoxidil into the scalp. It may also help improve the structure of the hair follicle (the cell wall), making the hair growth pathway less restricted.

Azelaic acid is typically prescribed for rosacea and some acne conditions. Recently, the potential effect of using azelaic acid in the treatment of androgenetic alopecia has been looked at and discussed. According to Kevin J. McElwee, an immunologist/dermatologist involved in research on hair loss and regrowth, "Studies carried out in France in the late 1980s were to assess the effects of zinc sulfate and azelaic acid on the human skin. The result of these studies demonstrated that at high concentrations, zinc could completely inhibit the activity of 5 alpha reductase. Azelaic acid was also shown to be a potent inhibitor of 5 alpha-reductase. Inhibition was detectable at concentrations as low as 0.2mmol/l and was complete at 3mmol/l. When zinc, vitamin B6, and azelaic acid were added together at very low concentrations, which had been ineffective alone, 90 percent inhibition of 5 alpha-reductase was achieved."

Copper peptides are a group of ingredients that have several companies clamoring and making serious claims about their hair-growth potential. According to a Reuters April 4, 1999, newswire story, the "ProCyte Corporation said that it obtained statistically significant results in an initial study of its hair growth compound, in a group of men, ranging in age from 18 to 40 years old, with male pattern hair loss. The early-stage Phase II clinical study of the company's investigational compound, trade-named Tricomin solution, enrolled 36 men with early to mid-stage androgenetic alopecia [male pattern balding]. Treatment with 2.5 percent PC1358 [alanine/histidine/lysine polypeptide copper hydrochloride] resulted in a statistically significant increase in the total hair count when compared to vehicle [placebo] treatment over the course of the study. Appreciable increases in total hair weight were not found over the treatment phase of the study." While this research is interesting, it has not convinced the FDA to approve copper peptides for hair regrowth. Of course, this hasn't stopped ProCyte and a company called Skin Biology from selling several of their product lines with forms of copper peptide. ProCyte owns Tricomin, and Skin Biology sells Folligen. (These are discussed further in Chapter Nine.)

There is a long list of oral medications being researched and used for hair growth. All of these drugs have serious side effects that should be taken quite seriously before treatment with any of them is considered. I mention three here, but for a more definitive discussion please check out the references listed below in "Hair Growth—Scams or Solutions?"

Tagamet (active ingredient cimetidine) is commonly used for acid indigestion and to treat stomach ulcers and other digestive discomforts. However, Tagamet has been shown to have an anti-androgenic effect, which blocks the binding of dihydrotestosterone, and that can thus reduce hair loss. Cimetidine has been used to treat hirsutism in women (excess facial hair), and studies in women with androgenetic alopecia have yielded promising results. Men, however, should not use cimetidine to treat hair loss because of its feminizing effects.

Aldactone (active ingredient spironolactone) is a hormone blocker specifically reducing the production of testosterone by the adrenal glands and thereby preventing DHT from having an effect. It is a serious drug and is not a consideration for men due to its feminizing effects.

Ketoconazole is a topical and oral antifungal medication. It is used topically to reduce the presence of fungus that might be triggering dandruff, as well as orally to reduce systemic fungal infections. It has been observed that oral doses of ketoconazole can lower serum testosterone and thereby reduce the presence of DHT. However, there are serious side effects to taking ketoconazole, including dizziness, nausea, and headaches. Due to the association of problems with taking ketoconazole orally, there are those who think that applying it topically, in the form of the antidandruff shampoo Nizoral, can produce the same testosterone-lowering effect as the oral dosage. However, there is no research of any kind demonstrating this to be the case.

Birth control pills for women experiencing male pattern baldness can be helpful for that condition, but not all birth control pills are equal. Diane 35 is the name of a birth control pill specially designed to deal with hair loss issues for women. Some forms of birth control pills can actually stimulate male pattern balding by increasing the levels of androgens (testosterone and DHT). Birth control pills like Diane 35 work by reducing the amount of hormones that stimulate reproduction, and thereby stop ovulation. When a woman stops ovulating, she stops producing estrogens, progesterones, and androgens. There are other intricate biological factors taking place with this kind of birth control but, in essence, this form of controlling hair loss is strictly for women.

Hair Transplants

Other ways of dealing with hair loss include hair transplants, scalp reduction, and grafting sections of scalp with healthy hair onto sections of scalp where the hair is gone. According to Dr. Sheldon Kebacher, president of the International Society for Hair Restoration Surgery (ISHRS), "the quality of hair transplants has significantly improved since I did my first one back in 1973. The current hair transplants involve strips of scalp removed from the back of the head that are then cut into tiny grafts creating one to three hair sections. Slits are then made around the top of the head where the grafts are inserted. This new technique prevents the appearance of noticeable plugs."

What is most impressive about hair transplants is their success rate. Kebacher said, "The hair transferred usually lasts up to 30 years with a failure rate of less than 1 percent. Some thinning can take place in those 30 years but the person would have some amount of hair coverage for the rest of their life."

What is most shocking is the price, which ranges from $3,000 to $20,000.

Why do hair transplants work? The area at the back of the neck for some reason isn't programmed to be affected by hair-loss patterns. That genetic dominance doesn't change when the hair is grafted from one section of the body to another.

Before you decide to consult a physician for a hair transplant procedure of any kind, keep in mind that *any* licensed physician in the United States and Canada is permitted to perform hair surgery. That means a doctor who was previously a gynecologist, without taking one course, could hang out a shingle tomorrow declaring him- or herself a hair transplant specialist. It is that easy, and it happens all the time. Because of this lack of licensing or course work requirements, it is easy to end up with disappointing and inferior results such as visible scarring, patching, fuzzy hair, or even more hair loss. Before you book an appointment, find out if the doctor you are considering is in good standing with the International Society for Hair Restoration Surgery; contact them through their Web site at www.ishrs.org, or contact the American Academy of Facial Plastic and Reconstructive Surgery: (800) 332-3223 or www.plasticsurgery.org.

Just in case: absolutely ignore those ads you've seen on infomercials that advertise cans of tinted hairsprays, the ones that color in bald spots and are supposed to look like hair, even close up. They don't look like hair, not even from a distance. They look like spray paint and wouldn't fool a child.

Hair Growth—Scams or Solutions?

The number of hair-growth products on the market is literally hair-raising. Sadly, very few are actually growing hair, though they are taking a lot of your money. Several products and product lines are making claims about hair growth, ranging from Nioxin to Proxiphen, Fabao 101, Hairgenesis, and dozens—perhaps hundreds—more. I address some of these in Chapter Nine. But, please, before you fall for the fraudulent or exaggerated selling tactics of any hair-growing product (even those products that can affect hair growth often exaggerate their claims), keep in mind the following information from www.keratin.com by Kevin McElwee: "Most alopecias are not a gradual progressive hair loss. Most, including androgenetic alopecia, develop in spurts and then stop. There may even be some improvement for a short time before the hair loss begins again. Someone using a hair-growth product might falsely attribute this slowdown or temporary reversal to the use of the [product they purchased].

"Second, people who want to believe will believe. When real drug companies test products for hair regrowth, they run at least two methods of analysis side by side. One method is entirely empirical evidence. They mark an area on the volunteer's head and count the hair density in the area before and after treatment to see if there is improvement. The other analysis method they run is more subjective. They give a questionnaire to the volunteer and ask how the volunteer tester perceives the drug is working. Most human trials of drugs for alopecia are classic double-blind studies involving a group that receives the drug and another control group that receives an innocuous placebo compound. No one knows whether they are using the drug or placebo. **Frequently what is found is that volunteers on the drug or placebo indicate they believe they have regrowth of hair, but when comparing their positive comments to the hair count/density data, it is revealed there is no actual improvement and there may even be a deterioration.** Call it optimism or an overactive imagination, it is an important factor for professional scam artists [because they can tell you a product works when it only appears to work due to a placebo effect]."

One of the more bogus claims for hair-growth products is that the hair loss is due to poor or decreased blood circulation. If this was legitimate, there are many more incredibly cheap ways to increase circulation than with expensive products. Any stimulation, from simple massage (you can do that when you are shampooing) or a topical application of a heating pad, will greatly increase circulation for free. As

McElwee points out, "If lack of blood circulation was the cause of androgenetic alopecia, then why would hair transplants work? In transplantation, hair follicles are taken from the back of the head and placed in the areas of supposed poor blood circulation. You would expect the transplanted hair follicles to wither and die in their new blood-deficient environment if the poor blood circulation environment hypothesis was correct. They do not, and hair transplantation is a very successful procedure when done properly."

This book can't address all the issues and controversies surrounding hair growth, which requires a book unto itself, but there are many sources that provide comprehensive information on this issue. Before you spend hundreds of dollars a year on products that can't do a thing or products that can generate only negligible to minimal hair regrowth, please check out the following sources:

• www.keratin.com (a comprehensive Web site from Kevin J. McElwee, an immunologist/dermatologist involved in research on hair loss and regrowth)

• www.follicle.com (a comprehensive Web site)

• *The Bald Truth: The First Complete Guide to Preventing and Treating Hair Loss*, Spencer David Kobren, Pocket Books, 1998

• *Disorders of Hair Growth: Diagnosis and Treatment*, Elise A. Olsen, ed., McGraw Hill Text, 1994

• *Baldness: A Social History*, Kerry Segrave, McFarland & Company, 1996

The Thin and Thick of Hair

Hair is primarily composed of keratin, a solid, resilient, strong, fibrous form of protein. Getting a bit more technical, keratin is made up of amino acids linked together in a chain. The keratin chains are held together by something called a peptide bond. The keratin in hair has a high sulfur content, which explains how perms work, but I get into that in the chapter on perms.

The outer layer of the hair shaft is called the cuticle. The cuticle is the protective coating for the hair shaft. This rather uninteresting structure is probably the most relevant one when it comes to the health and protection of your hair. As the cuticle goes, so goes the hair. When the cuticle is intact, you have healthy hair. When the cuticle is damaged, you have problems that cannot be cured. Disappointing, but accurate nevertheless. Most of what you can do to keep your hair healthy involves taking care of the cuticle. Later, when I discuss which hair-care products live up to their claims, I primarily look at how these products affect the cuticle. Hair products that claim they can restore, repair, and restructure have to not only get past the cuticle to help the inside of the hair, but also adhere to the cuticle in order to mend tears and holes in the cuticle or to shore up vulnerable spots that can allow the inside of the hair shaft to also become damaged. Of course all of that is only temporary, but it is the only way to create some feel of normalcy.

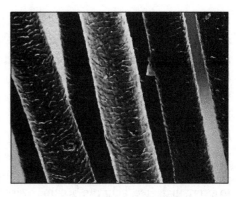

Bottom line: When the cuticle, the hair's first line of defense, is finally broken down, once the cuticle's seven to ten layers are eroded away, there is little hope left for the cortex and medulla, the heart of the hair shaft.

Under an electron microscope, blown up several thousand times, the cuticle resembles fish scales or layers of bark on a tree trunk. These overlapping layers form a tight barrier to the outside world's repeated attacks of washing, blow-drying, brushing, styling, and a number of other assaults we'll review later. Sadly, the cuticle is not, shall we say, as tough as nails, and it can only withstand our daily grooming rituals up to a point before it starts to break down.

The cuticle is composed primarily of *dead* protein called keratin. It also contains a large portion of *dead* amino acids, specifically cystine. (You'll hear more—actually, a *lot* more—about protein and different amino acids as they relate to hair and hair-care products.) **What is the cuticle protecting? The interior backbone of the hair, namely, the cortex and the medulla.** The cortex and medulla are also composed of protein, some cystine and other amino acids, water, and fats. Blown up under an electron microscope, the cortex and medulla have a porous, almost sponge-like appearance. The cortex and medulla are where factors such as the color, moisture content, elasticity, texture, and resilience of the hair reside. That's a lot for the cuticle to protect.

When the cortex and medulla are intact and healthy, the hair looks and performs the way it is supposed to (you may not like the way it performs, but at least it isn't damaged). When we try to change what the hair naturally wants to do with perms, hair dyes, styling tools, or even when we do simple things like shampooing and brushing, we start to break down the hair's bona fide inner strength. Regrettably, it doesn't take much to rip off pieces of cuticle and, given the demands of fashion, it is surprising we have any hair left on our heads. But what we do know about the cuticle can save our hair in more ways than one.

When the cuticle is healthy and intact, lying flat and tight against the hair shaft, the hair reflects light evenly, producing a wonderful luster and shine. When the cuticle is bruised, from chemical processes, heat, or any kind of manipulation, the edges of the cuticle begin to lift and separate from the hair shaft. Initially, that can have a positive effect on the appearance of your hair. When the cuticle is roughed up and the edges of the scales stand up, the hairs are held apart from one another, giving a fuller appearance. One of the reasons permed or dyed hair can appear thicker (if the hair is not overly permed or dyed and is not multiprocessed) is because the chemicals from the dye and perms cause the cuticle to lift. The same is true for hair that is backcombed or "ratted." Backcombing roughs up the cuticle, lifting the edges so the hairs grab each other at the overlapping, frayed edges, creating a pretty tough network that keeps the hair aloft. That's why backcombed hair can stay in place for a fairly long period of time. To an extent, none of this is a serious problem—but only to a certain degree. Hair can become overprocessed or overworked to the point of no return. When the cuticle is repeatedly mistreated, chips of cuticle are torn away from the hair shaft, literally peeling away like the layers of an onion until there is nothing left except an exposed core.

Hair Note: One way that hair-care companies use scientific information in convoluted ways to sell their products is with facts such as "the cortex and medulla are composed of protein, some cystine, amino acids, water, and fats." That sounds like you can add protein or amino acids to hair-care products to shore up and replace what may be lost due to damage. It just isn't true. Proteins have too large a molecular structure to get into the hair cortex or medulla. Amino acids are smaller and penetrate better, but they don't cling well to hair so they are easily rinsed or evaporated away along with the moisture on your hair. Fats are useful, but only in the way they can coat the hair as a conditioner.

Hair is exceptionally porous. **Water readily absorbs into hair; about 20 percent water is present even when the hair is dry, and that can go up to 75 percent (the maximum amount) when it is wet.** Too much water, though, can destroy any hairstyle, and the lack of water in the hair can do the same.

The Shape and Heart of the Hair

One strand of hair all by itself appears to be nothing more than a wiry string with muted, dull color. With the help of an electron microscope that same ultra-thin hair can be magnified to a thousand times its size, and the cuticle, resembling an overlapping shingled roof or fish scales, can be seen. Those shingles or scales are made out of protein. When the hair is cut in half and viewed under the same microscope, deeper inside are rings that look like the rings of a tree trunk. These rings are more layers of cuticle, about seven layers thick, depending on the head of hair. Past these cuticle layers lies the cortex, the heart of the hair. The cortex has long protein filaments, called microfibrils and macrofibrils, which run the length of the hair. These determine the strength, resilience, and moisture content of the hair. (The medulla is the innermost structure, but little is known about this part of the hair. Strangely, according to dermatologist Dr. Zoe Draelos, the medulla isn't even present in most hairs on your head when compared to hairs on other parts of the body.)

The form and shape of the hair are determined by even smaller components of the hair known as hydrogen and disulfide bonds. These bonds are part of the protein chain that keeps hair strong and helps it retain its natural shape. **Disulfide bonds are incredibly strong and not easily broken. Hydrogen bonds, on the other hand, are quite weak and change easily with humidity and wetness. Hydrogen bonds affect the temporary day-to-day, shampoo-to-shampoo shape of your hair.** The reason wet hair becomes longer and temporarily changes shape is because the hydrogen bonds have been broken. As the hair dries, the hydrogen bonds quickly reform and re-establish the hair's natural shape. Using rollers or blow-dryers on wet hair can change its natural shape temporarily because you've altered and reformed the flexible hydrogen bonds with heat. Once the hair becomes wet again (from water or humidity), the hydrogen bonds break and revert back to their original curl or lack thereof. **Hair's hydrogen bonds have a great memory unless you are there with heat in hand to convince those bonds to go in another direction than they normally would.**

Disulfide bonds are the backbone of your hair's shape, but they (unlike hydrogen bonds) are not so easily convinced to take on another form. Any permanent change in hair curl has to be done by breaking down these tenacious bonds. Because disulfide bonds are so strong, it takes potent chemicals to modify their shape. Permanent-wave or hair-straightening solutions (which actually use the same formulas; the hair is configured differently depending on what you want it to do) contain highly alkaline solutions that can fracture disulfide bonds.

Once the disulfide bonds have been broken, they are ready to be reformed, which is accomplished during the time the alkaline solution sits on the hair and the hair is molded to its new shape. If you curl your hair up in rollers or comb your hair straight and then soak it in an alkaline solution, the disulfide bonds will break and with time take on the shape of the roller or the straightened hair shaft. As soon as the alkaline solution is neutralized, the reforming process stops and the new shape is set. Remember, these disulfide bonds are stubborn. They want to go back to their original form. It takes a good deal of processing time and strong chemicals to get the disulfide bonds to do exactly what you want them to do, particularly if you have stick-straight or ultracurly hair. And don't think for one second that the process of reforming disulfide bonds is anything less than damaging to your hair. Even breaking down the hydrogen bonds and reforming them with heat is damaging to hair over time, but breaking the disulfide bonds is a heavy burden to put on anyone's hair, and you can't expect it to come out anything but damaged. So-called "gentle" perms do exist, but they are gentle because they have a lower pH, not because they contain natural or special ingredients. Regrettably, the lower pH also makes the product not very effective on perfectly straight or extremely curly hair if the goal is to straighten out the curls or put in tighter ones. For more information on perms and straighteners, see Chapter Six, *Perfectly Straight or Perfectly Curly*.

Understanding Hair Damage

Damaging the cuticle is the principal way in which we ruin all the things about hair that most of us want and envy—and, sadly, the cuticle is easily damaged. As the cuticle is chipped away, eliminating the hair's entire protective structure, you end up with a stripped naked, weak, shapeless hair shaft.

Split ends happen when most of the damage takes place on the ends of the hair. Since damage is almost always cumulative, it makes sense that split ends would be a typical problem—those ends have been around the longest and subject to repeated abuse.

Another typical problem is where hair breaks off in the middle and not at the ends. This is a result of either concentrated damage at that specific site, overextending the hair shaft beyond its capacity (particularly during styling), or a genetic weak link in hair growth.

For those who repeatedly perm and/or color their hair (especially if the hair is stripped (bleached) and then toned (adding another color after the hair has been stripped), the result is soft, mushy, dry, and brittle hair that breaks off in chunks. **This occurs when excessive overprocessing destroys most of the entire cuticle layer, leaving the hair shaft's cortex exposed.**

Sadly, it is actually all too easy to damage the hair shaft, yet we can hardly help ourselves. There are many things that make the cuticle fall apart, and most of the damage is not caused by the hair-care products we use. (Yes, that's ten points for the hair-care companies; on the whole, they are not making products that destroy hair. There are exceptions, but they are actually few and far between.) Most of the abuse is caused by what we do to our hair in the name of fashion and hygiene, and the havoc we wreak in the name of style is often irreversible and irreparable. What causes the damage? The answers will amaze and disturb you. They certainly disturb me.

In essence, hair is damaged by almost everything we do to it. Common, everyday actions can cause breakage, splitting, frizzing, and dryness. **Friction and heat are the primary sources of cuticle damage. Friction occurs when you rub your hair against itself; for example, when you towel-dry your hair, or when your loved one runs his or her fingers tenderly through your hair. When you move the hair against itself, especially roughly, you start breaking apart the cuticle. Brushing hair also tears apart the cuticle.** Every time the brush smoothes through your locks, separating the shafts from one another, little bits of cuticle are being chipped away. It is particularly damaging when the hair is being stretched, such as when you are trying to undo a knot or untangle a mussed hairdo. Blow-drying on the hottest setting, using hot rollers and curling irons, or turning your hair dryer to high fries off tiny, and sometimes large, parts of the cuticle every time, and the closer the heat, the greater the damage. Even shampooing causes damage when you massage the lather into the length of the hair by rubbing the hairs against each other.

Towel-drying the hair in a tousling manner by rubbing the towel over the hair (instead of just gently squeezing) damages the cuticle, but hair is already more prone to damage when it is wet than when it is dry. Yet, as many of us know, blow-dryers work best on wet hair. That's why your hairstylist rewets your hair after it's been cut: to blow it dry in a better, longer-lasting shape. Braiding hair, tying it back into a bun or ponytail, and rolling it up on curlers (especially the relatively new Velcro curlers) can all damage the hair. Environmental conditions can also diminish the health of your hair. Sunlight, wind, pollution, chlorine from pools, and dry heat can all take a toll. Don't forget that chemical processes such as perms and dyes can be damaging, and doing them over and over again or on top of each other is almost a guaranteed cuticle destroyer.

Those of us who dye or perm our hair understand the damage that occurs and, to a certain extent, accept it as part of the price of getting rid of gray or achieving straighter or curlier hair. **What some of us might not realize is that once hair has undergone a chemical process, the cuticle is softened and much more prone to damage.**

What are we supposed to do? Never touch our hair again? Sounds hopeless, doesn't it? But don't despair. It is neither hopeless nor impossible to change bad habits once you are aware of them. A total hands-off ultimatum isn't the answer. You just need a change of perspective and a new relationship with your hair. **Once you become aware of what you can do and what it takes to really have healthy hair, you can start protecting your hair immediately.** Keep in mind that the daily damage is cumulative and that it takes effort on your part to bring about. Luckily, the cuticle is seven to ten layers thick, there are a lot of hairs on your head, and your hair grows, replenishing itself with a new healthy base every month or two. You absolutely have some slack in the area between looking out for the welfare of the cuticle and styling your hair. Moreover, you don't have to buy products that promise to protect the hair (although some of them do help); there are better, more reliable solutions that require action, not money.

Stopping Damage

For all intents and purposes, taking care of your hair starts with taking care of the cuticle. Paying attention to the needs of this microscopic layer of protection will go a long way toward your having healthy hair and fewer bad hair days. You will need to change your ways, which can take some getting used to. For many of us, these may have become second nature but, with time, the old habits will become strange and the new habits will feel as natural as brushing your teeth.

Brush or comb your hair as infrequently and as gently as possible. Without question, brushing is one of the most damaging things you do to your hair, especially if you repeat it frequently during the day and use hard-bristled brushes. **Every time you brush through your hair, the spikes chip away at the cuticle. Be good to your hair and leave it alone as often as you can. That doesn't mean never brushing but, rather, brushing only when needed and using soft-bristled or soft-feeling brushes.** The farther apart the bristles, the better. If they are close together, they must have a soft, flexible feel. When you run the brush through your hair, take care to start at the base of your scalp, using as little force as possible. Avoid slamming the brush into your hair and driving it through to the ends. Brush your hair in sections starting at the top and working your way down, being the most gentle with the ends. If you want your hair to look its fullest, throw your head forward and brush from the nape of your neck forward, avoiding the ends. Then throw your head back and smooth the top and ends without digging into the hair. If you want to distribute the oil from your scalp throughout your hair, brushing it once in the morning, afternoon, and evening should take care of that. During the day you can also separate your hair with your fingertips, smoothing it with your hands.

Never use a brush on wet hair, and don't overbrush wet hair. Wet hair is more easily damaged than dry hair (in wet hair the hydrogen bonds have been broken and the hair is therefore in a more vulnerable state). It's best to use either a wide-toothed comb or a wide-bristled brush with rounded tips on wet hair.

Choose your brushes and combs carefully. Certain brushes and combs are more damaging than others. I list specific choices in the product evaluation section of this book but, as a general rule, the softer the brush or comb, the less it will damage the hair. If it tears and pulls at your hair as you brush or comb, it's hurting the cuticle. Combs with rough teeth, brushes with hard bristles, not to mention rubber bands, can tear and chip away at the cuticle, causing unnecessary damage.

When drying your hair, never tousle, twist, or wring it dry with a towel or with your hands; instead, squeeze it dry gently using either a towel or your hands. Friction erodes the cuticle. The less the hair is rubbed against itself or by or with anything else, the better off it will be.

Handle your hair as little as possible. Friction is the culprit here too. Rubbing one object or surface against another causes friction and fractures the cuticle. The less you interact with your hair, the better. If you have the habit of mindlessly running your hands through your hair (I know I do), try to develop another habit.

When blowing your hair dry, avoid applying heat directly to the hair. This rule is probably the hardest to comply with, so give yourself some slack if you're 100 percent good about keeping the nozzle of the dryer at least three to six inches away from the hair. Heat is the primary means of smoothing frizz or setting a curl, and we all know hair behaves better when you blow-dry it wet instead of waiting for it to dry and then putting in a style. There are many products that claim to protect hair from blow-drying, but they can only help in some situations and for some hair types. If your hair is already seriously damaged, or if you use high heat directly on your hair frequently and for long intervals, hair-styling/protecting products won't be able to protect the cuticle adequately, although they are better than nothing.

Perming and/or coloring hair causes damage. There is no way around this one. Even worse is perming and then coloring your hair (or vice versa); that causes terrible damage. Changing hair from dark brown to blonde is also extremely damaging. Once hair is damaged, there is no way to repair it. (I discuss all this at length in Chapters Five and Six.)

Use your blow-dryer, curling iron, hot rollers, or other heat implements as infrequently as possible, and try to use the least amount of heat to effect the style you want. Intense heat damages hair. There is no escape from this one either. The same way your skin gets burned with high heat, so does the hair. You may be tempted to ignore this warning if you use one of the many styling products or conditioners that claim they can coat the hair and reduce damage caused by styling implements. Unfortunately, that is not an accurate picture. These products do offer some protection, but how much is totally dependent on how thoroughly you saturate the hair and how hot your styling tool gets. High heat applied directly, along with brushing and pulling (a necessary element of using styling tools) for more than just a few minutes will wear down the product's ability to protect and will allow heat to easily get right through to the cuticle.

The following is an interesting letter (and my response to it) from the company that makes ThermaSilk, a product line making claims about protecting the hair from heat :

Dear Paula,

I recently saw your [newspaper] column syndicated by Knight Ridder and wanted to thank you for recommending ThermaSilk hair-care products. I admire your goal of providing consumers with straightforward information about cosmetic and hair-care products.

After reading your column, I am concerned that your readers may not understand how ThermaSilk works and, therefore, the benefit of the products. I know you would appreciate receiving factual information from scientists about beauty products, so I would like to take this opportunity to clarify and explain the technology behind ThermaSilk.

As a manager of microscopy and biochemistry at Helene Curtis, I have been involved for the last three of the five years of intensive research that has gone into creating the technology surrounding ThermaSilk products. When originally approached with the proposition of formulating a heat-activated hair-care product line that would improve the condition of the hair with heat, my first thought was that it couldn't be done. No one was more surprised than I was that we were able to find a way to make heat styling something that was actually healthy for your hair.

So how did we do it? In the case of our shampoos, we used a unique, patented combination of conditioning agents that are suspended as very small, positively charged particles in the ThermaSilk formula. First, the small size of these conditioning particles ensures a more even distribution on the hair. Secondly, as you might know, hair is negatively charged (i.e., source of static flyaway). The positively charged particles containing ThermaSilk's unique combination of conditioning agents are naturally attracted to the negatively charged surface of the hair. This allows more conditioning particles to deposit on the hair's surface and remain through the rinsing process. Once the heat of a styling appliance is applied, it causes the conditioning agents to spread along each hair strand, making the hair softer, smoother, and healthier.

Other shampoos may contain similar conditioning agents, but they are suspended as either significantly larger particles than ThermaSilk or the conditioning particles do not possess as much positive charge as ThermaSilk. The combination of the conditioning agent's smaller size and positive charge, along with the application of heat, is what really makes ThermaSilk different from other products.

ThermaSilk, like every Helene Curtis product, has gone through an extensive development and testing process to ensure that the product delivers on its promise. We used a number of commonly used as well as proprietary testing methodologies to confirm that ThermaSilk is truly heat-activated and that it works with heat to improve the condition of hair. For example, we tested and found that hair treated with ThermaSilk and then heat styled is significantly softer than hair that is treated with ThermaSilk and air dried. In addition, the tests revealed that hair that is untreated or treated with a standard non-conditioning shampoo becomes stiffer and less soft upon application of heat styling. The attached pictures from an electron microscope clearly illustrate the difference between ThermaSilk treated hair and non-ThermaSilk treated hair.

In your column, you raised questions about how ThermaSilk shampoos and conditioners could be heat-activated if the product is rinsed off hair before you heat style. All ThermaSilk shampoos and conditioners are designed for use prior to the heat-styling process. As I described earlier, as you wash and/or condition your hair, the smaller-sized, positively charged conditioning particles ensure a more even distribution and higher deposition of conditioner on the hair's surface even after rinsing. The heat of a blow-dryer or curling iron spreads the conditioners more effectively along each strand, which produces a higher level of conditioning.

You also expressed concerns about the effectiveness of ThermaSilk styling products if styling aids are applied after the heat-styling process is completed. To achieve ThermaSilk's heat-activated benefits, all of our styling products are meant to be applied before or during the heat-styling process, which is typically the time these styling aids are used. Even ThermaSilk's Shape and Hold Spray is uniquely formulated for dual usage on wet or dry hair. Attached are results from a 1997 study conducted by NFO Research Inc., which indicated that styling products such as mousse, gel, and shaping spray are primarily applied to wet or damp hair.

While many ingredients used in ThermaSilk can be found in other hair-care products, as I mentioned earlier, it's the science and technology behind how these ingredients are formulated that make the product unique. ThermaSilk products are specially formulated using different amounts of certain key ingredients and blending them in combinations different from other products. In fact, many of ThermaSilk's products have U.S. compositional patents, and we have filed for two U.S. and world patents to protect our formulation strategy.

Finally, we've conducted extensive research on the effect of heat styling on hair. We know that routine usage of blow-dryers and curling irons can dry out the hair and crack the cuticle, leaving hair extremely dry and coarse, but it should never degrade or scorch the hair. During standard heat styling, the temperature of a blow dryer or curling iron can reach between 90 degrees and 200 degrees Celcius. Hair, because it is such an excellent thermal insulator, only reaches an average temperature of between 50 degrees and 140 degrees Celcius when heat styled. In order to actually burn, the hair would have to exceed 250 degrees Celcius. ThermaSilk provides protection from the potential cracking, cuticle uplift, and excessive water loss associated with standard heat styling.

In closing, I hope that your readers will find this information helpful. Over its 70-year history, Helene Curtis has always held itself to the highest standards of product excellence. We know, especially with the wide array of hair-care products available today, that our products must live up to consumers' expectations in order to gain their continued support. This commitment has helped us create many of the hair-care industry's major innovations—including the first liquid shampoos, at-home permanents, self-adjusting conditioners, and, now, heat-activated hair-care products.

If you have any further technical questions regarding ThermaSilk, other Helene Curtis products, or hair care in general, I'd be happy to discuss them with you.

Sincerely,
Joanne Crudele
Manager, Microscopy & Biochemistry
Helene Curtis, Research and Development

Dear Joanne,

Thank you so much for supplying your information to me regarding ThermaSilk products. However, there are few points we disagree on. While I am certain your technology and formulation is excellent, the idea that conditioning agents adhere to hair is well established and not unique to your product. Silicone ingredients (a technology originated by Procter & Gamble) cling tenaciously to hair, and they can even do that when they are used in shampoos. You may have indeed found a way to make that molecular structure smaller and thereby more accessible to hair, but you didn't substantiate that in the information you sent me. [Actually the laboratory study from Helene Curtis indicated that propylene glycol and glycerin were the agents that improved heat distribution when coated over the hair—hardly special or unique hair-care ingredients.]

It is also well established that conditioning benefits are increased when mild heat is applied to the hair. Heat does help swell the hair shaft, and that allows the conditioning agents to get between the cuticle layers more easily. But, again, that would be true for lots of products.

This issue gets muddled by the way you use centigrade numbers. When those centigrade figures are translated to Fahrenheit, they are much more daunting. Styling tools can heat up to 120 degrees Fahrenheit [that's low to moderate heat for most rollers and blow-dryers] to over 350 degrees Fahrenheit on the top setting, well over the threshold for charring hair and skin [as a point of reference, remember water boils at 212 degrees Fahrenheit]. I personally have burnt my skin while using curling irons and blow dryers; now if that isn't "degrading" to the hair and skin I don't know what is. I think you were taking me too literally when I said hair can "burn" with the use of styling tools. Hair won't catch fire unless it reaches over 500 degrees Fahrenheit, but lots of serious damage can take place at temperatures far below that, and no cosmetic ingredients can prevent that.

We both agree that mild topical heat is not a problem, but that is not how many women use curling irons or blow-dryers, especially not nowadays with the new popular straight-as-sticks hairstyles and the new-wattage blow-dryers and heat-producing curling irons. If you meant your products were safe on very low, mild heat, that's one issue, but your ads don't state that and the consumer is left believing that your products can protect, and even be helpful, under any amount of heat.

One more point: It is one issue to "burn" hair, but it is another to boil or heat up the water content inside the hair shaft itself. When hair is wet, heat can cause water inside the hair to literally boil (it only takes 212 degrees Fahrenheit to get the water to a rollicking boil, and even lower temperatures can cause water to agitate in the hair shaft). This can burst the hair shaft and cause damage, something all the conditioners in the world can't address.

One final point. We both know that heat is only one source of hair damage; actual brushing and manipulation can be an even more significant source, and conditioning agents of any kind can only protect so much. Your conditioning agents are just fine and I do like the ThermaSilk products (I personally use your hairspray and shampoo), but I would never encourage my readers to rely on the ingredients to protect their hair from heat damage when using styling tools.

Paula Begoun

Scalp Facts

Your hair and your scalp are vastly different, yet intricately related. Oil production and dry scalp are probably two of the biggest headaches women have to deal with when deciding what shampoo and conditioner to use. Both oily and dry scalps can adversely affect the appearance of the hair on a daily basis. But even for someone with normal hair, a healthy scalp can play a significant role in the appearance of the hair over the long haul.

Like the skin on your face, your scalp goes through a shedding process. The lower layers of skin cells are alive and generally quite healthy and vital. Unlike other parts of your body that aren't protected by a dense covering of hair, the scalp rarely, if ever, has any sun damage, and that makes it some of the healthiest skin on your body.

As skin cells go through their life cycle, they transform, begin to die, and move toward the outside, changing shape and function along the way. By the time they get to the surface, they are dead and ready to fall off.

Emerging from the scalp via hair follicles embedded deep in the scalp are single strands of hair. Each hair follicle is connected to a sebaceous (oil-producing) gland, nerve endings, and blood vessels. Circulation at the base of the hair follicle feeds the developing hair cells, helping to make a stronger, healthier strand of hair. If for some reason the hair follicle gets plugged, whether from the oil produced by the sebaceous gland, from hair-care products (styling products or conditioning agents), or from dead skin cells that have not been shed, it can hamper hair growth. Please keep in mind that it is rare for the follicle to get plugged in this manner, because many companies make great sales points of generating fear around this issue.

Oil production is almost entirely controlled by hormonal activity. There is no way to stop oil production from the outside in. Oil-control products are a bit of a joke, because while some of them can clean away oil or absorb excess oil, none can change the stuff that is being produced internally.

For many reasons, oil production is both good and bad for hair. Oil is a problem when it makes hair look heavy, greasy, and limp, but mainly oil is good for hair because it functions to protect the hair from drying out. Essentially, a conditioner serves to reproduce what your own oil naturally provides. As the oil gland produces oil, it melts over the surface of the scalp and onto the hair shaft. On straight hair, the oil easily moves down along the hair shaft to the ends. On curly hair the oil follows the exact path of the hair, moving along the twists and curves. That convoluted path makes it difficult for the oil to make its way to the ends of the hair. Someone with straight hair and an oily scalp may experience far oilier conditions (meaning limp, greasy hair) than someone with curly hair and an oily scalp.

Struggling with oil production isn't easy because the oil you wash away is rapidly replaced. Using stronger surfactant shampoos isn't the answer because you can only remove the oil, and that is relatively easy for most shampoos to do. Trying to stop the oil with stronger products doesn't do a thing except dry out the hair and make matters worse.

The primary way to deal with almost all scalp types and to reduce damage to the hair shaft is to focus most of your shampooing attention on your scalp and not your hair. That doesn't mean treating the scalp roughly or overscrubbing it, it means gently massaging the scalp with your fingertips, gently moving your nails along the scalp. Not only does this help to remove dead skin cells, but the massaging action of your shampooing increases circulation. Gently increasing circulation is one of the only ways to help nourish the root of the hair follicle from the outside in to help maintain healthy growth. It won't produce miracles like helping grow hair where there isn't any, but improving circulation can be subtly beneficial. Don't be concerned that you won't be getting the length of your hair clean; despite the way products can build up on the hair, it actually gets pretty clean without much manipulation. Moreover, less manipulation of the hair shaft means less damage to the cuticle.

Likewise, given how much oil is usually present at the root of the hair, and by virtue of the root's state of health (it hasn't been around long enough to be damaged by styling tools, sun exposure, dyeing, or perming), it also requires less conditioner. As important as it is to clean the scalp more scrupulously than it is to focus on the length of hair, it is more important to condition the length of hair than the scalp. (I get into more of this in the section on conditioners.) Adding conditioner to the scalp is often like adding a moisturizer to oily skin on the face: it just makes matters worse.

So, regardless of the apparently close relationship between scalp and hair, it is essential to treat your scalp and your hair as if they were not at all related or even existing on the same head. Remember, the scalp is part of a living system, and the hair you see and need to maintain is dead. Scalp needs and hair needs are very different.

Genetic Destiny?

Many of us find that, regardless of how good we are to the cuticle or how diligent we are about taking care of our scalp, our hair still may not do exactly what we want it to do, especially in the areas of thickness, fullness, and density. Alas, what grows out of your head is genetically fated, and there isn't much that any hair product can do to alter your inherited traits. How full your hair appears mainly has to do with the number of hairs on your head and the size and curl of the hair shaft, which are predetermined at birth. Remember, the average head of hair has about 100,000 to 120,000 strands. Blonde and light brown hairs have a very thin, narrow shaft, while black, dark brown, and red hairs have the thickest (so even though blondes tend to have more hair, the hair itself is not as thick, and so gives the perception of having less hair). African hair is the thinnest and most fragile, both because of its thin hair shaft as well as the redundant twists and turns, with each twist being a potential break point. Asian hair, on the other hand, is rather thick and substantial, though most typically stick-straight.

If you have thin, fine hair; coarse, curly hair with a tendency to frizz; or thick, heavy hair with a mind of its own, all the products in the world, without the assistance of styling implements, can't do much to radically change its appearance and, even then, overworking the hair can eventually damage it and make matters worse. Perms can make hair look fuller by changing the shape of the hair, but constantly reperming your hair to maintain its appearance can fry it, making it stiff, frizzy, and shapeless. Coloring the hair can make it somewhat fuller by roughing up the cuticle and creating a bulkier appearance, but repeated coloring, especially if you are changing the color radically, can also cause irreparable damage. In short, you can, to some extent, change the hair you were born with, but big changes are more a figment of media-induced fantasy than reality.

The endless onslaught of seductive models with long, flowing, diligently coifed manes causes angst in many of us. We simply find it impossible to believe these women were born that way (believe it: that's why they're models and we're not). We also fail to recognize the energy and time it takes for a hairstylist to get hair to do what we see in the ad or commercial. If you haven't seen a photo shoot or a commercial taping, you probably aren't aware of the contributions of the camera person, the lighting crew, or any of a dozen details that culminate in an enticing image. Fans are strategically placed to blow the hair into billowing fullness; constant rebrushing and styling keep the 'do in place. **All the things we don't see are what really make those models look so good, and yet the ads suggest a product change can create those results. We want to believe it is really that simple, and the hair-care companies encourage us to.** This marketing influence is perhaps even more insidious for hair-care products than for skin-care or makeup products. True, it can cost $50 to see whether or not a new moisturizer will live up to the results tantalizingly reflected in the skin of sensually posed, pubescent models, and almost $30 for a foundation. For hair care, even the pricier lines may cost only $8 to $20, a reasonable-sounding amount to spend to see how well a product works. A veritable bargain. The difficulty lies in how much of these products we use and how often we change, hoping the next product will do the impossible.

I know I'm not telling you anything you don't already know from either experience or familiarity with ingredient lists. But with fashion magazines and hair-care companies incessantly telling you to expect the impossible, it is easy to fall prey to the advertising traps waiting to ensnare you.

What Causes Bad Hair Days?

Bad hair days can happen overnight. Perfect hair one day, nightmare hair the next, and you did nothing different. The scenario goes something like this: You wake up on a Tuesday and your hair is perfect; it moves just the way you want it to and goes into just the style and shape you have in mind, and you don't even try very hard. The next day, Wednesday morning, you wake up much as you did the day before, get dressed the same way you did the day before, everything is identical—except your hair now has a mind of its own and it has made up its mind to be spiteful and bad-tempered. No matter how you blow it dry or what styling products you use, it goes this way instead of that and, to add insult to injury, it moves stiffly and seems to have cowlicks that were never there before. What happened?

We know that the damage we inflict on our hair can cause styling problems. What we may not know is that conditioning agents and styling products can build up on the hair and eventually, seemingly overnight, cause the hair to feel heavy and limp. This recurring phenomenon is often the cause of bad hair days. It is also the reason that the myth about your hair adapting to hair-care products got started. It's not that your hair adapts, but that the ingredients in conditioners and styling products that like to cling to hair are not the easiest to wash off, and tend to build up. That buildup can greatly affect the appearance and quality of hair.

One thing that might be causing your hair confusion are your hormones. Increased estrogen production the week before you get your period can trigger increased oil production, making hair limp and dull. Hormones also affect how you see yourself, and the premenstrual blues can make any feature that looked fine the day before seem like an eyesore the next. Everything probably looks the same, but with PMS eyes, you can't see it. The significance of this should not be taken lightly. Often women waste more money on grooming products, fighting this time of month, when it has nothing to do with what really exists, but is a result of their own emotionally blurred vision. Depression and stress can cause the same misinterpretation of the facts. Realizing that you really haven't changed can help prevent your low spirits from getting even lower.

It's bad enough having your emotions and hormones play tricks on you, but the environment can also cause bad hair days. Humidity or dryness or a change in the weather can alter your hair, whether it's due to the change of seasons or a weather pattern moving through your area. Hair takes on moisture in the air with relative ease, and it also releases its moisture content to the air when it is dry outside. If you've ever gotten on an airplane when the humidity was high or at least normal, with your curls bouncing neatly in place, you may have noticed that by the end of the trip they've gone flat and dry. The lack of humidity in the airplane causes the water to be virtually sucked out of the hair, causing it to go flat and look dry. During the winter, dry heat at home and in the office can have the same effect. Dryness in the air can also cause static electricity, making hair go flyaway. On the other hand, increased relative humidity can cause naturally curly hair to swell and become more frizzy, more curly (where you don't want curls), and harder to control, while making thin or limp hair look even flatter and more limp.

Bad hair days are also affected by timing. **Hair behaves differently when it is dried at various degrees of wetness, and that behavior varies from person to person. Generally, if you start styling your hair when it is wet, you have a better chance of getting it to do what you want.** Perhaps your bad hair experience occurred on a day when you got to your blow-dryer after your hair had dried more than usual. Hair is finicky, and finding your hair's personal nuances can sometimes rescue bad hair days. For example, if you rewet your hair to style it the next day, consider getting the roots wetter than the ends. Roots are predominantly responsible for determining the movement, lift, and shape of the hair. How you sleep on your hair can set in a cowlick that all the heat in the world won't correct.

Damaged hair is particularly susceptible to all the variations of humidity, dryness, hormonal activity, and styling nuances; because damaged hair is so much more porous and the cuticle is rougher, these hazards are twice as likely to cause problems.

CHAPTER THREE

Hair-Care Basics

What Do They Mean When They Say . . . ?

What is most startling in the world of hair care is that the formulations are so incredibly repetitive. Despite the claims, the formula variations between shampoo, conditioners, and styling products is minor. Yet there is a great deal of marketing language to help create the illusion that amazing differences exist where there are none to be found.

What, then, is the difference between a product that builds body and one that builds volume? Are they one and the same or is there a difference? How *does* a product build volume or add body to the hair? Is a product designed for color-treated hair really very different from one designed for permed or damaged hair? What makes a product good for color-treated hair but not for dry hair, or vice versa? Can a hair-care product that claims to put curl back into the hair or to revitalize a perm really do that?

One of the more confusing aspects of the hair-care industry is trying to keep the terminology straight. I would love to straighten out all this industry lingo for you but, unfortunately, there is no easy way to do that. Product names and the results they allude to are not consistent from line to line or even within lines. If you buy a product claiming to clarify or deep-clean hair, it may contain ingredients that add more buildup, or be a formulation that can't deep-clean. A shampoo claiming to be good for oily hair may contain conditioning agents that will only add up to a greasy feel. One line may have a host of products claiming they can add volume to the hair, but those products may have nothing in common with those from a different line that claim to do the same thing.

As difficult as it is to wade through this morass of contradictions and inconsistencies, here are some general guidelines to help you get started.

Most products designated either separately or in combination for permed, color-treated, coarse, chemically processed, dry, damaged, porous, or sun-bleached hair tend to contain similar ingredients. These products all tend to be more emollient and conditioning than other product types. There is generally little difference in how any of these hair-care groups are formulated.

The reason these formulations can be the same and still function well is that although the cause of each of those hair problems is different, their effect on the hair shaft tends to be the same. Dry hair is a result of the hair losing its moisture content, often because damage has destroyed the hair shaft's ability to keep moisture in the hair, but it also can happen in a dry environment when you have healthy hair (in that case, your hair could be dry without being damaged). Either way, the product you use would remain the same, even if the source of the problem is different.

Products that claim to add body, volume, or thickness to the hair almost always contain lightweight water-binding agents such as glycerin, propylene glycol, amino acids, panthenols, and proteins, and a small amount of styling agents (film formers and plasticizing agents) such as acrylates, PVP, and PVM/MA (polyvinyl methyl ether/maleic anhydride). These styling agents are the same as those found in hairsprays or styling gels. The water-binding agents keep water in the hair to prevent dehydration and thus keep the hair swollen, helping to add a feeling of thickness. The styling agents cover the hair shaft with an almost imperceptible layer that adds to its thickness. That doesn't amount to much for a single strand of hair, but multiply this microscopic layer over the 100,000 hairs on your head and it can give a slight impression of feeling and looking thicker. It can also easily feel heavy—after all, an imperceptible layer is still a layer—and that buildup can feel heavy, not full. Another issue is that these volumizing products do easily build up, especially when these film-forming ingredients are in shampoos, because they never get washed all the way off before more are deposited on the hair shaft.

Many products in many different forms claim to reduce frizzies. They usually contain some form of silicone oil, emollients, film formers, and detangling agents. These ingredients put a tactile, emollient layer over the hair, binding the cuticle down and slightly sticking the hairs together without making them feel as bonded as with hairspray, gel, or mousse.

What about products that say they can add shine to the hair? Making the cuticle shut down tight gets a lot of attention from hair companies. When the cuticle lies flat, it has a smoother, more even surface that can reflect light. (Think of a lake. When the surface is smooth, you can see your reflection shining back at you. When the lake is rough and uneven, no more reflection.) How can you shut down the cuticle? Applying a shampoo, conditioner, or styling product with a low pH can make the microscopic layers of the cuticle close tight. Using a shampoo with a pH of around 3.5 to 4.5 is one way to do this; a lemon or vinegar rinse (both of these have a pH of about 3.5) at the end of your shampoo is another—but none of this is probably worth the trouble because hair's pH is incredibly fickle and the hair wants to return to its own pH. Even more material is the fact that most women who use styling products and tools end up roughing up the cuticle anyway, no matter what the pH happens to be. Another issue is that exceptionally damaged hair (from re-peated color treatments or perms) doesn't have enough cuticle left to work with.

Products that say they impart shine generally contain silicone or various oils, though silicone is by far the preferred ingredient for shine. Silicone is an out-standing hair-care ingredient, with properties that not only add reflection and sheen but an unbelievably sensual, silky feel. The only trick with these types of products is not to get carried away; too much can build up to a greasy mess that looks more wet and sticky than shiny.

Conditioners vary according to the amount of emollients, water-binding agents, detangling agents, antistatic ingredients, and oils they contain. When only a small amount of these are present, the conditioner is best for someone with normal, limp, fine, or oily hair. When more of these are in a conditioner, it is best for someone with any level of damaged or dry hair.

Styling products are the most redundant product grouping of all. The ingredi-ents that can help hold hair in place are limited, and these show up repeatedly in hairspray after hairspray and in styling gel after styling gel.

What's in All This Stuff?

Let's cut to the chase, shall we? The average hair product is 70 to 90 percent water. Thickeners and preservatives, which make the product look the way we expect it to, comprise another 5 to 25 percent. The remaining ingredients, totaling a paltry 5 percent, are what we think we are buying more of: collagen, protein, water-binding agents, and natural ingredients. It costs less than 50 cents a bottle or jar to make most hair products, and they're sold for $3 to $40 per item. And the products are so easy to develop—at least on the surface. That's why there are so many of them on the market. Yet, regardless of the formulas and the marketing, there are no secrets when it comes to whether or not a product works for your hair. You can tell immediately whether or not your hair feels clean, soft, defrizzed; is easy to style; and stays put.

One way to demystify hair-care products is to learn what's in them, what those ingredients can and can't do for the hair, and how they can affect your hair despite the claims on the label. Cosmetics companies can say practically anything they want on their labels, brochures, advertisements, and in their sales presentations. They can tell you that their product restructures, builds body, reconstructs, mends, restores, rebuilds, nourishes, or revives the hair, and they don't have to prove or verify any of it because hair products are cosmetics, and cosmetics, according to the FDA, don't have to prove their claims. Even if a hair-care company can substantiate a claim, often their results are evident only with the aid of an electron microscope that blows up a hair shaft a trillion times its original size. That's great from a scientist's point of view, but it might not have anything to do with how a product or a specific ingredient will affect your hair.

The labels of hair-care products are almost absurd in their descriptions and explanations of what their products will do for your hair—except for the ingredient list. Legally, the ingredient list is the only part of a cosmetic label that is strictly regulated. The more familiar you are with this part of the product, the less likely you are to be led astray by frivolous, flimsy, superficial information designed by marketing experts who want you to believe their products can do the impossible.

Once you make a habit of reading the ingredient lists, you will be shocked to learn that all hair-care products—from shampoos and conditioners to hairsprays and styling gels—have more similarities than differences. It's almost a bad joke. Yet even though becoming familiar with ingredient lists is essential to understanding exactly what you are buying, they aren't easy to decipher. Like their skin-care counterparts, the ingredients have complicated names, and the significance of the order in which they are listed may seem elusive. Another dilemma is that there is no way to accurately discern from the list exactly how much of an ingredient is being used. While a percentage point here or there might not appear to be a big deal, it can be when you are constructing molecules to penetrate the hair shaft or surfactant combinations to clean the hair.

The ingredient list is the best indicator of what you are buying. It is by far more accurate than anything else on the label. With that in mind, let's get a better sense of what we are putting on our heads.

Hair Note: Ingredients are listed in descending order. The first ingredient (almost always water) is present in the largest quantity. The next two to eight ingredients are usually about 8 to 2 percent of the product. Once you find yourself down to the fragrance or the preservative (about midway to the end of the ingredient list), you are at less than 1 percent of the contents. Below 1 percent, the FDA allows the ingredients to be listed randomly. When you are at or near the end of an ingredient list, or after any of the ingredients that follow the fragrance or preservatives, you are looking at negligible or token amounts of the stuff. If the fancy ingredients touted on the product are located down here, you are looking at what some cosmetics chemists refer to as the "fool's amount," or "nothing more than monkey dust." At this nominal level, there isn't enough for the ingredient to have an effect on the hair. Minuscule proportions of impressive-sounding ingredients are thrown in to convince consumers that they are getting what they want, and because most consumers don't look at the ingredient list or don't know how to interpret it, the company can get away with this chicanery. It isn't illegal, but it's extremely misleading.

The long list of plant extracts in the beginning of many hair-care ingredient labels may look appealing but the notion that this "tea water" is providing some benefit for your hair is just not true. If plant extracts could take care of hair, couldn't you just make your own "tea water" to create the same effect as the pricey stuff you're buying? There isn't a plant or group of plants in the world that can clean hair, make it feel silky soft, or keep it in place after styling.

Patented Secrets

Are there really secret formulas in hair-care products? After all, if you're spending $15 to $25 for a conditioner with impressive claims, you want to believe you're purchasing an exclusive product that justifies the exorbitant price. The salespeople and the marketing departments make much ado about patented or patent-pending formulas that only their line has access to. And when you look at the product label, there it is in black and white: "patented" or "patent-pending" formula. It must be special. You think to yourself, "Finally, something I can bank on," because you know that patent laws are very strict, and the cosmetics company couldn't be lying about this, particularly when it comes to patent infringement laws. Right? Well, yes and no.

A United States patent is a contract between an inventor (in this instance, a hair-care company) and the government. Once a patent is accepted, the inventor has exclusive use of the new ingredient, molecule, formula, package, or whatever for 17 years. In exchange for the government's protection of that restricted use, the inventor discloses to the government *all* the information concerning the product. After the 17 years are up, the patent is available to the world.

In order for an inventor or a company to get a patent, whatever they are trying to patent has to be new and different from what is already available. The Patent and Trademark Office examiners review the formula or new ingredient and decide if it is unique. In theory that should make patents pretty reliable when it comes to the concept of originality. It would appear, then, that with patented hair-care formulas, you might be getting a product that is verifiably special. But that is sometimes true only in theory. Due to the vast number of patents, and the copious paperwork that accompanies each one, it is almost impossible for the government to thoroughly analyze each one. Often, overworked patent officers merely acknowledge that a patent appears to be legitimate. If any further questions come up, say, a challenge to the patent, the patent officers know the courts are better equipped to handle the matter.

In any case, the fact that a formula has an exclusive patent doesn't tell you anything about how well the product works. It is not the patent office's responsibility to verify whether or not the patented formula or ingredient can do anything for the hair. There are millions of cosmetics patents, and not one has any meaning when it comes to effectiveness. Patents are granted for formulation procedures or for combining two standard ingredients in a new way—say, in alcohol instead of wax, or while heated instead of at room temperature. The variations are endless (which is why there are millions of patents), but the basic fact is that a patent doesn't speak to effectiveness, only to formula specifics.

Even when a patented product or formula actually does do something positive for the hair—in the instance of two-in-one shampoos, for example—it doesn't necessarily take much for another company to come up with a similar formula. Next time your hairstylist or someone selling hair-care products carries on about an exclusive patented formula, remember that a patent doesn't tell you anything about how well the product works, and it definitely doesn't tell you whether or not there is a similar product on the market that does a better job.

Hair Note: "Patent pending" means just what it sounds like: The company has filed for a patent but it has not been approved (and may never be approved). Companies like using the "PATENT PENDING" insignia because they want you to think their product is indeed unique, even though they might not have filed a patent yet or the patent has already been turned down.

Shampoo

First things first, and the first step is cleaning your hair. Get this step right, and you are halfway home. You will be relieved to learn that it is hard to get this step wrong. Most shampoos are kind to the scalp and do a good job of lifting oil, styling products, conditioning agents, mineral deposits, and dirt from the hair. For all their purported differences, all shampoos (especially the good ones) contain primarily water, *surfactants* (**SURF**ace **ACT**ive Age**NTS**), lather builders, humectants (ingredients that attract water to the hair), thickeners (ingredients that give the shampoo a pleasing consistency), and preservatives, along with whatever faddish natural ingredient or fragrance is added so you think you're buying something special.

Many shampoos (whether they are labeled as two-in-ones or not) usually contain varying concentrations of conditioning agents, and these range from quaternary ammonium compounds (antistatic and detangling agents) to panthenol, collagen, protein, elastin, dimethicone and amino acids, and film-forming or plasticizing agents (these are hairspray-type ingredients, and I talk more about these in the section on "Hairsprays, Spritzes, and Freezes") and a host of others. These emollients, water-binding agents, film-forming/plasticizing agents, and detangling agents are meant to stay on the hair, even after the hair is rinsed clean. Using a shampoo that contains conditioning, film formers, and emollients can have an impact on your hair that's both good and bad. The good part is that it can help the hair comb more easily and feel softer and smoother. The negative part is that they keep getting redeposited on hair, never really get washed out, causing a buildup, and making hair look flat and feel heavy.

In general, if you are concerned with dry scalp or irritation, you may want to *avoid* shampoos that contain drying surfactants (cleansing agents) such as sodium lauryl sulfate, TEA-lauryl sulfate, sodium olefin sulfate, and alkyl sodium sulfate, especially if they are the second or third ingredient in the shampoo. (**Reminder:** Don't confuse sodium *lauryl* sulfate with sodium *laureth* sulfate. They are not the same thing. Sodium laureth sulfate is considered a mild surfactant. Just to be clear, though I discuss this more later in this section, both ammonium lauryl sulfate and ammonium laureth sulfate are also standard surfactants used in shampoos and are considered to be gentle surfactants.)

As drying as some surfactants can be, there are lots of natural ingredients that can be drying and irritating to the scalp such as lemon, grapefruit, orange, menthol, peppermint, lime, balm mint, oregano, essential oils (which are really just fragrance, a major source of skin sensitivity), avocado, mango, papaya, and a long listing of other plant extracts. The more plants in a product, the more essential it is to increase the amount of preservative, which means a greater risk of irritation from those ingredients.

You cannot tell the quality of a shampoo (or any hair product, for that matter) by its thickness, color, or fragrance. Those are all emotional concerns and not in any way relevant to the product's performance. As pleasant-smelling as shampoos and other hair-care products can be, the fragrance serves no purpose. If anything, the fragrant ingredients in hair-care products (often listed as essential oils or plant extracts) can be skin irritants.

Shampoos do vary according to the hair type listed on the label; however, market segmentation tends to create more categories than are really justified by the slight differences between products. For example, even though there are different shampoos for color-treated, permed, dry, dehydrated, brittle, damaged, sun-bleached, and straightened hair, there is little to no difference between what each of these hair types needs.

Hair Note: You will notice as you go through this chapter that there is some overlapping of ingredients between shampoos, conditioners, and styling products. That is because each product type contains many of those same types of ingredients.

Surfactants and Lather Builders. The function of surfactants is to clean hair. Interestingly enough, surfactants do not lather. They have no foaming ability. Lather builders, on the other hand, do suds up into a bubbling mass over the hair. Despite the fact that lathering makes it feel like your hair is getting clean, lathering ingredients serve no purpose in the cleansing process. All the lather in the world won't clean one hair on your head! It is strictly the surfactants that clean the hair and scalp. Lather can indicate how well a hair-care product is working, though. When oil or styling agents build up on hair or are not removed, it will prevent lathering agents from working. Therefore the sign of good bubbles on the head can be an indicator that your hair is getting clean.

The surfactants that are most typically used in shampoos are sodium lauryl sulfate, sodium laureth sulfate, ammonium lauryl sulfate, ammonium laureth sulfate, cocamidopropyl betaine, cocoamphodiacetate, sodium cocoglyceryl ether sulfonate, and sodium lauryl sarcosinate. There are many more, but these are the most popular. Ingredients that create lather are cocamide MEA, lauramide MEA, lauric DEA, lauramine oxide, cocamidopropyl hydroxysultaine, and polysorbate 20, among others. In combination, cleansing agents and lather builders are the essence of every shampoo you buy.

There is much discussion in the industry about which surfactants are the most gentle or the most problematic. Sodium lauryl sulfate, TEA-lauryl sulfate, sodium C14-16 olefin sulfonate, and TEA-dodecylbenzene tend to be far more drying and potentially irritating to the scalp than other cleansing agents. Cocamidopropyl betaine, cocamphocarboxyglycinate-propionate, sodium lauraminodipropionate, disodium monoleamide MEA sulfosuccinate, disodium monococamido sulfosuccinate, disodium cocamphodipropionate, disodium capryloamphodiacetate, cocoyl sarcosine, and sodium lauryl sarcosinate are considered extremely gentle but do not have good cleansing ability. I discuss this more in the section on "Baby Shampoo".

Quaternary Ammonium Compounds. This wide range of ingredients, called "quats" for short, shares a unique molecular structure that is strongly attracted to hair. When one end of the quats grabs the hair, the other end sticks out, creating a lineup that resembles a temporary smooth surface, giving the hair a more even surface to help a comb or brush go through more easily. Found in shampoos, conditioners, and any product that claims to detangle the hair, these less than poetic-sounding ingredients are essential to having manageable hair. Quats you may encounter on the ingredient label may include guar hydroxypropyltrimonium chloride, dicetyldimonium chloride, dihydrogenated tallow benzylmonium chloride, behentrimonium chloride, behenalkonium betaine, benzalkonium chloride, quaternium 18, stearalkonium chloride, cetrimonium chloride, and on and on.

Humectants. Glycerin, sorbitol, glycols, mucopolysaccharides, hyaluronic acid, sodium PCA, propylene glycol, and glycosphingolipids, among others, attract and keep water in the hair shaft, giving hair bounce and a feeling of fullness. Humectants work in conjunction with quats and conditioning agents to keep static cling at a minimum and give hair a softer, thicker feel. These also help keep the hair's natural water content intact, particularly in dry climates. Glycerin and propylene glycol, among other glycols, are inexpensive but effective protective agents for hair.

Conditioning Agents. Conditioning agents such as collagen, protein, amino acids, silicone, panthenol, and triglycerides can end up in shampoos for most of the same reasons they are in conditioners: They help make hair easier to comb, softer, shinier, and more silky feeling. The only problem with most conditioning agents, except for silicone, is that they can't stand up under water and tend to get washed away. This is why conditioning shampoos rarely work well for damaged, dry, or coarse hair. The shampoo doesn't allow enough conditioning agents to be deposited to make that kind of hair manageable.

I wish there was more to tell you about protein and other conditioning agents, but there just isn't. Whether it is wheat germ triglycerides, silk protein, or some other enticingly named ingredient, it brings no added benefit to the hair shaft. It simply provides some amount of protective coating that is then washed away the next time you wash your hair.

Natural Ingredients. The list of fad ingredients showing up in hair-care products is almost too long for me to deal with, but I will do my best in the Product Review chapter. For now, just to pinpoint a few, let's take a look at tea tree oil, awapuhi, and hemp.

Tea tree oil (also called melaleuca) is getting a lot of attention these days from the hair-care industry, and showing up in all kinds of shampoos and conditioners. It comes from a seemingly exotic source (a tree of Australian origin), so the consumer assumes immediately it must be wonderful for the hair, and in fact it does have some reported benefit as an antibacterial and healing agent. That would be great for the scalp (it doesn't do anything for dead hair), except that the amount of tea tree oil used in shampoos and conditioners is too small to have an impact; it's even less effective when combined with water in the shower.

Awapuhi is just an extract of a ginger plant native to Hawaii. It sounds noteworthy, but there is no evidence that awapuhi provides any benefit for the scalp or hair, particularly in the minute concentrations used in hair products.

Hemp's infamous association with the marijuana plant is well known, but if you were hoping that would relax your scalp or hair, or offer some other improvement, think again. The amount of hemp used in hair-care products is negligible and used strictly to attract an unassuming shopper looking for something new and different. However, if enough hemp were used, there could be serious consequences. Hemp contains tetrahydrocannabinol (THC), the same active ingredient found in marijuana. According to Dr. Hugh Davis, Acting Head of Microbiology and Cosmetics at Health Canada, there is research showing that hemp accumulates in the body because of its long half-life, and that it has the same adverse physiological effects that smoking marijuana does (though it's not hallucinatory when absorbed through skin— where you get all the bad and none of the perceived positive). One study purports to find that cannabinoids may postpone puberty and have other negative hormonal effects. There are 60 known cannabinoids, only 3 of which have been widely studied.

This means that we don't even know what the other 57 components could do to potentially hurt your body when they are in a cream or shampoo.

Thickeners. These ingredients are responsible for the texture, appearance, and movement of the finished product for shampoos, conditioners, and styling products. There are literally hundreds of thickening ingredients used in hair-care products. Typical thickening agents used are cetyl alcohol, stearyl alcohol, hydrogenated lanolin, polyethylene glycol (PEG), glycol stearate, palmitic acid, and so on. All of these, and many more, have a soft waxy texture that creates the viscosity and weight of any product. For styling products such as gels, the typical thickening agents used in almost every product are carbomer and guar. These Jell-O–like substances create the appearance you associate with gels.

The list of thickening agents is too long to include in a book of this kind, but the effects these agents have are the major reason you find a product desirable.

Vitamins. Ah, the world of vitamins! When it comes to hair, even though we know it's dead, we somehow still want to believe vitamins can feed or nourish the hair. They can't. There is no research proving the effectiveness for hair. Panthenol and biotin are vitamin B derivatives that work on hair because of their consistency, not because of their nutrition value. Even if they could, vitamins are added in such tiny amounts they couldn't cover even one hair shaft of your hair, much less your whole head.

Preservatives. Hair-care ingredients are combined together in a very liquid solution. This wet environment is a perfect breeding ground for bacterial, fungal, and microbial contamination. It is therefore of primary importance that preservatives be used in all formulations to prevent this normal, though potentially harmful, growth from taking place. To that end, antibacterial, antifungal, and antimicrobial agents are included to help keep contamination to a minimum. The most popular preservatives used in hair-care products are methylparaben, propylparaben, phenoxyethanol, DMDM hydantoin, 2-bromo-2-nitropropane-1,3-diol, and imidazolidinyl urea.

Sodium Lauryl Sulfate

Speaking of shampoos . . . this is as good a place as any to tackle some of the major panics taking place on the Web and in other media publications over ingredients. I have been receiving more E-mails and letters than I care to count about the concern over sodium lauryl sulfate (SLS) and sodium laureth sulfate (SLES) being serious problems in cosmetics. I believe that this entire mania was generated by several hair-care and cosmetic Web sites, including Mastey, Aubrey, and Neways. These unethical companies generate this misinformation to showcase what makes their products special. But their scare tactics don't hold water. It seems that most of this entire issue is based on the incorrect reporting of a study done at the Medical College of Georgia. As a reminder, here is what is being quoted: "A study from the Medical College of Georgia indicates that SLS is a systemic, and can penetrate and be retained in the eye, brain, heart, liver, etc., with potentially harmful long-term effects. It could retard healing and cause cataracts in adults, and can keep children's eyes from developing properly. (Summary of report to Research to Prevent Blindness, Inc. Conference.)" It took awhile, but I was finally able to locate the doctor who conducted the study and delivered the final report. His name is Dr. Keith Green, and he is Regents Professor of Ophthalmology at the Medical College of Georgia, and received his Doctorate of Science from St. Andrews University in Scotland. Yes, Dr. Green is completely embarrassed by all this. Dr. Green told me, "My work was completely misquoted. There is no part of my study that indicated any development or cataract problems from SLS or SLES, and the body does not retain those ingredients at all. We did not even look at the issue of children, so that conclusion is completely false because it never existed. The Neways people took my research completely out of context and probably never read the study at all." He continued in a very perturbed voice, saying, "The statement like 'SLS is a systemic' has no meaning. No ingredient can be a systemic unless you drink the stuff, and that's not what we did with it. Another incredible comment was that my study was 'clinical,' meaning I tested the substance on people, [but] these were strictly animal tests. Furthermore, the eyes showed no irritation with the 10 dilution substance used! If anything, the animal studies indicated no risk of irritation whatsoever!"

When I asked if anyone has done any follow-up studies looking at SLS and SLES in this regard, Dr. Green said, "No one has done this because the findings were so insignificant." I was also curious to know if he or anyone in his family had changed the way they buy shampoos. Dr. Green laughed loudly, saying, "No one in my family has changed the way they buy shampoos, and they all contain either SLS or SLES." He added, "You may find it interesting to tell your readers that SLS and SLES have a natural source. The sulfates [ingredients like SLS and SLES] have been used for over 20 years by millions of people daily and weekly with no adverse effects. The sun is a far bigger issue for people to be concerned about when it comes to the health of their eyes than anything else!"

It is almost impossible for me to tackle every piece of misinformation floating around out there about ingredients and hair facts, but just to show how crazy it can get, let me point out two more interesting cases. Mastey has jumped on the cleanser-fear bandwagon too. In their on-line information they state that "Even though sodium laureth sulfate [and] ammonium laureth sulfate . . . are considered milder on the hair and skin, they may actually be worse for the body . . . [due to the] greater risk of exposure to harmful carcinogens, nitrosamines and/or 1,4 dioxane. These nitrates are capable of permeating through intact skin each time you shampoo." While there is research being conducted on the question of nitrosamine formation in all kinds of cosmetic products, from several different sources, there is no evidence proving the theory. The notion that nitrosamines can penetrate skin is not demonstrated anywhere. Of course, Mastey doesn't quote any sources, so their information can't be substantiated anyway. Whenever you see information on the Web supported by a study, but the exact source is not quoted, be very skeptical about taking it as fact.

Here is another Mastey fantasy about sodium lauryl sulfate: "In published studies, sodium lauryl sulfate (SLS) has been shown to deteriorate the hair follicle. It retards the growth cycle of hair, and increases the amount of time needed to regrow hair from a normal of 3 months to up to 24 months, prolonging the sleeping stage of hair growth and giving you the appearance of hair loss." Boy, if that were true, all it would take to reduce hair growth on your legs would be to wash with shampoos containing SLS! Absolutely this isn't the case, and once again notice that Mastey didn't quote any sources (that's probably because none exist).

DEA in Cosmetics

A report on *CBS Morning News* in April 1998 described the results of a study produced by the National Toxicology Program (NTP), "which found that repeated skin application to mouse skin of the cosmetic ingredient diethanolamine (DEA), or its fatty acid derivative cocamide-DEA, induced liver and kidney cancer." Besides this "clear evidence of carcinogenicity [only to mouse skin in high concentrations]," the NTP also emphasized that DEA is readily absorbed through the skin and accumulates in organs such as the brain, where it induces chronic toxic effects. The report went on to explain that high concentrations of DEA-based cleansing agents are commonly used in a wide range of cosmetics and toiletries, including shampoos, hair dyes, hair conditioners, lotions, creams, and bubble baths, plus liquid dishwashing and laundry soaps. "Lifelong use of these products thus clearly poses major avoidable cancer risks to the great majority of U.S. consumers, particularly infants and young children," the report noted. (That is a stretch—from high concentrations used on mice to long-term topical use by humans.)

If this made you nervous, you may well have been even more alarmed as the report continued, stating that "further increasing these cancer risks is long-standing evidence that DEA readily interacts with nitrite preservatives or contaminants in cosmetics or toiletries to form nitrosodiethanolamine (NDELA), another carcinogen as well that it recognized by federal agencies and institutions and the World Health Organization; NDELA, like DEA, is also rapidly absorbed through the skin.

In 1979, the FDA warned that more than 40 percent of all cosmetic products were contaminated with NDELA and called for the industry 'to take immediate action to eliminate this carcinogen from cosmetic products.' [NDELA is not DEA.] In two 1991 surveys, 27 out of 29 products were found to be contaminated with high concentrations of this carcinogen, results which were subsequently confirmed by the FDA. Based on this information, the European Union and European industry have both taken strong action to reduce or eliminate DEA and NDELA from cosmetics and toiletries. In sharp contrast, the FDA has taken no such action, nor has it responded to a 1996 petition from the Cancer Prevention Coalition to phase out the use of DEA or to label DEA-containing products with an explicit cancer warning. The mainstream U.S. industry has been similarly unresponsive, even to the extent of ignoring an explicit warning by the Cosmetics, Toiletries and Fragrance Association [CTFA] to discontinue uses of DEA. Such reckless intransigence is in strong contrast to the responsiveness of the growing safe cosmetic industry."

First, the European Union does not disallow DEA. They do have recommendations about concentrations, but it is not an illegal ingredient. Second, the CTFA does not agree that it warned consumers about DEA use in cosmetics. In a February 1998 press release, the CTFA said something quite different from the report CBS aired: "In 1986 the Cosmetic Ingredient Review [CIR—that's the independent arm of the CTFA that reviews cosmetic ingredients] found DEA to be safe when used as directed. The CIR is examining new information on DEA and will develop an up-to-date assessment of its safety. Since there is no evidence that products containing DEA have been unsafe for consumers, it would be unnecessarily alarming for the news media to suggest there is a [serious] health risk."

Also in response to the CBS news report, the FDA stated that "the NTP study did not address the link between DEA and human cancer risk."

Much like the CTFA, the FDA added, "Although DEA itself is used in very few cosmetics, DEA-related ingredients (e.g., oleamide DEA, lauramide DEA, cocamide DEA) are widely used in a variety of cosmetic products. These ingredients function as emulsifiers or foaming agents and are generally used at levels of 1 percent to 5 percent. The FDA takes these NTP findings very seriously and is in the process of carefully evaluating the studies and test data to determine the real risk, if any, to consumers. The Agency believes that at the present time there is no reason for consumers to be alarmed based on the usage of these ingredients in cosmetics. Consumers wishing to avoid cosmetics containing DEA or its conjugates may do so by reviewing the ingredient statement required to appear on the outer container label of cosmetics offered for retail sale to consumers.

"If FDA's evaluation of the NTP data indicates that a health hazard exists, FDA will advise the industry and the public and will consider its legal options under the authority of the Food, Drug and Cosmetic Act in protecting the health and welfare of consumers."

Because of all this hullabaloo, I can see why some people may want to avoid DEA in cosmetics, and it is easy enough to do so, but given the data, the entire issue does emerge as being alarmist. In essence, there is no real evidence demonstrating that people using cosmetics with DEA are any more prone to cancers than those not using them.

Carcinogens in Hair Care?

In a related matter, some of you may be familiar with research that warns against using cosmetics that contain triethanolamine, or TEA-lauryl sulfate, mixed in the same product along with formaldehyde-releasing preservatives such as imidazolidinyl urea, quaternium-15, 2-bromo-2-nitropropane-1,3-diol, or DMDM hydantoin. There is evidence that suggests these combinations can form nitrosamines in a cosmetic, creating a potential carcinogen (nitrosamines, as you may recall, are carcinogenic substances). There is also information from the University of Texas Health Science Center, School of Public Health, published in the journal *Environmental and Molecular Mutagenesis,* issue 28, looking at the cancer-causing potential of the cosmetic preservative methychloroisothiazolinone (Kathon). In bacteria cultures it did demonstrate mutagenic activity.

I find all this information very important, yet there is substantial disagreement among the cosmetics chemists I spoke to as to how significant a problem this is for the skin (or even whether it is a problem). After all, activity in vitro (on cultures in petrie dishes as opposed to live skin) is very different from activity in real life on people. Most all the researchers I spoke to suggested that going out of the house without a sunscreen or sitting in a bar exposed to secondhand cigarette smoke poses more risk to the skin than any combination of skin-care ingredients ever could. However, you should be aware that there are those who consider this a nonchalant attitude and to be merely an apology for sidestepping around a very serious question. As someone who has looked at this issue for some time, I actually understand both viewpoints and have no definitive position to share. While some companies would love to promote hysteria and then present their formulations as pure and untainted, there can also be concern that their products are not well preserved, with the resulting substantial risk of bacterial or fungal contamination.

Thus there is no absolute position for you to rush to and, as always, I leave the final decision up to you. All you need to do is check the ingredient list of any product you are considering to determine whether it excludes amines or Kathon as well as any of the other questionable preservatives mentioned above.

What About pH?

Cosmetic companies are notorious for bragging about the pH level of their products. pH indicates how acid or alkaline a formulation is. If a shampoo is too alkaline (a high pH), it can cause the hair shaft to swell and damage the cuticle; if the shampoo is more acid (a low pH), it can tighten the cuticle, helping the hair to feel softer and look shinier. When the cuticles are lying tightly against each other, the hair can better reflect light and the hair shaft is better protected from damage. When the protective layer of cuticle is swollen and expanded, the inner part of the hair is more exposed to damage. Plus, when the cuticle edges are lifted, they are also more prone to chipping and breakage, and with the cuticle lifted away, the hair is less capable of reflecting light.

Most hair-care products have a pH of approximately 5.5 to 6.0 (keep in mind that water has a *neutral* pH of 7). That is considered standard in the industry and is at or above the natural pH of unaltered hair, which is around 5.5. If a shampoo has a low pH, lower than about 4, it won't lather well, and there are those who think the cleaning ability of the surfactant in it is also diminished.

Regardless of the low pH imposed on the hair, the shaft is not interested in holding on to the artificially induced pH for very long. Much like skin, the hair will return to its own pH no matter what you throw on it. Nevertheless, a segment of the hair-care industry thinks that a lower pH is important. You can experiment with this one, but it is unlikely you will notice any difference in your hair, though you might feel it isn't quite as clean, or the products may prove to be more irritating and drying on your scalp than you would like.

Conversely, high pH can be quite damaging to hair. Though hair is inclined toward its own pH level, the effects of high pH on the hair are overwhelmingly negative and are impossible to reverse. **A hair-care product with a high pH swells the hair shaft, disturbing the cuticle layer and causing the interior of the hair shaft to be compromised. The hair's negative reaction to high pH and the difficulty hair has recovering from that assault is what makes high-pH hair-care products so terrible for hair.** The results of high-pH ingredients on hair are seen most clearly with hair dyes and perms. These products have a pH of 8 or 9 (as opposed to depilatory hair removers, which have a pH of 10, or water, which has a pH of 7), and that's enough to drastically and permanently alter the structure of hair. Yes, that means all hair dyes and all perms are a problem for hair.

Baby Shampoo

For all mothers out there looking to help clean, soften, and soothe your little one's skin, let me warn you about baby products. I know that the baby section in the drugstore and, increasingly, at cosmetic counters and in home sales companies, has adorable-looking shampoos, moisturizers, assorted cleansers, and sun products in pink and blue containers. You assume special care has been taken to use only ingredients that will be the most gentle to your baby's skin, but that assumption is not accurate. Think now about the wafting, appealing fragrances emanating from most all baby products, and therein lies a major problem, which is why I am leery of using baby products for anyone's skin, let alone babies'. Products for babies and young children are usually highly fragranced. That delicious, recognizable aroma you could smell a mile away is nothing more than added fragrance and can cause irritation. Moreover, baby products almost always have a pretty yellow or pink tint, which is contrived by coloring agents, another group of problematic skin-care ingredients for sensitive skin. If baby products were really more gentle than the stuff adults put on their skin, they would be fragrance free and contain no coloring agents. Sadly, few of those exist.

Cosmetics and hair-care companies know that mothers have an impulsive emotional pull toward scents triggering the image of their babies. That subconscious pull is hard for a marketer to ignore, given that their customers will gravitate to the fragrance generated by other perfume-laden products. In other words, hair- and skin-care companies don't have much impetus to take these problematic ingredients out. That means you, the consumer, as an advocate for your child, need to pay attention to this issue and choose fragrance-free and color-free products whenever you can!

When it comes to cleansing agents, the group of ingredients considered the most gentle are called amphoteric surfactants. As stated in the *Cosmetic Science and Technology Series,* volume 17, *Hair and Hair Care,* amphoteric surfactants do not cleanse or foam as well as other surfactants, but their one unique property is their very low irritation potential. Amphoterics are so gentle that they can even reduce the irritation potential of other surfactants known for their sensitizing possibilities, such as sodium lauryl sulfate. "The skin irritancy of sodium lauryl sulfate in the presence of cocamidopropyl betaine [an amphoteric surfactant] is reduced substantially."

This explains why Johnson & Johnson's Baby Shampoo was such a phenomenal success when it launched in the '60s. Johnson & Johnson's 1967 patent established the mild, nonirritating capacity for the amphoteric group of cleansing agents. As it turns out, the primary ingredient in Johnson & Johnson's baby shampoos is cocamidopropyl betaine. But this also explains why, when the mother tries to use baby shampoo on her own head, it doesn't work very well. The amphoteric surfactants just can't clean like other surfactants can, and given the styling products and conditioners most adults use, it is essential to have a shampoo with good cleansing properties. Nowadays most baby shampoos use a combination of cleansing agents to lower irritancy and improve cleansing, but they are still almost always more gentle than adult versions. Refer to the section above on "Shampoo" for a listing of typical gentle amphoteric surfactants.

Shampoo for Use with Well Water and for Swimmers

Whether you swim in a swimming pool or in the ocean, or you happen to live in a home that uses well water, you're likely to have hair problems that are difficult to contend with. Swimming pools can cause mineral buildup on the hair; salt water can cause dryness, breakage, and hard-to-remove tangles; and well water can deposit iron salts on the hair, turning it red.

We tend to blame the chlorine in swimming pools for turning blonde hair green, but chlorine isn't the culprit in this case. Chlorine does dry out the hair by breaking through the cuticle, staying put, and tearing at the cuticle every time you brush. But the green discoloration comes from the copper leached from city pipes into pool water. Salt water, if left to dry on hair and combined with wind and sand, can leave the hair in a tangled, dried-out, frazzled state (in addition to being sunburned). These hazards are especially significant for someone whose hair is already damaged. Damaged hair is more porous and therefore more susceptible to the invasion of salt, chlorine, and copper.

To battle swimmer's hair in both situations (pool or ocean), and if a swimming cap isn't in your fashion forecast, you might want to consider loading your hair up with silicone serums **each time** before you go into the water. The left-on silicone can cling to hair even in the presence of water and can act as a barrier to the copper in the pool and the salt in the ocean. When you're done playing in the water, if at all possible, be diligent about washing your hair (the silicone easily washes away with shampoo). It also helps to rinse the hair like crazy with fresh water **each time** you leave the pool or ocean water, the sooner the better. Do not, I repeat, do not comb or brush through the hair until you've shampooed and applied conditioner.

When you can wash your hair, or if you have a home using well water, be sure to use a shampoo that contains disodium EDTA. This chelating agent helps by attracting the minerals away from the hair shaft and making them easier to rinse away. Then apply a generous amount of conditioner to the ends. Never comb through your hair without the aid of conditioner. Trying to smooth out tangles after a swim without conditioner is just asking for damage. The cuticle is already in a vulnerable position—wet and laden with minerals—which makes driving a brush or even a wide-toothed comb through it a highly risky procedure that can easily rip apart the hair shaft.

Myth Busting: For some unknown reason, there is a myth circulating that wetting hair before swimming helps prevent chlorine and other drying minerals from affecting the hair. The story goes that once hair swells up with water, that prevents the minerals from getting inside because the water got inside first. There is no way water can prevent chlorine or other minerals from getting attached to your hair. After all, it occurs while your hair is soaking wet in the pool, right? Besides, minerals can't get inside the hair shaft; the molecules are too large. Minerals get attached to the outside of the hair, clinging to the layers of cuticle covering the hair shaft, and water can't block that from taking place.

Another myth I've heard is that applying conditioner before swimming is helpful to prevent problems. It won't. The conditioner would just be rinsed away. However, that wouldn't be the case if the conditioner contained conditioning ingredients that didn't rinse easily, like silicone. Silicone holds on to hair even with water pressure. A layer of pure silicone such as Aussie Shine or Citre Shine would give the most protection.

Dandruff Shampoo

See the section on dandruff in Chapter Four, *Hair Type*.

Conditioner

For all the claims about conditioners penetrating, restructuring, regenerating, and rebuilding hair, they have no ability to do any of that. Conditioners strictly modify the cuticle layer of hair—temporarily. The scaled layers of cuticle covering the hair shaft need to be held down tight to make the hair feel silky and soft. To that end, conditioners need to "glue" the cuticles down onto the hair shaft or fill in the damaged spaces, to bandage up the tears and breaks in the cuticle that make hair feel rough and dry. This bandaging is done by ingredients that have an attraction to the cuticle and the ability to bond with it. Cuticles are much like any dead, inanimate surface: Not everything wants to stay put on them. Only certain substances have the physical properties to attach themselves to the unique physical characteristics of the hair.

Why can't conditioning agents penetrate the hair shaft? Because the whole purpose of the cuticle is to protect its insides, and that means preventing things from getting inside. The cuticle layer and the cortex are there to keep the interior of the hair shaft intact and keep everything else out. Think about it this way: molecularly tiny hair-dye ingredients need a very elaborate, strong, chemical process to get the new hair color into the hair shaft and keep it there. It also takes a very elaborate, strong, chemical process to get your existing hair color stripped out of the hair's interior. Hair likes holding on to what it has and it doesn't want to let anything inside or let out what is naturally inside.

That conditioning agents can't get inside of hair isn't a bad thing because they do attach on the surface, where you need them. Conditioning ingredients migrate and cling to the hair's cuticle layers, helping to shore up what's there and fill in (temporarily) what might be missing, which is exactly what the hair needs. **In order to get as much of the conditioning agents to migrate over, around, and under the cuticles, you need to leave the conditioner on the hair for a while so the conditioning ingredients have more time to get where they need to be.**

A fascinating side note: Many conditioners contain an army of plant extracts ranging from citrus to ivy, thyme, horsetail, and on and on. It turns out these herbal extracts can interfere with the real conditioning agents attaching to the cuticle. Many of these plants block or dilute the ability of conditioning agents to perform their function efficiently.

When you buy a conditioner, you will find one or more of the components below on the ingredient list. They are found in different combinations in a long roll call of products whose names and descriptions defy the imagination: creme rinses, finishing rinses, deep conditioners, hair moisturizers, light conditioners, detangling conditioners, equalizing conditioners, reconstructors, and hair moisturizers.

Proteins. Proteins are large-chain molecules that cannot be absorbed into the hair shaft. Proteins are often partially hydrolyzed to help them cling better to hair. Regardless, proteins coat the outside of the hair, filling in gaps between the cuticles, which provides protection and a soft feeling. Proteins are a range of ingredients that include plant and animal by-products. Even though proteins are an elemental component of the hair's makeup, adding protein to hair-care products does not restructure or add to the hair's composition. To imply that any protein can somehow repair hair or permanently attach to hair is sheer alchemy and fantasy. Ironically, plant proteins, despite their desirability, don't cling well to hair, at least not as well as the animal by-product alternatives such as collagen or elastin (*Hair and Hair Care*, Dale H. Johnson, ed.).

Collagen and elastin are proteins that like to cling to hair. They serve several important roles in conditioning the hair. Both nicely coat the outside layer of the hair, filling in the gaps of the damaged cuticle and adding a slight feel of thickness to the hair. Collagen and elastin also have water-binding properties that are delivered mostly to the surface, which is good for the hair.

Collagen and elastin can be broken down with water (hydrolyzed), creating a smaller molecule form that has a better chance of getting in and around the cuticle. (We're talking a microscopic level of penetration, so don't get excited or carried away thinking hydrolyzed collagen or elastin will repair your hair or somehow mend it. They won't.) Unfortunately, very little of the specially treated collagen or elastin can penetrate and be absorbed, because after they have been hydrolyzed—partially broken down with water—they are more prone to being washed away. Hydrolyzed collagen and elastin work best when given time to penetrate a dry or slightly damp hair shaft.

Amino Acids. Hair is made of 22 known amino acids, including cystine, histidine, serine, glutamic acid, tryptophan, and proline. Proteins are assembled from amino acids, and in theory amino acids have a better affinity for hair because they are smaller and have a better chance of penetrating the cuticle layer and providing water-binding properties deeper in. But that's only in theory. Most cosmetics chemists feel that because amino acids are so small, they are also quite unstable and easy to rinse away, and therefore never get a chance to penetrate and do their thing.

Polysaccharides. Polysaccharides are used in conditioners because of their thickening and slip properties. Slip properties means that polysaccharides are excellent for grabbing on to hair, smoothing easily over the surface of the hair shaft, and staying put. They have a side benefit of helping to add viscosity to the product. Several types of polysaccharides are used in hair-care products, such as cellulose, glycosaminoglycans, hyaluronic acid, mucopolysaccharides, chitin, and chitosan PCA.

Nucleic Acids. In the human body, nucleic acids are part of a cell's genetic material that communicates genetic information within the cell. The appearance of nucleic acids in hair-care products is strictly for the purpose of marketing and sales pitches. Hair is dead and has no genetic coding to worry about! Even if hair was alive, you couldn't and wouldn't want to affect its genetic messages with a cosmetic.

Glycerin, Sorbitol, Propylene Glycol, and Butylene Glycol. These are all excellent water-binding agents. Helene Curtis has research revealing that glycerin and propylene glycol have a superior ability to glide over the hair shaft and stay in place. Their claims that this helps reduce heat damage are discussed on under "Stopping Damage," in Chapter Two.

Fatty Acids and Fatty Alcohols. These fatty (lipid) lubricants and emollients are often less oily or greasy than plant or mineral oils, and therefore give the hair a soft, velvety feel without feeling heavy or thick. A few of the more popular members of this group are cetyl alcohol, stearyl alcohol, triglycerides, myristyl alcohol, caprylic acid, lauric acid, oleic acid, palmitic acid, and stearic acid.

Vegetable Oils, Lanolin, Plant Oils, Castor Oil, and Mineral Oil. These oils do for the hair pretty much what they do for the skin: leave a protective barrier that prevents dehydration. They are also extremely emollient and oily, providing good water-binding ability but also a problematic texture on the hair. Their weight can slick down the cuticle of the hair shaft, helping give shine, but also adding a greasy feel. By the way, regardless of how exotic or earthy the oils may sound—such as geranium, lavender, jojoba, wheat germ, carrot, evening primrose, and babassu—they still function as oils, and they're no better than mineral oil or other less impressive-sounding oils such as safflower or canola.

Though there are positives to oils or lanolin in hair-care products, on balance there are more aesthetic negatives. The downside for all these ingredients is that they can leave a greasy, thick residue on the hair. This is particularly true in products designed for African-American hair that often contain large amounts of lanolin, petrolatum, and castor oil. All of these ingredients, by virtue of their sticky feel, also tend to attract dirt and increase the chance of styling products building up on the hair. The hair must be washed thoroughly, as these ingredients are hard to remove. **Products with oils and lanolin listed among the first ingredients are best used occasionally, if at all, and then only in styling products used on the ends of hair or over the most damaged areas and not all over.**

Vitamins. Remember, hair is dead and vitamins can't feed it. Can they prevent free-radical damage to the hair or scalp the way they have been said to on the skin? First, there is no real evidence anywhere that vitamins can prevent free-radical damage on the skin, let alone the scalp, and definitely not on the hair. (All the information about cosmetic ingredients preventing free-radical damage on the skin is theoretical.) Even if there were proof, a much larger amount of the vitamins would have to be present than is currently being used in cosmetics. Actually, you would need so much of these vitamins and have to reapply them so many times during the day that your hair (and skin) would probably be a sticky, smelly mess.

Panthenol, Biotin, and Other Derivatives of Vitamin B Complex Factors. Unlike other vitamins, the popular conditioning ingredient panthenol has an affinity for hair and is considered to have excellent penetration into the hair shaft. Does that mean it can mend hair or do any of a vast array of miracles, as claimed by hair-care companies? Can it really thicken hair up to 10 percent, stop hair loss, regrow hair, prevent damage caused by perms or dyes, or strengthen hair, as you've seen in brochures for hair-care products? All such claims are completely unsubstantiated. You can show panthenol to be effective on a hair strand when it's in a lab, but the way people use hair-care products is another story altogether.

The major problem with proving panthenol's effectiveness is that it converts to pantothenic acid on the hair. This is such a tiny molecule that once it is absorbed into the hair shaft it cannot be seen, so there is no way of knowing what it is actually doing in there, and no strength tests exist proving the hair is stronger because of panthenol. What panthenol can do is help give the hair a more substantial, smoother feel; keep moisture in the hair better if the hair is dry; improve movement if hair is stiff or brittle, and impart some luster to the hair.

Biotin, as several chemists and dermatologists told me, is one of those hair-care ingredients that have little function but women believe (and hair-care companies reinforce this belief) can help hair. Biotin has minimal ability to hold up under water and it doesn't cling well to the cuticle. It sounds strong but it hands up being a small weak molecule.

Quaternary Ammonium Compounds. See the description of these in the "Shampoo" section above.

Silicone. Ingredients like dimethicone and cyclomethicone are so vital to hair care and are used so widely in the hair- and skin-care industries that they deserve a book dedicated only to their function and use. These unsung hair-care marvels have an incredible capacity to cling to and spread over, under, and around the cuticle. Silicone's unsurpassed ability to maneuver effortlessly over the hair shaft and hold up under water pressure or styling routines makes it superior for smoothing out any of the cuticle's rough edges. Even more astonishing is silicone's luxuriant, velvety texture. Silicone is capable of imparting the most wonderful, silky-smooth feel to the hair. It is impossible to comprehend how awesome silicone feels unless you buy one of the new laminate or anti-frizz serums that have become so popular in styling products and feel it for yourself. Those types of styling products are usually pure silicone, which allows you to feel directly how sensational the texture is.

Not only does silicone provide temporary renewed smoothness to the hair, but the amount of research demonstrating its extraordinary safety (I can't imagine who could be allergic to these benign substances) fills several folders in my office. There almost isn't a downside, except that if you use too much of this stuff it can leave a greasy, rather than silky, feel on hair. There is more to say about silicone (see the section on "Two-in-Ones," this chapter), but for now, consider it your dry, coarse, frizzy, damaged hair's best friend.

Other oils such as mineral oil, petrolatum, and plant oils can perform similarly to silicone but they have a far more slick or sticky feeling and they also lack silicone's ability to spread evenly over the hair. Silicones have incredible movement, leaving a thin, even layer wherever you place them; other oils don't have this ability.

Balsam. The limited use of balsam these days makes even mentioning it almost unnecessary, but in case there are those who remember it as a popular conditioning agent in the 1970s and '80s, it may be worth a few quick comments. Balsam is a tree resin that has substantial ability to stick to the hair and coat it. Balsam also has a potent but pleasant fragrance. Why then has balsam fallen out of the limelight? Despite balsam's positive attributes, it has overwhelming negative points; specifically, it makes hair feel sticky and, due to buildup, can make hair brittle. It is best avoided in any hair-care formulation.

Thickeners and Emulsifiers. These types of ingredients are responsible for the consistency of any hair-care product you use. Thickeners can also function as emollients in hair-care products, but primarily they help produce the feel and texture of the formulation. Emulsifiers help all the ingredients stay mixed together. Without thickeners and emulsifiers you would find most all hair-care products to be a watery mixture similar to an oil-and vinegar-salad dressing.

Preservatives. These ingredients prevent the product from becoming contaminated with mold and bacteria (for more explanation see the section on "Carcinogens in Hair Care?").

Alpha Hydroxy Acids and Urea. Following the popularity of AHAs in skin-care products, hair-care formulators tried to capitalize on this favorable notoriety by adding them to shampoos and conditioners. However, high concentrations of AHAs in low-pH formulations (AHAs are effective in concentrations of 5 percent or greater in a pH less than 4), are never used in hair-care products, or should never be used, because if they performed on the hair the same way they performed on the skin (as exfoliants removing dead skin cells) they would denature and destroy the hair shaft—which is essentially nothing more than dead skin (keratin). It was once thought that AHAs could help with some dandruff or dry-scalp conditions, but the risk to the hair shaft itself is too great. If the AHA (such as glycolic or lactic acid) is at the end of the ingredient listing, it's there in such a small quantity that it would not have a negative effect on the hair.

Plant and Herbal Extracts and Other Hyped Ingredients. Honey, milk, plant extracts, herbs, and silk may all have a healthy, vibrant sound and may even have some benefit for the hair, but their value (if any) in shampoos and conditioners is lost in the rinse or the formulation. How can plant extracts and milk cling to hair under water pressure? They can't. Besides, the amount of these ingredients is usually negligible to almost nonexistent. Just for the record, it is my opinion and the opinion of countless cosmetics chemists I have interviewed that these types of ingredients have no benefit in hair-care products and are there mostly for enticing the consumer (who always thinks natural ingredients are best).

Film Formers. This vast range of ingredients are typical styling products found in hairsprays and styling gels. They keep hair in place by literally placing a microscopically thin layer of film or plastic over the hair shaft. This can help add a feeling of thickness to the hair and volume, smooth down frizzies and split ends, and reduce static and flyaways. The downside of these unsung hair-care heroes is that they have a stiff, sticky side. That can be a problem for a product's perceived performance. These ingredients also tend to build up on the hair. (See the section on "Hairsprays, Spritzes, and Freezes" for more detail.)

Rinse-off or Leave-in Conditioners

On the surface, all conditioners leave the hair easier to comb, moisturized, protected from assault with blow-dryers, and smoother to the touch, using practically the same ingredients. Because they are so similar, leave-in and rinse-off conditioners perform those functions equally well. Yet there are significant differences in consistency, emollience, and formulation between leave-on and rinse-off conditioners.

Leave-in conditioners have a far thinner, less emollient texture than rinse-off conditioners. Leave-in conditioners also omit most of the emollient ingredients, such as fatty acids, fatty alcohols, and thickening agents found in rinse-off conditioners. Because leave-in conditioners don't include heavy lubricating emollients or thickeners that can weigh down hair, they are often recommended for women with thin, limp, or fine hair, to add body and control. Leave-in conditioners often contain a small amount of styling ingredients such as PVP, PVP/VA, and acrylates/acrylamide copolymer to help give the hair form and an impression of thickness by holding hair slightly in place (as opposed to falling limp). This is a crucial distinction that can affect hair negatively. These hairspray/styling type ingredients place a light, slightly sticky substance on the hair that can build up, leaving the hair with a brittle, stiff feeling. Of course, most leave-in conditioners don't advertise this problem, and unless you know how to read an ingredient list, you would never know what was making your hair feel unpleasant. Because of this problem, leave-in conditioners with film formers are best for someone who wants only minimal or extremely light, controlled styling and who washes her hair on a regular basis with a strong enough cleanser to wash out the buildup. Leave-in conditioners that don't contain these ingredients vary for different hair types.

Two-in-Ones

A shampoo and conditioner all in one was the ideal product for the new woman of the 1980s, who barely had time to cook dinner and feed her family, much less spend time grooming her hair with a battery of products. With this in mind, Procter & Gamble was in the right place at the right time with new research proving that you could wash your hair and condition it with the same product. Procter & Gamble's Pert (and, later, Pert Plus) two-in-one shampoo/conditioner was launched, and today Pert and its own spin-offs (ranging from Pantene to Vidal Sassoon, among others) make up almost 20 percent of the shampoo market. Now almost every line has a shampoo-and-conditioner-in-one to sell, but most of them are based on Procter & Gamble's landmark research.

The conditioning agent in Procter & Gamble's two-in-one products is silicone (specifically, dimethicone). As I mentioned, silicone has an amazing attraction to the hair shaft and the spaces between the cuticle layers. Not only does silicone want to nestle in between damaged, lifted cuticles, but it is relatively impervious to the force of rushing water trying to wash it down the drain. If anything, the water drives the dimethicone deeper into the cuticle while the shampoo is being rinsed away. From this perspective, two-in-ones work quite well, particularly for someone with normal to moderately dry or slightly damaged hair. **Where two-in-ones come up short is for someone with seriously damaged or dry hair or someone who has an oily scalp but still needs conditioning on dry or chemically treated ends.**

For someone with coarse, dry, or chemically treated hair, two-in-ones just don't have a wide enough variety of conditioning agents to deal with the resulting damage. While silicone does have a beautiful feel and texture, many other conditioning agents that don't hold up well in shampoo formulations can also help improve hair quality.

For someone with an oily scalp, two-in-ones pose a placement problem. Because of the way two-in-ones work, you can't control how much and where the silicone conditioning agent gets deposited on the hair. Shampooing takes place all over the head, which means the silicone is going to be left in places where you might not want it, like near the scalp where more emollients or a coating of any kind is not required or wanted. Instead, you need a conditioner you can put on just the ends, where it is needed.

Another problem with two-in-ones is the issue of buildup. The very action of two-in-ones means that the conditioning agent (silicone) is deposited every time you wash your hair. Even though the surfactants can wash some of that away, it is impossible to deposit more without leaving some of the old behind. It is unrealistic to expect two-in-ones not to have a problem with buildup. However, there are some hair types where buildup of silicone is not necessarily a bad thing. Two-in-ones do work great for those with completely normal, healthy, straight to wavy hair, regardless of the length, if there is no great need for fullness. If anything, the constant depositing of the silicone conditioning agent can help hair lay flatter against the head. For that very reason two-in-ones also work well for short hair, where the need is to have less fullness rather than more. (Interestingly, two-in-ones sell very well in Asian countries where the appearance of flat, smooth hair is preferred.)

Masks, Packs, and Hot-Oil Treatments

These supposedly intensive, specially formulated conditioning treatments are nothing more than standard, and sometimes relatively unimpressive, conditioners, just like the one you use every day in the shower. It takes only a quick look at the ingredient listings to notice how identical to regular conditioners these specialty treatments are. The principal difference between regular conditioners and specialty hair treatments is that the latter cost far more than conditioners, even though you get far less of them. The other difference is that specialty hair treatments are intended to be left on longer, and they are more effective when you use them along with a hair dryer using minimal heat (less than 100 degrees Fahrenheit). Can you do the same thing with the conditioner you use every day and get the exact same results? Absolutely!

Every time I've gotten my hair dyed at a salon, I'm told that I need to have a hair mask treatment or buy a hair mask to use at home to undo or prevent any damage from the chemical process. It simply isn't true. There are no ingredients in these hair-care products that can perform any function over and above that delivered by a traditional conditioner.

Perhaps most shocking are the hair masks that contain clay! What is that doing in a hair-care product of any kind? Clay is a drying substance with no other function. Plus, as the clay dries, it can actually chip away at the cuticle. Whose idea was this, anyway?

Speaking of hair treatment, you may have read that mayonnaise or vegetable oil right out of your cupboard and heated up is good for the hair. Almost without exception, hair-care products are infinitely superior to anything you can cook up in your kitchen because most hair-care products are designed to be water soluble. Mayonnaise and vegetable oils must be thoroughly washed out of the hair, and that it isn't easy to do, which means you would have to repeatedly lather up to be sure you got all the food off your hair—and that excessive washing damages hair.

Hot-oil treatments have developed a revival over the past few years. These specialized conditioners first came on the scene in the late 1950s to help counteract the damage caused by Marilyn Monroe wannabes turning their dark tresses blond. In some ways the concept wasn't so bad: Put conditioning agents, most of them being some kind of oil, on the hair and then sit under a hair dryer to help expand the hair shaft and allow the oils to better get in and around the cuticle layers. Although this does work, there is a downside that makes the outcome not so desirable. The downside is that high heat—much over 120 degrees Fahrenheit (which is only a few degrees hotter than most hot tubs)—in the long run causes damage!

Laminates, Serums, and Hair Polishers

Laminates, hair serums, hair polishers, and hair smoothers are names of products designed to smooth away frizzies and add shine to the hair. They come in small bottles and look like a thick, viscous oil. The major, if not the only, ingredient in all these products is silicone, usually in the form of dimethicone, cyclomethicone, and phenyltrimethicone. As you get more familiar with ingredient lists, you will notice dimethicone, cyclomethicone, and phenyltrimethicone showing up in just about every cosmetic product you use. Can silicones eliminate frizzies? To some extent they can, but definitely not even remotely as well as they appear to do in advertisements for these products. What these laminates, serums, and polishers do superbly is add a gorgeous silky feel to the hair, along with a highly reflective shine.

The prices for these products are astounding, ranging from $6 for 4 ounces to $20 for 1 ounce. This disparate price range is nothing more than marketing chicanery, because these ingredients and formulations are so standard and basic, it is almost laughable.

In the past I have written that silicone is an oil, and I must correct that misinformation. Silicone is a "fluid" and is not technically an oil. That means when you use it, you may think that what you're seeing and feeling has an appearance and texture similar to oil, but it still is not an oil.

Pomades and Greases

These are the original frizz busters. Regardless of the packaging or the company's impressive name on the label, they are a rather greasy mix of petrolatum, wax, mineral oils, lanolin, plant oils, castor oil, thickeners, film-forming/plasticizing agents, fragrance, and preservatives. Why would you want this grease or wax in your hair? That's a good question, because not many people do or should. It isn't for everyone. People with oily scalps or limp, thin, or short hair are not likely to be interested. Still, when accompanied by good styling techniques, pomades and greases can keep together ends that would normally fly away, smooth down coarse hair, and impart a lustrous shine with minimal sticky after-feel. However, this stuff can build up on the hair and should be kept away from the scalp at all costs. Pomades and greases are truly for the ends of hair only.

Spray-on Shine Products

Shine and luster in a bottle is what these products claim to be. They may also have some conditioning and detangling agents mixed in as well. Generally these products contain dimethicone, phenyltrimethicone, or cyclomethicone (see the "Laminates, Serums, and Hair Polishers" section above) to deliver shine and a silky feel to the hair; quats (see the "Shampoos" section) to help detangle the hair; and a number of different conditioning or water-binding agents such as panthenol, proteins, or glycerin (see the "Conditioners" section) to protect the hair shaft. Some of these spray-on shine products also contain plant oils, but you will notice, these are at the end of the ingredient list and silicone is almost always at the beginning. When it comes to imparting shine and incredible texture, there isn't a plant oil or a grease that can compete with the silicones. On occasion, these products may also throw in a sunscreen just for good marketing measure, but without an SPF number it is only a gimmick, and there is no way to know how much or how long your hair will be protected, if at all, from the sun.

Styling Gels and Mousses

Here's where things start getting sticky (pun intended), but hopefully not too sticky. Gels, spray gels, mousses, volumizing sprays, curl revitalizers, molding muds, styling lotions, and sculpting sprays are ingeniously formulated products designed to both help the hair and make it stay put in ways it wouldn't otherwise be able to do.

Mousses, with their lighter-than-air texture, spread easily through the hair, melting into place and providing soft styling control and fullness. Styling gels are clear, viscous substances that move easily through the hair (but not as easily as mousse) and tend to offer more control and potential for fullness. For the most part, spray-on gels are diluted versions of the thicker gels, providing a softer degree of hold. Curl revitalizers and volumizing sprays are relatively light, almost like water, with a small amount of conditioner and styling ingredients. Sculpting and molding gels tend to be stiffer, giving ultimate control over where the hair finally ends up.

What these products all share is a tendency to dry slowly and provide movement to the hair for a period of time until the liquid dries. Regardless of the nuances (and there are an almost limitless number of names and formulas), what these products have in common, line to line, is pretty much the same array of ingredients. Often the only difference between products is the price, not the ingredient list.

Regardless of the extraordinarily elaborate claims companies make about their styling products, there are only a limited number of ingredients that can mold and hold in this film-forming, plasticizing manner, and they are not unique or rare in the least. These standard film-forming/plasticizing ingredients showing up in styling product after styling product are called polymers. If you've skimmed almost any styling product label (other than pomade-type products and some softer-hold type products), you've probably seen the ingredients PVP (short for polyvinylpyrrolidone), PVP/VA copolymer (VA is short for vinyl acrylate), acrylates/vinyl isodecanoate crosspolymer, acrylamide/ammonium acrylate copolymer, acrylic/acrylate copolymer, vinyl acetate, polyvinyl acetate, and styrene/acrylamide copolymer.

All of the above are varying forms of polymers. Polymers are long molecular chains of synthetic compounds, usually of high molecular weight (meaning they can't be absorbed into the hair or easily broken down), with millions of repeated linked units, yet each is a relatively light and simple molecule. It is the linking and lightweight nature of polymers that makes them so hair-friendly. Polymers can bind to the hair, creating a consistent film between and around two or more hair shafts, with barely any detectable weight, and give the hair strength, resilience, and hold.

Alone or in combination, all of these styling ingredients provide a profusion of product choices. But again, as you get used to reading the ingredient list, you'll notice that beneath the surface of the marketing language lies a glaring similarity between styling products, regardless of price range or designer image.

Hair Note: Detangling agents (quats) are sometimes included in styling products, but not often, because they do the opposite of what you want the hair to do when you are trying to get it to stay in place. Detangling agents are meant to separate the hair, while styling products are meant to keep the hair together. For appearance's sake, styling products once in a while contain conditioning agents, although their benefits are lost. The polymers, resins, guars, and cellulose form a film over the hair, preventing the conditioning agents from connecting with the hair shaft, which means it is difficult for them to have any real, positive effect. They may sound desirable in styling gels and mousses, but in these types of products they're wasted.

Hairsprays, Spritzes, and Freezes

While styling products are meant to be worked through an entire head of hair to give it form, shape, and style, hairsprays and their counterparts are meant to dry in place very quickly, holding the hairstyle you created relatively still, preventing it from returning to its natural or normal appearance, and, most important, keeping humidity out. Hairsprays work by building consistent, continuous bonds between hair fibers. Hairspray ingredients are identical to those in other styling products, only with less water and generally higher concentrations of film-forming/plasticizing agents such as acrylates, acrylamides, styrene, crotonic acid, and methylacrylate copolymer. (Plasticizing agents help make film-forming ingredients more pliable. If these weren't included, your hair would have a brittle, stiff feel.)

What about holding power? Generally I found that hairsprays, and most styling product labels, tell the truth about how well they hold the hair. If the label says "SUPER HOLD," it means super hold; if it says "SOFT HOLD," it will do just that. There are exceptions, but I get to those in the product reviews.

Should you use aerosol hairsprays or nonaerosol hairsprays? That decision is one of personal preference. The major difference between them is the way the spray is dispersed. Aerosols discharge a featherweight mist, while nonaerosols are apt to go on more heavily. It takes a skilled hand to get nonaerosol sprays to go on lightly and sparsely. The heavier the spray, the more likely it will flake off in white or clear chunks.

The issue of aerosol or nonaerosol is really more an environmental concern than an aesthetic one. Aerosol hairsprays use volatile organic compounds (VOC s) to disperse the hairspray ingredients over the hair. VOC s negatively impact the earth's atmosphere. Hairsprays containing ethanol alcohol (listed as SD alcohol, followed by a number), hydrocarbons, isobutane, and butane release vapors into the air that generate ozone in the lower atmosphere. While other human-made pollutants deplete the ozone in the upper atmosphere, emitting VOC s into the lower atmosphere produces an additional ozone layer that traps heat and ultraviolet radiation nearer to the earth's surface, adding to the levels of smog in cities caused by automobiles and other industrial pollution. California and New York have been the leaders in setting environmental standards for VOC s, and since 1998 they have not allowed the sale of any hairspray containing more than 55 percent VOC. It is not known whether the rest of the states will follow suit. Eventually hairsprays will most likely have to be formulated without any VOC s whatsoever. As a result of this legislation, new hairspray formulas are being worked on. Many hairsprays use perofluorcan as their propellant because it does not affect the ozone. In the meantime, if you notice changes in the hairsprays you're buying, they are changes for the better, at least for the environment.

Hair Note: Aside from environmental concerns, is alcohol a problem in hair-care products such as gels, mousses, and hairsprays? It all depends on who you ask. Cosmetics chemists feel alcohol is essential to help a styling product, usually hairspray, dry in place without leaving the hair overly wet, which would destroy a skillfully arranged style. Consumers and many stylists feel alcohol is a problem in any hair-care product, particularly if the hair is damaged, excessively dry, fragile, brittle, chemically treated, or naturally very porous, because it can be drying. Both points of view are valid, although I side with the cosmetics chemists on this one. The amount of alcohol in hair-care products is probably not a problem for most hair types. In reality, alcohol in hairsprays evaporates too quickly to impact the moisture content of the hair. But if you have any concerns about the condition of your hair, I would encourage you to avoid alcohol or any other drying agents in your hair-care products. In the long run, alcohol will probably be eliminated from styling products anyway, because of environmental regulations in regard to alcohol's effect on the ozone. In a few years this concern will be history, as cosmetics chemists are forced to design these products with minimal or no alcohol.

Sunscreen in Hair-Care Products

It is unquestionable that hair needs to be protected from the sun! Sun damage destroys hair by breaking down the bonds that keep hair's structure intact. Where brushing and combing chip away at the outer cuticle, the sun destroys the interior of hair, which explains why hair color fades with sun exposure. Yet despite this desperate need for protection, sunscreens in shampoos and conditioners are nothing less than a waste of time and money. There is no way that these formulations can provide adequate sun protection for the hair. Shampoos and conditioners are meant to be rinsed out and, consequently, there is no way to know how much, if any, sunscreen has remained behind. In fact, because of the water-solubility of most sunscreens, they are probably rinsed away almost immediately.

Leave-in hair-care products that contain sunscreen are a better bet, but only slightly. Although the sunscreen's ability to stay on the hair shaft increases with a leave-in product, there is no way to know or measure whether any of the sunscreen still remains on the hair after brushing or styling. What's foremost, when considering this issue, is that hair-care products are not allowed to have SPF numbers because the FDA does not consider hair-care products with sunscreen safe or reliable for sun protection. Without an SPF number, there is no way to determine how long the hair shaft will be protected if any sunscreen is indeed left behind. If you can't know the SPF, you have no idea if the product is an SPF 2, SPF 8, or SPF 15. Moreover, with the skin, we know that sunscreen must be reapplied after swimming or long exposure to the sun, but what about the hair? After two hours of bike riding, are you going to reapply your leave-in conditioner with sunscreen and get your hair all gooped up all over again?

I'm not saying that sunscreen ingredients can't protect the hair from sun damage, because they can. There are plenty of studies in which a swatch of hair is covered with sunscreen ingredients, then placed under UVA/UVB light, and after a period of time measured for deterioration. The sunscreen ingredients absolutely prevented damage. However, until there is a solution to the application and adherence issues, it is a huge mistake to rely on sunscreen in hair-care products. Until the FDA gives its SPF blessing to hair-care products, wear a hat when spending long periods of time in the sun. That's the only real way to prevent sun damage to your hair.

Here is an interesting correspondence I received, along with my reply to Redken concerning the issue of sunscreen in hair-care products:

Dear Paula,

First of all, if you are going to say that Redken's Color Extend Shampoo and Conditioner do not work, you might have at least called us to ask for our claim substantiation. You know that Redken "knows better," as you have visited us before, and we take our products very seriously. The two products are covered by two United States patent applications, one of which is a composition for depositing sunscreens and other lipophilic ingredients on the hair.

Second, for a reader who has not seen the products, your comments might lead them to believe we claim an SPF value, which of course we do not. There is no SPF value for hair, not because sunscreens have no effect, but because there is no established methodology. However, Paula, to suggest the sunscreens cannot have a protective effect on hair condition or color is just plain wrong. Laboratory studies with Color Extend Shampoo and Conditioner demonstrated the deposit of sunscreens on both normal and damaged hair and the amount increased with the number of use cycles. We should of course agree that the deposition from a shampoo or conditioner is less than the amount obtained by drying a product into the hair. Simulated shampoo/conditioning tests coupled with irradiation exposure demonstrated less lightening of color-treated hair. The hair condition of color-treated hair as measured by compatibility studies showed the products produced a protection against further irradiation damage.

The products were evaluated by an external investigator in a randomized double-blind study with consumers who regularly color their hair and shampoo at least three times per week. Evaluations at weeks two and four by the consumers rated color protection, softness, shine, and manageability all above 75 on a scale of 0–100.

Last but not least, the products have been on the market for about one year, and our post-market surveys indicate salon and consumer satisfaction. I cannot believe professionals and consumers continue to purchase products that do not work.

Your comments this time, Paula, are not your best effort and we would appreciate the opportunity to have your readers see our response.

David Cannell, Ph.D.
Senior Vice President
Redken Research & Development

Dear Dr. Cannell,

Your letter and feedback were greatly appreciated. I will be certain to use the full content of your letter in my next newspaper column and newsletter. I do indeed respect Redken's expertise and I'm fairly certain your association with L'Oreal has only expanded your range and scope. Although I understand your concern about my information and analysis, we disagree on several points.

In terms of your comments regarding how Color Extend is marketed in regard to SPF content, I regret if I led anyone to believe there was a claim being made for an actual SPF value, because there is not. However, while Redken does not directly indicate an SPF value (it would be illegal to do so), it is my strong impression that the consumer is nonetheless certainly being led in that direction. Six of the salons I visited and all five salons I called in different regions of the United States explained in varying degrees how Redken's Color Extend products could protect against sun damage because they were as "effective as any SPF product you would put on your skin, only this is for the hair." Plus, the copy on your product sure sounds like you're talking about reliable sun protection for the hair.

You are correct in suggesting that I did not contact your company directly to inquire about your research or methodology regarding sun protection; however, I am very familiar with many studies looking at the issue of sun protection for hair. Both Procter & Gamble and Clairol have very impressive laboratory studies proving sun protection (preventing amino acid and protein breakdown) for the hair. Given the similarity in formulation, I assumed yours would be no less impressive. Yet translating any of that into actual, real-life protection, given varying routines and intervals of cleansing and conditioning the hair, styling techniques, how often hair is brushed, types of dye used, length of time in the sun, as well as many other considerations, is just not possible, and is the primary reason the FDA has not attributed SPF to any hair-care product.

In terms of the studies you conducted on real women and their perception of how they felt about using the Color Extend products, I would love to see the actual study and methodology. I'm curious how the double-blind test was handled; in other words, what product formulations were used in your comparison model? If you would send the actual study to me, I would be glad to review those results as well, but I can't comment or expect a consumer to rely on studies that are not available to them.

One more point: Your comment that consumers would not continue to buy products unless they worked is somewhat ingenuous, don't you think? Do you really believe that everything being sold for an extended period of time has automatic consumer value or is worthwhile? Cigarettes are continually sold, slasher movies rake in huge dollars, and I bet there are lots of hair-care companies selling products we would both rate as being less than wonderful or effective. Additionally, *Consumer Reports* rates a multitude of varying products, which have been on the market for years and years, as being far less than beneficial and often dangerous. Length of time doesn't prove anything except that uninformed consumers can, at the very least, waste their money or, at the very worst, cause themselves harm.

For now, until the FDA and the cosmetics industry develop a consistent, dependable SPF system for hair-care products, I consider any product for the hair or skin without an SPF to be incapable of providing reliable sun defense. I stand by my opinion that a woman relying on any hair-care product (as opposed to a hat) to protect her hair color from sun damage is making an unwise decision.

[As this book went to press, I still had not received any information back from Redken regarding their "randomized double-blind study." I doubt that it will be forthcoming. I sent my request to Dr. Cannell on August 10, 1998, just two weeks after I received his letter.]

Naturally Bad

In the world of natural ingredients, all things are considered bright and beautiful. Many women believe that if they use a product labeled "NATURAL" or "PURE," their hair will become pure and naturally beautiful. Nothing could be further from the truth: Natural doesn't assure quality or even safety. But that doesn't stop consumers or the cosmetics companies.

Many natural ingredients pose problems for the skin. While I can't stop the craze for natural ingredients, I keep trying because I know how much money women are wasting on these products. I thought it might be a good idea to provide a list of the more popular, but possibly irritating or photosensitizing, natural ingredients found in cosmetics.

All of the following can cause skin irritation and/or sun sensitivity: almond extract, allspice, angelica, arnica, balm mint oil, balsam, basil, bergamot, chamomile, cinnamon, citrus, clove, clover blossom, coriander oil, cottonseed oil, fennel, fir needle, geranium oil, grapefruit, horsetail, jojoba oil, lavender oil, lemon, lemongrass, lime, marjoram, melissa, oak bark, papaya, peppermint, rose, sage, thyme, and wintergreen.

The label might say "pure and natural" but you could be buying a purely irritating product. It won't irritate the hair shaft, because the hair is dead, but if it rinses off onto the face or makes contact with the scalp, you can have problems. Even if natural ingredients were all beneficial to hair, they would only work with leave-in products. In a shampoo, most of them are rinsed down the drain.

You may have noticed lately that several cosmetics lines are using descriptive terms to identify either the source or the purpose of the ingredient. For example, Aveda lists polyquaternium-10 as "plant cellulose" and polyquaternium-16 as an "antistatic agent." Aveda and other companies that provide this more specific, apparently consumer-understandable information are only disclosing what they want you to know about their ingredients. Polyquaternium-10 (and -16) are not plant cellulose, as the description implies; rather, they are *derived* from plant cellulose. That is not just a technicality. How it is derived isn't quite as pure-sounding as it reads. Very *un*natural ingredients are used to take the plant cellulose and turn it into polyquaternium-10. Does that change the acceptability or effectiveness of the polyquats as antistatic agents or surfactants (cleansers)? Not in the least. It is just another way in which the cosmetics companies help encourage the consumer to think more highly of natural ingredients than is necessary or warranted.

The pressure from consumers to have natural-sounding ingredients is so powerful that there is a new bit of deception taking place on ingredient labels. For example, rather than listing mineral oil or petrolatum in a product, some companies list the trade names instead, namely, Protol and Protopet. Because many consumers erroneously believe mineral oil and petrolatum are bad for skin, cosmetics companies use these names to cloak the real ingredients on the label.

One more point: The next time you hear a hair-care company proclaiming that their products are natural, give them a skeptical nod of your head and then read the ingredient list. The amount of plants used in any hair-care product is negligible in comparison to the chemical-sounding ingredients. Concentrating on natural ingredients is a way to let yourself be duped.

You may also find recyclable packaging an intriguing notion when it comes to the hair-care products you buy. It is, but at this stage of the game, the promises of recyclable or ecologically friendly don't hold up in the landfill. According to *Drug and Cosmetic Industry* magazine, Sebastian tried to be the first on the market with containers that were supposedly biodegradable, meaning they would break down in landfills after two years. Research by solid-waste disposal experts exposed the fact that even after ten years there was little evidence that any breakdown occurred. As of yet, there are no authentic claims of truly environmentally friendly packaging available, especially when it comes to plastic bottles. (However, boxes and brochures may indeed be made from recyclable paper and, for now, that's as close as we can get.)

Allergic Reactions

When it comes to hair products, as opposed to cosmetics, the chance of allergic reactions is greatly reduced for the obvious reason that very little of the product actually stays on your skin for very long. Conditioners and shampoos have minimal contact with the scalp because of the copious amounts of water being used at the same time. Furthermore, because hair is dead as a doornail, you can put all kinds of irritating ingredients on it that would normally wreak havoc on the skin and never be aware of the difference. The problems start when the ingredients in hair-care products come in contact with the skin. Hair covered in conditioning or styling agents can come in contact with your hairline, face, neck, or shoulders, and that can cause irritation, allergic reactions, or breakouts.

Hair-care ingredients found in most styling products, pomades, and conditioners (especially ones designed for damaged, dry hair) can cause skin problems, including breakouts and allergic reactions (*all* styling products contain ingredients that can be fairly strong skin irritants). While it is essential to experiment with products to find which ones won't be a problem for you, hair-care products are so similar that changing products may not be of much help. The best option is to be careful about what gets on your skin.

Be sure when you apply hairspray that you do not get any on your face. If you are using styling products, you often wear your hair brushed forward, and you are breaking out in the areas where the hair touches the face, consider either wearing your hair off the face for awhile or temporarily not using the styling products, and see what happens. The same is true for shampoos and conditioners. Conditioners don't often contain irritating ingredients (although there are several nowadays with some of the irritating ingredients I mentioned in the above section called "Naturally Bad" that can cause allergic reactions), but they almost always contain emollients and conditioning agents that can clog pores. A great option to take to avoid problems is to be careful when rinsing off conditioner; be sure to bend forward or backward to avoid getting it on your skin.

You can use the same trick of rinsing off shampoos away from the skin, but that won't help the scalp where the cleansing agents must do their job. There is a definite concern that some surfactants and other irritating ingredients can cause allergic or irritating skin reactions on the scalp. In any case, if you have a particularly sensitive skin or scalp, or notice flaking or irritation, you may want to avoid shampoos containing sodium lauryl sulfate, TEA lauryl sulfate, ammonium lauryl sulfate, and alkyl sodium sulfate, when they are the second or third ingredients in the shampoo, and avoid all of the irritating ingredients listed in the section "Naturally Bad."

You Gotta Have a Gimmick

You've probably noticed that many hair-care lines have divided their products into increasingly segmented groupings. L'Oreal has hair-care lines for colored hair (Colorvive), permed hair (Permavive), and dry hair (Hydravive). Each grouping is further broken down into hair types, such as dry/delicate, normal/healthy, and fine/thin. Talk about getting specific! Every line has its own angle, with divisions forming over ingredient choices, such as chamomile versus ginger or proteins versus panthenols; scalp type versus hair condition; or conditioning goals such as more curl, less curl, smoothness, wave, and fullness. Regardless what the products tell you, there is little basis for these other than creating marketing niches. Dry, permed, color-treated, or damaged hair has similar needs. Hair that is thin, limp, fine, fragile, or delicate has similar needs. Sure enough, when you read the labels on products designed for dry, permed, color-treated, or damaged hair, they almost always share a comparable ingredient list. Product segmenting may seem helpful, but it ends up being more confusing than useful.

Similarly, specific ingredients alone do not guarantee the value of any given product. Panthenol may be a good conditioner but, by itself and without the addition of quaternary ammonia compounds, emollients, and other conditioning agents, it won't perform the way you expect it to. Awapuhi and burdock root may sound healthy, but they (along with myriad other natural-sounding ingredients) won't produce healthy hair all by themselves; they are nothing more than window dressing for the other, more chemical-sounding ingredients that make hair-care products effective. Proteins in conditioners may sound like they will help reinforce hair but they actually do so poorly and unreliably. Focusing on one or two ingredients is a waste of time and energy when shopping for any hair-care product.

Hair Wands

Speaking of gimmicks, there are several product catalogs selling a device called the **Ionic Hair Wand** *($39)*. They claim that when this product is stroked through the hair, it "bathes each strand in ions, which adds body and volume; calms dry, brittle, or windblown hair; . . . removes such odors as cigarette smoke; . . . [and] reduces bacteria on the hair and scalp, while removing particles such as dandruff flakes; . . . [and it] actually smoothes the hair by causing hair cuticle shafts to lie flat. It also unifies the charge, so hair strands no longer clump together."

If you've taken one or two chemistry courses, you'll realize that there is enough scientific lingo here to sound almost convincing, but just almost, because you would also have enough information to know that other parts sound almost laughable. I guess you can put a price on anything, including static electricity, which is the issue at hand for the Ionic Hair Wand. Ions are nothing more than groups of atoms that have a positive, negative, or neutral electric charge. They can't repair anything, despite the claims in the catalogs selling these implements. Hair itself has a negative electrical charge and is attracted to things with a positive charge. (Two positives repel each other and two negatives repel each other, but a positive and a negative cling together.) Hair becomes flyaway when positive ions (static electricity) are conducted through the body (electricity can pass through people) and build up. The negatively charged hair responds to this positive charge moving through the body and out the top of the head by standing on end. If you diminish or eliminate the static charge flowing up through the hair (i.e., stop the flow of the positive ions), your hair will calm down. It's just that simple. Of course, if the air is cold, the second you shuffle over a carpet or some other fabric, static electricity will be generated again. And if the wand isn't nearby, your hair will take off again.

The information for this device also asserts that damaged or roughed-up scales on the hair shaft can be smoothed down by the wand's ion output. I assume that the same static charge that makes hair lift can get under the scales and make them lift, and that negating that charge can reduce some frizziness. However, other things can also cause the hair to be frizzy, including humidity, curly hair growth, and the thickness of the hair, and none of these can be affected by ions.

The question of whether dandruff and bacteria will jump off the hair and scalp and grab the wand is much more suspect. The catalog deals with that by stating that the wand can reduce (not eliminate) those things. If the electrical charge of the dandruff and bacteria is different from that of the wand, I suppose they would be attracted to the wand and cling to that instead of to the hair or scalp. However, you would never get all the bacteria and dandruff off the hair or scalp, nor would you be changing the environment under the skin of the scalp (where the wand's ions can't reach), which is causing the dandruff in the first place. I have no idea how the ions would work to remove cigarette smoke!

CHAPTER FOUR

Hair Type

Normal? Oily? Dry? Damaged?

Searching for hair-care products in hopes that they can do the impossible is literally a headache for your hair and pocketbook. If you are still under the false assumption that hair-care products can prevent or reverse damage, you won't make wise decisions about taking care of your hair. Reducing the risk of damage is the first step to choosing the right products. When you have those new habits firmly in place, you've gone a long way toward taking great care of your hair.

Now, the next step is determining your hair type and then dealing with it. In order to do that, it is essential to understand the relationship between the scalp and the hair. We tend to treat the scalp and the hair as if they were the same, or at least closely related, when often the way they respond is completely unrelated. Before you wash your hair, it is necessary to differentiate between what the hair and the scalp require separately and then make sure that each is getting what it needs. Your scalp type, the condition of your hair, and what you want the final results to look like determine what you should be using.

Before we go over specific product choices, let's take a closer look at the four traditional categories of hair type: normal, oily, dry, and damaged (generally meaning chemically treated or overstyled). Although these categories are useful, they are too narrow to take into consideration many of the subtle distinctions and variations that exist, and they don't explain how to actually use products. For example, your hair can be oily in places (mostly at the root for curly hair, or all over for straight hair, or just on the scalp) and dry in places (the ends of longer hair, all over for bleached blonde hair). The same is true for the scalp. It can be partly oily but still have dry flakes, be itchy and oily, or be dry.

In addition, the hair and scalp are not static; seasonal changes can affect the hair, as can hormonal changes. Hair can be normal in the summer and dry in the winter, or it can be cooperative or uncooperative depending on the amount of humidity in the air. If you dye your hair you could have dry, damaged ends with frizzies and an oily scalp. Moreover, hair care is greatly influenced by the movement of your hair. Straight hair has very different needs from wavy hair, curly hair, or kinky hair.

Often the hair and scalp types we think we have are really a result of the products or implements we use and not the true state of our hair. We might complain that our hair is flyaway and unmanageable or that our scalp is dry, and then go to the store wondering which products will correct the problem. What we don't realize is that the issue may not be about using different products but may require a simple change in habit. Flyaway hair can be caused by overbrushing, using a conditioner that isn't emollient enough to coat hair, or using a wash-out conditioner instead of a leave-in one.

A dry scalp might not really be dry, but could be the result of overwashing the hair or not rinsing it well enough, leaving irritating detergent or plant extract residue on the scalp. An oily scalp might not be as oily as it appears but, rather, the conditioner you're using may be making the scalp feel greasy or thick. Before we can ever decide what our hair needs or doesn't need, we must first determine what kind of hair and scalp we really have and how what we are presently doing affects them.

Aside from the differences between hair and scalp, the quality of hair on any one head is not uniform. If your hair is layered, the shorter hair on top is most likely at a different stage of fitness than the longer ends. The longer ends have been putting up with blow-dryers, brushes, weather, swimming pools, and styling products for a longer period of time. The new hair on top is not in need of the same attention or product usage as the ends. Combination hair of this kind is as typical as combination skin, yet the hair-care companies virtually ignore this condition.

Normal hair (usually straight or wavy) and normal scalp . This is the dream head of hair. If your hair feels soft to the touch, has good body and manageability (and doesn't require a conditioner to feel that way), and has not been color-treated or permed, and if your scalp is neither dry nor oily, then you have "normal" hair. This hair type needs minimal attention. However, normal hair can quickly become damaged hair if you overuse styling implements or drastically change your hair color. Also, overwashing can dry out the scalp.

It is easy to get seduced by perms or extreme changes in hair color, especially when you have healthy, normal hair. You're told it will just bring a little more life to your hair—and no damage. I've seen it happen over and over. A woman with beautiful, healthy hair is convinced that it could be *more* beautiful (we are so easily convinced we can be more beautiful with help from the cosmetics industry) with a few highlights or changing the color to a few shades lighter. Now the normal hair is damaged and conditioner is mandatory, with no return to normalcy until the hair grows out; all for the sake of a "beautiful" change. Sometimes the best policy is to do as little as possible.

A shampoo for normal hair or a shampoo with a minimal amount of conditioner does just fine for this hair type.

Oily hair (usually straight) and oily scalp or dry ends (usually curly or kinky hair—may or may not be color treated) and oily scalp. Technically, hair itself is not oily; but when the scalp produces too much oil, it slides down the hair shaft, causing the hair to become heavy and matted. This is especially a problem for those with straight hair and an oily scalp because the oil has a straight path down the hair shaft with no resistance. Curly hair, on the other hand, has more twists and turns, so even though the scalp is producing the same amount of oil as is the scalp of someone with straight hair, the person with curly hair experiences it far differently.

The major questions most women have concerning their oily hair is how often you can wash it and how you stop the oil. Essentially, you can wash your hair as often as you like. The only problem is washing with strong shampoos that contain strong detergent cleansing agents, or with cleansers that contain irritating ingredients. Both of these elements can dry out the scalp and hair. What you can't do is stop the oil from being produced. Shampooing or trying to dry up the oil won't stop or alter oil production in the least. You cannot control or change oil production from the outside in. Oil production is generated by hormonal activity, which cannot be influenced topically. So wash your hair as often as you like with shampoos that contain gentle cleansing agents (they will be enough to clean hair without causing dryness). **But it is essential to never use shampoos with conditioning agents (especially those designated as two-in-ones), because these deposit ingredients that add to the greasy feel of the hair, especially on the scalp.** If the hair is hard to comb after washing, then use the lightest-weight conditioner possible and keep it away from the scalp.

If the hair length is dry, that does require a conditioner, but absolutely use a separate product. Only condition the ends or dry sections and, as much as possible, never place conditioner on the scalp or anywhere near the root area close to the scalp.

Short hair and oily scalp. This kind of hair can be a blessing because a simple shampoo with minimal to no conditioners, used as often as you want, is probably all you need. You probably produce enough natural oil to have enough of your own built-in conditioner. Since your hair is short, even if you color your hair, you probably won't need a conditioner because you are constantly cutting or trimming away the damaged length. If you do need a conditioner, use the least amount possible and keep it away from the root area and scalp.

Dry hair (regardless of cause) and dry, itchy scalp (usually with straight, fine, or thin hair). This type of hair is very tricky because if you apply an emollient conditioner all over, it can make your hair go limp, although it will help moisturize the dry scalp. But if you avoid an emollient conditioner or shampoo, your scalp can flake and your hair can be flyaway. And a two-in-one product won't provide enough conditioner to the dry hair. Another problem is the fear of overwashing. Someone with dry hair and dry scalp can go several days between shampoos, but that causes dead skin cells and styling products to build up on the hair, making it look dull and shapeless.

Shampooing at least twice a week to prevent buildup and using an emollient conditioner that rinses well off the scalp and hair is the best way to go. Avoid greasy conditioners and hair treatments near the scalp, even though they promise to take care of the dryness. If a product contains lanolin, vegetable or plant oils, cocoa butter, mineral oil, castor oil, or petrolatum among the first four to five ingredients on the ingredient list, it is considered fairly greasy. These ingredients are also difficult to wash out of the hair and tend to sit on the scalp, trapping dead skin cells. Shampoos and conditioners need to be rinsed off well. Massage your scalp gently but thoroughly when shampooing and conditioning, but don't overmanipulate the hair.

Do not use leave-in conditioners; they are rarely emollient or moisturizing enough for this kind of dryness. Instead, apply a drop of silicone serum before styling (see the section on "Laminates, Serums, and Hair Polishers" in Chapter Three *Hair-Care Basics*) to the very dry ends of the hair. This will make a big difference in the feel of your hair.

The best way to deal with the dry scalp is to treat it as you would dry skin anywhere else on your body. Consider using a lightweight moisturizer such as Lubriderm, Cetaphil Moisturizer, or Eucerin Lite on your scalp at night if you plan to shampoo the next morning. It may seem a little strange at first, but it can make a real difference in the condition of your scalp, particularly during the winter. When you shampoo in the morning, take extra care to massage and wash the scalp, rinsing generously.

If your scalp feels itchy, a little over-the-counter cortisone cream massaged into the scalp the night before you wash your hair the next morning can easily take care of that problem.

Dry hair (regardless of cause), and dry, itchy scalp (usually with wavy, curly, coarse, or kinky hair). In many ways this hair type is easier to care for than the one above because wavy, curly, coarse, or kinky hair doesn't get as limp or heavy with the application of its much-needed emollient conditioners. To this end, the only difference from the hair type above is that you can be more liberal with emollient products and less concerned about weighing hair down, and you can also be a bit more generous with the laminates, serums, or hair polishers. All the other suggestions still pertain.

All hair types and combination scalp . If your scalp is both oily and flaky at the same time but the flaking is not caused by dandruff (see the following sections on dandruff or the information on dandruff in Chapter Three), you've got a tricky condition to contend with. It might be caused by overwashing, which causes dryness, or by not washing often enough, which causes buildup of skin or styling products. The flaking can also be caused from irritation or an allergic reaction to the hair-care products you are using. Or it can be a result of seborrhea or psoriasis. As a general rule, it is best to use a shampoo that contains minimal to no conditioners and to be sure to gently massage your nails over your scalp to help exfoliation when shampooing. A lightweight conditioner that you use all over but carefully rinse out won't weigh the hair down and should help. If you have hair that's more coarse or dry, generously apply conditioner to those areas, avoiding the scalp.

If you suspect that any of the flaking is a result of allergic reactions or irritation from the products you're using, change to one of the products recommended in Chapter Ten for itching or allergy problems. It will take some experimenting to find which solutions work for you. It can help reduce the itching to massage an over-the-counter cortisone cream into the scalp the night before you wash your hair.

All hair types and flaky dry scalp. If the flaking is caused by dandruff or you suspect some other scalp dermatitis, see the following sections on "Is It Dandruff?," "Seborrhea," and "Psoriasis." If the flaking is not related to any of those disorders, there can be several causes and solutions. The flaking may not be related to a dry scalp, but could be a buildup of styling products coming off in sheets. Cutting back on the amount of styling products you use and keeping them away from the scalp will take care of the problem if it is related to buildup.

If your scalp is truly dry and it isn't a result of irritating ingredients in your shampoo or conditioner, be sure you use a conditioner designed for dry scalp and/or dry hair and gently massage it into the scalp, avoiding the ends so as not to weigh down the hair. Always rinse well; residue from shampoos can cause irritation and make matters worse. Two-in-one shampoos can be a good option for this hair type, as they avoid overconditioning normal hair but provide enough conditioner for the scalp. It may also help to use a skin moisturizer such as Nutraderm or a 5% AHA product such as Alpha Hydrox's Sensitive Skin Cream the night before if you plan to shampoo in the morning. Doing this on a regular basis can really make a difference in the condition of the scalp. Styling products should be kept at a minimum to decrease the chance of them flaking off and adding to the scalp flakes you already have.

Dry hair ends and oily scalp. If the entire hair shaft is dry and the scalp is oily, it is usually because the hair has been overprocessed or styled to death. In that case, you should first get a haircut to eliminate broken ends, which will help the appearance of your hair almost immediately. Cut back on curling irons, blow-dryers, and extreme changes in your natural hair color or you will only continue the cycle of dry ends. Use a shampoo designed for normal hair, one that contains no conditioning agents. Wash your hair no more than two or three times a week; washing every day can cause a rebound effect, making the scalp more oily. Besides, washing the hair too often also means more blow-dryers and curling irons, further damaging the hair. Select an emollient conditioner for dry, damaged hair and use it only on the ends, being sure to leave it on for as long as possible, then rinsing well. The longer the conditioner is left on the hair, the better the chance for the conditioning agents to get deposited on the hair shaft or absorbed into the cuticle. Before you style your hair, saturate the ends with a protecting spray (this should be separate from your styling gel or mousse).

Fragile, dry hair and dry scalp. This combination is typical of African-American hair. For specific details and a thorough discussion of this unique hair type, please see Chapter Seven, *For African-American Women*.

Fine, thin hair and normal scalp. Follow the basic guidelines for normal hair and normal scalp. It's best not to use overall conditioners or two-in-one shampoos for this hair type, as they can weigh down the hair. Lightweight spray-on conditioners containing proteins, water-binding agents, and a small amount of styling ingredients can be applied after washing to help with combing and to add a feeling of fullness, but you control where you need it and how much. *The less product the better for thin hair, to avoid weighing it down.* It is tempting to get caught up in using more and more products in the belief that the volume will add up too, but thin hair can only take so much before it begins to fall. (Many products make claims about adding body, but you can't add body without risking adding weight to the hair.)

Chemical treatments such as perms or hair color (not both; choose one or the other) can add body and fullness because of the swelling effect these chemical processes have on the hair shaft. However, in time, with repeated coloring and perming, the fullness can change to damage very quickly. What styling products you choose always depends on the kind of look you want, but, as much as possible, you are better off with lightweight styling products to keep the hair from getting weighed down.

Fine, thin hair and dry scalp. Follow the basic guidelines for normal hair and dry scalp. Chemical treatments such as perms or hair color (not both; choose one or the other) can add body and fullness. If you choose to perm, do not let your stylist select small rods. Large rods will add body and smoothness; small rods can make kinks and frizz.

Fine, thin hair and oily scalp. Follow the basic guidelines for normal hair and oily scalp. Chemical treatments such as perms or hair color (not both; choose one or the other) can add body and fullness. If you choose to perm, do not let your stylist select small rods. Large rods will add body and smoothness; small rods can make kinks and frizz.

Coarse hair and dry scalp. Follow the basic guidelines for normal hair and dry scalp. It is almost impossible to overcondition coarse hair, so don't be afraid to use these products generously; let them stay on as long as possible and then rinse. Hair laminates and serums are dream products for this kind of hair.

Avoid leave-in conditioners—they tend to make hair brittle because they usually contain styling agents such as acrylates, acrylamides, or PVP. Pomades and greases are an option for this hair type, but be careful. They can get greasy and tacky, leaving a slick, messy finish, when what you really want is a soft, smooth appearance. Use them sparingly and only on the areas where they're needed, not all over. In general, avoid styling gels and hairsprays that leave a hard finish on the hair; they may hold better, but they can make the hair feel coarser and rougher.

Coarse hair and oily scalp. Follow the basic guidelines for normal hair and oily scalp. Applying frizz busters or spray-on and leave-in conditioner on just the parts of the hair that are coarse or frizzy can leave a softer, smoother finish on the hair as long as these products don't contain any styling agents (such as acrylates, acrylamides, and PVP). In general, avoid styling gels and hairsprays that leave a hard finish on the hair; they may hold better, but they can make the hair feel coarser and rougher. Because of the oily condition of the scalp, it is best not to use pomades or greases.

Chemically treated, damaged hair, regardless of scalp type. Essentially it is best to choose a shampoo for your scalp type and a conditioner for your hair. Pay particular attention to the ends. Do not overwash or manipulate the hair too much. Be good about protecting your hair from exposure to the weather and sun by wearing a hat if you are going to be outside for long periods of time. Don't trust products that contain sunscreen to protect your hair from environmental damage. Until the FDA decides to regulate SPF (sun protection factor) ratings for hair products, they can't do what they claim.

Overuse conditioner and keep it on the hair for as long as possible. Hair laminates and serums work beautifully to make hair feel silky-soft. Pomades and greases can help ends look smooth.

Sparse hair. Little can be done to handle sparse hair, at least when it comes to shampoos, conditioners, or styling products. If sparse hair is being caused by breakage (from overperming or radical changes in hair color) or by hair loss, you must address those problems first before you take any other course of action. Some women color visible scalp areas with makeup, such as mascara or eyebrow pencils that match the hair color. Other women experiment with the hair extensions advertised in infomercials, but these take quite a bit of effort and time, with extremely mixed results. These clip-on hair extensions don't work well when the thinning is obvious at the top of the scalp.

Is It Dandruff?

When it comes to hair trauma, almost nothing is as annoying as dandruff or dandruff-like conditions. No matter how much you clean your hair, the flakes fall from your scalp in a virtual snowstorm, leaving your shoulders messy and your scalp looking greasy and matted. What a pain! There is a difference, however, between authentic dandruff and dandruff-like conditions. Dandruff-like conditions can happen for several reasons: When dead skin cells build up on the scalp and don't have the opportunity to slough off, which can be due to overuse of conditioners, infrequent hair washing, inadequate rinsing after shampooing (which can leave a flaky residue on the scalp), using a shampoo that has cleansing agents that cause your scalp to flake, and/or a buildup of styling products on the hair shaft. Each of these things, or several in combination, can cause the scalp to flake, and that can look a lot like dandruff.

Dandruff-like conditions can be easily dealt with. Avoid heavy, concentrated conditioners and use them sparingly, if at all, near the scalp. These can build up on the scalp and hold down dead skin cells, causing excessive accumulation. After shampooing and conditioning, be sure to rinse well for at least a minute or more. Even if your hair and scalp are dry, don't go long periods of time between shampooing. If you have dry flakes, shampoo at least twice a week, concentrating your attention on the scalp. Give yourself a thorough scalp massage and gently use your nails to help exfoliation. Sometimes you only need to change the shampoo you are using to stop the scalp from flaking. Depending on your scalp's sensitivity, some surfactants or several in combination can cause flakes.

Styling products that leave a white film on the hair should be avoided. There are fewer and fewer of these on the market, but hairsprays, mousses, and gels can cause buildup that looks like dandruff.

Dandruff-like conditions can also be seasonal. Dry heat and cold temperatures outdoors can leave the scalp hungry for moisture, yet you may not want to wash your hair too often for fear of drying out the scalp and hair even more. Shampooing infrequently is not the answer. You wash your face to keep the skin clean and remove dead skin cells, and you must do the same for your scalp. Unlike the skin, however, you can't apply a moisturizer to your scalp to cope with dryness. Washing twice a week and then conditioning the hair is the best way to correct the problem. Concentrate the shampoo on the scalp, the conditioner on the ends, rinse well, and put off chemical treatments for as long as possible. You may also want to consider an overall once-a-week hair treatment (be sure to cover the scalp) that you then wash out well. Following all these suggestions should make a big difference.

Hair Reminder: It is problematic to use keratolytic agents (a type of chemical exfoliant) on the scalp because of the risk of getting them on the hair and negatively affecting the cuticle. Chemical exfoliants like glycolic acid, lactic acid, and beta hydroxy acid (salicylic acid) are great at removing layers of dead skin cells that need to be removed to prevent buildup in cases of dry skin, clogged pores, or blemishes. But due to the fact that hair is technically nothing more than dead skin, chemical exfoliants can denature and degrade the hair shaft, causing dryness and damage.

Genuine Dandruff

How can you tell if you really have dandruff (or seborrhea, which is identical to dandruff, only more severe)? Dandruff is generally not seasonal, although it can become worse during the winter, probably because the scalp gets dryer and adds to the flakes that are already there. Dandruff is not caused by dry scalp; in fact, the scalp may be oily. There are many theories about what causes dandruff, but the leading researchers in the field feel strongly that dandruff is caused by a yeast organism (specifically *P. ovale*) that normally exists on the scalp but tends to grow out of control and penetrate the scalp in some individuals. That would explain why antimicrobial agents can have such a positive effect on the condition, why dandruff tends to be so persistent, and why it isn't affected significantly by the drier seasons. Primarily, you can tell when you have dandruff because it does not respond to any of the above suggestions for dandruff-like conditions such as changing shampoos or styling products or using a moisturizer or cortisone cream on the scalp. Essentially, it isn't easy to get rid of the microbes causing dandruff.

Dandruff shampoos use one or more of the following ingredients to deal with the problem: zinc pyridinethione (found in Head & Shoulders), coal tar (Denorex), selenium sulfide (Selsun Blue), and ketoconazole (Nizoral—available in both prescription strength and over the counter). Although their effectiveness is not as substantiated as the ones I just mentioned, sulfur, resorcinol, and salicylic acid products are also available.

Tea tree oil (technical name, melaleuca) is being used in some new dandruff formulations. Tea tree oil is distilled from the Australian plant *Melaleuca alternifolia*. Topically, tea tree oil can be a decent antimicrobial agent, similar to benzoyl peroxide, but not as effective. The other problem with using tea tree oil is that, because it's a cosmetic ingredient and not a pharmaceutical, there are no specific quantities identified as being the right amount to use, meaning that companies can throw in as much or as little as they want. In most of the products I've seen, I doubt enough tea tree oil is being used to make a difference. If you do want to give this option a try, remember that tea tree oil, like all antidandruff or antiseborrhea products, must be left on the scalp for several minutes to gain results.

Zinc pyridinethione, sulfur, selenium sulfide, and ketoconazole act as potent and proven antimicrobial agents, helping to decrease the amount of yeast present. These are considered the optimum way to control dandruff because they don't just tackle the symptom, they attack the organisms that are the underlying cause of the problem.

Some antidandruff and antiseborrhea shampoos contain salicylic acid. This helps exfoliate dead skin cells, but the risk is that it could also eat away at the hair shaft, causing damage and creating brittle, dry hair.

Coal tar slows the creation of skin cells, thereby reducing the number of flakes present on the scalp. This is helpful for many and is often the only product needed to keep the problem under control. One possible problem with coal tar is that some people consider it carcinogenic. However, it should be mentioned that studies conducted by the Mayo Clinic indicate that topical application of coal tar does not increase the risk of cancer. For those individuals with psoriasis (which is not caused by the presence of yeast; it is strictly a hypergrowth of skin cells) and persistent dandruff that is not curbed by antifungal shampoos, coal tar shampoos may offer the only relief.

The problem with all these active dandruff ingredients is that they have some fairly irritating, sensitizing, and drying side effects. Moreover, ingredients like selenium sulfide and sulfur, in the amounts used in dandruff shampoos, tend to have a terrible smell and can damage hair.

What a dilemma! The very ingredients that can help dandruff can also cause scalp problems and make hair hard to manage! To reduce the drying effect these products can cause, it is often best to add a conditioner for the length of your hair, or to alternate your dandruff shampoo with a regular shampoo. Fighting dandruff can take some experimentation, so be patient. Also, don't think you are better off fighting the problem with hair-salon products than drugstore products. Most all of the major dandruff research is being conducted by the pharmaceutical industry or the major hair-care companies, not the smaller contract manufacturers.

In the product-review chapter of this book, I discuss specific recommendations. However, in general the best option for those with true dandruff or other dermatitis scalp conditions is to start with products that contain zinc pyridinethione, such as **Head & Shoulders Dandruff Shampoo for Normal Hair** *($5.99 for 25 ounces).*

If zinc pyridinethione isn't effective, the next step is to consider **Nizoral** *($9.99 for 4 ounces),* because it is now available over the counter at most drugstores. It is worth a shot to see if this one may work best in treating those stubborn, day-in and day-out flaking-scalp problems. Don't expect Nizoral to be the ultimate cure. It isn't. In a study published in the May 1996 issue of the *Journal of Cosmetic Dermatology,* Head & Shoulders was found to be as effective as 2% ketoconazole, which is the prescription-strength version of Nizoral. The over-the-counter version now being sold contains 1% ketoconazole, which has been shown to be as effective as the 2% prescription form.

If you find Head & Shoulders and Nizoral aren't effective, the next step would be a product like Selsun Blue, which uses sulfur, or a coal tar shampoo such as

Denorex Extra Strength Medicated Shampoo *($9.89 for 12 ounces)*, **Ionil T Thera-peutic Coal Tar Shampoo** *($7.99 for 4 ounces)*, **Neutrogena T/Gel Shampoo, Original** *($11.99 for 16 ounces)*, or **Zetar Medicated Antiseborrheic Shampoo** *($16.39 for 6 ounces)*.

Reminders: Don't avoid washing your hair. Twice a week is the minimum. A clean scalp has an easier time shedding unwanted skin cells. However, it may be necessary to wash only once a week or once every other week with a dandruff sham-poo to reduce or stop the flaking. When the flaking is minimized, alternate the dandruff shampoo with a shampoo for your scalp type, which can be anything from normal to dry. (Avoid shampoos for oily scalp or hair, even if your dandruff is accom-panied by an oily scalp. Shampoos designed for oily hair can be too drying for someone with dandruff or a dandruff-like condition.) If that works for you, it is also a way to minimize the risk of irritation or dryness that can be caused by dandruff shampoos. Don't avoid conditioner; use it as you normally would after you wash with a dan-druff shampoo.

A few words of warning: If you color your hair, avoid dandruff products that contain sulfur or selenium sulfide. These ingredients can strip hair color. Many dandruff shampoos use irritating, drying ingredients such as menthol, sodium lau-ryl sulfate, and TEA lauryl sulfate, which do not help deal with the cause of the dermatitis; for example, **Head & Shoulders Refresh** *($3.99 for 15.2 ounces)*, which adds mint to the basic formula. I know that sounds refreshing, which a lot of consumers will love (I'm sure that is why it was added), but mint serves no purpose in the fight against dandruff.

Regardless of how you go about dealing with dandruff, stay realistic about what works and be prepared to experiment to find what is best for your head. Nothing is guaranteed when it comes to handling dandruff, and as natural as tea tree oil sounds, it doesn't provide any more benefit than ingredients that sound more chemical.

Seborrhea

According to the American Academy of Dermatology patient information sheet on seborrhea, there are distinct differences between dandruff, seborrhea, and sebor-rheic dermatitis. "Dandruff appears as scaling on the scalp without redness. Seborrhea is extreme oiliness of the skin, especially of the scalp and face, without redness or scaling. Patients with seborrhea may later get seborrheic dermatitis. Seborrheic der-matitis has both redness and scaling." What makes seborrhea different from typical oily skin is that the increased oil production has a thickened, viscous discharge as opposed to just an "oil slick" over the skin. At the hairline this overproduction of sebum can form small, firm mounds called whiteheads. The size of the eruption, the texture of the oil, and the tendency toward flaky skin are what differentiate seborrhea from acne.

Seborrhea's excessive yellowing sebum and thickened scaling are possibly triggered by a yeast organism present in the hair follicle. Seborrhea can occur at any age, but typically it is seen in infants (when it is called "cradle cap") or in older people. The most effective treatment is applying low-strength cortisone cream or hydrocortisone to the affected areas along with frequent use of nonprescription shampoos or topical medications containing coal tar, zinc pyrithione, ketoconazole, selenium sulfide, sulfur, and/or salicylic acid. The recommendations for this condition are the same as in the dandruff sections above.

For patients who do not respond to this treatment, there are several other effective medications that a dermatologist can prescribe.

Psoriasis

The most common type of psoriasis that occurs on the scalp is called plaque psoriasis. This type of psoriasis is a chronic, recurring disease of the skin, identified by the presence of thickened, rough skin covered by silvery white scaly areas. Often papules are present, which are small, solid, often inflamed bumps that, unlike pimples, do not contain pus or sebum. These bumps are usually slightly elevated above the normal skin surface, sharply distinguishable from normal skin, and red to reddish brown in color. The extent of the disease varies from a few tiny lesions to generalized involvement of a good deal of the entire scalp. Counting all the various forms of psoriasis, it affects over 6 million people in the United States alone. For most people it tends to be mild and unsightly rather than a serious health concern.

No one really knows exactly what causes psoriasis, although recent studies suggest it may be related to an immune system disorder. To put it simply, psoriasis is the recurring growth of too many skin cells. A normal skin cell matures in 28 to 45 days, while a psoriatic skin cell takes only 3 to 6 days.

Sadly, there is no cure for psoriasis or scalp psoriasis, but there are many different treatments, both topical and systemic, that can clear it for periods of time. Experimenting with a variety of options is essential if you wish to find the treatment that works for you, but all require a doctor's attention.

Of the various therapies available to treat scalp psoriasis, it is generally best to start with those that have the least serious side effects, such as topical steroids (cortisone creams), coal-tar shampoos, and exposure to sunshine. If those methods are not successful, you can proceed to the more serious treatments that involve oral medications. More often than not, successful treatment requires a combination of methods.

Natural sunlight can significantly improve, or even clear, psoriasis. Regular daily doses of sunlight taken in short exposures with adequate sun protection are strongly recommended. Sun protection is vital not only to prevent sunburn, which may make psoriasis worse, but also to reduce skin damage from the sun's ultraviolet radiation. This outdoor approach to treating psoriasis is often referred to as climatotherapy. Some people travel to Florida, Hawaii, the Caribbean, or the Dead Sea in Israel (where special clinics offer treatment solariums and supervised medical assistance) to use swimming and natural sunlight as their psoriasis treatment; other people believe immersion in salty, mineral-laden water may also have some unknown benefits. In some countries, medical plans actually cover trips to these types of sunny climates and mineral spas for subscribers with psoriasis.

When you can't get to sunshine, medically supervised administration of light from UVB lamps may be used to minimize widespread or localized areas of stubborn and unmanageable psoriasis lesions. UVB light is also used when topical treatments have failed, or in combination with topical treatments. The short-term risks of using controlled UVB exposure to treat psoriasis are minimal, and long-term studies of large numbers of patients treated with UVB have not demonstrated an increased risk of skin cancer, suggesting that this treatment may be safer than sunlight. (Sunlight has both UVA and UVB radiation; UVA causes skin cancer, while UVB mainly triggers sunburn.) UVB treatments are considered one of the most effective therapies for moderate to severe psoriasis, with the least amount of risk.

Using coal tar to treat psoriasis is a very old and effective remedy. These topical medications are available both over the counter and by prescription; the difference is in the potency and amount of coal tar the medication contains. Coal tar can be combined with other psoriasis medications (e.g., topical steroids) or with sunshine (ultraviolet light). However, coal tar can make the skin more sensitive to ultraviolet light, and extreme caution is advised when combining its use with UV therapy (or exposure to the sun) in order to avoid getting a severe burn or causing skin damage.

Anthralin, another topical prescription medication, has been used to treat psoriasis for over a hundred years. It has few serious side effects but can irritate or burn the normal-appearing skin surrounding psoriasis lesions. Anthralin also stains anything it comes into contact with. It is prescribed in a range of concentrations, and there are a variety of regimens for its use, but the negative side effects make it a less than desirable option.

Calcipotriene, a synthetic vitamin D3 analog, is used to treat mild to moderate psoriasis. It is a prescription medication with few side effects. It is not the same compound as the vitamin D found in commercial vitamin supplements. Calcipotriene is sold in the United States as a topical, odorless, nonstaining ointment and cream under the prescription brand name of Dovonex.

More serious systemic medications such as Methotrexate, Tegison, Accutane, Soriatane, Cyclosporin, and oral steroids are also used to treat psoriasis, but each has pros and cons that need to be researched and discussed at length with your physician.

Discovering whether any of these will work for you, alone or in combination, takes patience and a systematic, ongoing review and evaluation of how your skin is doing. As is true with all chronic skin disorders, success requires diligent adherence to the regimen and a realistic understanding of what you can and can't expect. It is also important to be aware of the consequences of the varying treatment levels. For example, continued long-term use of topical cortisone creams can cause skin thinning, stretch marks, and built-up resistance to the cortisone medication itself, so that it actually becomes an ineffective treatment. Exposure to sunlight without adequate protection (particularly from UVA radiation) can cause skin cancer. Oral steroids can have serious withdrawal effects, including increased bouts of psoriasis. Accutane causes birth defects if a woman becomes pregnant while taking it.

For more information on the current status of available treatments, visit www.psoriasis.com or write to the National Psoriasis Foundation (NPF) at 6600 Southwest 92nd Avenue, Suite 300, Portland, OR 97223; send e-mail to 76135.2746@compuserve.com; or phone (800) 723-9166 (toll-free).

Thin to Thicker

Regardless of the condition of your hair, the desire to have it be something it isn't generates a good many of the purchases we make. If you have thin, fine, or even normal hair thickness, the aspiration to have it be thicker is overwhelming. A horde of hair-care products want you to believe they can do just that with all sorts of natural ingredients. Can any of these products deliver? Yes and no. Sorry, that really is the truth. Most all hair-care products making claims about generating thicker, fuller hair contain the same basic combination of ingredients, namely, film-forming ingredients, the kind found in hairsprays. These ingredients coat the hair with a thin (hopefully), pliable layer of plastic. It's just that simple and it isn't vaguely exceptional or natural. Film-forming ingredients can create the feel of thicker hair, but they can also easily lead to buildup if you don't get the stuff out every time you wash your hair. To that end, it's best to alternate your "hair thickening" products with a plain shampoo that cleans well and doesn't contain any conditioning agents.

Curly to Straight

This is a styling issue only, because there are no shampoos or conditioners that can make hair straight. Please refer to Chapter Eight for details on how to get this coveted, smooth look.

More Myth Busting

What you believe can affect the health of your hair. If you are misled or lied to, you will not only waste money but also choose the wrong products for your hair type. I want to address a few hair-care myths that most women, maybe yourself included, have accepted without question. Let's separate fact from fiction.

You need to change or alternate shampoos because your hair adapts to them. The hair and scalp can't "adapt to" shampoos. Hair is dead, so it isn't capable of adapting or becoming used to something. What can happen is that the conditioners, emollients, and slip agents found in many shampoos can build up on the hair shaft over time, making the hair limp, sticky, or dull. That buildup is easily washed away with a new shampoo. The cycle starts all over again when the new shampoo's conditioning and styling agents start building up.

Shampoos containing conditioning agents, emollients, and slip agents are formulated in such a way that the detergent cleansers lift the dirt and oil away from the hair, allowing the water to rinse them away while leaving the conditioners behind. Cosmetic chemists do a great job of devising shampoos that clean the hair but allow conditioners to stay put despite the pressure of cascading water. It is the nature of these shampoos that they cannot adequately remove the very conditioners they contain because the conditioners in them are designed to do just the opposite—stick to the hair. When you change to a new shampoo, that new formulation cuts through the previous shampoo's conditioning agents, leaving the hair feeling new and full again. However, the cycle begins all over again if the new shampoo now contains different conditioning or styling agents that can once again build up on hair. It is this endless rotation that leads women to believe that their hair adapts to shampoo.

Changing shampoos is a simple way to remove the buildup, especially if you choose a shampoo that contains no conditioning agents. I should mention that not all cosmetics chemists agree with this theory about changing shampoos. Some believe it is more a factor of perception or change in weather conditions than a result of the products you are using. Given consumer perception and the information I've received, I still side with the notion of changing.

You need to change or alternate conditioners because your hair adapts to them. The truth about this one is pretty much the same as it is for the shampoos above. Hair *can't* become resistant to conditioners, but conditioners can build up on the hair—especially when the conditioners are designed for damaged, chemically treated, or dry hair and are used in conjunction with shampoos that contain conditioning agents. A shampoo with conditioners might not wash out the buildup every time you shampoo. Repeated use of the same conditioner and a shampoo with conditioner can impart a sticky, heavy, or dull appearance to the hair. You don't need to throw out the conditioner; you just need to use a shampoo without conditioning agents that will cut through the residue and thoroughly clean the hair. The same is true for leave-in conditioners. Because they get left on and aren't rinsed off, those ingredients tend to cling better to hair and are somewhat more difficult to shampoo out, especially if you're using a shampoo that contains conditioning and styling agents.

I know a particular shampoo will be gentle enough for my dry, fine hair because it says on the label I can wash my face with it. Some facial cleansers contain the exact same detergent cleansing agents as shampoos (facial cleansers just eliminate the ingredients that produce copious lather). Simply because a shampoo can be used on the face doesn't mean it should be used on your hair. Besides, facial cleansers that contain the same order of ingredients as a shampoo are often quite drying for the face. Being able to use a product on your face doesn't say anything about how well it will clean your hair or whether it is really gentle. Moreover, truly gentle shampoos might not be able to clean the buildup that can occur from using conditioners and styling products.

You need to lather twice to make hair look and feel clean. Absolutely not. If anything, overwashing the hair can dry it out, and the more you handle your hair, the greater the chance of roughing up and damaging the cuticle. Shampooing the hair twice may be necessary for women who use a lot of styling products, or favor heavy or waxy conditioners, or have extremely (and I mean *extremely*) oily hair, but that's it. In those situations, the ingredients and oils can be hard to break down, and a second lather may be just what it takes to get through the debris. Other than that, the only reason hair-care companies suggest shampooing twice is to sell more shampoo!

Shampooing oily hair can make it oilier. I need to correct previous statements I've made about this issue. I have wrongly stated that irritation can stimulate oil production. There is little evidence of that being the case. Rather, it is your hormones that trigger your oil glands to be overproductive, and there is literally nothing you can do from the outside in to stop or change that activity. Unfortunately, products for the face that absorb oil don't work on the scalp without causing the hair a great many problems.

My hair is oily, so it is best if I wash with a shampoo designed for my hair type. Shampoos for oily hair often contain stronger detergent agents than are really necessary for an oily scalp or hair condition. Strong detergent agents can dry out hair and that can add to your problems. Of late, shampoos for oily hair have been throwing in ingredients like peppermint, menthol, balm mint, eucalyptus, orange, grapefruit, and lemon. None of these ingredients have any effect on oil production. However, because they are all serious skin irritants, they can cause an itchy, flaky scalp or other skin irritation or allergic reaction.

Everyone needs to use a conditioner. The only reason to use a conditioner is if your hair is dry, you have difficulty getting a comb through it, your scalp is dry, or you use a lot of styling tools, such as blow-dryers and curling irons. If none of that is true and your hair naturally feels soft and smooth, then there is very little reason for you to use a conditioner. Contrary to what the advertisements would have you believe, conditioners are not automatically necessary for all heads of hair. In fact, using a conditioner when you don't need one can make your hair limp, heavy, and difficult to style.

The longer you leave a conditioner on, the more effective it will be. Depending on the ingredients, this is entirely true. There is plenty of evidence that certain ingredients can penetrate the cuticle better when left on longer.

I should mention that there is discussion in the world of hair care about the permeability of the hair shaft. Can ingredients penetrate beyond the cuticle into the hair shaft? Given that hair can absorb water, why not other elements? If hair wasn't permeable, then humidity couldn't get in and change the hair's appearance, hair dyes couldn't get inside and become permanent, and perms wouldn't change the curl status of the hair. The question that leaves experts arguing is, how much benefit is derived from the absorption of amino acids, panthenols, biotin, and the like?

What we can be fairly certain of is that these microscopically tiny ingredients are absorbed to some degree. However, this information is derived from using pure forms of these ingredients on hair in a laboratory setting. The amount of these ingredients used in shampoos and conditioners is negligible, and given the way the products are rinsed off or manipulated during the styling process and then in exposure to the elements, it is almost impossible that they have any effect on hair whatsoever. Besides, what most of us know from our own experience is that even the most expensive hair products in the world won't change damaged hair, and those lovely ingredients are gone the next day when you wash your hair.

I have oily hair, so it is best for me to avoid conditioners. If you have oily hair it is because your scalp is producing oil and the oil accumulation is making its way down the hair shaft. Other than that, hair itself is not oily, which means the hair length farthest away from your scalp can be dry or damaged. In that case, you do need a conditioner, but you should use it on the ends only and be careful not to get it anywhere near the scalp.

The scalp needs toning, just like the skin. What a hoax! Most of the toners and astringents for the scalp contain many irritating and drying ingredients that can cause irritation, skin sensitivity, rashes, and dryness. Witch hazel, alcohol, peppermint, balm mint, menthol, orange, grapefruit, and lemon are the typical "toning" ingredients in these products, and they cannot in any way control oil. By the way, toning is a dubious cosmetic term that has no real meaning. None of these products can't firm the skin, change the size of a pore, or stop oil. Whatever the cosmetics and hair-care industries do mean by toning may be clear to them, but it's a mystery to the rest of us.

Hair needs to be squeaky in order to tell if it's really clean. All the experts I've interviewed said hair doesn't have to squeak to be clean. Instead the reason hair squeaks is because of calcium deposits left on the hair by hard water, not because it's clean. It turns out most households in the United States have hard water. The reason we've come to associate squeaky hair with being clean is because the times hair doesn't squeak can mean detergent residue has been left on the hair. Most women feel it's important to hear their hair resonate through their fingers after washing for it to be really clean. I'm torn between what the experts tell me, what I personally feel, and what other women repeatedly tell me. When I can't hear my hair squeak after I wash and condition it, I almost always feel it doesn't style as well or look as full.

Because of the disparity between scientific evidence and what I've heard from women and hairstylists, I would say this is a personal decision, or at least one you will have to experiment with for yourself. Nonetheless, because most people live in hard-water areas, and the expense of putting in a water softener system can be steep, your hair might squeak whether you like it or not.

Lots of lather means the hair is getting thoroughly clean. I know this may be shocking—it still shocks me—but lather is unrelated to the cleaning ingredients in shampoo. Lathering ingredients are added to shampoo for the emotional appeal they provide. They have no effect on cleaning. Why do we associate the amount of lather with clean hair? Because the amount of lather you get while shampooing is directly affected by the amount of oil and debris on the hair. The more oils, conditioning agents, or styling-product residue on the hair, the less lather will be produced when you shampoo. So the hair may be clean, but the lather ingredients were deactivated by the presence of the oil and other stuff you want to wash away. That is why hair generally lathers better the second time you wash it, because then it really was clean from the first go-around.

Baby shampoos are milder and gentler, so they are the best to use for my dry scalp and dried-out ends. No way! Baby shampoos do leave out ingredients that can sting the eyes (to some extent), which is nice, but they are also formulated with cleansing agents that are less drying and irritating and also have less cleaning ability. Children are obviously not using styling products, applying emollient conditioners, perming or coloring their hair, overusing blow-dryers or curling irons, or doing any of a number of other problematic things that adults inflict on their hair. If you want to handle adult hair issues, adult shampoos and conditioners are the only way to go.

Brushing the hair 100 times is good for the hair. Nothing could be further from the truth. Brushing the hair roughs up the cuticle, eventually chipping it away and exposing the cortex, leaving the hair porous and frayed.

Even though two hair-care products list the same ingredients, they are not the same product because the quality of the ingredients varies. Most cosmetics companies would like you to believe that you can't tell anything from reading the ingredient list because the quality of the ingredients is what counts. Having spoken with many raw-ingredient manufacturers and cosmetics chemists from most of the major hair-care companies and contract manufacturers, I can assure you that the quality of the ingredients is fairly consistent. There are only a small number of raw-ingredient manufacturers, and they are not in the business of producing inferior materials for companies looking for a bargain. Every time I have asked an expensive hair-care line to show me proof that their ingredients are of a better grade or quality, I'm told they can't reveal their sources. Sources aren't a secret; if they were, the ingredient manufacturers couldn't earn a living. If a company can't substantiate a claim, then they have made it up, knowing that most consumers will fall for the line and won't press for details.

Products within a line are designed to work together, so it is best never to mix products from other lines. Do not assume that hair-care products from the same line are all wonderful or that all of them will be compatible with your hair. Experiment with what works best for your hair's needs, not the needs of the hair-care line selling you products. All of my research indicates that women mix products all the time anyway, and they are generally more or at least equally as satisfied as women who stay line-loyal.

Cutting your hair makes it thicker. Cutting hair does *not* make it thicker. However, because damaged ends can feel sparse, look thin, and may lie in a fuzzy layer, cutting them off can make your hair look newly thick. And it can stay looking and feeling healthy if you don't start re-torturing the ends. Also, depending on the talent of your hairstylist, a specific hairstyle can make the hair appear thicker through layering or stacking.

Hair can be double-processed without causing damage, or hair can be double-processed if you wait a few weeks between treatments. In other words, you can perm and color your hair at the same time or a few weeks apart and not worry about excessive decomposition of the cuticle or hair shaft. Well, nothing could be further from the truth (although some hairstylists would like us to believe otherwise). And why shouldn't they? A perm and a color job add up to a lot of technical work, not to mention the intensive hair treatments the hair will need to endure your fashion indulgence. As I explain in Chapters Five and Six on hair color and hair relaxers, both of these treatments require a strong alkaline base to effect a permanent change in the length of hair. That process causes the hair shaft to swell, making it more porous and damaging the cuticle. Doing that to the hair twice is twice as damaging. Waiting doesn't heal hair. Damaged hair cannot be repaired. Nothing can restore the hair from the effects of one chemical process, much less two.

You can double-process the hair if the products being used are gentle and don't contain any harmful ingredients. If it were possible to find gentle dyes and perms I would agree with this statement, but the basic characteristics of dyes and perms (those that create lasting change to the full length of hair—until the roots start showing) are damaging to the hair. What you have to put the hair through to change its color, cover gray, and straighten or curl it is damaging to the hair. Doing both is doubly damaging. Products often claim they will be less damaging to the hair because they don't contain peroxide or ammonia. What they often don't tell you is that the ingredients used instead don't sound like peroxide or ammonia but they do the exact same thing to the hair as peroxide and ammonia would do. You may not recognize their names, but they are just as damaging.

You can protect your hair from chemical damage by using a good conditioner or conditioning treatment before you color or perm your hair. That would be a great idea, but if you layer conditioning ingredients on the hair it will block the effectiveness of the perm or hair color. That will reduce damage but it will also reduce the effectiveness of the perm or color treatment. If you wash the conditioner away, then the protection is also washed away.

If you dye your hair a different color from your eyebrows, you need to dye your eyebrows. Not all blondes have blonde eyebrows, so it's not necessarily more natural to have blonde eyebrows to accompany a head of artificially blonde hair. Another problem, particularly for women with dark brows who prefer low-maintenance beauty regimes, is that eyebrow growout can look strange. There are ways to cope when the brow does grow out and the roots become evident, such as brow powders, brow coloring gels, and mascara, but in general there is little reason to go through the hassle unless the difference in hair color is very light blonde with dark brown brows.

The best way to make limp, thin hair full is to perm it. To some extent that's true—perming can make hair look markedly fuller—but perming the entire head, especially on small rods and on a regular basis (to keep up with growout), is not a viable solution if you want full hair that looks good. When perming was all the rage in the 1980s, we saw plenty of evidence of what happens when thin, fine hair gets permed on a regular basis or when small rods are used to set in curl as opposed to fullness. Hair can't easily handle repeated perms without risking a frizzy mess. Growout can look terrible, and re-perming only makes matters worse. A root perm can be an option (only the root area is treated with perm solution, while the rest of the hair is protected with conditioner, creams, or oils), but it takes a very savvy hairstylist to do it well.

Taking vitamins can make hair stronger and healthier. If you started taking special vitamin supplements for your hair, it would take months for the effect, if any, to show up. Hair has to grow to be affected by a new addition to your diet. So the promise of instant hair health with any vitamin supplement is sheer nonsense. Additionally, there are no definitive studies indicating that taking any vitamin changes the texture or appearance of the hair. Trace minerals and drugs can show up in hair analysis after the hair is chemically broken down and treated, but this doesn't mean you would be able to detect a difference between the months you took the vitamin supplements and the months you didn't.

How to Begin Shopping

Now that you have a solid idea of what hair is all about, you need some guidelines to help narrow down the selection of products to choose from and to better understand how your buying habits may be affected by some intrinsically flawed beliefs. The main goal is to never leave the store with something you don't want, don't like, can't afford, can't fully identify, or that doesn't work. There is no other way to be a better consumer when it comes to hair-care purchases. From my point of view, the worst thing consumers do is overbuy or buy something because they believe what an advertisement, product label, or salesperson told them. One way to prevent that, or at least start changing it, is to consider my recommendations in Chapter Ten, following the product review chapter of this book, and try to keep them in mind the next time you read or hear an overblown testimonial about the latest, unequaled hair-care product. The following list is a good starting point if you hope to keep your budget and sanity intact while maintaining the health and welfare of your hair.

1. **You must be willing to change some of your beliefs about hair care.** A hair-care company does not necessarily have your best interests at heart. If you are willing to buy a product that is overpriced or doesn't work, they will keep selling it, because there is no reason for them to change. It doesn't matter that hair can't be repaired or reconstructed by a conditioner or that hair can't be restored by a moisturizing pack or treatment. As long as people buy these products, why should the hair-care companies stop selling them?

2. **Every hair-care line has good and bad products.** Actually, most hair-care lines have fairly good products. The confusion is caused by labels that give misleading information about which products are best for specific hair-care needs. And all lines have their share of useless, overly perfumed, unreliable, and *overpriced* products that can't live up to the claims on the label. They also have products that work, but these products are often still overpriced. Also, just because a product works doesn't mean it is worth $20; there are absolutely $3 or $5 equivalents available elsewhere.

3. **Give up line loyalty.** It is great when you find a line you are comfortable with. For example, you might like Sebastian styling products and conditioners or Joico's treatment pack and shampoos. But that doesn't mean that every other

product in those lines is also guaranteed to please you or be good for you, or that you need more of what the line offers. No matter how enthusiastic salespeople are about their terrific line, they are not unbiased bystanders; they have a vested interest in what you decide to buy.

4. **Do not buy impulsively or quickly.** That statement speaks for itself, but it isn't always easy to do! There you are at the salon, the stylist has just finished making you look brilliant, and the premium products he or she used are staring you in the face. With just this small additional purchase of $35, you think, you can get your hair to look the same between visits. Stop and breathe. Consider what you already have at home. Try to remember how I rated the products you're looking at. It would also be beneficial to remember the last time you bought the products recommended by a hairstylist and then ask yourself whether or not those really made a difference before you jump in and buy again.

5. **Hair-care advertisements may be alluring and interesting, but they are ads, not documentaries.** Just because the ads are sensual doesn't mean the products featured in the ads are, and it doesn't mean they'll make *you* more sensual. Accept seductive ads for what they are—seductive ads, not reliable sources of facts.

6. **Don't pretend you are above being affected by cosmetics advertising.** All advertising, especially cosmetics advertising, is a very, very powerful stimulus in our lives. Hair-care advertising, like any advertising, is designed to make us buy a specific product or be attracted to a specific company. Whether we like it or not, advertising strongly affects the way we make decisions. It is unwise to ignore the fact that advertising sells products, and sells them very well, because the hair-care companies wouldn't keep throwing money at something that produced no financial return. The next time you think you are not being affected by cosmetics advertising, think again.

7. **Hair-care products are not a bargain just because they are less expensive than products offered by other areas of the cosmetics industry.** Because hair-care products are so much less expensive than those found in the rest of the cosmetics industry (particularly skin-care products), and because you need fewer products to maintain your hair than your skin (at least for some women), it is easy to consider the price of a $15 hairspray or $20 shampoo a mere pittance in comparison to the $75 moisturizer or $100 antiwrinkle creams the skin-care industry sells. Still, it all adds up. A savvy hairstylist or salesperson can sell you a line of hair-care products for $40 before you know it. When you consider how often you have to make these purchases and realize that there are excellent products available in less expensive price ranges, it may give you pause.

8. **When it comes to hair-care products, there are no miracle ingredients, trade secrets, exotic ingredients, patented secrets, or salon-tested formulas that will permanently repair your hair.** If there were a magic potion, it wouldn't stay under wraps. Every line would get their hands on it. Chemists are capable of analyzing a product's ingredients and duplicating whatever they want. Sophisticated technologies make reproducing a product's components, even when they are patented, as easy as assembling a jigsaw puzzle when all of the pieces are included. And speaking of patented secrets, this is an oxymoron. U.S. patent law is very clear: In order for an ingredient or group of ingredients to be patented, the exact components and precise formulation details must be disclosed in full. It doesn't take much for a hair-care company to figure out an alternative to a patented formula; and if that's not feasible, they can buy the licensed right to use the formula.

9. **Truly superior shampoos, conditioners, styling products, and special treatments can be found in inexpensive lines.** Formulations vary, and some products are better than others, but on the whole I found just as many great products at the drugstore as I did at the hair salon—and just as many bad ones. Marketing creates mystique, not reality.

10. **Shopping for hair-care products in a salon may feel more elegant than shopping at the drugstore, but that is a perception about the environment, not the quality of the products.** The elegance lies in the pampered feeling you get from the earnest, helpful information and advice the salon stylist provides. If that environment is important to you, it is essential that you should also expect the products you buy to live up to their claim. Do not hesitate to return a product that doesn't live up to its claim—regardless of what the claim is. If your frizzies do not go away, if your hair is not reconstructed, if the hair gel does not keep the curls in, and the hairspray that promised to be soft feels stiff and hard, take it all back for a refund!

CHAPTER FIVE

Hair of a Different Color

Real Color

The hair roots or follicles contain pigment cells that, depending on your genetic background, create a black pigment called melanin or eumelanin and a reddish pigment, produced by a separate gene, called heomelanin (or sometimes called phaeomelanin). The greater the amount of pigment sent to the hair, the darker the hair becomes. If the amount of pigment is reduced, the hair color turns brown and then reddish or blond. Color changes with age. Most children who have blonde-whitish hair turn into brunet adults. The shades of hair color are influenced by how light bounces off the hair proteins, but basically depend upon pigment contained within the hair shaft cortex, or center.

Eumelanin is the pigment found in brown or black hair and, to a far lesser extent, in blonde hair. Heomelanin produces red hair, while a mix of eumelanin and heomelanin produces red highlights in hair. A mix of minimal amounts of eumelanin and heomelanin creates a blonde-red mixture, or "strawberry blonde." When pigment is significantly diminished, the hair appears gray, and when the pigment is completely absent, the hair is white.

From Light to Dark

"Does she or doesn't she? Does she or doesn't she? Does she or doesn't she? Only her hairdresser knows for sure," echoes a deep male voice in the well-known 1956 Clairol television ad. What a powerful message that must have been back then. An attractive, elegantly dressed woman lights a candelabra, pausing long enough to admire her image in the mirror, then strokes her perfectly formed blonde waves. What the candelabra was for is anybody's guess; maybe Clairol thought all women longed for candelabras in the '50s. What they really wanted was a product that could get rid of the gray and leave the hair looking natural and lustrous.

Before that ad appeared, only 7 percent of the female population in this country dyed their hair; today, depending on whose statistics you use, that number is somewhere between 50 to 75 percent. Imagine, half to three-quarters of the female population dyed or color-treated their hair in some way this year. That number is simply amazing.

The question now, as it was back then, still is: How do you get your hair to look like what all the ads over the past several decades have been promising? That's what you're about to find out.

Hair Note: Throughout this book, I use the words "color" and "dye" interchangeably to refer to a change of any kind in the natural color of the hair as the result of applying any salon or drugstore product. I've been told that "dyeing," like the word "beautician," is an old-fashioned term and that "coloring" is the more current term. Well, it might be more current, but it is also a way to imply that the consumer won't be doing anything radical or damaging to her hair if she "colors" it rather than "dyes" it. There are some hair-coloring processes that aren't at all damaging, such as the temporary and semipermanent methods, but the mid/intermediate/demi/level 2 and permanent hair dyes, no matter how gentle they sound, do damage the hair. Furthermore, cosmetics chemists call those little molecules affecting hair color "dyes," so I will too.

Why Color?

Without question there are unmistakably positive reasons for coloring hair. Hair dyes and color treatments can make the hair appear thicker, can enliven otherwise drab hair, and can create the perfect hair color. But by far the biggest reason most women (and men) dye their hair is because they don't want to be gray. In days gone by, the desire to be blonde drove the hair-color market; today it is mostly the desire to be anything but gray.

When those gray strands start popping up, no matter how a woman feels about any other issue surrounding age, she is not happy about the prospect of becoming gray. Case in point: How many coloring products are on the market to change your hair *to* gray? None, although a small handful brighten gray or reduce the yellow cast of the gray you already have. How many coloring products are there to change hair to a precise or distinct shade of blonde, brown, black, or red? Hundreds! Being gray is the same as being old in our culture, and to baby boomers that is about as acceptable as being wrinkled or overweight.

While cosmetics companies love to merchandise their products to all the over-40 baby boomers, they have also targeted another segment of the market that is just as likely to spend money on how they look, namely 20- and 30-year-olds:

For those under the age of graying (assuming that you aren't graying prematurely) there is a huge incentive to change color. While baby boomers want to cover gray without making any radical changes to their hair, women between the ages of 14 and 35 want to play with color the way they might try on a trendy, fun outfit. For those younger women, color is about making a statement, being glamorous, adding flash and excitement.

Hair Color for African-American Women

A much smaller but growing portion of the hair-color market involves dyes for the ethnic market. Previously, women of color usually only accented their natural dark tresses with deeper or subtle tones of red, amber, or copper. Rarely did you ever see a woman of color with a blonde or a red 'do. Recently, celebrities and models such as Beverly Johnson, RuPaul, Jada Pickett, and T-Boz have started sporting golden and red locks (well, RuPaul's aren't exactly golden or red or real, but that's another story). The problem is that celebrity hairdos often end up in the mainstream, and that translates into a lot of women dyeing their hair blonde or red. Regardless of race, anytime you make an extreme color change you are running the risk of seriously damaging your hair. This is of greatest concern to African-American women, who already have fragile hair that is often chemically treated or harshly styled with blow-dryers, curling irons, and hot combs, which adds up to extremely damaged hair. Adding color to this type of hair almost guarantees compounding hair problems to the point of breakage. (See Chapter Seven, *For African-American Women*, for more information.)

The exception to this is for women of color with short, natural, nonstraightened hair. This virgin hair can handle the transition from being dark to being dyed a light color far more easily. That doesn't mean there is no damage, it just means there is less damage to get the color you want.

Drugstore vs. Salon Hair Color

Whether we are hiding gray strands, improving otherwise lackluster natural hair color, or simply treating hair color as a fashion statement, the vast majority of us are spending our money on hair color from the drugstore rather than paying to have it done at the hair salon. That's one reason this is one of the most intimidating, worrisome segments of the beauty business. Intimidation and worry are caused by knowing that your color choice might be wrong and unavoidably permanent.

As you wonder what it would be like to be a redhead or to add a touch of auburn to your rather plain brown hair, there is always the underlying fear that the color could turn out green or your hair could look more like straw than silky, flowing tresses. You can buy a lipstick, foundation, mascara, shampoo, conditioner, hairspray, or styling gel, and if you get it wrong, just wash it off and start over again tomorrow, no worse for wear. Altering your hair color may not be the same story. A semipermanent dye that washes out with six to 12 shampooings might be completely harmless, but living through several shampoos with bad hair is not a thrilling idea. More to the point, the mid/intermediate/demi/level 2 and permanent hair dyes, which are part of you until they grow out or you cut them off, are damaging to the hair, don't wash out at all, and need to be bleached out and redyed to get the wrong color out. Now that's serious!

Hair-care companies would love you to believe that coloring your hair won't hurt the hair, or at least not very much, but there is no way around it. All the claims about botanicals, proteins, collagen, amino acids, moisturizing ingredients, panthenol, or any other ingredient in hair-coloring products can't change the way dyes get into the hair and stay there. That process is damaging, plain and simple.

The hair-color section of almost any drugstore features a dazzling cavalcade of boxes lined up in neat, orderly rows and offering hundreds of colors and various levels of staying power. Every color in every product grouping has a different woman on the front panel looking exceedingly pleased, almost smug, about her beautifully coifed, vibrantly colored, natural-looking hair. On your own, with two dozen different product options lying before you, it seems almost overwhelming to assume you can ever get this one right. As surprising as it seems, though, many women do, and you may be pleasantly pleased to learn that statistics indicate that women who color their hair at home are as pleased (or displeased) with their results as women who have their hair dyed at a salon.

For this book, I focus mostly on hair-coloring products available at the drugstore. The sheer number of professional hair-coloring products, the varying ways they are blended by each stylist, and each stylist's training, talent, and experience limits an individual assessment of their work. Hairstylists can perform coloring techniques that would be impossible at home. For example, a stylist can dye your hair a particular color and then put in a corresponding highlight with a foil. I would never in a million years suggest a woman try that at home herself.

Suffice it to say that beyond the difficulty of some special techniques or turning dark hair blonde, there are many reasons to get your hair colored at a hair salon, including the pampering, the mess (it's theirs and not yours), the trust between you and your hairstylist or technician, and the benefit of your stylist's experience. It is great to just have the stylist make the decisions and do the work while you sit back and read a magazine.

However, there are many other reasons to consider doing the simpler processes at home yourself, of which the most compelling are the savings in time and money. If you get your hair dyed six to 12 times a year at a salon, you could save $400 to $1,200 or more doing it at home. What you might not know is that the hair colors you buy at the drugstore are superbly formulated and almost foolproof. **In many** regards, and except for the salon's ability to mix different colors together, there is little to no difference between the hair-coloring products used at the hair salon and the ones sold at the drugstore. In fact, all the major drugstore color lines make hair-coloring products widely used by salons. So much for exclusivity.

Which one to choose? There is a quagmire of confusing product choices (it's almost impossible to discern differences) and misleading information. Conceivably the most confusing part of the whole hair-color business is that the names of the products are meaningless. What does Ultress or Castings mean, anyway? What is Nice & Easy as opposed to Clairesse, and is L'Oreal's Excellence less preferred than L'Oreal's Preference? Does Lasting Color really last or does Revlon's ColorStay do a better job? To make matters worse, and supposedly to help us understand what kind of hair dye we are purchasing and how long it will last, the companies have created phrases like "harmonizing color," "tone-on-tone," "oxidation" and "nonoxidation," and "permanent" versus "intermediate" or "midcolor," "level 2," or "demi color"— but what does any of that mean? Thanks for the help, guys, but thanks for nothing.

As I watched women shopping for hair-coloring products and talked to women who have their hair colored at the salon, it became clear that the primary issues were how long the color might last (whether or not it washes out), how the chemicals impact the hair shaft, and what kind of results you could count on. At the drugstore, most products have a color guide on the back of the package to help you understand the dye's impact on your natural hair color and how long the color can last—which is helpful, but it doesn't adequately explain product limitations or distinctions. It doesn't illustrate what kind of coverage you can really expect for gray, it is almost impossible to clearly see the color swatches on the card, and it doesn't warn about problems of hair becoming too ash, red, or copper (and that's always a risk). In any case, this still isn't what I would call a user-friendly situation. In order to go safely into the arena of hair color, you need to be armed with a cheat sheet and some straightforward facts so you can make informed decisions.

"Natural" Hair Color

No matter how I battle the inane use of the word "natural" to sell skin- and hair-care products, this term remains the selling point consumers are attracted to most. It all makes me want to scream. I have fantasies about becoming some sort of *superwoman* and having the power to eliminate all the bogus claims circulating through the cosmetics industry, starting with this one. When it comes to hair color, there are several product lines, especially those available on the Internet or from some designer lines, claiming to be the essence of natural and pure and using only vegetable dyes to alter hair color. It just isn't true. One such product, **Vita Wave from Nature to You**

Hair Color, Gentle, Safe, Organic *($15.90)*, represents all of these to a T. Vita Wave makes polyester look natural. With ingredients like hydrogen peroxide, dihydroxyethyl, nonoxynol-9, sodium sulfite, resorcinol, and EDTA, this product isn't even remotely natural. What is more frightening is that the pH of the developer is between 11 and 12! That is not gentle by anyone's definition. Rather, this product—and all those like it—are standard, highly alkaline, very unnatural hair dyes that can be just as damaging to hair as every other hair dye on the market. Actually, there are a handful of hair-color products with pHs of 10 at the drugstore that are less damaging to the hair. (The lower the pH, the closer to a neutral pH of 7—water is a pH of 7—the less damage to hair, though this also makes the product less effective.)

Here is a run down of the varying drugstore versions and their pHs. **Clairol Balsam Color** *($2.99)* pH 11; **Clairol Hydrience** *($6.99)* pH 11; **Clairol Lasting Color by Loving Care** *($6.39)* pH 10; **Clairol Miss Clairol** *($6.29)* pH 10; **Clairol Natural Instincts** *($6.99)* pH 11; **Clairol Nice & Easy** *($6.29)* pH 10; **Clairol Revitalique** *($6.59)* pH 11; **Clairol Ultress** *($7.69)* pH 11; **Dark & Lovely** *($3.99)* pH 11; **Garnier Nutrisse** *($6.99)* pH 11; **Garnier Belle Color** *($5.99)* pH 11; **L'Oreal Casting** *($7.39)* pH 11; **L'Oreal Excellence** *($6.99)* pH 11; **L'Oreal Feria** *($9)* pH 11; **L'Oreal Preference** *($8.99)* pH 11; **Revlon ColorSilk** *($3.79)* pH 11; **Revlon ColorStay** *($6.99)* pH 11; and **Revlon Super Lustrous** *($8.99)* pH 11.

Other than the dye-types listed below, the actual variation between products in each grouping is minimal. Promises of gentler, more natural, luminescent, glowing, shimmering, longer lasting, or more anything color are marketing language and don't translate to variations in chemical performance. Color differences between products do exist and some lines have more red or ash shades, but that has nothing to do with a special, unique formulation. The best analogy I can think of is that a crayon is a crayon is a crayon, but a chocolate brown crayon doesn't look the same as a red crayon does.

To make this point crystal clear, according to the February 15, 1999, issue of *The Rose Sheet*, a cosmetics industry insider newsletter, Clairol brought a case of false advertising against Revlon. The newsletter stated that Revlon ColorSilk and Frost & Glow claim that their permanent hair colors repair hair on the inside and out and produce healthier hair/highlights every time you color. Clairol maintains that isn't true. The article noted that Clairol's complaint to the National Advertising Council said, "Revlon's claims that its products can improve hair health cannot be substantiated 'when, in fact, the hair coloring process causes irreversible damage to hair.' Consumers could be deceived by Revlon's marketing claims. Since hair is not living tissue this process [dyeing hair] cannot be reversed. Hair exposed to permanent hair coloring products suffers permanent damage and consequently is less healthy than it was before treatment."

Cancer and Hair Dyes?

Does dyeing your hair cause an increase in certain cancers? That question has been studied and evaluated by the FDA, the National Cancer Institute (NCI), and the National Institutes of Health (NIS) but, regrettably, there is no absolute consensus from any of these agencies on whether or not a risk really exists. In fact the research is confusing and conflicting. According to the NIS, "A recent study looking at the use of permanent hair dyes and cancer did not find an association between such use and hematopoietic cancers (cancers of the blood or lymph systems). The study, by a team of researchers from Brigham and Women's Hospital in Boston, involved more than 99,000 women." At the same time the NIS acknowledges that "The new study's findings differ from the results of at least eight earlier studies which indicated that women and men who dye their hair frequently may be at increased risk for hematopoietic cancers. The early studies showed an association between hair dye use and increased risks for multiple myeloma (cancer of cells in the bone marrow), non-Hodgkin's lymphoma (cancer of the lymph system), and leukemia (cancer of blood-forming cells) in both sexes, and ovarian cancer in women."

According to the FDA, "In 1978, FDA proposed to require a warning on the labels of hair dyes containing the compounds 4-methoxy-m-phenylenediamine (4MMPD) or 4-methoxy-m-phenylenediamine sulfate (4MMPD sulfate), two coal-tar ingredients. This followed findings by researchers at the National Cancer Institute in Bethesda, Maryland, that rodents fed either of the chemicals were more likely to develop cancer than animals not fed the substances. . . . Some researchers say that extrapolating results from ingested hair dye studies to absorbed hair dye use cannot accurately assess cancer risk because the compounds being tested are altered or are absorbed differently in the gut than they are when applied to the scalp."

The issue of *Environmental Health Perspectives*, volume 102, number 6–7, for June–July 1994 quoted a study published in the February 2, 1994, *Journal of the National Cancer Institute* that stated "[A] study, conducted by the American Cancer Society, found that women who used black hair dye for more than 20 years had a slightly increased risk of dying from non-Hodgkin's lymphoma and multiple myeloma. Researchers surveyed 573,369 women who completed questionnaires about their use of permanent hair dye. Surprisingly, women who dyed their hair showed a slightly reduced risk overall of dying of cancer than women who never used dyes." Isn't that confounding?

What does all this mean for the consumer? In essence it means there is no definitive proof one way or the other. According to the FDA, "The findings so far are inconclusive. The studies raise some questions about the safety of hair dyes, but at this point there's no basis for us to say that hair dyes pose a definitive risk of cancer. In the final analysis, consumers will need to consider the lack of demonstrated safety when they choose to use hair dyes." I agree. There is nothing definitive about any of this information and research. I wish there was something more conclusive to tell you but there isn't. However, what is absolutely certain is that the products claiming to use natural dyes to permanently alter hair color and thereby eliminate any risk are lying. They aren't natural or they couldn't permanently alter hair color.

Color Categories

Essentially, there are five primary types of hair-coloring options available, whether you buy them at the drugstore or get your hair done at the hair salon. These five categories are: temporary, semipermanent, mid/intermediate/demi/level 2 (sometimes called longer-lasting semipermanent, shorter-lasting permanent, or in-between color), permanent, and gradual or progressive dyes. Within each of these categories are further divisions.

Temporary hair colors are available in shampoos, conditioners, and mousses, and generally, but not always, wash out after one or two shampoos.

Semipermanent hair colors come in cream, gel, shampoo-in, and mousse solutions that are left on the hair for up to 20 minutes (or less) in order to deposit the color on the exterior of the hair shaft. These take six to eight shampoos to wash out.

Progressive hair colors most frequently refer to those products containing lead acetate. Lead acetate gradually accumulates on the outside of the hair shaft or just under the cuticle, altering the hair shade with a blanket of color. For men this is considered an easy way to completely cover gray with a simple shampooing and without a radical overnight change. There's also no need to worry about growout, because the color fades gradually when you stop using it. However, lead acetate can also give a strange greenish cast to the hair that is far less than natural in appearance.

Technically, within this group of progressive colors are also a group of regular permanent and mid/intermediate/demi/level 2 hair colors that are shampooed in for five minutes and then rinsed off. The repetitive, five-minute applications are meant to gradually build up the color on the hair. What takes place is some amount of processing with each successive shampoo. Unlike lead acetate–based progressive colors that cover the outside of the hair shaft, these are standard dye products.

If you wondering if men can use a dye product aimed at women, the answer is an indisputable yes. Why don't men use women's products? Because most men are unwilling to go through the 20- to 50-minute process time, preferring the ease of getting rid of gray in the least amount of time possible. Can women use men's products? Again the answer is yes, but with a caveat. These kinds of progressive permanent or intermediate dyes only work when the hair is short. If you constantly shampoo in the color over longer hair eventually it will saturate the length of hair with too much color and you will no longer get the color you want.

Mid/intermediate/demi/level 2 hair colors are shampoo-in type products, similar to permanent hair dyes, and are left on the hair for up to 45 minutes. These products contain only enough dye to make subtle changes in your hair color, but they will cover gray. You can't use mid/intermediate/demi/level 2 hair dyes to go from brown to blonde or even dark brown to light brown. But because you can't make a drastic change in your hair color, there is little risk of getting a terrible color, and any change (growout), except for the gray, is virtually undetectable.

Permanent hair colors are available in creams, lotions, and gels, and are shampooed into the hair and left on for up to 45 minutes. There are shampoo-only, single-process, double-process, and special-effects permanent dyes. They can make a considerable, permanent change in hair color and only require touch-ups based on fading and growout.

Each category has a specific, identifiable performance record with its own set of pros and cons. Add to that the technical nuances and your personal expectations of what you want from a product, and the subject gets complicated.

Temporary Hair Color

Temporary hair colors or color rinses are designed to be short-lived. The colors are deposited directly on the hair shaft and, because they don't penetrate the hair shaft, they are washed out the next time you shampoo your hair. Do not expect temporary hair colors to hide gray if you are more than 10 percent gray. They offer a sheer, translucent veil of color over the hair, but that's about it. The color of the dye you see in the container is the color your hair will get. These are meant to be a fun, noncommittal way to improve hair color or add subtle highlights, similar to trying on a see-through blouse (not exactly what you would call a full cover-up).

Temporary hair colors are a way to try minor color variations in your hair without risk. They are also a good way to neutralize the yellow in white and gray hair or tone down the brassiness in certain shades of blonde and frosted hair for a day or two. They can also stretch the time between mid/intermediate/demi/level 2 or permanent hair colorings. Temporary dyes can help to slightly disguise growout. Some temporary hair colors are formulated with conditioners so they are less likely to cause frizzies or dryness. Despite this, the coating of dye over the hair shaft can be somewhat drying or could cause the hair to become flyaway.

The number of temporary color-enhancing shampoos that have popped up on the market over the past two years is amazing. ARTec, Alberto Culver, Aussie Intermissions, Clairol, Color Plus, Garden Botanika, Halsa, L'Oreal, Mastey, Paul Mitchell, Redken, Revlon, and Sebastian, to name a few, all have shampoos with color additives. These interesting products offer some outstanding color choices that can cling to the hair shaft and effect a small, subtle degree of change. Different hair types can have more or less success with these shampoos, but in general, porous or lighter shades of hair, such as blonde or red, will show the most change and darker shades the least. How do you know what color you'll end up with when using these products? As is true with any temporary hair color, **the color you see is the color you get.** There are no secrets with these products.

Even if you do not normally use a conditioner, it is best to do so when using color-enhancing shampoos because of the way the dye is deposited on the hair shaft. One of the drawbacks of color-enhancing shampoos, besides dryness and flyaway hair, is that the dyes do not stand up well to the entire shampooing, so coverage can be uneven or disappointingly inadequate and poor. A few companies have tried to correct this problem by creating conditioners with temporary colors added to them. Conditioners are a better vehicle for wash-in, wash-out colors because they contain no detergent cleansers, and the conditioning agents, like the dyes, are meant to be left on the hair shaft. The only negative is that someone with an oily scalp or normal, thin hair will not be happy putting a conditioner all over the head or on the scalp. Conditioners with temporary coloring agents are best for someone with a normal to dry scalp and/or normal to coarse hair.

A new addition to the hair-color market (which is growing daily) are styling products with color. It is a fun, extremely uneven way to add a hint of color or shine or sparkle. These tend to be messy (although the color does wash off the hands) and sticky to use (just like any mousse), and the color has a minimal effect on the hair. However, if you don't mind the overall effect of mousse on your hair and the other negatives, these do happen to add a nice vibrant shine and depth of color.

The best uses for temporary hair color are to blend away a very tiny percentage of gray hair, deepen faded hair color in between using more permanent types of hair color, subtly brighten or highlight your own natural hair color, and reduce ash or red tones in the hair, both natural and those caused by intermediate/demi/level 2 or permanent hair dyes.

Hair Note: Lighter shades of hair will pick up temporary hair color more noticeably than darker shades, much the same way a white surface shows color more vividly than a black surface.

TEMPORARY HAIR COLORS: **Revlon Roux Fanci Rinse** (32 shades) and **Revlon Roux Fanci Mousse** (16 shades) are more substantive temporary hair colors. These two products can add potent hair color that takes several washings to remove and can leave unwanted residue.

There are also a vast range of extremely temporary color-enhancing shampoos and conditioners listed in Chapter 10, *The Best Products.* Those listed all tend to work equally well and can be used over any kind of hair or with any other hair-color treatment or with perms. The more porous, thin, damaged, blonde, or red the hair is, the more likely it is to grab the color.

Plant-Based Temporary Dye

Plant-derived hair colors such as henna come and go from the hair-market scene, but because they are natural and the public believes natural must be better, they never completely go away. Henna is by far the most popular temporary vegetable dye available; others are available but they are insignificant and offer minimal or unpleasant color. Produced from a shrub indigenous to North Africa and the Near East, henna has the requisite exotic background that is so intriguing to cosmetics consumers. Over several uses henna deposits a stain on the hair, creating only a reddish orange shade (and not a very attractive shade, either). Depending on your own hair color, henna can eventually turn more orange than red. Henna also has a few other problems. It tends to leave a sticky film over the hair that can dry out the hair shaft, which can be a problem for most hair types. However, someone with fine, thin hair may want to try a product with colorless henna powder to add some thickness to the hair. Be careful, because henna buildup can cause hair to be heavy and hard to manage. For the most part, henna should probably be avoided. (If you are using a henna product and it works for you, that's great. However, it might not contain much henna or perhaps you are using it once in a while instead of on a regular basis.)

Do not use henna products for at least a week or two before using a different hair-color product or perming the hair.

HENNA PRODUCTS: **Aveda's Madder Root Color Conditioner, The Body Shop Henna Cream Shampoo, Egyptian Henna,** and **The Body Shop Henna Wax.**

Hair Note: A clear, noncoloring form of henna is sometimes added to shampoos and conditioners in the name of improving the feel of the hair. It can add a certain amount of thickness to the hair, but when used repeatedly it can build up and become heavy and sticky. If you want to try a clear, noncoloring henna conditioner or shampoo, consider using it every other time you shampoo or once a week, to prevent hair problems.

Semipermanent Hair Color

Formulated to stay on the hair for six to 12 washings, semipermanent colors are more substantial than temporary hair colors. While temporary hair colors coat only the outside of the hair shaft, semipermanent hair colors have some ability to embed themselves into the top layers of the cuticle, although the primary effect is more of a hair stain than anything else. The actual dyes used in semipermanent products are preformed, meaning they don't require peroxide or ammonia to be assembled, developed, or embedded into the cuticle. Despite the dye's slight capacity for making its way into the cuticle, temporary hair colors only make your hair a little brighter or darker, adding subtle highlights of red, copper, or ash. Do not expect them to make the hair much more than a fraction lighter. Semipermanent products can only camouflage up to 20 percent gray. That means if more than 20 percent of your hair is gray, semipermanent colors won't hide it even a little. If you are graying in clumps, these products will also be ineffective. Semipermanent hair colors are for blending or veiling gray. When there is too much gray in one area, the veiling is less convincing. Much like temporary hair colors, which are gone after one shampooing, semipermanent colors fade with each washing so there is no discernible growout. Instead, the color fades away until your own color is revealed.

Semipermanent hair colors do not contain any peroxide or ammonia, so they cause no serious damage to the hair shaft; however, the dyes can cause some detachment of the cuticle, resulting in minor damage and possible dryness.

The best uses for semipermanent hair color are to blend away a tiny percentage of gray hair, test the effect of a new, subtle change in hair color (almost imperceptible for darker hair shades) before using a mid/intermediate/demi/level 2 or permanent hair dye, brighten or faintly highlight your own natural hair color (soften or intensify ash or red tones in your own hair color), or make your permanent or mid/intermediate/demi/level 2 hair color last longer between touch-ups.

Hair Note: Just as with temporary hair colors, lighter shades of hair will pick up semipermanent hair color more noticeably than darker shades, much the same way a white surface shows color more vividly than a black surface.

SEMIPERMANENT HAIR COLORS: **Clairol Glintz** (16 shades), **Clairol Loving Care Color Creme** (24 shades), **Clairol Silk & Silver** (three shades), **L'Oreal Avantage** (20 shades), **L'Oreal Exuberance** (12 shades), and **Revlon Rev Up** (12 shades).

Men's Hair Color/Progressive Dye

Simply put, men don't want anyone to know they are coloring their hair. Grecian Formula is probably the best-known men's hair-coloring product. **Grecian Formula** is a progressive hair-coloring product and, because of its popularity, its product line has been expanded to include **Grecian Cream** and **Grecian Plus** (a foam-in product). All of Grecian Formula's products contain lead acetate (a metallic dye). After several washings or applications, the lead acetate gradually accumulates on the outside of the hair shaft or just inside the cuticle, altering the hair shade with a blanket of color. For men this is considered an easy way to completely cover gray with a simple shampooing and without a radical overnight change. There's also no need to worry about growout because the color fades gradually when you stop using it.

While the change in color over time may in some regards be subtle (though a greenish cast to the hair is an inevitable, noticeably unattractive side effect), the change in hair quality is far from subtle. Metallic hair dyes can dry out the hair, leaving it brittle and stiff. But aside from the aesthetic problems, there are more serious questions with regard to these products.

There is controversy over the lead acetate used in progressive dyes. After the first edition of this book was published, Combe Incorporated, the makers of Grecian Formula, provided me with extensive information demonstrating the safety of lead acetate. The following is an excerpt from my communication with the company:

Dear Ms. Begoun,

Thank you for your willingness to review materials in Combe Incorporated files that discuss the lead acetate issue [you posed regarding our product Grecian Formula and its safety]. Enclosed are documents that substantiate the safety of lead acetate in hair dye preparations.

A significant scientific paper, which was published in the April/May 1980 issue of *The Journal of Cosmetic Toxicology*, details a six-month clinical study performed at the Universities of Munster and Gottingen by Professor Fritz Kemper and Helmut Ippen, respectively. The study was performed at the request of the German government in connection with an application by a Combe affiliate for approval of lead acetate hair dyes in Germany. Fifty-three human volunteers used a lead acetate hair dye for six months, with one group using the products at levels higher than is customary in order to create an abuse exposure. Every known biological parameter affected by changes in blood and urine content was monitored. It was determined that no lead acetate was absorbed from the usage in the study. Subsequently, the Kemper-Ippen study formed the basis for the European Community countries [to accept the use of lead acetate in hair dyes], which culminated in the approval for all member[s,] as set forth in an EC Cosmetic Directive that was published in 1990.

An earlier safety study was performed in Scotland under the supervision of Dr. Michael Moore and Sir Abraham Goldberg. That study was of particular significance because Dr. Goldberg is a world authority on lead toxicity. The study, published in Volume 8 of *Food Cosmetic Toxicology* (1980), also concluded that there was no toxicologically significant absorption, even under certain extreme conditions. On the basis of that study, the U.S. FDA permanently listed lead acetate as a safe color additive for hair dye use.

Fredrick G. Giel
Associate Counsel to Combe Incorporated

Dear Mr. Giel,

I have reviewed at length the extensive material you sent me regarding the studies supporting Combe's position that lead acetate is not a problem for use in hair dyes. After further checking with several other sources, I am convinced that lead acetate in the amounts used in Combe's Grecian Formula products [and other lead acetate-based dyes] is safe to use for both men and women. The source I used for my position that lead acetate is a problem for the scalp was speaking of much higher concentrations and had no supportive documentation in regard to hair dyes, and her contention should not have been extrapolated to your products.

Separate from the health issues, when it comes to creating a desirable color, far better options may be found with traditional mid/intermediate/demi/level 2 or permanent/level 3 coloring products (see the following section) that are used in shampoo-in type products. When used in a shampoo-in-and-rinse-out-after-five-minutes kind of product, the color builds up gradually with each application and can cover a good amount of gray over time without radically changing natural hair color. The differences between the men's products and those for women are how they are applied and how long they are kept on. Men's products also have a limited color selection with less drastic changes offered. The application process for men is always done all over the head with no sectioning or root application as women do for touch-ups. Men who keep their hair short don't have to worry about getting the ends too dark or too bleached if they are always cutting off the damaged length (this would be true for women with short hair as well), which is why the repeated shampoo-in process can work.

Like all mid/intermediate/demi/level 2 and permanent/level 3 coloring products, these shampoo-in colors are fairly permanent, meaning they don't wash out and when the roots grow out, they show the original hair color. See the following section for more information about this type of progressive hair color.

Mid/Intermediate/Demi/Level 2 Hair Color

Forgive this long section header, but these are the various names companies attribute to their "not quite, but almost" permanent hair dyes. These are the newest and fastest-growing segment of the hair-coloring market at both the drugstore and the hair salon. Mid/intermediate/demi/level 2 hair colors are often called longer-lasting semipermanent, shorter-lasting permanent, or in-between colors because they are as permanent as permanent dyes but they have lower concentrations of peroxide and dye, which allows for only subtle changes in hair color.

In the long run, mid/intermediate/demi/level 2 hair colors have more in common with permanent hair dyes than with semipermanent hair dyes. However, there is only enough dye in mid/intermediate/demi/level 2 hair dyes to change the natural color of your hair a shade or two, thus the association with semipermanent hair colors.

Mid/intermediate/demi/level 2 dyes last as long as permanent dyes do, that is, until the hair grows out and the roots show up, but mid/intermediate/demi/level 2 dyes cannot produce as great a change as permanent dyes. Mid/intermediate/demi/level 2 colors contain a small amount of hydrogen peroxide, while permanent hair dyes contain twice as much, though mid/intermediate/demi/level 2 dyes do contain the same amount of ammonia or ammonia-type (alkaline) ingredients that permanent hair dyes do.

Mid/intermediate/demi/level 2 dyes cover up to 25 to 50 percent gray. That means if more than 50 percent of the hair on your head is gray, mid/intermediate/demi/level 2 dyes won't work. If you are less than 50 percent gray but you are graying in clumps or in concentrated areas, mid/intermediate/demi/level 2 hair color also won't work. You need to consider the next step—permanent hair color.

Mid/intermediate/demi/level 2 hair colors are considered the baby boomers' answer to dealing with newly arriving gray hair. With only minor changes you can cover the gray. The mistakes you might make won't be major, because these products aren't capable of radically changing hair color. They can only alter the color a shade or two, so strangely colored hair is almost impossible.

Mid/intermediate/demi/level 2 hair colors *do* contain a small amount of peroxide and a mild alkaline base (and even when the label claims it contains no ammonia, a different alkaline ingredient such as ethanolamine is used), which can cause some damage to the hair shaft.

The best uses for mid/intermediate/demi/level 2 hair colors are to match your natural hair color and give it more depth, cover up to 50 percent gray, highlight your own hair a shade or two, and lengthen the times between permanent hair-color treatments.

Hair Note: All of the products in this group of hair colors claim boldly on the package that the color will last through 24 shampooings. That is incredibly misleading. These are not wash-out dyes; the color stays in the hair shaft *permanently,* period. You have to consider coloring your hair again after you see growout (meaning the gray roots are showing up). Growout happens after four to six weeks, which is what 24 shampoos add up to, because on average most women wash their hair four to five times a week. Mid/intermediate/demi/level 2 dyes don't fade any more than permanent dyes. The difference is the amount of color change you can obtain. Because mid/intermediate/demi/level 2 dyes change the hair color only a shade or two, you won't notice different-colored roots, aside from the gray. That is a nice benefit of mid/intermediate/demi/level 2 dyes, but it has nothing to do with the permanence of the color. Mid/intermediate/demi/level 2 dyes are permanent, regardless of what the packages seem to assert.

MID/INTERMEDIATE/DEMI/LEVEL 2 HAIR COLORS: The choices in this group are **Clairol Lasting Color** (14 shades), **Clairol Men's Choice** (seven shades); **Clairol Natural Instincts** (25 shades); **Clairol Natural Instincts Exotic** (eight shades); **Clairol Natural Instincts for Men** (seven shades) **L'Oreal Castings ColorSpa** (18 shades); and **Revlon Super Lustrous** (22 shades).

Permanent/Level 3 Hair Color

As the name implies, these traditional hair-coloring products permanently change your hair color to almost any color or shade you want it to be. Black to blonde, red to brunette, and gray to brown are just a few of the awesome color possibilities, but, most importantly, they cover almost any amount of gray hair. Permanent hair colors (which includes the stripping of hair color known as bleaching) are also known as oxidative colors, and contain about 20 to 30 percent (by volume) hydrogen peroxide in an alkaline base with a pH of about 10 to 11.

Permanent and bleaching hair-coloring products come in different forms, such as gels, foams, shampoos, and lotions. No form has any particular advantage over another. This is a matter of personal preference. I find the lotions easiest to work with, but I know other women who swear by the cream formulas. Given that you will be dyeing your hair more than once, this is an area you can experiment with for yourself.

In trying to choose which product line to consider, think about the color you want and ignore claims about the color being natural or gentle, or having a hair-strengthening formula. All of that marketing language is completely bogus. All hair-dye products in each category are shockingly similar and all have virtually identical instructions. They perform equally well, with the major difference being color choice. In the long run, color choice and experimentation should be your main considerations in making a final selection, because all of the other stuff is nothing more than gimmicks trying to get your attention regardless of the facts.

Permanent hair-coloring products rely on three basic methods of application: shampoo in, single-step process, and two-step process. Shampoo-in products are the easiest and quickest, and can be used on dry, damp, or wet hair. With this type of product, the hair tends to slightly fade and grow out after four to six weeks. When you color your hair again, the dye is again shampooed in over the entire head all at once.

Shampoo-in permanent hair colors are the standard for men's coloring products. The most popular are **Combe International Just for Men** (eight shades) and **Clairol Men's Choice** (seven shades). Because most men keep their hair short and because these products are less potent than other permanent dyes, they can be reapplied in subsequent applications all over the head without the need to do roots first and then the hair length. Ease of application, quick processing time (most of these products require only five minutes on the hair), and small color selections make it an uncomplicated purchase for men whose comfort level with cosmetics is somewhere between embarrassed and pained.

Single-step permanent hair colors (shampoo-in and root application) involve a first-time application for virgin hair with an overall shampooing-in of the hair dye, which is left on for approximately 20 to 45 minutes. Subsequent colorings require sectioning the hair, applying the color only to the roots, and letting the roots process for the longest period of time—anywhere from 15 minutes to 35 minutes into the treatment. The dye can then be pulled through via a shampooing motion to the length of the hair, letting the color develop there for a shorter period of time, say five minutes or less, to refresh the previous color and prevent hair from becoming too dark. This type of permanent hair dye is stronger (meaning it has more dye saturation) than the shampoo-in type permanent dyes, and offers more control over obtaining the exact hair color you want, with some fading depending on your hair type and color choice. Lighter shades of hair dye, especially red shades, fade more easily than darker shades.

As the hair grows out, the gray or natural color of the roots becomes apparent if you have changed your hair color by more than two shades or if you were covering gray. That means the roots require the same amount of processing time the hair needed the first time you colored it, while the length needs less processing time because it has already been dyed and is close to the color you want.

Sectioning the hair and gauging the different processing times of the roots and the length of the hair makes this type of at-home coloring precarious to use yourself. Sectioning the back of the hair can be extremely tricky, and determining how long to leave the color on the length of the hair is a matter of judgment. Balancing the processing time of the roots and the ends is at first a bit of a guessing game, but it does get easier with experience and a strand test. For some hair color, especially if you don't have a problem with fading, it isn't necessary to pull the color through to the ends each time; you can just color the roots and then shampoo it out when you're done.

Both shampoo-in and single-process hair-coloring products are best when you are trying to cover between 60 to 100 percent gray, and/or you want to change your hair color by more than two shades.

Double Processing/Two-step permanent hair colors/Bleaching and Toning, and **Tone on Tone** are all variations on a theme but essentially do the exact same thing. First, the natural or existing hair color is lifted and stripped out of the hair with 20 to 30 percent volume peroxide. The next step adds the color you want your hair to become. (Hair can be stripped—bleached—without the second step, but that can leave the hair looking a straw-white color of blonde.)

Regardless of the terminology, this form of changing hair color is best done at a salon. If you do decide to attempt this at home, do it only after you've established the right color and process timing at the hair salon. Two-step hair color is mostly used when you want a radical change from any shade of brown or black to any shade of blonde (even someone with light brown hair must go through this routine to become blonde), or from red or blonde to black (though not very many people ever go in that direction). Either way, this process requires bleaching (stripping) out your natural hair color (step one) so that when you apply the dye (step two) it has a clear path with no dark or opposite colors to get in its way.

Two-step processing is very damaging, and there is no way around that. A dramatic change from dark to light may constitute a fashionable glamour statement or supposedly have more sex appeal, but up close, especially after a few applications, the hair looks and feels like straw instead of soft, healthy hair. If you also use blow-dryers, curling irons, rollers, brushes, and/or styling products, you compound the damage even more. Now if you want to run your hand through your tresses, you are likely to get stuck or break off brittle strands by the hundreds.

For that reason, I strongly suggest that radical color changes be handled at first by your hairdresser or not done at all. There are just too many things that can go wrong along the way, such as the timing, the mess, judging the color saturation, applying the color evenly, and choosing the right color. But don't think that getting your hair blonded at the hair salon is any less damaging than doing it yourself at home, because it isn't. As I said before, changing the hair color radically, and doing it repeatedly, is damaging, period. What the stylist can provide is a better color tone, more accurate processing time, and more options for becoming blonder without dyeing the whole head of hair, such as frosting or foiling.

Highlighting is a process that requires selectively choosing which hair will be altered. This can be a one- or two-step process. The one-step process is a bleach that strips away the natural hair color, leaving varying degrees of lighter color depending on the processing time. That can be all you need to achieve the color you want. But this can also be a two-step process, where the hair color is lifted (bleached) and stripped out completely, and then a second color (often called a tone) is applied to create a specific, more controlled color to the hair.

The original method for highlighting (which is still employed with at-home kits) is with a plastic cap placed over the entire head through which strands of hair are pulled and then bleached. This fairly painful pulling process reduces accurate placing of the color and prevents application of the dye close to the root areas, making the highlights look like two months of growout as soon as you are done. This immediate appearance of growout, inaccurate color placement, and the discomfort are primary reasons hair foiling became the preferred method of adding highlights.

In foiling, little strands of hair are separated from larger sections, placed on foil, painted with bleach (depending on the color you are going after), and then wrapped up in a little foil packet. Foiling is a more sophisticated, subtle-to-dramatic way to place highlights throughout the hair, even closer to the root, and can be accomplished only at the hair salon.

One more technique for placing highlights (or streaks of color) through the hair is called hair painting, and it is the only blonding method I would even begin to suggest you try at home. Hair painting involves using a bleach that is artistically or, depending on your point of view, randomly applied to the hair. Back in the '70s, hair painting (streaking) often meant bold stripes of silver or gold strewn through the hair. Now streaking can range from butterscotch to caramel, honey, red, auburn, and beyond, controlled by the amount of time the bleach or one-step color is applied to the hair. Regardless of the color, the effect is the same: obvious lines of color running through the hair. Hairstylists love calling this look "natural" and they use all kinds of adjectives to convince the consumer that it is. I've heard such phrases as "natural, but *pushed* natural"; "what the sun would do to your hair" (what the sun does is damaging, and so is any kind of bleaching); and "it is fashionable to have the roots show through." It just depends on whether or not you want to believe the trend-makers' defense of an obvious fashion statement.

Hair Note: The darker the hair, the less likely that frosting or streaking (bleaching) will produce natural blonde highlights. Darker hair can be pushed to shades of reddish copper or golden brown, but that's about it. In general, highlighting works best on dark/medium brown to blonde hair.

A small, special group of permanent, at-home coloring products can effect an understated change for women with a deeper shade of blonde hair who want it to be a shade or two lighter. These dyes use a mild lightener (dye color) with hydrogen peroxide (bleaching agent) and are done in one step. They only lighten one or two shades, so they are really for someone whose hair is already light. If this applies to you and you only expect to be one or two shades lighter than you already are, you may want to consider trying **Chattam Labs Sun-In, Clairol A Touch of Sun,** and **L'Oreal Summer Soleil,** all good options. These products use a less severe bleaching process than products that can turn a brunette's hair blonde, but they still cause damage. Any amount of stripping away natural hair color is damaging.

SHAMPOO-IN AND SINGLE-STEP PERMANENT HAIR COLORS: **Carson Dark & Lovely** (11 shades); **Clairol Balsam Color** (17 shades); **Clairol Hydrience** (38 shades); **Clairol Miss Clairol Creme Formula** (24 shades); **Clairol Nice & Easy** (37 shades); **Clairol Ultress** (33 shades); **Clairol Revitalique** (32 shades); **Garnier Belle Color— owned by L'Oreal** (20 shades); **L'Oreal Excellence Creme** (32 shades), **L'Oreal Feria** (38 shades); **L'Oreal Preference** (45 shades); **Revlon ColorSilk** (28 shades);

Revlon ColorStay (24 shades); **Revlon ColorStay Naturals for Men** (seven shades); **Soft-Sheen Optimum Care** (eight shades).

SPECIAL EFFECTS AND TWO-STEP PERMANENT HAIR COLORS: These are very tricky products to use at home yourself. They either cause too much damage, due to the two-step process, or are difficult to apply artfully on your own. **Highlighting: Clairol Frost & Tip** (two shades); **Clairol Hydrience Creme Highlights** (two shades); **L'Oreal Frost & Design** (two shades); and **Revlon Frost and Glow** (two shades). **Hair Painting Kits: Clairol Hair Painting** (two shades); **Clairol Nuances** (two shades); and **L'Oreal Brush-on Highlights** (one shade). **Two-Step Blonding: Clairol Born Blonde** (four shades) and **L'Oreal Super Blonde** (one shade). **Special Duo Highlighting** (adds two colors to the hair instead of one): **L'Oreal Accenting** (six shades).

Mixing Types of Hair Dye

Hair dyeing is about experimenting and finding which combination works for you. It is also about being flexible, knowing that problems will occur and having a game plan to make changes as needed. One of the best ways to go about this is the creative mixing of the different types of hair dye. Just because you've been using a permanent/level 3 dye doesn't mean you can't use an intermediate/level 2 dye to soften a color or reduce the appearance of highlights you don't like.

For example, if you've been dyeing your hair with a permanent dye and you're starting to feel that the ends are getting too dark or a shade of ash or red you don't want, rather than trying to go over that color with a permanent/level 3 dye, you can go over the ends with an intermediate/level 2 dye or a semipermanent hair color. This trick helps to reduce the brassy or red tones without radically affecting the actual hair color.

Keeping this in mind can make the dye experience at home or at the salon a great experience. Don't assume that your hairstylist will automatically think of these options either—your participation and influence can go a long way toward getting a great color.

How Does It All Work?

In order for mid/intermediate/demi/level 2 or permanent/level 3 hair dyes to work, they all require the same brilliant chemical process to take place. First, hydrogen peroxide in some amount lifts the existing color from the cortex. Second, the ammonia base (almost always at a pH of 10 to 11) swells the hair shaft, allowing total penetration of the hair dyes. Third, once the dyes enter the hair shaft, they interact with the hydrogen peroxide and the color molecules; it's this interaction that creates the color you expect (that's why they are called oxidative hair dyes). Although there can be some fading with permanent hair colors, especially red dyes, for the most part, once you get started you are committed to the result. If you choose a color that's different from your natural hair color, you will end up with totally contrasting roots after two to six weeks, depending on your hair's growth rate. The only way to go back is to strip out the mistake and put in a color you think is more to your liking.

On a microscopic level, the dye molecules in permanent hair colors are capable of becoming a limitless variety of tones, hues, tints, and intensities. Cosmetics chemists with computer simulation programs have concocted thousands upon thousands of potential color combinations for the hair. The dyes are a matter of pride for each of the companies that make hair-coloring products. Whether the product is a cream, lotion, gel, or foam, the molecular structure of the dye itself is what determines the outcome. Depending on who you talk to, each of the major companies producing permanent hair-coloring products has a reputation for the color tone you can expect. L'Oreal is supposedly known for the blue or violet quality of their dyes, Clairol leans toward the drab or golden shades, while Revlon is reportedly in between, neither too blue or too golden. In general, it is almost always suggested you go a shade or two lighter than your hair color is currently to soften the hair color. Going dark can look severe and fake. (Later in this chapter, in the section called "Strand Testing," I go over the best ways to get the right color for your hair at both the drugstore and the hair salon, regardless of the product you buy.)

Some permanent hair-coloring products claim to contain no ammonia. Although that may sound healthier for the hair, the claim is somewhat misleading. In order for a permanent (or mid/intermediate/demi/level 2) hair color to work, it must contain ingredients that can raise the pH of the product enough to swell the hair shaft, allowing for penetration of the hair dyes. If the pH is too low, say, under a pH of 9, you won't get an acceptable penetration of the color. Permanent hair dyes need to be around pH 10 or 11, to work, and at least a pH of 10 if you want to make an extreme change in hair color. Ammonia hydroxide is one of the ingredients that can raise the pH level of a product. The so-called nonammonia-based permanent hair colors simply use a different alkaline ingredient, such as ethanolamine, to raise the pH of their product, and that can cause the same amount of damage to the hair shaft as ammonia. It is true that ammonium hydroxide or ammonium has a stronger odor than ethanolamines, but that doesn't translate to being better for the hair. A high pH is damaging to hair no matter what ingredient produces it.

It takes only about 1 percent ammonia to raise the pH of the dye to an acceptable level to help the color penetrate the hair shaft. The more the hair shaft swells, the better the penetration of the hair color and, because the hair shaft is more expanded, the fuller your hair appears afterward. If your hair is already coarse and frizzy, a more swollen hair shaft only makes things worse. But if your hair is thin, fine, or limp, that extra swelling can add welcome volume. Unfortunately, it can also add extra damage.

The only real benefit of nonammonia-based hair colors is their more pleasant odor. Ammonia has a distinctive aroma that leaves much to be desired!

Reminder: Hair-coloring products from the salon to the drugstore often make sweeping claims about their mid/intermediate/demi/level 2 and permanent formulas being natural and pure. I've heard every description, from botanical-based to containing absolutely no peroxide and no ammonia. **You are supposed to believe that the presence of plants and the elimination of peroxide or ammonia means there will be absolutely no damage or, at the very worst, minimal damage to the hair. Well, it just isn't possible.** According to all of the cosmetics chemists I interviewed, there is no way to get permanent (or mid/intermediate/demi/level 2) hair dyes deep into the hair shaft without an alkaline-based product and some amount of hydrogen peroxide. Ammonia is one ingredient that can raise the pH of a product, but there are others (with names you don't recognize, such as ethanolamine, so you won't know to be concerned) that provide the same effect and the same possible damage.

Hydrogen peroxide or some other oxidative ingredient is necessary to remove a little or a lot of your own hair color (depending on the shade you want your hair to become) and essential for oxidizing the dyes inside the hair shaft, and that can be damaging. No way around it. Ask to see the ingredient list. I promise you there will be a long list of very unnatural-sounding ingredients with a few plants thrown in for effect.

Critical Rules

Before I try to decipher the world of hair color for you, I want to list a few critical rules that apply to all hair-coloring products.

If your hair is damaged, naturally porous, or chemically treated (especially from perms or sunlight), it will take **less time** for the hair to grab the color. The healthier or thicker the hair, the **more time** it will take to grab the color. Texture is one way to judge how porous your hair is. Curlier, coarse, fine or fragile, and already processed or damaged hair tends to be more porous, while straighter, thicker, heavier hair tends to be less porous.

If you've been using henna or metallic dyes (lead acetate–based, progressive dyes), **never** apply any color treatment until you've gone several washings after you last used a product containing henna or until the metallic dye area has been cut off. The layer these coatings leave on the hair can interfere with the dye's ability to penetrate into the hair shaft. **Never** add color to bleached hair or strip hair color without specific advice from a stylist or from the company whose product you decide to use. These kinds of chemical processes are extremely hard on hair and the effect can be relatively unpredictable without experience.

Always do a strand test to be sure you will be getting the color you want. No matter how resistant you feel about this process, do it anyway; it will save you from struggling through several weeks or months of bad hair days.

Follow the directions of the product you are using *exactly*, or at least closely (I mention exceptions later). If you have any questions at all; if you are making a radical change in your hair color, changing products, or coloring over a different type of product; or if you just want someone to talk to about the products you are using, thinking of using, or thinking of changing to, call the company's consumer hot line for help.

As I state several times throughout this book, **it is best not to both dye and perm the hair,** even if you wait between treatments. You can do one or the other, but doing both greatly increases the risk of badly damaging your hair. (Exception: If you have extremely strong, resilient hair, you can consider doing both, but don't expect the texture of your hair to feel anything like normal, especially after additional perms and dyes.)

Mid/intermediate/demi/level 2 and permanent red or lighter brown or blonde hair colors (especially red) **can fade,** regardless of what you do to prevent it from happening. Cosmetics chemists are not 100 percent sure what breaks down the dye from the hair shaft—it could be caused by sunlight, plain air, or even shampooing— but regardless of the reason, some fading is part of the struggle of hair coloring.

You can't make dark hair color lighter without bleach—not even one shade lighter! Whether it is your natural color or a dyed shade, if you want to lighten the color any amount, you must strip (bleach) out the darker shade you are trying to change. You can't change a dark shade of hair color, natural or dyed, to a lighter shade without this fundamental step.

Understanding tone variations is a significant part of getting the shade you want. Color theory is what hair color is all about and those nuances establish whether the shade you get looks rich and vibrant or fake and contrived.

According to the FDA, "reactions to **hair dyes can severely harm the eye** and even cause blindness. Inadvertently spilling dye into the eye could also cause permanent damage. [The] FDA prohibits the use of hair dyes for eyelash and eyebrow tinting or dyeing even in beauty salons or other establishments."

There is also a high incidence of **allergic reactions to hair dye products.** Before getting started it is essential to do a patch test on your arm or behind your ear to be sure you don't have problems.

Strand Testing

In the varying color categories, the differences between salon and drugstore products are truly subtle and open to debate. What is not debatable is the necessity of performing a strand test if the consumer is to get the color she wants. It is of vital importance with any hair-coloring product, but without question it is fundamental for mid/intermediate/demi/level 2 and permanent dyes. If you don't want to play Russian roulette with your hair color, a strand test before you go about coloring your entire head of hair is the only way to protect your interests.

Strand testing is recommended on every box of hair color I've ever seen, at the hair salon as well as at the drugstore, and yet is probably the step most overlooked by consumers and hairstylists. I understand the reluctance to take the time for this tedious procedure. Not only do you have to go through an entire coloring process on a small section of hair, but for permanent and mid/intermediate/demi/level 2 products it is recommended that you cut a tiny section of hair from your head to perform the test. What woman wants to do that? Yet there is absolutely no better way to avoid problems. A strand test is essential, but it isn't necessary to cut the hair from your head; there are two other viable options you should consider. You can collect strands of hair from your brush for several days and tie them off with tape, and use that to check the color you want to try. You can also section off a tiny section of hair directly on your head and perform the strand test there. (I have had bad hair colors that cost me $200, $45, and $4.95, and all could have been prevented with a strand test that nobody, including me, wanted to do.)

Admittedly, seasoned hairstylists can get away without strand testing. But for a lot of women who have left salons with colors they didn't want, a strand test could have made all the difference in the world!

L'Oreal, Revlon, and Clairol all have consumer hot lines that field hundreds of thousands of calls a year (the phone numbers are listed below), with the overwhelming majority from women who didn't get the color they were hoping for. When asked if they had done a strand test, the overwhelming response was "No." Why? The excuses ran the gamut, but essentially they amount to "didn't have the time," "didn't want to," "didn't think it was really necessary," and "didn't want to cut off part of my hair." What all these women have in common, besides not doing a strand test, is that they now have bad hair color. With help from the consumer hot lines or a trip to the hair salon, you may be able to get close to the color you want, but there is no way to do that without causing more hair damage. If you or your hairstylist is not willing to do the strand test, you may have to pay the piper the next time you want to dance.

Hair Note: Don't be alarmed to read that hundreds of thousands of women a year call consumer hot lines for help with drugstore hair-color products. When you consider that millions of women are coloring their hair at home every year, a few hundred thousand questions and complaints amount to only a fraction of the total picture.

Consumer Help Lines:
• Clairol (800) 223-5800
• L'Oreal (also owns Garnier products) (800) 631-7358
• Revlon (800) 4-REVLON

Reminder: Follow the directions as precisely as you can. The recommendations and procedures are exact. Do yourself a favor and follow them exactly, with only minor adjustments, as I explain in the "Avoiding Disasters" section below. **Also, if you are planning to change from dyeing your hair at the salon to dyeing your hair at home, you will want to start paying attention to your stylist's technique so you can copy it at home. But if your stylist processes your hair with heat, say, for 20 minutes, then you will want to double the length of time, to about 40 minutes, if you do it at home without heat.**

Getting the Color You Want

Before you select a specific hair-coloring product, particularly one of the mid/intermediate/demi/level 2 or permanent hair dyes, it is best to understand some common terms and approaches that can help determine what color to use on your hair. The first thing to ascertain is the hair color that you're starting with. Your own **base color** is the cornerstone in establishing how a particular dye color will affect your hair and no one else's (not Cindy Crawford's, Heather Locklear's, or any other celebrity gracing the ads for a hair product). If you know your natural hair color, you will have a clearer idea of how to choose an appropriate new color.

Your base color is determined by the level, depth, and tone of your hair. The **level** is the actual color of your undyed hair. To some extent you have a pretty good idea if you have blonde, brown, red, or black hair. The **depth** of your hair color is identified by whether it is light, medium, or dark. Once you have a sense of the level and depth of your natural hair color, such as dark brown, medium brown, or light brown, you need to determine the **tone** of your hair color. Tone refers to how warm or cool the color of your hair is. **Warm** is the amount of red, copper, auburn or gold that appears in your hair. **Cool** is the amount of ash or the muted, drab shade of your hair. (*Cool* is synonymous with *drab* in the world of hair color.)

Tones in all hair-coloring products affect the highlights that radiate from the hair. Before you choose a hair color, you need to determine not only what color you want your hair to be, but what tone you would like it to be. That can be relatively simple, but it does take some forethought. There are no real rules for this one but, ordinarily, the more extreme the color choice, the more fake it will look. It is also generally well accepted by every hairstylist I interviewed that darker (meaning black or dark brown hair colors) were not suitable for older women (meaning women over the age of 40).

In terms of choosing which shade and tone would look best on you, the general rule is that warm shades are best for someone with warm (sallow) skin tones, and cool tones are best for someone with cool (blue) or fair skin tones. Some people recommend that you choose the tone according to the color highlights found in the eye. As clever as that sounds, there are no words for how limiting and silly it really is. If you have blue eyes, you are never going to have red highlights in them unless your eyes are bloodshot. Most brown or black eyes aren't going to have any highlights, and lots of eye colors have multiple hues in them. What do you do then? Eye color has nothing to do with choosing any cosmetic color, and that includes hair color.

The depth of color has to do with how much processing time you will need. If your own hair color has a strong saturation of darker colors, it will require longer processing time; the less saturated, the less processing time you may need.

After you've done your best to choose a level, depth, and tone of color that you think will be perfect, the tone may sometimes appear to be more red, yellow (brassy), or drab than you were hoping for. Trying to achieve soft, warm (golden) highlights in your hair can pay off in red highlights. In trying to correct for this, you may over-compensate with an ash color, only to discover that the highlights look more green than ash. And the same can happen in the other direction: A fear of going too ash can leave you with highlights that look too pink. How to compensate? This takes experimentation. Start with colors that have the least amount of red or ash tones (in other words, neutral) and see what happens. Color commitment only lasts from application to application, so don't overreact if it isn't exactly right the first few times. Jumping in and redyeing your hair immediately will damage the hair more. Remember, the less often you process your hair, the healthier it will be.

Try some temporary steps and wait until the next time you color your hair. For example, if you use a mid/intermediate/demi/level 2 or permanent hair color and you feel the color looks too red, you can use either a temporary or semipermanent hair-coloring product, especially a color-enhancing shampoo, to reduce the red cast to the hair. An ash or drab shade can reduce the red color. The same is true if you feel your hair appears too yellow or brassy. A temporary or semipermanent color in a violet or cool tone can reduce the yellow or brassy color.

Setting down guidelines for choosing hair color is as difficult as selecting makeup colors, because the options are so vast. Nonetheless, my strong suggestion is to start within a shade or two of your own hair color.

Warning: When you redye your hair, the roots are still your primary consideration if you are matching your hair color or staying close to your actual hair shade. The roots are always dyed first, and then the color is pulled through to the ends for a shorter period of time. The ends are processed for five minutes if you are staying with the same or a similar color, 15 minutes if you are changing color or using a new product.

Keeping the Color You Want

What makes hair color fade? In reality, the least of your worries is the shampoo or conditioner you're using. Exposure to the sun and air plays a vital role in lifting color from your hair. Sun damage causes the actual structure of the hair to break down, and that allows the hair-dye molecules to break down and degrade. Despite the influences of damage and sun on the hair, the truth is, no one is exactly sure why some dyes fade faster than others or why some hair types lose color faster than others. As one cosmetics chemist explained to me, if he knew what caused hair color to fade and if he could find a way to stop it, he would be a rich man sitting in the Bahamas sipping Mai Tais.

Protecting your hair from the sun can help (that means wearing a hat, because sunscreens in hair products are useless), but that doesn't guarantee much. You could stay inside and not touch your hair until new growth required another dye job and it would still fade slightly, especially if you have chosen a radical change in hair color or if you used any shade of red. In other words, fading is inevitable.

A host of products proclaim their ability to keep your hair color around longer than if you were to use other products. "Color Hold," "ColorStay," "No Fade Shampoo and Conditioner," "Protects Hair Color," and dozens more promise: "Use me and you won't lose your hair color." Except for the color-enhancing shampoos and conditioners, and other temporary or semipermanent coloring products, they are nothing more than fairly ordinary (but usually good) shampoos and conditioners. Do these "color-fast" shampoos eliminate ingredients that other shampoos don't? No! However, as a general rule, it would be best to avoid hair-care products that contain any strongly sulfonated oils such as sodium lauryl sulfate, TEA lauryl sulfate, triethanalomine, or alkyl sodium sulfate, whether or not you color your hair, but especially if you do. These are stronger detergent cleansing agents and dry out the hair or swell it, making the hair prone to loosing its color more easily or just feeling drier and more damaged.

What conditioner to choose is wide open. There are no conditioning ingredients that are unique to color-hold products and no conditioning agents that you should avoid. All the phrases about hair-care products aiding color stability are a marketing artifice, used to attract a specific type of consumer. They do not indicate a unique formula.

Shampoos and conditioners that contain dye colors are a horse of a different color. These add a topical layer of dye colors to the hair, giving the impression that there is a tad more color, but these cover poorly to not at all over roots or gray hair.

Some of the suggestions in the following sections can prevent poor product application, which can result in the color not grabbing well, but that is a usage problem, not an issue of fading.

Getting Rid of the Color You Don't Want

It is inevitable that at some point you may find the dyed hair color you have isn't the color you want. Then you need to get some of the old color out. There is truly no way to go about this without some amount of bleaching or "stripping" out the color. Removing hair color you don't want, either your own or dyed color, requires either hydrogen peroxide to "lift" out the color, or a sulfite to strip out hair color. These two ingredient types are the only ones that can perform this function on hair.

There are products like Schwarzkopf's Igora Modulat Color Corrector System, an expensive service performed at salons, which claims it can "reverse your [dyed] color without affecting your natural shade or damaging your hair's condition." Schwarzkopf also contends that "in the past, unwanted color could be corrected in only one of three ways: 1) cutting off the tinted area, 2) covering it with another shade, or 3) removing hair color with harsh bleaching products that often damage the hair shaft." Schwarzkopf claims its product can eliminate the dyed color you don't want with less bother and damage because it "shrink[s] the oxidized artificial color pigment molecules in the hair, so they can simply be shampooed out. The hair's natural color is left unaffected by the process." Regardless of how the dye color is broken down, the process of getting a substance into the hair shaft to do this would still be damaging. Either mode is a chemical process that could hurt the hair. (I should mention that I did try to get the ingredient listing from Schwarzkopf to verify my suspicions, but they were unwilling to provide it. Because this line is not sold to the public, they do not have to provide ingredients on the label. The only information they did send was that this was a sulfur-based product. I thought that would be the case. If it didn't contain bleach, then a sulfite is the only other option.)

What can you do at home? You can create something called a soap-bleach shampoo cocktail. To lift out some of the color, combine one packet of bleach powder to 2 ounces of shampoo (you can add an ounce of water for longer hair to help with spreadability). You mix this up and then shampoo it in and over the areas of hair where you want to reduce the color problem. Watch closely for any lifting, meaning the hair turning lighter as the wrong color leaves. You can wash it out and reapply it as often as you need to. After you're done with this step, you can apply a mid/intermediate/demi/level 2 color to lay down the color you really wanted in the first place.

Another option is **Metalex** *($10.50 for 8 ounces)* from Clairol. This hard-to-find product claims to remove problem overtones that occur from hair dyes depositing too much ash, red, copper, or lavender. Clairol claims its product can do this without "chemicals." It actually ends up working similarly to Schwarzkopf's for far less money. Metalex contains sulfonated oil, and that "strips" hair color just as the Schwarzkopf product does.

Doing It Yourself

Having colored my hair both at hair salons and at home myself, I am acutely aware of the pros and cons of both. Obviously, the main premium of getting your hair colored at a salon is that you don't have to do it yourself. Someone else is putting up with the mess, application worries, timing, cleanup, stained towels, rinsing, and final styling. The stylist also takes the fall if there are any problems, and problems are almost guaranteed. At home all the details are yours and yours alone. You may have seen statistics quoting that 70 percent of women who color their hair at home are disappointed with the results. That is a bogus statistic being generated by companies who sell hair-salon products. The truth is, statistics indicate that women are equally disappointed about the results of a dyed hair color whether it is done at home or at a salon.

If you decide to do this at home, it is important to get an application system in place. That can make everything go more smoothly with less room for error. Women who are about to attempt coloring their hair at home or who already do but don't have a comfortable system down yet might want to try the following modus operandi:

- If you have **permed hair, do not consider highlighting** or an extreme hair color change. That is only asking for trouble.
- Don't proceed with an all-over hair color until you've done a **strand test and a patch test for allergic reaction.**
- If you are highlighting or hair painting, preselect the areas you want to color. Having a game plan ahead of time can prevent mistakes and disappointments.
- **Assemble everything you need.** You can keep a carrying tray with all the things you need on it, including hair clips, extra plastic gloves, a comb with a pointed end (typically called a rat-tail comb), a small portable clock, hand mirror, comb, portable radio, scented candle, magazines, an extra package of dye in case you run out, and, depending on the product type, a small pair of scissors. A comfortable chair you don't mind getting stained will ensure you have a place to sit other than the edge of the bathtub or the toilet seat. Purchase a **hose extension** for your sink or tub so you don't have to get your head under an awkward faucet.
- Now that you are organized, the following steps will help get the job done efficiently and pleasantly.

- **Make sure your hair doesn't have a buildup of styling products on it, particularly waxes or pomades that heavily coat hair and can prevent the dye from penetrating.**
- Choose the bathroom with the **best light and largest mirror.** For mid/intermediate/demi/level 2 and permanent hair dyes, use the bathroom with the best ventilation. Even nonammonia products can have unpleasant fumes.
- Set up a small **portable clock** on a shelf that is clearly visible.
- Take four to six towels that won't cause you stress if they get stained, and arrange them on the floor and over the countertop.
- Take a large portable mirror (an inexpensive, lightweight one is best) and place it directly across from the mirror you will be facing so the back of your hair is clearly visible with only minor head adjustments.
- Apply **Vaseline or thick cold cream** to your hairline; this prevents the dye from staining your skin or causing irritation on the face.
- Put on an **old lightweight outfit** that won't cause you stress if it gets stained.
- Use a pair of **good latex gloves** from the drugstore. The plastic gloves that come packaged with hair dyes tear easily.
- Before you get started, inform your family or roommates that you are not to be bothered for the next hour or so and they better use the bathroom now if they need to.
- Light the **scented candle** (this isn't for lighting purposes; the candle is to keep the chemical scent at a minimum and set a pleasant mood), turn on your favorite radio station, set the chair in the most convenient position, and get ready to begin.
- If this is a touch-up application, **section the hair** with clips into five or six different areas to keep your product application organized. Release one area at a time and work only with that section, separating the hair into quarter- to half-inch parts. **Apply the color to the roots using a finger to spread the color up on the gray areas.**
- If this is a first-time application, start with the same sectioning process but work the color through to the ends.
- Be patient with the back area. That's what the mirror behind you is for. You should be able to apply the product and see what you are doing. It takes a while to get used to working with the mirrored image, but it is better than not seeing at all what you are doing. (Because the back area can be so tricky to do, consider having a friend help with this area.)
- Processing time varies, so **check it in 15-minute intervals.** That means wiping the hair color off of a strand of hair and checking to see if the color level is what you want.
- When you are done, if this is a touch-up, you may need to **pull the color from the roots to the ends** of your hair to obtain a color touch over that area too.

Hair that is already dyed rarely requires as much processing time as the roots, which are virgin growth. For some hair types, pulling the color through to the ends can saturate that area with too much color. If you are noticing that the length of hair is becoming darker than the root area, do not pull the color through.

- When you are finally ready to rinse the color out of your hair, take your time and try not to splash. **Rinsing thoroughly is essential.** Keep a hand towel nearby to wipe away any drippies that may get on your face or near your eyes.

- **Keep a chart** of everything you do to your hair and what the results were. Write down how long you kept the dye on the roots, how long you kept it on the ends, the name and color of the product you used, and how you felt about the results. That way, you will have a clear record of what you need to change or want to keep the same next time.

Avoiding Disasters

Fundamental obstacles can get in the way of obtaining the color you want. If any of these apply to you, be very careful about the next step you take when it comes to dyeing your hair.

Problem: The ends of your hair turned out darker than you expected.

Possible Reason: Hair that is damaged and, as a result, more porous can grab more color than virgin or undamaged hair. How can you tell if your hair is damaged? If you use heat styling implements every day, if you have been dyeing your hair on a regular basis for more than two years without trimming it every few months, if you spend a lot of time outdoors without covering your hair, or if you have a lot of split ends, you can be reasonably certain your hair is quite damaged and porous. Generally this kind of hair grabs too much color at the ends because the hair that has been around longest is always more damaged than the newer hair nearer the roots.

Solution: Before coloring your hair, heavily condition the ends that are damaged or get a haircut that trims off the ends. Conditioning agents can coat the hair shaft and prevent some absorption of the dye. You may also want to pull the color through the ends of your hair for the least amount of time, no more than five or ten minutes of the processing time, or skip this step altogether and just redo the roots but not the length of hair. You can also color the length of hair with a lighter shade of a mid/intermediate/demi/level 2 hair color to help bring out more of the highlights.

Problem: The overall hair color is darker than you expected.

Possible Reason: Aside from the explanation above, if your hair isn't damaged, you may have chosen the wrong color. Lighting in drugstores isn't the best, and we are not always as familiar with our actual hair color as we would like to think. This is one of the major shortcomings of shopping for a hair color at the drugstore. However, this can also be a problem at the hair salon, even with a very experienced hairstylist.

Color swatches are only representations of hair-color potential. Your hair's condition could be another factor. As I've said before, more porous and damaged hair absorbs more color. Also, your natural color or previously dyed color affects the color you put on each time, making the correct processing time more difficult to determine.

Solution: If you can live with the color until the next time you color your hair, work with it then and go a shade or two lighter, being sure to do a strand test. If you can't live with the color, consider seeing a hairstylist who can remove the offending hair color and hopefully add the right one. But stripping out the color is the last and least desirable move to make, because it can be so damaging to the hair. You can also follow the instructions in the section on "Getting Rid of the Color You Don't Want."

Problem: The ends of your hair turned out lighter than you expected.

Possible Reason: If your hair is seriously damaged, the color has no place to penetrate and be trapped in because the cuticle is entirely gone and the cortex is open and completely porous. When hair is this damaged, it can't grab the color, so the ends may remain lighter or darker depending on the original color of your hair and the color you were going after.

Solution: The only solution for this is to cut off the damaged ends or the entire damaged length, or to wait patiently for the hair to grow out. All the conditioner in the world cannot rebuild (or even fake the appearance of) a cuticle and cortex this damaged. If there is no place for dye to be deposited, it will just rinse right off your hair.

Problem: The hair color you used went on unevenly.

Possible Reason: If you used heavy conditioning treatments a shampoo or two before you colored or if you have heavy styling gels or hairsprays on your hair, you may have inadvertently placed an occlusive layer over the hair, blocking the penetration of the dyes. Conditioning agents such as dimethicones, proteins, collagens, elastins, mucopolysaccharides, hyaluronic acid, some oils, and petrolatum coat the hair shaft. These potent blocks keep moisture in the hair and keep things that can damage the hair out. Hair colors are one of those things conditioners can keep out. The same is true for styling products. They are designed to coat the hair shaft.

Solution: Unless your hair is very damaged, do not condition your hair, especially with heavy conditioners, for one or two shampoos before you plan to color your hair. Do not use heavy styling products a day or two before you plan to color your hair.

Another Possible Reason: You may have applied the dye unevenly.

Solution: Make sure you are sectioning your hair and applying the product in a continuous line along the part, spreading it with your finger so it expands up evenly on the growout.

Problem: The hair color you chose seems to have given you too many red highlights.

Possible Reason: Most women with medium to dark brown and black hair, and some women with light brown or blonde hair, have naturally red pigments in their hair they weren't aware of. As a result, they may end up with reddish highlights they weren't counting on when they color their hair. This occurs most frequently with shampoo-in or single-step hair-coloring products. There just isn't enough peroxide in these products to lift the natural reddish color out of the hair. You may have also chosen a color that provides red highlights when you really didn't need any.

Solution: If you want to avoid red highlights, be very careful to choose hair colors described as ashy or golden. That should take care of the problem.

Problem: The hair color you chose has too many ash or drab highlights.

Possible Reason: If you chose a lead acetate progressive dye product, it can leave a greenish cast on the hair. For other dyes, you may have chosen a hair color that was too drab. This often happens when you overreact to the concern of making your hair too red and then decide on a color with a strong ash tone.

Solution: Avoid drab colors. In the meantime, use a semipermanent or mid/intermediate/demi/level 2 dye that has just a hint of red or a neutral tone. That can help improve the situation. The next time you dye your hair, think about colors with a bit more red or copper colors.

Problem: You followed the directions exactly, took time to match your natural hair color exactly, yet a good deal of the gray you were trying to cover was still there when you were done.

Possible Reason: You used the wrong type of hair-coloring product. Temporary hair colors barely cover any gray; semipermanent hair colors realistically cover no more than 10 to 20 percent gray, and even then not well. Mid/intermediate/demi/level 2 hair dyes can only cover up to 50 percent gray, and that depends on how you are graying. If you have concentrated patches or areas of gray, you need to use a permanent hair color.

Solution: Rethink your product choice and consider a permanent hair color next time you color your hair, but wait about two weeks to a month before you jump in and do another chemical process on your hair. You may also not have left the color on long enough. Most product instructions recommend the shortest amount of time. Healthy hair may take longer to grab the color than the minimum time listed. Of course, you did remember to do a strand test, didn't you?

Problem: You finally gave in and used a permanent hair color to cover the gray, but it didn't work and the gray is still evident.

Possible Reason: Permanent hair color can be a big step for some women, and the fear of causing damage may have made you overly cautious so you didn't leave the color on long enough. Gray hair can be pretty resistant, so be patient.

Solution: Let the dye stay on for up to 50 minutes to cover the gray. What would work best is for you to leave it on for the same amount of time as the strand test took to develop the color you want.

Problem: The color you chose looked a shade or two lighter than your hair color on the box, but you ended up with a color much darker than you expected.

Possible Reason: If your hair is porous, damaged, previously color-treated, thin, fine, or permed, it can grab the color quickly, making it darker in spite of the color on the box.

Solution: Certain hair types require shorter processing times than others, and you probably didn't do a strand test. If you did and still didn't get the expected results, you may have tested an area of hair (usually from the nape of the neck) that was healthier than the rest of your hair and produced a different outcome. If your hair is naturally porous, damaged, repeatedly color-treated, thin, fine, or permed, you will want to reduce the amount of time the color stays on your hair. Keep in mind that different sections of hair can have different timing requirements. You may want to consider *two* strand tests if you think this may be your particular circumstance.

Problem: Your hairline always ends up darker or too red after you dye your hair.

Possible Reason: The hair around your face may have a finer, thinner texture than the rest of the hair, making it more susceptible to grabbing the color.

Solution: If you don't want to change the color of the hair at the hairline (given that there's no gray in this area), you can protect the hairs around your face with a thick face moisturizer, thick hair conditioner, Vaseline, or a cold cream like Abolene. The goal is to cover the hair with something that will keep the dyes off that area, and one of those should do the job. If the hairline has gray that you want to cover, apply the hair dye over this area 15 minutes after you apply it to the rest of your hair. The fine hair in this area probably needs less time to process.

Problem: The hair around your face shows gray roots sooner than the hair on your head.

Possible Reason: Gray hair has no rhyme or reason; it grows wherever it wants to. Some women gray at the crown first, some at the hairline, while others gray randomly in strands all over the head. If you gray at the hairline, it will be more obvious as soon as you have any growout.

Solution: There is no reason not to dye just the hair around your hairline as soon as you see the gray, particularly if you are doing it at home yourself. That's true for any area that shows gray faster than elsewhere, such as a specific heavy patch of gray. Simply apply the hair color to the precise spots only and process as usual without pulling the color through to the ends. However, you can also use brow mascaras over the hairline, or pencils like Origins **Change Your Locks** *($14)*. This pencil is applied wet and nicely covers the gray at the hairline.

Problem: For some reason your permanently dyed hair is fading, but you don't want to dye it again for another two weeks.

Possible Reason: The more porous, damaged, or gray the hair is, the more likely it is to fade. This is especially true in the summer or for outdoor enthusiasts, but it can happen any time of year if your hair is very gray. Gray hair and shades of red dye, and some shades of blonde fade more quickly and may require a longer processing time than you have been using, or a stronger depth of color (instead of a soft strawberry blonde, go with a more vivid red shade). You may also be grayer than you think, and that may require you to use a longer processing time or a stronger dye (permanent/level 3 instead of mid/intermediate/demi/level 2). Additionally, dyed hair just tends to fade. There is no way around this one.

Solution: Color-enhancing shampoos, temporary colors, and semipermanent colors are great ways to extend the time between recoloring your hair, and they can conceal the fading. But be careful not to use these products in the last shampoo or two before you color your hair again. The dyes from these temporary coloring products lie on the hair shaft and can block the absorption of your normal hair-coloring product. Also, if your hair has become grayer over the years and you've noticed increased fading, you may want to do a strand test and see if your hair now requires a longer processing time.

Problem: Your hair is extremely damaged from being dyed blonde and you don't want to damage it any more, but it is in desperate need of coloring.

Possible Reason: Hair gets damaged mostly by brushing and by styling with blow-dryers or curling irons, but absolutely the most harmful thing you can do to the hair is to repeatedly dye it with a two-step coloring process. Turning darker hair blonde, particularly if you are keeping it long, destroys hair when done repeatedly to maintain the color.

Solution: There isn't an easy solution for this problem because there is no way to prevent further damage to the hair when you use a two-step dye on it. You can try temporary or semipermanent dyes until the damage grows out, but those products have extremely limited coverage. Growing out the damage and starting again is sometimes the only answer. Otherwise you will just be compounding the problem, never allowing the healthy roots to come out and shine. Your only options are to cut off the damage and go short. Then when you redye your hair, consider a less dramatic hair-color difference.

Problem: You hate the hair color you ended up with when you dyed your hair.

Possible Reason: You either went after too extreme a change or you misjudged your natural hair color or the color of your dyed hair versus the color of your roots. Often women think their hair is darker than it is or they choose a darker color because they think it will look more dramatic or cover gray better. It's also possible you left the color on too long.

Solution: This is a difficult situation, because you'll want to run out and try another color to get rid of the one you hate. But you can't just dye the hair a different color over a permanent hair color. First, the wrong hair color must be removed or lifted with bleach, and then a different color can be added. Review the section above on "Getting Rid of the Color You Don't Want."

While you are getting used to the process of dyeing your hair, it is best to start out with mid/intermediate/demi/level 2 dyes to get a sense of how different colors look on your hair. These semi-noncommittal hair dyes wash out after a period of time, so the risk of making a mistake is minimal. Once you find the color you are most comfortable with, you can start using permanent hair colors. You did remember to do a strand test, didn't you?

Problem: You tried dyeing your hair red, but it just looks brown.

Possible Reason: If your hair is damaged or porous, the hair might not have been able to hold on to the red dye.

Solution: Next time you dye your hair, choose a color that has more red in it. Be sure to do a strand test so you know exactly how this new color is being taken up by the hair.

Problem: You've been coloring your hair at the salon and you want to change to a drugstore product.

Possible Reason: It's getting too expensive or too difficult to schedule. You've also noticed that your friends who color their hair at home look pretty good, and you're tired of the expensive coloring mistakes that happen at the salon.

Solution: First, ask your stylist what coloring product and color he or she has been using on your hair. With that information in hand, you can call the consumer hot line of the drugstore product you are thinking of trying. This is the best way to avoid mistakes. Revlon, L'Oreal, and Clairol all have highly trained advisors who will direct you to the right product, color, and instructions for your specific situation.

Problem: Whenever you color your hair, you end up with dye under your fingernails or on your skin.

Possible Reason: Keeping those gloves on is difficult when you're trying to do two things at once. Also, the gloves often tear and you might not notice until you are almost done.

Solution: You can double up on the gloves, wearing two pair, instead of one, or—even better—use plastic or latex gloves you buy at the drugstore instead of the gloves that come packaged in the hair-coloring kits. If you still have problems, there are products on the market designed to lift the color off the skin or from under the nails, such as **Revlon Roux's Clean Touch.**

How Much Gray Coverage?

If you want to color your hair to cover gray, you should know how much gray you have before selecting any hair-coloring product. The percentage of gray affects the coverage of the various kinds of hair color.

How do you know how gray you are? Single gray strands that pop up individually in no discernible concentration mean you are probably somewhere between 5 and 15 percent gray. Temporary and semipermanent hair dyes are perfect for you and can create an incredible highlight effect by turning the gray a lovely shade of copper or golden brown. If you have a discernible amount of gray woven through your hair but it still appears to be random and in no specific concentration, you are probably about 20 to 40 percent gray, and mid/intermediate/demi/level 2 hair colors should cover the gray nicely, with no discernible growout. If your gray hair is quite noticeable, or grows in clumps or in one area more than another, you are probably more than 50 percent gray. At this point the mid/intermediate/demi/level 2 hair colors won't work to cover your gray, and you will need to turn to a permanent hair color.

Most-Asked Questions

Can I mix colors to get the exact shade I want? You can only mix colors from within the same line an although it can be tricky, some women are quite good at it. Absolutely *never* mix colors between product lines! The nuances between lines can negatively react to cause a hair disaster.

Do conditioners or botanicals in hair dyes make them better for my hair? Conditioners in hair dyes can make the hair feel better after being processed, but a product that contains conditioners isn't inherently better for the hair than one that doesn't. Botanicals don't improve a hair-coloring product in any way, and the little fragrance packets that are mixed in are useless and don't improve the end results. In order for a hair color to do what it has to do, the dye must get into the hair and stay there. That process takes chemicals, and those chemicals can damage the hair. Hair-color manufacturers do not use ingredients that block the chemicals that allow penetration of the hair dye. The only way to prevent the damage from the chemical assault on a hair shaft is to keep the chemicals off, not add natural ingredients to the mixture.

How can I keep my hair color from looking fake? Most pros suggest going one or two shades lighter instead of darker. Darker hair colors tend to look unnatural and fake. Also, the more dramatic the change, the less realistic the hair color will look. If it's too light or too dark, going too long between color treatments makes the roots stand out, which always makes any hair color look fake. In some circles, roots are considered a fashionable alternative to, and I quote, "looking like you're a slave to fashion." Now that's a creative rationale if I've ever heard one! I'm not in the circle that believes roots look natural.

Why do I have to turn gray in the first place? It's genetically predetermined. There is nothing you can do to slow or change the inevitable.

How can I be more blonde without using anything extreme on my hair? It depends on what you mean by extreme. If you just want to be one shade lighter than you are, semipermanent dyes are the most gentle way to achieve that result. If you want to become two shades lighter, mid/intermediate/demi/level 2 dyes are the best choice with the least impact on the hair. If you want to change your hair color by several shades in order to be blonde, even with special effects, there is no way to achieve that without a good deal of damage. That much change requires stripping, bleaching, or removing your own natural hair color from the cortex, then adding the blonde color you want.

The light in drugstores is terrible; I feel like I'm poking around in the dark trying to match my hair color. Is there anything I can do to discern the color better? Great question, but I don't think the answer is too great. It is probably best to shop for a new hair color only during the daytime. Take a few color possibilities that you are interested in and ask the store clerk if you can take the boxes outside and check them in the daylight. Other than that, there is no way to compensate for store light—or the light in the hair salon either. If your hairstylist is choosing a new color for you, check the hair samples in the daylight.

CHAPTER SIX

Perfectly Straight or Perfectly Curly

What About Perms and Relaxers?

No one will be shocked when I say that permanent waves (and hair relaxers, which are essentially permanent waves with a different name and shaping technique) are not permanent, because they do not affect new growth. Ultimately, this impermanence isn't a problem because you can just have another perm to take care of the growout. As easy as this sounds, in the long run, it isn't easy on the hair at all. I hope that by the end of this chapter I will have convinced you to consider a perm or hair relaxer only as a last resort for creating fullness and curl or removing curl and making hair straighter. Any chemical process that permanently alters hair is damaging. The condition of your hair is dependent on the cuticle and cortex being undisturbed and whole. When you permanently reform the shape and texture of the cuticle and cortex, you inevitably end up with damage. Drastically altering the shape and texture of the hair (taking very straight or very curly hair and processing it) means you end up with drastic damage. There is no way around this one no matter what the pros say to defend themselves.

If you decide to try a permanent wave or relaxer, then my heartfelt suggestion is to get it done at the hair salon and not at home. It's not that permanent waves or hair relaxers from a salon are any better than the ones you buy at the drugstore—these products are all the same whether they are purchased at a drugstore or performed at a hair salon. The issue is one of risk during the processing procedure and how the hair is manipulated. Wind the hair too tightly around the rod for the curly perms, and you can loose chunks of hair; comb hair in the wrong direction for a relaxer, and you can also destroy hair, or leave the chemicals on too long, and you can end up with burns and hair loss. Seeing an experienced professional reduces your risk immeasurably over doing this yourself.

How They Work

Your hair's natural, permanent shape is held tightly in place by the arrangement of the hair's protein structure in combination with an extensive, complex matrix of other lipids, fatty acids, and other organic and inorganic matter. Protein is assembled like a twisting ladder throughout the hair shaft. Disulfide bonds are the strongest links of this protein ladder. These disulfide bonds hold the hair in its normal configuration. In order to change the shape of your hair, the disulfide bonds must be broken, reformed, and put back together. Reforming and putting the bonds back together isn't the difficult part of a perm; rather, what's so troublesome for the hair is what it takes to break the disulfide bonds.

Disulfide bonds are incredibly strong and difficult to break down. It takes serious chemicals to modify their shape. However, after the disulfide bonds have been softened and split, they are then capable of being reformed. Varying substances are used to achieve the desired results. Permanents meant to curl hair or relaxers needed to straighten hair use similar to identical formulations.

Salon or Home Products?

I know many of you would love me to recommend the perfect at-home permanent-wave or hair-relaxer kit or the exact method for getting foolproof results, but the truth is, there aren't any. Permanent waving is hard on the hair whether it is done at the salon or at home, but doing it yourself is riskier because so many details go into creating an attractive perm that it is hard for even the most experienced technician to get all the elements right. What makes the process so difficult? Each of the following factors has to be handled very carefully: choosing the kind of permanent wave best for your particular hair type, timing the processing just right, choosing the right rods and winding the rods into the hair using the correct amount of tension, handling the endpapers, saturating the rods evenly, neutralizing the hair thoroughly, and rinsing with solutions other than water before neutralizing. Like I said, it's complicated.

But one more warning before you make a final decision. Perhaps the most important thing an ethical hairdresser can do is to honestly explain when you are not a good candidate for a perm. If you have damaged hair, particularly if it has been dyed from black or brown to blonde, is blonded from sun exposure, or is extremely thin and fragile, you are not someone who should be having a perm. It cannot be stressed enough that perming and hair relaxing is ultimately damaging if you both color and perm your hair, even a few weeks apart from each other. All the permanent-wave kits on the market (and the ones at the salon) say you should **never** perm hair that has been double-processed, streaked, highlighted, colored with metallic dyes, or sun-damaged. I think they stop short of saying not to perm over permanent or mid/

intermediate/demi/level 2 dyed hair because that would exclude more than 36 million women, leaving a very tiny group of women to buy their products. But the absolute truth is that perming or relaxing is hard on hair, and it is ruinous if you also color it. You may not want to hear this, but it will save you a lot of heartache if you know when not to perm.

After mulling all this over, if you still think you have a knack with hair, can time all the chemical components correctly, and can implement the combing or rolling portion properly, you may indeed want to consider doing this process at home.

Are there less dire risks if you have healthy, non-color-treated hair that isn't porous, too curly, or too straight? Yes, the risks are greatly reduced (assuming, of course, the processing was done right). However, once you have your hair relaxed or curled, it is no longer healthy and you then run the same risks the next time around.

Types of Perms

There are three types of permanent waves, known as acid perms, cold (or alkaline) perms, and neutral perms. All three versions use the same steps and formulation requirements, and they are all based on sulfur chemistry. The first step is to place the hair in the position you want it to be. If you want the hair curly, rods are used to wrap the hair; if you want the hair straight, weights are used to hold the length of the hair elongated and horizontal. The wave solution (reducing agent) is then applied to break down the disulfide bonds. After a period of time, that solution is rinsed off to stop the action of the reducing agent. Finally, a neutralizing ingredient (oxidizing agent) is applied to relink the disulfide bonds.

In the various formulations that go into the making of permanent waves and hair relaxers, the ingredients sound a bit daunting. But remember that the varying components are actually not as significant as the resulting pH of the product.

Alkaline perms (also known as cold waves) use reducing agents like thioglycolic acid, sodium thioglycolate, or ammonium thioglycolate. Sodium thioglycolate is considered to be more damaging than the relatively more gentle ammonium thioglycolate (see *Hair and Hair Care*, edited by Dale H. Johnson).

For thioglycolic acid, using the term *alkaline perms* may sound like a contradiction. After all, how can an acid ingredient like thioglycolic acid produce an alkaline solution? Despite the acid name, the pH of the perm is still high. In order for the thioglycolic acid and the other alkaline perming ingredients to affect the disulfide bonds, the final solution is always alkaline, with a pH of 10 to 14. Most all hair relaxers for women of color are this kind of perm, with a pH of 13 to 14.

Acid perms utilize a derivative of thioglycolic acid called glyceryl monothioglycolate. This ingredient is effective at a lower pH of around 8 to 9. It is the difference these two or three pH points makes that contributes the names *acid* to glyceryl monothioglycolate (which is effective at a pH of 8) and *cold or alkaline waves* to thioglycolic acid (which is effective at a pH of 9 to 10).

While the lower pH of the acid perm is indeed less damaging to the hair than the alkaline version, the acid type is also less effective.

Neutral or bisulfite perms are even milder and less effective than acid perms. Bisulfite perms use sodium sulfite to effect a change in the bonds of hair. Bisulfite does break down the disulfide bonds of hair at a lower pH than both the acid and cold-wave perms, but due to the mildness of these perms, they don't work very well and are inadequate to make much change in the shape of the hair.

For hair relaxers, the difference is generally the level of pH used. Relaxers usually involve the use of sodium hydroxide, ammonium hydroxide, or guanidine hydroxide, with these products having a very high pH of 13. Obviously, these reducing agents are far more aggressive and far more damaging to the hair, but they are also far more capable of changing a very tight curl to a looser version.

There are hair relaxers that make claims of being effective at extremely low pHs (see the section in Chapter Seven, *For African-American Women*), but their low pH of 3 to 3.5 does not affect the shape of hair in any way like the higher-pH products do. Plus, the notion that a pH of 3 isn't at all damaging to hair is not substantiated (there is very little research on this issue). A pH of 3 is quite acid and can theoretically denature hair.

How to Choose

The more resilient the hair, the stronger the perm needs to be, and the stronger perms are alkaline or cold-wave ones. But a stronger perm that is not watched carefully or is used on damaged, porous, or color-treated hair can cause frizzy, broken-down, mushy hair. If you just want extra body, softer curls, or less-than-complete straightening, you can use a more gentle perm such as an acid or bisulfite perm. All at-home perm kits are grouped by hair type or shape preference (soft curl, tight curl, or straightened): thin, fragile, or color-treated; hard-to-curl; normal; and soft body wave are the most typical classifications. These categories are fairly accurate determinants of how your hair will react with the permanent-wave solution.

Alkaline waves are the best choice for perm-resistant hair (such as stick-straight hair or thick, heavy hair), resistant gray hair, Asian hair, generally hard-to-perm fine hair, and normal, healthy hair. Types of alkaline or cold-wave perms are: **Ogilvie Conditioning Home Perm and Lilt Foam** and, in the salon market, **Helene Curtis Luxuriance, Tressa Full Cycle,** and **Zotos Design Freedom.**

Alkaline perms that incorporate heat are used for even more stubborn hair than the types listed above. These include **Precisely Right by Ogilvie** (available at drugstores) and, in salons, **Zotos Feels So Lively, Matrix Therma Vantage,** and **Helene Curtis Even Heat.**

There are no acid waves available at the drugstore. It isn't clear why this is so, but perhaps it's due to their odor or reduced performance. Acid waves are milder than alkaline perms; because they work at a lower pH, they cause less swelling of the hair during the perm process, thus reducing the chance of damage to fragile or thinner hair types. The acid waves available at the salon are **Helene Curtis Quantum; Zotos Acclaim; Tressa Clientage, Pliance,** or **Full Cycle;** and **Matrix Opticurl.**

Bisulfite perms are rarely used and there are actually very few of these on the market. They don't take well and the result is minimal curl or hardly any straightening. If you are interested in bisulfite perms, **L'Oreal Curl Free** and **Ogilvie Whisper Wave** are options. (See the review for Copa hair-straightening products in Chapter Seven, *For African-American Women.*)

Alkaline or cold-wave perms are by far more popular than acid waves due to the quality results they provide. Alkaline perms and alkaline relaxers create the results most women are seeking. Acid perms are far less effective, but if the consumer isn't looking for extremely straight or extremely curly hair, they are an option to consider. Bisulfite perms are even less effective than the acid waves and therefore far less useful for those looking to change the structure of their hair.

For hair relaxers, see Chapter Seven, *For African-American Women.*

The Process

Once a product type is chosen, depending on the final results desired, the hair is either combed straight or curled around rods to fashion it in the intended shape. To say that the wrapping process for permanent waves or the combing method for hair relaxers is of vital importance is absolutely an understatement! Keep in mind that wrapping the hair around the right-size roller is critical. Winding the rods and papers evenly and symmetrically—not too tight or too loose—all over your head, or alternating the various-size rods to get the best look for your hair type and haircut, is a complicated, precise creation. For hair relaxers, the combing procedure is crucial, and combing in the wrong direction can cause problems.

After the hair is prepared, the reducing solution is poured over the hair and left there for a period of time, allowing the disulfide bonds to become malleable. Time is the key here. Some hair is stubborn and doesn't take to the solution very well, requiring more processing time, while other hair is more pliant and easier to reshape, requiring less processing time. For those with earlier damage, the hair soaks up the alkaline solution like a sponge, causing the hair to practically dissolve. This is particularly true for African-American women who repeatedly perm their hair (and color it) and then use high-heat curling irons to create straight hairdos. This amount of damage is a disaster in the making.

When the processing time is up, a neutralizer is used (often hydrogen peroxide or potassium bromate formulated at a low pH) to stop the reducing solution from doing its thing on the hair. Now the disulfide bonds realign, hopefully into the new style dictated by the size, placement, and number of rods used or the combing method used for the now-straightened contour of the hair.

The Rods

OK, you've decided you can handle all the steps I've listed and you still want to do your perm at home. You must consider other issues I haven't discussed yet. There are different techniques for rolling the rods. You can do a root perm if you want fullness at the roots only and not all over. In that case, only the root of the hair is rolled and the rest of the hair is covered in a thick cream or conditioner to prevent contact with the solution. You can create a spiral or ringlet effect if you place the rods at an angle to the head instead of parallel. The number of rods used is also a factor in the perm you get. Too few rods, and the hair will not take on an attractive shape or the perm will not hold well. Do you want me to go on? OK, but only a few more warnings.

The thickness of the individual strands of hair plays a major role in how fast the perm solution is absorbed by the hair. The thicker the hair shaft, the more time is needed for processing; the thinner the hair shaft, the less the processing time. If the hair is also porous, the processing time must be reduced because porous hair absorbs the chemicals faster.

No matter how you look at it, perming is complicated, and I just don't have the heart to send you to the drugstore to risk your lovely tresses. It is enough of a risk at the hair salon.

Checking and Timing

Once you have chosen the right perm for your hair type and the type of results you desire, placed the right rods uniformly on your head with the endpapers wrapped correctly, and applied the solution evenly, you must check the perm at ten-minute intervals to see how it is taking the curl or how the straightening process is being set in (this is true both at home and at the salon). Undo a rod and test curled hair for buoyancy, or manipulate straightened hair to test for retention.

Some perm products are designed with their own internal "stopwatch." These products complete the processing of the chemical reactions within a set period of time. This is done to minimize the risk of overprocessing the hair, which can mean disaster. However, the inherent problem with this kind of product is self-evident: How does the product know when your hair is done? If the product's preset processing time is 30 minutes but your hair needs 20 minutes or 40 minutes, you're out of luck.

Many hair-care companies make a great to-do about how you can use products to prep the hair before or after you perm or relax. The truth is, you can't prevent damage other than by using products judiciously and with skill. However, after you're done, it absolutely helps to reduce dryness by using emollient conditioners, although none of these will change or alter the damage one iota!

CHAPTER SEVEN

For African-American Women

Somewhere in the Bible it say Jesus' hair was like lamb's wool, I say. Well, say Shug, if he came to any of these churches we talking 'bout, he'd have to have it conked before anybody paid him any attention. The last thing [folks 'round here] want to think about they God is that his hair is kinky.

Alice Walker, *The Color Purple*

A Different Point of View

When the first edition of this book was published, I was surprised at the response it received. Women were either thrilled with the information, finding it confirmed what they already suspected was true, or appalled that I would suggest some of the things I did. I am used to hair-care companies being disturbed by my research and conclusions, but why would women take me to task for what the scientific literature proves to be true? It was like someone was shooting the messenger.

For women the world over, hair is a very emotional issue. I want to be very respectful of this. I will do my best to present the information in as straightforward and nonjudgmental a way as I can. However, there is nothing I can do about the genetic fragility of African hair. Nor can I do anything about the fact that trying to change extremely curly, fine hair to straight hair can cause serious damage and balding. I also can't change the fact that braids and tightly woven braids or cornrowing can cause hair loss and bald spots. I wish it were otherwise, but the evidence is clear to anyone in the African-American community, and it is poignantly clear to the dermatologists and hairstylists who have to deal with the aftermath of these contemporary hair fashions.

The Kitchens

For African-American women, the term "kitchen(s)" is well known. If a black woman has long hair, more often than not, the hair at the nape of the neck tends to be a jangled, tangled group of knots that is almost impossible to comb through. This snarly area is referred to as the kitchens. How did it get this name? While many black women knew the term, it took some time to find someone who knew the history behind it. According to several women I spoke to, the term *kitchens* seems to have originated from how African-Americans used to style their hair before the advent of electricity. Hairstyling was done in the kitchen in order to conveniently use the stove to heat up the curling irons, combs, and hot oil that were used to smooth through and straighten hair. The most difficult part was struggling with this area of hair at the nape of the neck. For young children the notion of going to the kitchen and getting your hair done was a painful one, especially when you got to the back of the neck.

The kitchen was also associated with other disagreeable hairstyling techniques. In many ways, going to the kitchen for hair care could even be frightening. Using hot oil with a hot comb was a popular way of mechanically straightening black hair prior to the turn of the last century. The hotter the oil, the longer it would stay hot on the hair. Hotter temperatures help make the hair as straight as possible when a hot comb is run through it. To say the least, this wasn't an easy process. Hot oil could easily drip onto the skin, causing serious burns. If it got on the scalp, a frequent occurrence, it would leave a scar that could prevent hair growth in that area. It was clearly a matter of history and slang that coupled the location of the kitchen as a hair salon with the most frustrating part of styling hair.

What makes this folklore significant is the notion that African Americans have been grappling with their hair for quite some time. As writer Veronica Chambers in the June 1998 issue of *Vogue* explained, "Because I am a black woman, I have always had a very complicated relationship with my hair . . . the politics of hair and beauty in the black community [is that] . . . 'Good' hair is straight and, preferably, long . . . 'Bad' hair is thick and coarse, a.k.a. 'nappy' and often short."

It is not easy to follow fashion trends and the pressure to have hair that is 180 degrees from what is predetermined genetically. It is especially arduous when obtaining the desired results can cause damage and the upkeep generates a lot of trouble and inconvenience. As Chambers described it, "The sound of a hot comb crackling as it makes its way through a thick head of hair makes me feel at home; the smell of hair burning is the smell of black beauty emerging like a phoenix from metaphorical ashes." Chambers's article continues to explain why she finally eschewed hair straightening or cropped hairdos for dreadlocks.

Suffice it to say that the natural state of black hair is currently not an acceptable fashion statement for women of color. Even if it were, unless black hair is kept short, it isn't easy to work with. Meanwhile, the quest for smooth hair can be a never-ending problem that causes hair to become brittle, broken, and mushy, and scalps to be dry, flaky, and itchy. Over and above the issues of hair and scalp problems, there's the excessive amount of time, trouble, and expense it takes to deal with the styling. I doubt there is going to be a return to the short "Afro" anytime in the near future, but hopefully there are some beautiful alternatives to straight hair that just might be an option for women of color. It definitely can save hair, time, and money while reducing the number of products necessary to take care of the destruction that chemical processes leave in their wake.

The following information is not meant as a treatise on fashion or style. Every woman needs to decide for herself what she is comfortable with and how she wants to approach her beauty needs. Through a good deal of research, I've uncovered some fascinating hair facts and I try to present that information as concisely as I can. What you determine for yourself is certainly a personal decision, but hopefully that decision is based on reality and not the hype and hope concocted by an industry that has, more often than not, avoided telling consumers the truth about its products.

Struggling with Nature

Most African-American hair is exceptionally fragile and delicate. Each bend, curve, and coil of African-American hair is a weak link that is likely to break even before it's been touched, let alone styled. Unlike any other hair type, it is prone to breakage and damage whether or not braids are twisted into the tresses, hot irons are pressed through to flatten out the kinks, or straightening products are used to permanently generate smooth, shiny locks. Of course, any of those procedures make matters worse. To facilitate and atone for the damage caused by the straightening process, the ethnic hair-care market is overflowing with product choices. The statistics are nothing less than mind-boggling. African-Americans buy more than 37 percent of all hair-care products, even though they comprise only 15 percent of the population and wash their hair, on average, no more than once every seven days (compared to Caucasians and Asians, who wash their hair an average of four to five times a week). With all that buying power and product selection, there should be a plethora of great options for creating attractive hairstyles for African-American women. Yet nothing could be further from the truth, at least in terms of healthy hair options.

Many of the products and hairstyles designed for African-American hair are unsuitable for that kind of hair. Even if the chemical processes used to straighten black hair weren't severely damaging, they would still be intolerable for African-American hair. African-American hair can barely survive simple brushing. Yet the ads in magazines aimed at black women suggest that all it takes is a change of shampoo, conditioner, perm, or relaxer for the hair to appear resilient and bouncy, without any negative side effects. That is absolutely not the case, and in fact it is physiologically impossible. In truth, the options are limited; there are no perms or relaxers that can make fragile African-American hair smooth without causing serious damage (and there are assuredly no all-natural or even partly natural ones either). To top it all off, a great number of the products designed to correct or at least alleviate the damage caused by hair straightening, such as pomades, greases, and oils, can create even more problems.

Somewhere along the way, the cultural myth that greased-up, oiled, slicked-down hair was healthier hair became the norm for many black women. Too often, product after product for black hair is just another version of grease or oil. Yet all the grease, oil, and emollients in the world won't produce longer, thicker, or healthier hair. It simply is not possible. If anything, just the opposite is true. Grease and oil can clog hair follicles. What happens when follicles get blocked? The circulation is literally choked off and, as a result, the natural hair growth can become stunted. The products used most frequently by black women to handle the consequences of hair straightening or hot combing are the very ones that can hamper hair growth, causing the hair to eventually become more fragile, weak, brittle, and damaged.

Shampooing and Conditioning

To complicate matters, because black women typically wash their hair once every seven days, the grease and oil often sit on the scalp for long periods of time. The oil holds down the skin cells that would normally be shed from the scalp, which, along with the grease, can cause a flaky, oily-looking scalp. The need to shed those skin cells is even greater when the hair has been chemically straightened. Any chemical process can temporarily dry out (actually burn) the scalp, which results in more skin cells that need to come off. But what usually takes place after a chemical process is the application of hair treatments that grease up the dried-out scalp and fried hair. Just when the scalp needs to breathe and exfoliate, it gets suffocated with grease.

When I read ingredient lists on many specialty hair-care products designed for African-American women, I just want to cringe. Petrolatum, lanolin, waxes, oils, wax-like minerals, and emollients fill almost each and every one. While those can be good for the hair shaft (though there are lighter-weight ingredients, such as silicones, that can produce the same effect with far less stickiness or greasy feel), they are terrible for the scalp.

Strangely, despite the need to effectively remove these emollient conditioners from the scalp, the fact is that most shampoos designed for women of color are usually mild, so as not to dry out the hair or scalp further. That means the emollients in the hair-treatment products are not getting washed off properly. Leaving any amount of grease on the scalp for long periods of time causes problems for hair growth.

Perhaps the most disastrous beauty advice directed at African-American women is to wash their hair as infrequently as possible. If it weren't for this dilemma of choking off the hair follicle, I would agree that less is better, because the more often you wash the hair, the more often you have to restyle it with curling irons, hot combs, and blow-dryers, and the more you style and manipulate hair, especially African-American hair, the more you damage it (which is the very reason for the reduced frequency of shampooing).

Unfortunately, the trade-off isn't a viable option. Taking more time between shampoos might leave a style in place longer, but if the hair-care products used are loaded with grease, and many of them are, it renders the hair sticky and greasy with split ends sticking out in a fuzzy mess, makes hair mat together in sections, and creates real potential for increased dandruff-like flakes. Washing the hair at least once every three to four days is probably the best way to keep the scalp and hair healthy, along with choosing a hairstyle that requires the least amount of manipulation. Hair that is washed more frequently and styled carefully can have more movement, look less matted and greasy, and stay healthiest in the long run. Styling carefully is the crux of the matter, and that means you must rethink how the hair is handled.

Before You Relax

The first thing you need to know is that smoothing out tightly curled hair is relatively safe when the hair has some strength to it. Most African-American hair types can't really survive an extreme straightening process for which the goal is to get the hair "Whitney Houston" straight. Any chemical straightening process that takes longer than 20 minutes is excessive for most hair types. Also, many hair relaxers for African-American women have extremely high pHs, somewhere between 12 to 13. This can burn the scalp and skin and fry the hair if left on too long. Damage may not be evident the first time the hair is straightened, but any subsequent straightening after several weeks of growout will leave the hair begging for mercy. Add styling with overly heated hot combs and curling irons to that and, in time, you won't have even a close facsimile of the soft, bouncy, smooth hair you were hoping for.

I know I'm not telling the African-American women reading this book anything they haven't heard before or don't know from experience. But while the idea of only using a chemical process that takes no longer than 20 to 25 minutes and preferably contains lower pHs (usually found in perms for Caucasian or Asian hair) instead of highly alkaline perms is hardly new, it isn't mentioned or followed very often. It is the only alternative to the same old merry-go-round of burnt, greased-up, stiff-looking hair.

That means that a texturizing perm, as opposed to a hair-straightening perm, is the safest, healthiest, and easiest alternative for fragile African-American hair. Texturizing perms can create curls with fullness, length, softness, and bounce, and cause the least amount of damage. If you decide to go this route, remember to have a texturizing perm only once every three months; any more often than that and you're back at the beginning with baked-to-a-crisp hair. I know this isn't an easy suggestion. To get to the point of doing a texturizing perm, you must grow out the damage you already have or cut it off and let it grow out. You can't do a texturizing perm over a straightening perm. The hair will rebel and break off. Growing out damaged hair is a painful experience for any woman, but once you get through it, the hassle of struggling with your hair may be over forever.

To help minimize the possible risks of perming, you should evaluate your hair for yourself. Before you choose a perm, pull out three strands of hair from the root from various areas of your head. Hold the hair tightly between two fingers and tug gently. If two of the three strands break, your hair is in no condition for any kind of perm. Another variation of this test that can help determine what kind of perm your hair can handle is to take a strand of hair and run your nails over it in a pinching fashion, as if you were curling a ribbon. Again, if two of the three strands break, your hair is in no condition to be permed. If the hair curls easily in a wave or curls up tightly, you can handle a stronger, high-alkaline solution (but leave it on for no more than 20 minutes). If your hair doesn't curl up much or feels inelastic, you should use a gentler perm.

Judging the length of time of the application is perhaps the most critical part of any relaxing process. To avoid damage or scalp irritation, regardless of the product, follow these guidelines:

•   If you have fine or previously damaged hair, leave the solution on for no longer than 13 minutes.

•   If you have medium strength or slightly damaged hair, leave the solution on for no longer than 15 minutes.

•   If you have coarse, resistant, and minimally damaged hair, leave the solution on for no longer than 20 minutes.

No Lye Is a Lie!

Well, at least it's a fib, depending on which products you're referring to, but even when it's true, it is meaningless for helping a consumer know if the product she's getting is going to be less damaging than another.

Lots of perms and relaxers claiming to be lye-free and, therefore, more gentle for the hair are being promoted at salons and drugstores these days, with a large number aimed at African-American consumers looking for hair relaxers. The issues here are twofold: First, is the product really "lye-free?" and two, is it better to use a lye-free product? Actually, it turns out that the lye-free claim is more a matter of marketing language than it is of any benefit to a consumer.

Traditionally and technically, lye-based perms have used sodium hydroxide. The purpose of sodium hydroxide is to raise the pH of the reducing solution since a high pH is the best and most effective way to relax hair. However, there are lots of ways to significantly raise the pH of a product without using sodium hydroxide. No-lye products often use calcium hydroxide mixed with guanidine carbonate to do the exact same thing as sodium hydroxide. Chemically, calcium hydroxide is a form of lye, and it can be irritating and damaging to hair. I know lye-free products sound like they should make your hair happier, with less damage and dryness, but that is not automatically the case!

The history of using sodium hydroxide perms and hair relaxers has not been a pleasant one because they almost guaranteed damage and scalp irritation. What African-American woman wouldn't love to believe she could have straight hair without any negative side effects. Because sodium hydroxide is perceived by the consumer as being bad for hair, the hair-care industry created a bit of a ruse to make things appear nicer, even though the pH of the product still needed to be high to be effective. It turns out that lye-free relaxers have the same high pH as most sodium hydroxide relaxers!

Don't let the hair-care industry confuse you with this one. There is no benefit to hair in a lye-free perm if the pH is high! High-alkaline perms, even though they work better than lower-pH perms, still damage hair, and misrepresenting the ingredients won't change that. The following list of hair-straightening products and their pH might curl your hair, especially the product with a pH of 14 marketed toward children!

African Pride Miracle Deep Conditioning No-Lye Relaxer System ($5.29) **pH 13; At One with Nature Botanical Strongends Sensitive Scalp Relaxer, Regular with Herbs and Moisturizers** ($6.99) **pH 14; Dark & Lovely Beautiful Beginnings No-Mistake No-Lye Children's Relaxer System** ($5.99) **pH 13; Dark & Lovely Plus Ultra-Deep Conditioning No-Lye Relaxer System** ($6.99) **pH 12; Gentle-Treatment No-Lye Conditioning Creme Relaxer, Regular for Fine or Normal Hair** ($6.99) **pH 13; Luster's Pink Conditioning Super No-Lye Creme Relaxer** ($4.99) **pH 14; Raveen No-Lye Conditioning Creme Relaxer with Multiple Conditioners** ($6.21) **pH 14; Revlon Creme of Nature No-Lye Creme Relaxer System** ($2.79) **pH 13; Revlon Fabu-Laxer Multiple Conditioning No-Lye Relaxer Kit** ($4.29) **pH 13; Soft & Beautiful Just for Me No-Lye Conditioning Creme Relaxer, Children's Formula** ($5.99) **pH 14; Soft & Beautiful Super No-Lye Conditioning Relaxer** ($7.52) **pH 14; and TCB Naturals No-Lye Relaxer, Regular with Olive Oil, Aloe, and Henna** ($5.99) **pH 14.**

The Rio Hair Disaster

A number of African-Americans are aware of the class action lawsuit against Rio Hair Naturalizer System. For those who aren't familiar with this saga, here's what happened: Going back two or three years, many women saw an infomercial for a do-it-yourself-at-home-hair relaxer called Rio Hair. The commercial claimed that, with supposedly no chemicals (it was all natural) and no muss or fuss, Rio Hair could transform tightly curled African-American hair into silky Caucasian-like hair without any kinks, dryness, breakage, oil buildup, or any of the other hair problems that can plague black women.

For any African-American woman who has coveted Oprah's bouncy, smooth, flowing locks; Phyllicia Rashad's curl-free tresses; or Janet Jackson's sexy mane, this infomercial was nothing less than mesmerizing. Even more difficult to ignore was the parade of apparently satisfied African-American women smiling as they shook their soft, pliable 'dos. How could this work, particularly sans chemicals? Is there actually a blend of plant extracts or vegetable oils that can "de-corkscrew" ultra-tight curls like no other products have before?

The answer was and still is an incontrovertible "No, it isn't possible"; there aren't any natural ingredients that can produce results like the ones shown on television. Not only did Rio products contain almost exclusively a concoction of very unnatural ingredients, the pH of the relaxer was between 1 and 2, enough to eat through hair and scalp, which is exactly what it did. The rest is FDA history.

The following information is from the FDA: "Two types of hair relaxers, valued at almost $2 million, were destroyed last fall after thousands of consumers reported problems with them. It was the largest number of complaints [the] FDA had ever received about a cosmetic product."

The destruction was one of several measures the hair products' distributor, World Rio Corp. of Los Angeles, agreed to take in a consent decree entered in the U.S. District Court for the Central District of California on September 1, 1995.

In 1994 and early 1995, more than 3,000 people reported to the FDA that their scalp itched or burned and that their hair broke off or fell out—and, in some cases, turned green—after using the Rio Hair Naturalizer System and Rio Hair Naturalizer System with Color Enhancer.

Based on the complaints and an FDA investigation, the agency alleged that the hair products were being illegally sold in the United States because the adverse effects experienced by consumers were consistent with those seen with harmful substances. The company's labeling was false. The products' labeling listed an acid pH level of 3.4, but FDA and California State analyses of the product have found a pH range below 2. In addition, FDA that alleged the labeling falsely described the products as "chemical free," even though the ingredient labels listed substances commonly recognized as chemicals.

"On Jan. 23, 1995, at FDA's request, U.S. marshals seized the entire lot of products at Product Packaging West in California. On Jan. 24, an investigator with FDA's San Francisco district office went to Addressing and Mailing to inspect the firm and found more than 8,000 cases of the Rio hair relaxers, worth about $500,000 in retail value. FDA notified the State of Nevada Division of Health, which, in turn, embargoed the products, thus preventing their sale."

Relying on the hair-care industry to give you the whole story about any product is rarely wise. Rio Hair is perhaps the extreme, but it is not the only case of blatant misinformation, lack of information, or misleading explanations about chemical content or product performance.

There are always downsides to permanently altering the hair. The more gentle the product, the less effective it is. The more caustic, the more damage it causes; but the potential for straighter hair is better. Until that changes—and there is ongoing research looking at this issue—buying into exotic claims of all-natural ingredients that give you perfect hair is about the same as trying to buy the Brooklyn Bridge.

Now There's Copa

Now, **Copa Natural Curl Release System** (*$19.95 for one application*) is the new miracle hair-straightening product being sold to African-Americans, and when you hear the claims stated in the brochure, your hair will stand up and curl: "Copa Natural Curl Release System is not a straightener, but naturally releases tightly curled hair. Curl release is not instantaneous, but a natural process which requires some patience as the Copa system works naturally with your hair's chemistry and texture. Depending on the type of hair you have (and how permeable it is) it can take from one to five applications to achieve the level of curl control you desire. In our testing, the average number of applications required was three. With each successive application you will see a difference." Doesn't that sound a lot like Rio (which also said you could perm your hair several times one after the other to receive the desired results without causing damage)?

Copa is very aware of the similarity between its product claims and that of Rio's because they take some effort to pinpoint the major differences between the two companies: "Copa uses sodium thiosulfate and Rio used acid and cupric chloride; [Rio had a] different active pH (Copa at 3.5, and Rio as low as 2; and Copa and Rio have different reactions in the hair (Rio [affected] the disulfide bonds directly and Copa has salt bonds)."

First, Rio did not use "acid." Rio used ammonium chloride, centrimonium bro-mide, and sodium thiosulfate, quite similar to Copa. Rio did have a very low pH, but the hair doesn't have something called salt bonds; the only molecular bonds that affect hair shape are disulfide bonds. If you don't break those and re-form them, you can't change the shape of hair, period. And there is nothing natural in the least about sodium thiosulfate. Rather, according to the *International Cosmetic Ingredient Dictionary and Handbook,* sodium thiosulfate is the salt form of thioglycolic acid and is "used in hair waving and hair straightening products and in depilatories." So much for being special and different.

Copa's pH of 3.5 is indeed more gentle than Rio's, but it is still low and can denature hair. The real point is that you can't gently straighten your hair. As I ex-plained above, the lower the pH, the less effective the hair-straightening product is. There is no way around this one.

For more information about Copa call (949) 474-9677.

Whatever Happened to Curly Perms?

There was a period during the 1980s when curly perms for African-Americans were all the rage. Curly perms used a process where the hair was first straightened with an alkaline hair relaxer before it was then wrapped around rods to create soft, tendril-like curls rather than stick-straight hair. The concept was great because the curls required less aftercare than straightened hair. Straightened hair requires styling tools to create the desired look, while curly hair has minimal need for any further styling time. Using fewer styling tools also means there would be less additional damage to the hair. A curly perm was a truly carefree style but, unfortunately, it had its problems, which caused the market to slowly decline to the point where this hairstyle is rarely seen. What went wrong?

Curly perms require a two-step process, and that means more damage. Each successive perm was like adding two treatments to the hair. That produced a lot of damage and dryness, despite the ease of styling. In order to maintain the softness of the curls, a good deal of hair conditioning was required. These rich, emollient products easily built up on hair, producing a notoriously greasy, oily look that eventually became fodder for African-American comedians. A major problem for curly perms also happened at the salon level. According to *Hair and Hair Care,* edited by Dale H. Johnson, "to offer economy to the hairstylists, manufacturers packaged the professional perm components in bulk sizes. The large, bulk-size cremes and lotions containing ammonium thioglycolate could not be packaged air-tight and they started to decrease in pH. . . . Therefore, at the salon level, permanent-wave products were subject to inconsistent performance." The demise of curly perms was also a result of a major fashion change for African-American women. Sleeker hairstyles became popular as more African-American models and actresses appeared in the media wearing smooth, flowing coifs.

Braiding, Cornrowing, and Weaving

Hair straightening isn't the only precarious hair fashion for African-American women. Braiding (including extensions), cornrowing, and weaving designs into the hair may be alluring, but the expense, time, growout, maintenance, and potential harm to the hair make it almost a life-altering project. On the surface, braiding appears to be a pragmatic, utilitarian option because it can be washed and requires no styling between weaves. As long as the braids aren't put in too tightly, which puts pressure on the follicle that can make the hair fall out before its time and causes thinning or bald spots, the ease of maintenance is a benefit. However, all too often, the weight of the braids and the tension put on the connecting hair causes hair to fall out. Eventually, the effects can be seen in a continually receding hairline and bald spots.

Over the past several years, there has been a trend in black hair fashion for braiding extensions to become even thicker, longer, and, therefore, heavier. This extra weight only compounds the problem of hair loss.

Again, for African-American women this is not new information—the results are blatantly obvious. Yet for some reason there is an overwhelming feeling that this is the price you pay to be fashionable. I do not set trends, but I frequently ask women to think more critically about how they allow themselves to become a slave to fashion styles that are either harmful or at the very least expensive and time consuming. What are we willing to give up, and why are we willing to give up so much, for a hairstyle? I can't answer that. This one is for the individual to think about and decide for herself what direction makes the most sense.

Back to Basics

Regardless of the hairstyle you choose, all of the following suggestions can help prevent breakage and further damage.

- As much as is realistically possible, avoid brushing the length of your hair.
- When you do brush, use the softest-bristled brush you can find. If it tugs at your hair the least little bit, it is not a good brush for your hair. Concentrate your brushing efforts on the scalp and minimally on the ends.
- Use your fingers to gently separate strands of hair and distribute the natural oil of the scalp through the hair with short, gentle, stroking motions.
- Do not run a brush through the entire length of your hair all at once.

- Massage your scalp twice a day. You can do this with your fingers or a very soft brush. Section the hair and gently stroke the scalp, then move on to the next section.
- The less pressure on the scalp, the better. Avoiding tying your hair back in tight buns or ponytails. If you set your hair on rollers, don't wind them too tightly.
- Roller sets are safer for African-American hair than heat-producing tools. If you do use rollers, set them in hair that is just beyond damp but not yet dry. This will afford a shorter setting time. Avoid rolling hair up tightly.
- Consider sleeping on a satin pillowcase instead of a cotton one. The cotton fibers cause friction, grabbing the individual hairs and breaking them.
- When drying the hair, avoid using a terry-cloth towel. The hooked weave can catch on African-American hair and break it off. Try using a towel with a smooth surface.
- When you wash your hair, concentrate on the scalp and wash in one direction only. If you tousle your hair, it can easily become knotted, making styling more difficult and encouraging breakage.
- Rather than styling the hair perfectly straight, consider a looser natural curl as an option. It takes less effort and can save your hair.
- When using a blow-dryer and a round brush, keep the heat moving over the hair; avoid keeping the heat in one place for too long.

Hair Note: A popular myth making the rounds is that pulling or tugging on the hair shaft somehow improves circulation. Where this came from is anyone's guess, but it is potentially damaging to the hair. Tugging on the hair can pull it out or break it, that's all. The only thing that improves circulation is gentle massage.

Keeping the Hair in Place

Avoid styling products that contain ingredients that clog pores and are hard to wash out, such as cocoa butter, lanolin, palmitic acid, stearic acid, myristyl myristate, and isopropyl myristate. If you do use pomades or rich cream treatments, use them sparingly, concentrating the application on the hair shaft, not the scalp. It is a waste of time to concentrate hair treatments on the scalp alone. The corkscrew shape of black hair makes it very difficult for the oil or emollients to make their way down the hair shaft. In straight or wavy hair, the oil produced by the scalp has a clear path, with few turns that prevent the hair shaft from being lubricated. In tightly curled hair, the oil has to go around each twist, which takes almost forever, leaving the top of the head treated and the ends of the hair dry.

Speaking of oils, many different kinds are being touted as hair-treatment miracles for African-American women. Almond oil, jojoba oil, mineral oil, palm oil, castor oil, plant oils of all kinds, and petrolatum are just a few of the many options. As interesting as those all sound, none of them are any more reliable or effective than a vegetable oil you can pull out of your kitchen cabinet. Safflower oil, olive oil, or canola oil can be used for a great lubricating effect. If you want to try an oil treatment, do it *before* you wash your hair. Carefully covering the length of the hair and avoiding the scalp, smooth the oil downward over the hair in dabbing motions. Remember, rubbing the hair damages it. You can even use a cotton ball if you want. When you've coated the hair in a thin layer—not saturated, just coated—you can take a plastic cap and cover your head with it. Wait at least 20 minutes (the longer the better; several hours or more, if you can), preferably under heat, to help the oil soak in as much as possible. Then shampoo your hair as recommended above.

What about the countless product choices for African-American women? If you overlook the greasy pomades and so forth (as you definitely should), there is no discernible difference between hair-care products for African-American women and the rest of the lines. I think you would find it shocking how similar hair-care products are, regardless of who they are supposedly designed for. I get into that more in the product reviews, but in general, when there are differences in products, it is usually in favor of adding grease to damaged hair. Definitely the black hair-care market has more products like that than other lines.

CHAPTER EIGHT

Getting It to Do What You Want

A Matter of Technique, Talent, and Tenacity

A great haircut, the right styling products, and good styling tools are, without question, indispensable assets to having a head of hair that looks and behaves the way you want it to. Well, almost indispensable. If your hair falls into place with just a shake of your head or a simple scrunching to arrange curls and then you're done, you probably need read no farther for assistance. However, for most of us, it takes a lot more effort than that. Where most of us get snared is in the search for the right products. Yet all the best styling products in the world are worthless without the ability to proficiently handle styling implements. Knowing how to use a blow dryer, brushes, and a curling iron is integral to getting your head out of bad hair days . . . at least most of the time. Finding a hairstylist who is willing to help teach you how to use styling tools is the wisest investment you could ever make. Learning the techniques, developing your own skill and talent, and then practicing until you get it right is the totality of great-looking hair. Of course, the kind of environment you live in (humid or dry) can have a huge effect—but we get into that later.

Styling aptitude is of vital consequence for your hair, but your haircut is the structure and framework that everything else is based on. Exactly how those locks of yours are trimmed, shaped, layered, or patterned is the basis for how your hair will look. Telling you exactly what haircut, style, silhouette, or hair color would look good on you is not within the scope of my work. But I can help point you in the right direction so you have an idea of how to get the look you want or need.

Which Hairstyle to Choose?

Most women love looking at fashion magazines. The dazzling, alluring pictures are always exciting and fun to peruse. Admiring these photos is one thing, but basing a hairstyle choice on pictures of celebrities or models with great heads of hair more often than not has *nothing* to do with your lifestyle or what your hair can actually do.

It rarely even has anything to do with the model or celebrity in their real life! Before hair is coifed, celebrities and models usually don't have perfect or even great-looking hair. Without the aid of an expert stylist, their hair is hardly worth looking at or emulating. What a picture represents is almost never reality. Model or celebrity pictures are just this: pretty pictures created by makeup artists, hairstylists, good lighting, and expert photography—not what you would call low maintenance or easy to reproduce on your own. To find a haircut appropriate to your needs in terms of time and convenience, celebrity and model pictures are probably not all that helpful.

So how do you get an idea of what hairstyles are workable for you? Look for someone you know who has a similar or identical hair type, face, and body shape, who also has a haircut you admire. It would also be wise to select someone who is successfully on the career or social track you aspire to. Why is it better to emulate someone you know when it is so much more interesting to take the lead from someone famous or drop-dead gorgeous? You may think you want to look like a particular celebrity, but her style may be completely inappropriate for what you want to do in life. Also, to assume that how a hairstyle or dress looks on her has anything to do with how it would look on you (unless you look like that person) requires a leap of faith most of us would be foolish to make.

Talking to Your Stylist

Perhaps the most important tool for getting the look you want is recognizing how to make decisions about your hair and communicate them to your stylist. That isn't as easy as it sounds, because your hairstylist may have an agenda different than yours. Some hairdressers are inspired by the latest trends being presented by high-tech hairstylists working for companies such as Sebastian and TIGI. One way salon-only hair-care companies get the attention of hairstylists is by producing hair shows or semiannual hair books that showcase the most outrageous or difficult-to-maintain styles. These also keep hairstylists interested in the latest styling products. Sometimes hairdressers like change to satisfy their own artistic needs instead of *your* needs. While the latest hair trends may be right for you, I encourage you to reconsider whether or not that is really the direction you want to go. Trendy frequently translates into high-maintenance and short-lived. It can also mean that your hair becomes more noticeable than you are! A hairstyle that keeps you coming back to the hairstylist every four weeks can look more like art than hair, or is only reproducible with a number of hair-care products and a great deal of time. That may be good for the hairstylist, but it isn't good for you. In my opinion, the most important elements in getting a great cut are convenience and/or what is appropriate for your career.

In this regard, your best friend is still your hairstylist, but find one who is willing to listen to you and create a workable, professional hairstyle. How do you find a good or, better yet, great stylist? That is an important question, but the answer isn't necessarily easy to implement. For a consumer it means asking questions, and we are not always good about being assertively inquisitive.

What makes a good stylist? Ah, now there's a loaded question! It depends on your tastes. Probably the best definition of a good stylist is one who has the training and experience to work with your head of hair. On your part, that means research.

How do you find a trained and experienced stylist? Through referrals, credentials, training, and experience. Referrals are probably the most typical way we choose a stylist. A friend whose hair you admire goes to this wonderful stylist and the friend can't say enough about how much she loves this person and how she wouldn't go to anyone else. Or you read a fashion magazine and discover an article that hails the talents of a local stylist. Those are probably the two most reliable ways to choose a hairstylist—certainly more reliable than using a stylist because a hair salon ran a special for $25 off a perm and cut.

So why do referrals sometimes end up badly? You may have admired your friend's perfectly beautiful blunt cut, but you need a carefully blended layered cut; or the stylist may be a whiz at blunt cuts but can't handle the difficulties of a layered cut. If personal referrals are going to work for you, look for someone whose hair is similar to yours. Similarly, the fashion magazine recommendation can also be a good referral option; frequently a stylist gains some recognition in your city (and that rarely happens accidentally), but, alas, what that stylist sees for you might not be what you want. Sometimes it's your lack of communication skills or willingness to be assertive about what you want, or maybe your inability to hear what the stylist is telling you about the limitations of taking naturally tight, curled hair and making it straight in a humid climate.

If referrals haven't panned out for you or you simply don't know anyone with hair like yours that's cut in a style you admire, then the only way to gauge a stylist's ability before you sit down in the chair is to check out his or her credentials and training. That means finding a stylist who has attended advanced hair schools or seminars—not just beauty school, but training above and beyond. How do you find that out? You ask. "What training besides beauty school have you had?" is a more than valid question, and the answer you get is significant. A stylist whose only training is from beauty school has only rudimentary knowledge of what it takes to cut, style, color, or perm hair, and choose products for a client. It would be like going to a physician who just graduated from medical school; a doctor who hasn't done a residency has no experience. You want a stylist who has had at least some advanced training and does continuing education above and beyond the beauty school's state licensing qualifications.

Hair Note: <u>Don't try to save money on a hairstylist.</u> You can save lots of money on product choices and coloring your hair at home by following some of my advice, but don't save money on a hairstylist. That doesn't mean you have to spend a fortune (and just because a stylist charges $50 and up for a cut doesn't indicate whether he or she is automatically going to be proficient or best for you), but it does raise your chances. That means avoiding those places that advertise $10 or $20 haircuts. Some women have hair that can look great with a bargain haircut, but not many. Accomplished stylists charge more; it is an issue of skill having more value. For your head of hair, that is one area worth the expense.

Hairstyle Basics

Although I said I am not going to discuss hairstyles, I want to go over a few of the basics to help you formulate some ideas when you start thinking about a change in the way you wear your hair. There aren't many rules, but here are a few I encourage you to consider:

Bangs that are too long or too thick de-emphasize the eyes, accentuate the nose, and generally make your face look smaller. If you wear long, thick bangs that conceal your forehead and eyes, the next feature in line is your nose. Lighten up on the bangs and make sure they don't ride heavily below the eyebrow.

Parting your hair in the middle is another way to give the nose center stage (although it isn't as bad as dense bangs). A center part divides the face severely in half. This median line creates a linear movement down the face. The next feature that lines up with this central lineup is the nose. Center parts also tend to look childish or pubescent, instead of sophisticated and polished. Either no part or a side part will correct these problems.

Brushing hair away from the center of the face is, nine times out of ten, the best fashion advice. This is a hard one to convince women of because so many stylists love brushing hair into the face. Yet when fashion designers or advertisers showcase their latest looks or products, or when hair designers want to advertise their newest products, the models almost always have their hair blown away from the face. Let's say you don't want that flowing, windblown look. Even a short, styled hairdo can be brushed off the face or at least arranged in a way that doesn't hide the sides of the face. Hair that lies directly on the face cuts the cheekbone in half, making the face look rounder and fuller (so much for the hollowed-out cheekbone look), and if you wanted your eyes to look bigger, you've just cut off at least an inch of length. Style the hair away from the face, upward and out. Your hair will not only look fuller, but your facial features will look softer and more defined.

Extremely short hair looks best on thinner women with great bone structure. The same is true for extremely long hair. Layering is good for someone with hair that is neither too thin or too thick. If the hair is too thin, layers hang obviously off the head in steps; if the hair is too thick, the layers can lift away from the head like a balloon. Full is good, but too full and you'll look like "Here comes the hair!"

Bilateral haircuts, where one section of hair is short and the other long, and etched haircuts, where one section of hair looks radically different from the other, are fashion statements you should avoid. They are trendy and hard to maintain, and make the hair look like it's been "cut." They are too severe and prevent a soft, flowing look, making the head look like sculpted artwork.

Farrah Fawcett bangs from the '70s are out of style (and will remain so for eternity, I hope). Flipped-back bangs were fun once, but so were go-go boots and Nehru jackets; those days are long gone.

If you want hair to look fuller, cut your hair to just about the shoulders. Never allow your hair to get so long that it breaks at the shoulder with some hair falling forward and some falling back. If hair falls just above the shoulders, the buoyancy created from the hair resettling just above the shoulder will almost always make the hair appear fuller.

Making It Look Like the Hairstylist Does

Why can't you get your hair to look like it does just after you leave the salon? You use the same styling products your hairdresser uses, the same blow-dryer (the new one with the cool-air button), and soft brushes that can hold onto the hair. Yet, even so, it doesn't look the same. There are three basic reasons why the hairstylist is capable of doing what you aren't, and they are, as I mentioned above, technique, talent, and tenacity. Hairstylists are trained to make your hair look good; cutting and finishing hair is their primary occupation. Talent is an intangible factor, but you know it when you see it! Finally, stylists not only spend more time on your head than you do (which makes a vast difference both in the final appearance of your hair as well as in how long the style will stay in place), but they are also in a better position to get the right angle, pressure, and heat direction on your hair. Standing over your own head is something you simply can't do. That's why a salon style has incredible movement and durability versus an at-home effort that falls out or is still fuzzy after you're done.

Because of all those varying elements, it's almost impossible to get your hair to look just like the stylist gets it to look. That's the bad news. The good news is that there are some tricks of the trade that can get you closer. It just takes patience and experimentation to find out which techniques work best for you. The suggestions that follow will minimize damage but maximize style. Please notice that in most cases, as you might expect, less is more.

Never overuse a styling product. Too much or too many styling products that are too heavy or stiff (or even lightweight ones) can make the hair limp, heavy, stiff, greasy, and/or hard to manage. Almost without exception, the less you use, the better. *Rule of palm:* Apply only enough gel, mousse, hair serum, or heat protection to *minimally* cover your palms and fingers in a thin layer. Then smooth this in an even layer through your hair or just in the areas where your hair needs it.

What should you do with spray-on styling products? Be careful. Although spray-on products are generally formulated to be lighter than those you spread with your hands, you aren't touching your hair as much, so it's harder to tell how much product you've applied and whether or not you've gotten it through the thickness. Spray-on gels don't guarantee thinner coverage. If you are trying to beat the frizzies, it is essential to cover every hair on your head, but if your hair is fine or limp, less coverage is better than more.

Use different products for different needs. Your hair may need a gel all over but you may need a pomade or wax for the ends or the more damaged parts of your hair to lie smooth, and a hairspray to keep it all in place when you're done.

Hairstyling products often don't mean what they say, so don't take them seriously. Styling products labeled as "firm," "medium," or "soft" hold aren't always accurate. Following my recommendations from Chapter Nine, *Product Reviews*, always consider the lighter-weight styling products for all over the hair, and then firmer- or heavier-hold products on stubborn areas only.

Gently move your wet hair into the shape you want it to be, with the least amount of brushing, combing, or manipulation. The less brushing, the less damage. A vent brush or a wide-toothed comb is best for arranging wet hair.

Do not blow-dry hair that is sopping wet. Do not begin styling your hair with a blow-dryer or any other styling tools when it is wet. Either let your hair air-dry for a period of time first or blow-dry some of the moisture out, using a diffuser or a medium heat and medium air setting, before you begin to create a specific style. This is called rough-drying (even though you should never do it roughly). To rough-dry the hair, use either direct heat that you quickly move over the hair (including the root area) or a diffuser, always working the hair in the pattern or movement you want it to go. You can begin to use your fingers to scrunch your hair if you are going after a curly, natural look.

Use your fingers instead of a brush when you first begin to remove moisture from your hair. Never try to style wet hair with a brush. Using your fingers instead of a brush can prevent a lot of cuticle damage. It is very important to avoid dragging a brush through wet hair until most of the real moisture is gone. Wait until your hair is somewhere between not damp but not yet dry; that's the time to pick up the brush and start setting the style in place.

First style the roots by lifting and moving them against the direction you want them to go. When you are ready to work in a specific style, pay attention to the length of the hair last. For the most lift, direct the heat on the roots first, either with your fingers **lifting** the roots away from the scalp in a **forward angle** or **in the opposite direction** of where you want it to go. This will set in a good deal of fullness. You can also do the same thing by turning your head upside down and blowing the hair dry underneath first. From this position it is best to start on a low heat and low air setting so you don't blow tangles into the hair.

Treat the length of hair differently than you treat the roots. The roots get blown in an angle up and away from the head or slightly against the direction you want the hair to go. The length of hair is blown dry as much as possible in the direction of the cuticle, down along the hair shaft. Blowing against the downward movement of the hair shaft can make the hair fuzzy or encourage frizzies by roughing up the cuticle.

Aim the heat on the length of the hair in the direction you want the hair to go, following the hair. As basic as that sounds, I've seen women at the gym just get the heat on their hair without any rhyme or reason. Blowing heat on the hair without controlling it with your fingers or a brush can cause tangles (by roughing up the cuticle), which can cause damage when you try to smooth them out of the hair. If you want the hair to curl under, move the heat along the top of the hair shaft in a downward motion, following the brush or your hand. To prevent damage, avoid holding the heat too long in one place.

If your hair is thin, blow it dry on a lower setting. High heat can blow the life out of hair. To maintain some amount of thickness and fullness, and to prevent blowing out all the hair's natural movement, use lower heat.

If your hair is coarse or frizzy, blow it dry on a hotter setting. It would be great if low heat could shape, but it can't. Altering the natural shape of your hair, particularly going from curly to straight, requires high heat, and the higher the better. Heat helps mold and reform hair. If you want to blow-dry away the frizzies or smooth coarse, kinky, or curly hair, higher heat is the only way to accomplish this. I know this is more drying and damaging to the hair, but there is no way around this one if you are going after a specific style.

After you're done rough-drying your hair, work systematically, blow-drying each area of your hair. In essence, you are making sure you are not laying dried hair over wet hair, which can destroy the smooth or softly curled style you were trying to create. Wet hair can make a style go flat or frizzy. It may be helpful (though more time-consuming) to securely clip sections of hair so they don't get in the way of the hair you are working on. But always be sure your hair is thoroughly dry if you want a style to last the entire day.

The right brush can make a tremendous difference in the finished look of your hair. For styling purposes, a vent brush is best for creating the most fullness, but it isn't great at smoothing out frizzies when your hair is coarse. A round, circular-bristled brush is best for making hair smooth and even. A round brush with pliable wire bristles inserted into a metal base can grab hair better and is good if you aren't adept at getting a bristled brush through your hair. On the other hand, wire bristles aren't the best for smoothing coarse hair. When using a brush, be patient. Keep the brush moving through the hair in tandem with the blow-dryer. Roll the hair up into the brush, hold the dryer on this position for a few seconds, take the blow-dryer away from the hair and allow the hair to cool, then pull the brush through the hair, following with the blow-dryer along the length of the hair. Some blow-dryers have a button that provides a shot of cool air on the hair. Heat temporarily severs the molecular bonds that give the hair its shape, so you can mold it into the shape you want; cool air resets those bonds to keep the new shape in place. To get this technique down, have your hairdresser take you through a lesson, even if you have to pay for the extra time.

A good blow-dryer is lightweight and produces a concentrated gust of high heat. In general, if a blow-dryer doesn't yield high enough heat, it won't be able to smooth or form the hair. If a blow-dryer is too heavy, you won't be able to hold it in position (usually up and over your head) as long as is necessary to get the hair completely dry while styling. Too much power and it will be hard to control your hair. The new blow dryers have a cool trigger (a fast way to apply cool air without changing settings) that can help keep the smoothness or curl in place.

Heat is everything. I know I've already said, this but let me repeat: hot, direct heat is the best way to reconfigure hair. Almost everything you've read about blow dryers says to hold them anywhere from 6 to 9 inches away from the hair. Although that is a great way to reduce damage, it is completely unrealistic. No hairstylist in her right mind would bother with such a time-consuming ordeal, and you've never seen it happen. Holding the blow-dryer that far from the hair triples or quadruples the amount of time it takes to style your hair. Does this damage the hair? Yes. Does it help that the stylist keeps the brush and blow-dryer moving over the hair when they do hold it close? Yes, but not much. **To minimize damage when working on your own, try to never hold the blow-dryer in one spot for more than a few seconds.** Spray-on styling products or rich conditioners can reduce the damage from high heat but, all in all, this part of hairstyling has more cons than pros. The only advantage is that your hair gets done quickly, but when time is of the essence, that's everything. It is a necessary evil, because there are no real solutions for the negative side effects.

Hair Note: If you're in a hurry, which most of us are, and you don't have the time to make sure your entire head of hair is dry before you leave the house, concentrate your blow-drying efforts on the front of the hair. The back can fall or frizz a little bit without causing a serious bad hair day, while the front is the one area of focus you can't ignore.

Hair diffusers are good for setting in curls. You still need to rough-dry the hair first, scrunching the curls as you go to save time. When the hair is no longer damp but not yet dry, start concentrating the diffused air equally on the root and the length of your hair. Directing your attention on the length only can make the hairstyle go flat. Also aim the diffuser equally on the top of the hair as well as underneath. If you center your efforts only underneath, the top of the hair will look fuzzy.

Use your fingers as much as possible to separate and move the hair. The less you use brushes, the less you damage the hair.

When using regular rollers, set the hair when it is nearly dry to prevent long drying periods. Spray the hair with a mist of hairspray, spray gel, or volumizing spray (which is nothing more than a lightweight hairspray with more water), then roll it up, but not too tightly. You don't have to roll the whole head to get the benefits of curlers.

Smaller-circumference curling irons and hot rollers are great for setting in soft curls. The trick is to use them when the hair is completely dry as a finishing tool, not for creating the primary shape and movement of the hair. If you wish, use a light styling spray to get the style to last longer. Do not use firm-hold styling products with any heat-producing implements. They can make the hair sticky and brittle. Firm-hold styling products are best for natural air-drying, not heat styling.

Larger circumference curling irons and flat irons are great for straightening hair. These tools are standard for making hair look stick-straight.

Tools of the Trade

Great technique means little without the right tools. Poor tools leave your hair open to more damage and make your style look second-rate. You will be relieved to know that there are more good styling tools than bad. If that's true, you may be wondering, why doesn't a specific brush or curling iron work for your hair? Because it might not have anything to do with the quality of the implement, and everything to do with the type of hair you have. A brush that is great for coarse, thick hair may be the worst for thin, straight hair, while a brush that can smooth away frizzies might make some hair types go limp. Even the size of the styling tool can make a huge difference. A small circumference brush mak hair curlier, while a large-circumference brush smooths out the curls. Purchasing the right styling tool means knowing your hair type and knowing which brush, curling iron, blow-dryer, or hot rollers work best with that kind of hair.

Do you have to spend a lot of money on styling implements? Absolutely not. There are great options available at the drugstore. Unfortunately, at least when it comes to brushes, you can't often touch or feel the bristles to help you make a decision about how the brush will work in your hair. Brushes at the drugstore aren't packaged with identifiable or differentiating names, so there is no way I can recommend a specific brand.

When it comes to blow-dryers, there are great ones to be found at the drugstore and, in many ways, for at-home use they are superior to professional blow-dryers. The same is true for hot rollers and curling irons. The following sections will help you find the right tools for your hair type.

Brushes

The number of brushes that exist, and the wide array of types and sizes they come in, is nothing less than astonishing. But to begin with, there are three basic kinds of brushes: half-round and vent brushes, circular or round brushes, and flat or paddle brushes.

Half-round brushes are basic for styling and brushing through the hair. As the name implies, the bristles go only halfway around the brush. Generally this all-purpose brush is difficult to get wrong, but there are brushes of this type that have very pointed, sharp, or stiff plastic bristles. That can hurt the scalp and chip away at the cuticle. If the bristles are too soft, they won't smooth through hair. **Vent brushes** are recognizable by their wide bristle spacing, rubber-tipped ends, and, often, large spaces in the base of the brush. Vent brushes and standard half-round brushes generally have rubber handles and bases with plastic bristles inserted in a plastic cushion. They are great for arranging wet hair or brushing through already styled hair to refresh it. They can also work well when the goal is to blow fullness into the hair, particularly thin, limp, or fine hair. Because they allow heat to blow through the brush (and then through the hair) instead of capturing the heat, which helps smooth hair, they are a poor choice for eliminating frizzies. When it comes to blowing hair dry, it is best to use vent brushes in conjunction with natural-bristled round brushes (see below). Use a vent brush during the rough-drying stage and a natural-bristled round brush for the smoothing stage of the drying process.

Brush Note: It is best when the handle and base of half-round brushes are made out of rubber, because this material reduces static. Regardless of the brush type, always avoid nylon-bristled brushes unless they have rubber tips. Nylon is just too scratchy and stiff to be good for the scalp or hair.

Round brushes are easily recognizable because the bristles go all the way around the brush. Round brushes come in varying widths to accommodate a tighter or smoother curl, and offer different types of bristle density. Large natural-bristled round brushes are great for smoothing out frizzies and adding fullness to the hair. The smaller the width of a round brush, the better it is for shorter hair or, if you use it on longer hair, the tighter the curl it produces. If you have fine, thin, or limp hair, the softer-bristled round brushes work best. If you have thick, coarse, or extremely frizzy hair, a firmer-bristled brush is best. Bristles that are too stiff can break or increase damage to the hair. Round brushes should have enough flexibility to move through the hair, but be stiff enough to grab the hair and hold it while you move a blow-dryer over it.

Round brushes also come with wire bristles attached to a metal cylinder. These are slightly less effective at blowing out frizzies for coarse hair, but great for adding fullness to thinner hair. The metal part retains heats from the blow-dryer, working somewhat like a curling iron. Some round brushes have rubber bristles with rubber tips, which can be good for someone with thin, fine, or limp hair as a way to add fullness and waves. Because this type of brush tends not to grab and hold the hair well, and the rubber doesn't retain heat, it also tends to blow in frizzies.

Flat or paddle brushes are another tool for straightening long, wavy, or curly hair. These generally come with wire or nylon bristles set into a rubber cushion (similar to a pin cushion) on a wide, flat oval or square base. Paddle brushes grab hair well and are best for straightening out stubborn curls, rather than smoothing out frizzies. To smooth out the hair and get rid of frizzies, use a paddle brush in conjunction with a round natural-bristled brush.

Velcro Rollers

We all know that the days of sleeping in brush or plastic dry rollers are long dead, right? Not only is it uncomfortable and unattractive (which is important if you aren't sleeping alone), it is bad for the hair. Aside from being an intimacy blocker, rollers, especially if you wind them up too tightly and leave them in for long periods of time, can put too much pressure on the root of the hair, causing it to fall out before its time. Additionally, the kind of friction caused by hair rubbing all night against rollers can cause serious damage to the cuticle. Never mind the mess and the bother, dry rollers are just obnoxious. No beauty regime should be so time-consuming (could you imagine any man going through that kind of rigmarole?) or that bothersome.

To combat some of the bother, someone came up with the idea of Velcro rollers as a way to roll up the hair without clips or pins. Unfortunately, depending on your skill and patience, the concept is better than the delivery, because Velcro rollers are just as bothersome and time-consuming as any other kind of roller. Although they claim to stay put without the aid of clips, if you have long, thick hair, that just isn't true. Unless you have short, thin hair, Velcro rollers can easily get tangled if you aren't careful with exactly how you put them in or take them out. If you are curious to give them a try, they are definitely an option, but buy one pack first and try them out before investing more money in a complete set.

Hot Rollers

Over the past ten years, hot rollers have taken a back seat to curling irons and blow-dryers. Hot rollers are considered less convenient because they have to sit in the hair for awhile, while curling irons do their job immediately. There are few models available to choose from, but still, all in all, when you do have the time, hot rollers are a relatively quick, easy way to smooth out frizzies and put in soft or tight curls. To get the most mileage out of any hot roller, be sure you smoothly and evenly roll the rods into neatly parted hair sections. Too much hair, bunched up hair, or loose ends give you the worst results from any hot roller set.

Dry-heat rollers are more efficient and faster than steam or damp-heat rollers. Steam rollers are a viable option if you have more time. The roller and hair must dry completely before you remove the rollers so you don't get frizzies. Because of the moisture they provide and the soft sponge part of the curlers, steam rollers are considered less damaging than dry-heat rollers, but they are also more time-consuming to use.

Curling Irons

A hairstyling staple for decades, curling irons are a fast, relatively easy way to style hair once it is has been dried. It takes some practice, but there are some great curling irons on the market that make experimentation easy. Most of the better ones come with variable heat settings and tips that don't get hot. Variable heat means you can learn how to use it on the lowest setting, which reduces the chances of burning yourself or destroying your hair. The cylinders also come in a range of sizes; the wider the cylinder, the smoother the curl and the easier it is to use.

Hot-air styling brushes and curling irons are situated somewhere between curling irons and blow-dryers. They look like curling irons, but the metal cylinder extension blows diffused, low-force hot air out of the center instead of just generating heat. Unlike curling irons, the heat is practically instantaneous, although the metal cylinder cools off immediately once it is turned off. These tools are an option for smoothing out the hair. Unlike hot rollers and curling irons, which should not be used until the hair is completely dry, hot-air styling brushes and curling irons can be used when the hair is still slightly damp. The diffused air helps dry the hair, and the metal cylinder heats up enough to ease away the frizzies—just don't expect the same smoothness you can achieve with a regular curling iron.

Blow-Dryers

Blow dryers are the most fundamental of styling tools. A good blow-dryer is the cornerstone for getting the style you want as well as getting your hair dry in an efficient manner. Though you need a superior blow-dryer, the best blow-dryers for in-home use are not the same as the professional ones your hairstylist uses. You and your hairstylist have different needs. Perhaps one of the most critical elements to take into consideration is weight. If a blow-dryer feels heavy in the store, it will feel like a ton when you've been holding it over your head for 15 minutes or more. Hairstylists can use a more heavy-duty blow-dryer because they stand over your head, keeping their elbows at their sides.

Two more crucial components for a blow-dryer are the heat settings and the amount of wattage. Most blow-dryers have between 1,200 and 2,000 watts of air speed. Most stylists consider 1,500 to 1,875 watts essential in order to concentrate enough air and enough heat to get the hair dried and styled. Closer to 2,000 and you can literally blow the life out of your hair. Check the heat settings; if they are hard to figure out or difficult to manipulate, you won't use them, and they are essential for blowing your hair dry. Full air with medium or high heat is great for rough-drying, medium to full air with high heat is best for smoothing out frizzies, and low air with high heat is great for setting in curls.

Many blow-dryers have a cool-shot button in the handle that delivers a blast of cool air to the hair. If you have the time, this is a decent way to set in the style, because when hair stays hot it is vulnerable to changing form until it cools.

Be sure the cord of the blow-dryer is at least 6 to 9 feet long. Any shorter and you won't have the flexibility you need to reach your head from all angles after you've plugged the dryer into the wall socket. Some blow-dryers are designed to stay on only if you depress a trigger on the handle. When you release the handle they turn off, preventing accidental immersion in water while on. Although this safety device makes sense, it can be extremely difficult on your hand and arm to keep the trigger depressed the entire time you're styling.

A straight-nozzle blow-dryer is the only kind to consider. The long, vent-style blow-dryers might be OK for men's hairstyles, but they won't give you the control and concentrated heat you need to smooth and shape hair with a brush. Some blow-dryers come packaged with attachments such as diffusers, combs, and pick-like implements. For the most part the only useful attachment is a diffuser, which is great for gentle drying or setting in natural curls. Combs and pick-like implements can't replace fingers or natural-bristled and vent brushes. As a rule, the brush moves through the hair and the heat moves down and over the brush. When the heat blows through the hair, you can get frizzies.

Most blow-dryers nowadays come with 1,875 watts of power at the maximum setting. This can be good for quickly getting the hair dry and styled, but remember, it can be overdone and make hair look lifeless. Be careful with this much power, and use the top setting only in conjunction with a brush or a diffuser.

Hair Tips from Top to Bottom

These are just reminders, a summary of the more salient points discussed throughout the entire book. They aren't the whole story, but they are standard operating procedure for getting your hair to behave and survive the latest hair fashion. If you want to convince your hair to do what it would rather not do, these concepts are basic.

When you wash your hair, take more time washing your scalp than the ends of your hair. Hair ends don't get all that dirty (unless you've got large doses of styling products layered over them), but the scalp can get oily, with dead skin cells that need to come off. In addition, the scalp almost always can benefit from a massage, which will increase healthy circulation and help the hair developing in the follicles.

Conditioners that claim to be deeply penetrating only work if there's enough time and heat for them to be absorbed into the hair shaft. Most women who apply a conditioner in the shower never leave it on for longer than a minute or two. That's fine, but don't expect the hair to soak it up. If you have damaged hair, it is very important to leave the conditioner on for as long as possible. The same is true for shampoos that contain conditioning ingredients.

Too much conditioner or conditioner that isn't thoroughly rinsed out can make hair go limp. A shampoo that contains conditioners and a conditioning agent can cause too much buildup on the hair, making it heavy and lifeless. Generally, a shampoo with minimal or no conditioner at all is best, and then use your conditioner only where you need it, not necessarily all over or near the roots and scalp.

Be careful to thoroughly rinse shampoo out of your hair. Leaving traces of detergent cleansers behind can make hair sticky and flat.

The longer you leave a dandruff shampoo on your hair, the more effective it will be.

Apply shampoo and conditioner by first spreading it over your hands and then smoothing it over the hair. Placing one big dollop in the middle and then working it through the hair wastes product and roughs up the hair more than is necessary.

When in doubt, use products designed for your hair type. Unless you have truly normal hair, undesignated products, even those that promise to reconstruct or rebuild your hair, are not for everyone.

Every now and then, take your brush and comb into the shower with you and give them a good shampooing. Styling products, conditioners, and your own oil can cling to brushes and combs, transferring some of the grime back to your clean hair. Get the excess hair out and go for it. For a more thorough cleansing, or if you have dandruff, soak them in a solution of diluted bleach; about three tablespoons to a quart of water should be enough to kill whatever may be lurking around.

When using a blow-dryer, hair is easier to style and control when it is damp but not wet. When it comes to blow-drying, hair can be fickle. It takes some experimentation to find out how damp your hair needs to be to get the best smoothness.

Never use a curling iron on wet or damp hair. The heat from a curling iron can easily exceed the boiling point of water. The water content in the hair shaft can actually boil from the application of a hot curling and cause serious breakage and damage.

When blowing your hair dry, go after the roots first. Drying the roots up and away from the direction you want will achieve fullness and create the foundation for the rest of the hairstyle. Once the roots are done, you can smooth or curl the rest of the hair. If you leave the roots until last, they may already have dried in a direction you didn't want them to go, making them harder to shape. The length of the hair is easier to manipulate even if it is somewhat dry.

Wet or damp hair is more vulnerable to losing its shape. It is best to blow your hair all the way dry and not leave any wetness, not even a little. Unless partial natural movement is what you are after, blow the entire head completely dry in order to keep the style in for as long as possible.

If you have the time, alternate using hot air and cool air while blow-drying. Heat forms the curl or smoothness, and the cool air helps keep it there.

To help prevent hairspray from flaking off in white specks, apply it at least 6 inches away from the hair. A concentrated blast can make the polymers and resins go on too thickly, causing a stiff, matte bond that can lead to flaking.

Getting It Straight

For those of us with naturally curly hair, the 1960s and '70s were nothing less than a nightmare, because straight hair was the only acceptable fashion statement for years. Anyone with thick, twisting locks subjected herself to sleeping in oversize rollers (orange juice cans were all the rage) or ironing her hair with a real iron on an ironing board! It was sheer torture. (African-American women had a brief respite during the '60s, though, when their natural spirals were the way to go.) Total relief came with the '80s, when natural 'dos were the style of the day. Finally, those with straight hair had to subject themselves to damaging, utterly fake-looking perms, while those with homegrown curls merely tousled their locks and were on their way. There is justice in the world. But, alas, as is always true with the fickle fates of fashion, thanks to Jennifer Aniston and Courteney Cox of *Friends* fame, we are back to straight hair as a major fashion. Ultra-smooth is in, and has been for awhile, and even Julia

Louis-Dreyfus, Nicole Kidman, and Minnie Driver, whose manes are normally lush and tumbling with twists and turns, now boast stick-straight hair. Hence the market is filled with straightening balms to accomplish the seemingly impossible.

The primary thing to keep in mind is that getting this to work for your hair is only possible if you blow-dry your hair completely dry, and if you do that by dividing your hair into smaller sections. For extremely curly hair a large-barreled curling iron is essential. Regardless of the tool, **every section of your hair must be thoroughly dry; the slightest amount of moisture will cause your hair to frizz and curl.**

- First you need to use a good emollient conditioner on the length of your hair. Depending on your hair type, leave-in or rinse-out is just fine. Leave-in is best if your hair is hard to control or very thick and frizzy.

- Towel-dry well by dabbing and blotting; avoid tousling or rubbing, which can damage the hair shaft.

- To the frizziest part of your hair, apply the thinnest amount possible of a silicone product. This adds a silky feel and helps start the smoothing process.

- Then apply any of the new hair-straightening balms or gels on the market. Everyone from Sebastian to Paul Mitchell to L'Oreal has a version. I list all the options in Chapter 10.

- Next, use your blow-dryer all over to remove the excess moisture. Be sure to get the underneath part of the hair, where water loves holding on. If you are going to use a curling iron, be sure all the moisture is removed first or you can literally boil the water content of hair and cause serious damage.

- Use a ponytail holder or big banana clips to partition your hair. Start with the bottom layer and work your way up. If you have full hair, be sure to lift the roots up and get the heat concentrated in that area, over every section. If you have flatter hair, pull the roots down and concentrate the heat there.

- The best tools are wood-handled, round-bristle brushes or metal-framed round brushes with plastic handles. Both wood- and metal-framed round brushes work well, but the metal-framed brushes help heat the hair more, which can make it straighter. The larger the brush, the straighter your hair will be. Flat brushes tend to make hair frizzy, so they work best on hair that tends to be naturally smoother. You may have to brush several times over each section, following the blow-dryer as you use the brush to smooth out the hair. Be sure to apply heat to the hair on top of the brush and the underside to get each small section entirely dry, and get the heat evenly distributed over the hair. You need to be patient on this step, because this is the only way to go about it.

- A pomade or hair wax can be used over the frizziest areas to get control.

Hair Note: For some unknown reason, silicone has been getting called on the carpet as a hair-care ingredient. Some industry experts, and I use the term "experts" loosely and sarcastically, assert that silicone attracts dust, is hard to shampoo off hair, and is bad for women with thin hair. What a joke! Silicone is no more likely to attract dust or be difficult to shampoo off than a horde of common hair-care ingredients, including standard thickening agents and film formers that show up in 100 percent of all hair-care products.

The final twist (or untwist): tension and heat are the keys to getting hair straight. The tighter you pull your hair and the better able you are to get heat on it, the straighter it will be. The reason stylists can get your hair so straight is because they are in the perfect position to get the necessary tension to make hair behave, and their styling tools generate intense heat. Another trick stylists use is to keep the blow-dryer moving instead of leaving it in one spot. Aiming the heat at the roots and making sure the roots are going in the direction you want—up for more fullness, down for straightening—is the best way to get control of your locks. Another styling essential is to move the blow-dryer down along the hair shaft instead of back and forth.

Product Application

You're looking at all the varied product options for styling hair—gels, laminates (silicone serums), pomades, styling sprays, and hairsprays—and wondering which to apply when. That's a good question. The only universally agreed upon order of things is that hairspray is applied last when you are done styling. When to apply all other styling products depends on what hairstyle you are trying to create and your own personal preference. For example, if you have particularly coarse, curly hair, and you are trying to get it to appear straighter and smoother, it may be best to first apply a silicone serum all over the hair to get the silky-smooth feeling down first. Then you can apply a styling gel, styling spray, or mousse to begin the styling process of blowing the hair dry and/or using a curling iron. When you are done with that, over stubborn ends you can then apply a pomade or styling wax to get those areas tamed. On the other hand, some stylists like applying the styling gels, sprays, or mousses first and then applying the silicone serum. It all depends on what works best for your hair.

For those with fine or thin hair, layering styling products can be a problem. A leave-in conditioner with hairspray-type ingredients (film formers) may be enough without the need of any other styling product, though you can add a styling spray over stubborn areas. But be careful. Fine, thin hair gets weighed down easily by styling products.

Fighting Humidity and Desert Heat

Hair loses its shape when there is too much moisture in the air or when there's no moisture in the air. All the hair products and hair tips in the world can't convincingly counteract what I call Hawaii hair or Arizona hair. Hawaii hair refers to what happens to hair when it is bombarded by high humidity. Some very stiff, firm-hold hairsprays can keep humidity off the hair, but then you sacrifice movement and your hair looks like a helmet. Arizona hair occurs when extremely dry air robs moisture from the hair shaft. You can load up the hair with conditioning agents, but then you end up with heavy, limp, or greasy hair. Myriad products try to combat all this and their claims could fill a library, but the end result, as you can see from my reviews, is limited. You can only fight physics and biology to a point with hair care products and styling tools. For the most part, genetics and the environment, more often than not, end up winning.

CHAPTER NINE

Product Reviews

The Process

You may well be wondering how I go about deciding what distinguishes a terrible product from a great one, or a good product from a fantastic one. Above all, you need to know that I do not base my decisions on my own personal experience, or let my personal feelings about a particular company blur my judgment. In other words, just because I happen to like the way a shampoo or conditioner feels on *my* hair doesn't translate to how anyone else will feel or experience that product. Rather, I base my decision on the individual product's formulation, using published research about the ingredient(s) being used and their possible resulting interactions with the hair. **Further, every styling product reviewed in this book was tested for feel, texture, performance, weight, and function.** Whether or not I think a company is absurdly overcharging for its products or is exceedingly dishonest in its claims and literature, and no matter how unethical I find it, that won't prevent me from saying its product is good for a particular hair type (though I do often say, "This is a good product but what a shame the price has to be so absurd and the claims so offensive and deceptive!").

I also asked the following questions to see if a product could hold up to its claims, based on established research: (1) Given the ingredient list, could the product do what it promised? (2) How did the product differ from other products? (3) If a special ingredient or ingredients were showcased, how much of them were actually in the product, and was there independent research verifying the claims for those ingredients? (4) Did the product contain problematic preservatives, fragrances, coloring agents, plants, or other questionable ingredients? (5) How far-fetched were the product's claims? (6) If a product said it was good for sensitive skin or scalp, did it in fact contain irritants, skin sensitizers, or drying ingredients?

I wish I had the space to challenge and explain every single exaggerated claim and lofty explanation that accompanies the products listed in this chapter, but there is just not enough room (or time) to tackle that prodigious task. For this book, I chose to include all the information I could to provide you with as much information as possible to help you understand the sales pitches so you can focus on a product's quality, realistic performance, and "feel," and not on the deceptive marketing and advertising practices.

For those of you who are familiar with my reviews, you may notice that I am much more cautious about hair products that contain any amount of irritating ingredients, particularly those containing lemon, grapefruit, mint, peppermint, menthol, camphor, eucalyptus, ivy, fragrant oils, overly drying detergent cleansing agents, and an excessive amount of useless plant extracts. These can all cause a flaky, itchy scalp—and some of them can dry out and damage hair.

My reviews of hair-care products, with a few exceptions, are organized in the following categories: shampoo, conditioner, styling products, and specialty products such as hair masks or special conditioning treatments.

The Ingredients for Hair Care

While I want to emphasize to what extent hair-care products are portrayed in a misleading, disingenuous way, I also want to underscore what great products *do* exist for all hair types. That's why it is difficult for me to describe my elation or enthusiasm about any product without always being careful to let you know what can you can really expect from it, and how out of line the price often is for what you are getting. Just because I think a formula can be amazing for extremely dry hair doesn't mean that I concur with its claims about repairing the problem.

Every hair-care product was first evaluated on the basis of what it contains and then on how it performed. This was especially true for every styling product included in this book. All styling products were tested for whether or not they were greasy, sticky, stiff, or flaky. But the ingredients are always the basis for whether a claim can be verified. Remember that the amount of any ingredient in a product always corresponds **to the order in which it appears on the ingredient list.** Also, when ingredients are located from the midpoint to the end of the ingredient listing, there are only trivial traces of them. Incidentally, by comparison, with prepared foods when an item has less than a given measurable amount of calcium, for example, the label has to indicate that, based on the RDA, I assume; it appears that in cosmetics, they can list even traces, since there's nothing corresponding to RDA. So people who come to trust food labels may think cosmetic labels are handled the same way—and they aren't!

In the product reviews, when I do describe a product's contents, I frequently use the phrase "contains mostly," often followed by one or all of the following terms:

anti-irritant
chelating agent
coloring agent

conditioning agent
detangling agent
detergent cleansing agent
dye agent
emollient
film former
fragrance
lather agent
plant extract
plant oil
preservative
propellant
silicone
slip agent
thickener
vitamin (antioxidant)
water (tea water or plant juice)
water-binding agent

It was easiest to summarize groups of ingredients by using these general terms, but they need more explanation before you read the reviews.

Hair Note: When reading ingredient lists, remember that the closer a specific ingredient is in the list to a preservative (such as methylparaben, propylparaben, ethylparaben, imidazolidinyl urea, or quaternium-15) or a fragrance (listed often as an individual essential oil like lavender or bergamot oil, or simply as fragrance), or the closer it is to the end of the ingredient list, the less likely it is that any significant amount is present in the product.

Also, some ingredient groupings such as thickener, conditioning agent, and emollient can overlap in function. All of those are technically interchangeable, but I refer to a specific type of ingredient by what it is most typically known for in a formulation. The same is true for detangling agents and film formers, whose functions can also overlap, though when these do specifically overlap I often list them in the summary as **detangling agent/film former.** This is also the case for some lathering agents and detergent cleansing agents. Often these are listed in conditioners or styling products, but the amounts used show they are meant to function as emulsifiers, ingredients that keep other ingredients mixed together. I did not indicate these in the product summaries.

For products in which an ingredient is included primarily for its cleansing ability I use the general term **detergent cleansing agent.** Ingredients in this category include sodium lauryl sulfate, sodium laureth sulfate, cocamidopropyl betaine, sodium cocoyl isethionate, sodium cocoamphoacetate, TEA-lauryl sulfate, cocamide DEA, ammonium laureth sulfate, and ammonium lauryl sulfate, to name a few (though these tend to be the most typical). Because sodium lauryl sulfate, TEA-lauryl sulfate, and sodium C14-16 olefin sulfate (and the far less used sodium dodecyl sulfonate and alkyl benzene sulfonate) are very strong, drying, or irritating detergent cleansing agents, I warn against using a product that contains these ingredients when they appear in the first part of its ingredient list. For those who dye their hair, using a product with sodium C14-16 olefin sulfate, sodium dodecyl sulfonate, or alkyl benzene sulfonate can potentially strip hair color.

Lather agents are ingredients added to shampoos strictly for the purpose of creating a healthy dose of foaming suds on the hair. Most women don't feel their hair is getting clean unless this foaming effect happens, yet the amount of foam is completely unrelated to the effectiveness of the detergent cleansing agents, and lather agents are added strictly for aesthetics and consumer appeal.

Conditioning agents or **emollients** are designations I give to a number of ingredients that are known for their ability to coat hair and help improve its feel, thickness, smoothness, and tensile strength. Some are better at this than others, but they are not the ones you immediately notice on an ingredient label. Proteins, amino acids, collagen, elastin, and other hair-healthy-sounding ingredients do an OK job, but they don't perform quite as well as you might expect, given their names. However, the range of other conditioning and emollient ingredients, from panthenol to quaternium, do a very good job and help a conditioner provide the feel you want for your hair.

Silicone is an exceptionally hair-friendly ingredient that shows up repeatedly— it's in almost 80 percent of all hair-care products being sold. This standard conditioning agent deserves special mention because of its unique properties and benefits for hair. Technically speaking, silicone's chemical components are related to fluid technology, and that gives it an exquisite, silky, somewhat slippery feel on the hair. Its popularity in formulations reflects its versatility and the finish it gives products. It is also a cheap ingredient, and standard to all kinds of cosmetics in all kinds of price ranges. It is by far one of the fundamental conditioning and shine agents used in hair-care products. It can cause buildup when overused, but just the tiniest amount can give a phenomenal silky combability to hair.

Castor oil and mineral oil are also typical conditioning ingredients that show up in many hair-care products. Castor oil's unique properties warrant a little explanation of how it affects a product's performance. It's a seed extract (there is actually a castor bean plant), an oil that, when dried, imparts to hair a shiny, smooth feel that can be greasy and have a slight sticky feel. It is the combination of shine and stickiness that makes this an interesting styling agent for stubborn frizzies or curls. Mineral oil gets a bad rap in the cosmetics industry for being harsh or unnatural, when it is neither. As an oil, mineral oil is one of the most benign of all cosmetic ingredients, rivaling even water in terms of lack of irritation potential. It is also natural, because the original source is earth mineral. Regardless, for the hair it is a good conditioning agent, providing slip and conditioning effects on dry hair.

When I use the term **thickener** to describe an ingredient, the word refers to those components that add texture, thickness, viscosity, spreadability, and stability to a product. Thickeners are also vital for helping to keep other ingredients mixed together. They also have a waxlike texture or a creamy, emollient feel, and can be great lubricants or conditioning agents. There are literally thousands of ingredients in this category, and they are the staples of every hair-care product out there.

A wide range of technical- and chemical-sounding ingredients are used in shampoos and conditioners to help hair be more combable, and I refer to these as **detangling agents.** This group of ingredients is primarily known in the industry by the abbreviated name of "quats," from such typical agents as quaternium 18 or polyquaternium. Their unique molecular structure allows quats to cling to hair in a way that helps a brush or comb glide easily through the hair. There are a handful of detangling agents that also function as film formers (see the next description). When that takes place the ingredient is indicated as a **detangling agent/film former.**

Film formers are ingredients such as PVP, acrylates, acrylamides, styrene, crotonic acid, vinyl acetate/crotonates, vinyl neodecanoate copolymer, methacrylate copolymer, and polyglycerylacrylates, among many others that are the backbone of any styling product. This small but essential group of plastic resins holds hair in place with relative combability and firmness. These are also used in volumizing or thickening shampoos and conditioners as a way to uniformly coat hair and add a feeling of thickness. What all film formers share in common is that they impart varying degrees of stiffness and have a sticky feel on the hair. There is no way around this one, because there are no film formers (and definitely not one plant extract) that can hold hair in place without some firmness and a sticky feel. They also add weight to hair, which those with fine and thin hair may find heavy or flattening. What is most shocking about this group of ingredients is their redundancy. The same film-forming agents show up in product after product after product in all price ranges. Despite what you may emotionally think of less-expensive products, the ingredients they use to hold hair in place do not differ from those in the expensive ones.

Water can be given an elevated status by using an assortment of exclusive-sounding adjectives—deionized, purified, triple-purified, demineralized—to describe what is actually just plain water. These terms indicate that the water has gone through some kind of purification process, which is quite standard for cosmetics and nothing special in the least. You will also find phrases such as "infusions of" or "aqueous extracts of," followed by the name of one or a long list of plant extracts; I use the term **tea** when that type of concoction is listed. That means you're getting nothing more than a tea concocted from a group of plants, or **plant juice** mixed with water. Is there any benefit to plant water? The hair-care industry would love you to believe there is— but water is water! The kind of water used does not affect the hair or the scalp, unless you happen to be allergic or sensitive to the myriad bouquets thrown into the product. Even if the tea or plant water could be effective for hair care, after it is combined with other ingredients, its original status is all but lost.

It is impossible to list all the individual **plant extracts** used in hair-care products. As far as the world of hair care is concerned, if it grows, it can improve hair. Yet there is no consensus on which plant is the most amazing and there is no research demonstrating any hair-friendly properties for plants. Of course, that's not what the various hair-care companies want you to believe. As far as they are concerned, plants from ginger to hemp, mango, pineapple, sambucus, horse chestnut, dandelion, oak bark, lemon, grapefruit, coffee, and on and on and on can all have the most astonishing merits. For hair, it is all meaningless. What is more significant for hair care is that the plant extracts thrown into hair-care products to impress the consumer can often be a problem for the scalp. Plant extracts, regardless of their claimed quality, can often cause irritation, allergic reactions, or skin sensitivities. None of that is good for the scalp.

Plant oils (other than those called essential oils) are almost always beneficial as conditioning agents. The debate about whether or not sunflower, canola, olive, avocado, almond, or any of a myriad of other oils or blends of oils is superior is a marketing game to showcase a product; it has nothing to do with common sense about hair.

Some plant oils, often referred to as essential oils, are highly fragrant, volatile oils and because these are almost always irritants or photosensitizers, I indicate it when this is the case. However, I attribute no superiority to one over another, because none exists. Essential oils are nothing more than a way to get fragrance into a hair-care product. The hair-care industry knows that many women are aware that fragrance can be a strong source of skin irritation and sensitivities, so they use the term "essential oils" as a way to add fragrance to a product without saying "fragrance." Women may know that fragrance ingredients are bad, but they still want their products to smell nice. Caught between a rock and a hard place, the cosmetics industry came up with the phrase "essential oils" as the way around the dilemma. But the notion that plants can save the hair is sheer fantasy and has no legitimate substantiation.

Vitamins in hair-care products are useless. Not only are they unable to feed dead hair, they also don't cling well to the hair shaft—so they aren't effective as conditioning agents either. Ingredients like panthenol and biotin do have vitamin origins, but their effectiveness for the hair has nothing to do with nutrients; they cling to the hair shaft, improving feel and tensile strength just like any other conditioning agent.

For the scalp, vitamins would be rinsed off or brushed away before they had a chance to be effective. For skin care, most vitamins do perform well as **antioxidants,** but in hair-care products they just can't stay around long enough to provide that function. Antioxidants are an overly hyped area of skin and hair care. While there is impressive research pointing to the effectiveness of antioxidants in petrie dishes and some minimal information about topical application of antioxidants in lab animals, there is no substantiation of their effect on human skin. If anything, we don't even know whether or not any antioxidant, whether it be vitamin A, vitamin C, or vitamin E, to name a few, is really worthwhile for skin. Antioxidants providing benefit for skin is all theory, and that doesn't translate to good hair or skin care.

Anti-irritants and soothing agents are ingredients known for their ability to reduce inflammation. A small group of ingredients, such as bisabolol, allantoin, burdock root, aloe, licorice root, and green tea, can perform this function. These ingredients work much better in skin-care products than hair-care products because they need to be left on the scalp to have an effect. In shampoos and conditioners, where they are typically found, the product would be rinsed off before it ever had a chance to have an effect.

Slip agents help other ingredients spread over or penetrate the hair's cuticle. These include propylene glycol, butylene glycol, polysorbates, and glycerin. They are as basic to the world of hair care as water.

Water-binding agents are known for their ability to help the hair retain water, but they have only minimal effectiveness because they are so easily rinsed or brushed away. These ingredients range from the mundane glycerin and propylene glycol to the more exotic hyaluronic acid, sodium hyaluronate, mucopolysaccharides, sodium PCA, collagen, elastin, proteins, amino acids (of which there are dozens), cholesterol, glucose, sucrose, fructose, glycogen, antioxidants, phospholipids, glycosphingolipids, and on and on. For the most part, they all work equally well and there is interesting research pointing to glycerin and propylene glycol as being the most effective for clinging to hair. Looking for a specific one is a waste of your time and energy. They are all what they are: good water-binding ingredients.

In the same way that the film formers mentioned above are fundamental to any hairstyling product, **propellants** are essential to aerosol hairstyling products from mousses to hairsprays. Propellants such as butane and propane allow a product to dispel its contents over the hair in an aerated mist or a foaming lather. Whether you choose to use an aerosol or regular hairspray is a personal preference. Some prefer the aerosol version because it sprays a fine, even mist, as compared to a regular spray that tends to concentrate the mist more and to cover less uniformly.

It is typical for aerosol and some nonaerosol hair sprays as well as hairstyling gels to use alcohol as the main ingredient (but not stearyl alcohol or cetyl alcohol, which are just benign thickening agents), and it is usually listed as SD alcohol, isopropyl alcohol, or denatured alcohol. As drying as alcohol can be for the skin and hair, in hairsprays or styling products, the alcohol evaporates before it has a chance to negatively affect the hair. In this regard alcohol is a blessing for the hair because other liquid alternatives would quickly wreck a hairstyle! In gels and spray gels, the alcohol is slightly more problematic for hair, but not much. It truly evaporates before it has much chance to affect the hair in any way other than to help the styling ingredients set faster on the hair without oversaturating the hair with more water.

When **fragrance** is listed in the ingredients, I indicate this simply by stating it as such. Fragrances are used in cosmetics either to mask the smell of a product's ingredients or to add a specific fragrance. My strong recommendation is that all hair-care and skin-care products not contain fragrance. Fragrances of all kinds, including essential oils, are irritants, and more often than not serve absolutely no function for hair or scalp. Especially for hair-care products, trying to find those that are fragrance-free is almost impossible. Except for KMS Puritives and my skin-care products (Paula's Choice), there are no other options I know of. Please keep in mind that unscented products are not fragrance-free. "Unscented" simply means that a product uses a masking fragrance to reduce the "natural" odor of the ingredients, as opposed to adding a fragrance that creates a distinctive aroma.

There are **preservatives** that some people feel are more problematic than others. I have not included specific warnings for preservatives such as quaternium-15, 2-bromo-2-nitropane-1,3-diol, phenoxyethanol, or dmdm hydantoin. While there is research indicating that these ingredients pose a higher potential for irritation than other preservatives, more recent data strongly dispute that conclusion. After discussing this matter with several cosmetic chemists, I have concluded that all preservatives can be a problem for many different types of skin, so it would be unfair and misleading to pinpoint one specific preservative as a problem. If you are concerned, you can easily avoid any of these ingredients. However, as several cosmetic chemists warned me, a reliable preservative system is better for the skin because without it microbial contamination of a product can cause more problems for the eyes, lips, skin, and scalp than the risk of a reaction to a preservative.

On a related matter, some of you may be familiar with research that warns against using cosmetics that contain DEA, triethanolamine, or TEA-lauryl sulfate mixed in the same product along with formaldehyde-releasing preservatives such as imidazolidinyl urea, quaternium-15, 2-bromo-2-nitropane-3,1-diol, or dmdm hydantoin. There is evidence that suggests these combinations can form nitrosamines in a cosmetic, creating a potential carcinogen (nitrosamines, as you may recall, are carcinogenic substances). There is substantial disagreement among the cosmetic chemists I spoke to as to how significant a problem this is for the skin (or even whether it is a problem). They suggested that going out of the house without a sunscreen or sitting in a bar exposed to secondhand cigarette smoke poses more risk to the skin than any combination of skin-care ingredients ever could. However, you should be aware that there are those who consider this nonchalant attitude to be mere apologetics for and sidestepping around a very serious question. As someone who has looked at this issue for some time, I actually understand both viewpoints and have no definitive position to share. To that end, I leave the final decision up to you. All you need to do is check the ingredient list of any product you are considering to determine whether it excludes amines as well as the questionable preservatives mentioned above.

Coloring agents are mentioned when pigments are added to products to change the products' color. The term **dye agent** is used when hair colorants are added to affect the actual color of the hair. These types of dye agents are found in color enhancing shampoos, conditioners, and occasional styling products.

Antimicrobial agents are ingredients to fight off the presence of certain microbes that may be causing dandruff or other scalp dermatitis. More often than not I refer to these by name; most typically they are zinc pyrithione, coal tar, or tea tree oil. Occasionally I use the more general term "antimicrobial agent."

Chelating agents are ingredients added to shampoos to prevent minerals from binding together in the product and preventing hardening or a coupling of ingredients. When chelating agents are listed higher up on the ingredient listing, they are present in sufficient quantity to prevent most minerals in tap water, ocean water, or pool water from binding to the hair.

The Ratings

The following are the rating symbols for the products reviewed in this book. These simple but succinct (and albeit cute) symbols graphically depict my approval or disapproval of a specific product:

☺ This smiling face indicates a great product that I recommend highly and that is also low in price. It means the product is definitely worth checking into and potentially worth buying.

☺ $$$ This symbol designates a great product that I would recommend without a doubt were it not so absurdly overpriced, either in comparison to similar products or in relation to what you are getting for the money.

☻ This neutral face indicates an OK but unimpressive product, or an OK product that can cause problems for certain hair or scalp types. I often use this to portray a dated or old-fashioned product formulation. Depending on your personal preferences, products rated with this face may be worth checking out, but are nothing to get excited about.

☺ **$$$** This symbol indicates an ordinary, boring product whose excessive price makes it ludicrous to consider.

☹ This symbol reflects a product that is truly bad from almost every standpoint, including price, performance, application, texture, potential for irritation, scalp reactions, stiffness, or sticky feel.

Prices: Because the cost of drugstore and salon products fluctuates from store to store, and because hair-care companies often change prices, the prices listed in this book may not be up to date or match what you find when you are shopping. Use the prices as a basis for comparison, but realize that they may not precisely reflect what you will find when you go shopping.

Up-to-date information: My staff and I struggle to make sure all the information we have is accurate and current. **However, hair-care companies frequently and without notice change or reformulate their products, sometimes in a minor way and sometimes extensively.** To keep abreast of these changes that cannot be kept current in a book, I report all revisions and new product launches that occurred after this book went to press in my newsletter, *Cosmetics Counter Update*.

Foreign names: For the most part, I give only the English names of foreign-produced products. The French and Italian names are pretty, but they don't tell you anything about the product if you don't speak the language.

No endorsements: Neither the information nor the evaluations included in any of my work are to be misconstrued as endorsements, nor do they represent a particular company's sponsorship. None of the companies listed paid me for my remarks or critiques, and none supplied products. All the "Best Choices" are just that, choices, with the final decision up to you.

Order of presentation: The cosmetics are listed alphabetically by brand name, so the order in which they appear does not represent my preference. There is no implied winner among any of the cosmetics companies included; no one line has all the answers or the majority of great products. Almost every line has its strong and weak points.

The Criteria

Each product category had different elements that I considered essential for establishing a single product's desirability. These criteria were very specific and not something everyone would automatically agree with, particularly the people who sell the products. But then again, I don't expect them to agree with me very often anyway. (Although they tend to strongly agree with me when I recommend one of their products, they vehemently disagree when I suggest that one of their products doesn't live up to its claims.) I assigned each category of products the following specific standards and guidelines.

Shampoos for normal to oily hair needed to be practically free of emollients and oil, as well as lacking irritating ingredients that could possibly cause a rebound effect. **Conditioners** for normal to oily hair had to have a minimal amount of conditioning agents and no heavy waxes or oils. Shampoos and conditioners designed for coarse hair needed to contain smoothing agents. Shampoos and conditioners claiming to be good for dry, damaged, chemically treated, or fragile hair needed to contain conditioning agents, emollients, detangling agents, silicone, and water-binding agents, all in the first part of the ingredient list, well before the preservatives and fragrance. (If they were listed after the fragrance or preservative, the amount would be negligible and have minimal effect on the hair.) If a company made claims about plants and their effectiveness on the hair but would not supply any substantiation, those assertions were considered invalid.

Styling products needed to live up to their claims about hold, stickiness, and allowing the user to run a brush through her hair after using them. If a product claimed it was unique or superior and the ingredient list read the same as any other product in the same category, the claim of superiority was considered unsubstantiated.

All products were rated comparatively to other products of their own kind on the market. Shampoos, conditioners, and styling products were all rated as to how they were either similar or dissimilar to other products in their category. Styling products were grouped by subcategories in this general order: gels, mousses, hairsprays, and specialty products.

Even though shampoos and conditioners are usually labeled to be purchased together, they do not have to be used that way. Sometimes, using shampoos and conditioners that are seemingly designed to work together can cause problems. Too much of one ingredient isn't always best for hair. A shampoo that contains the same conditioning agents as the conditioner can make hair heavy and limp. For this reason I primarily grouped the products in each line by type; all the shampoos are listed together, then the conditioners, then the styling products, and then the specialty products.

I think you will be shocked when you notice how stunningly similar products are from line to line. The differences lie not in spectacular ingredient lists but, rather, in amounts (how much protein or panthenol does a product really contain?) or specifics (is the detergent cleansing agent one that can strip color from the hair?).

Important warnings:

1.   Any shampoo with conditioning agents, silicones, or film formers can cause buildup on the hair with repeated use. I tended to only specifically point this out if I thought the concentrations of these were enough to make it a more apparent problem.

2. Any conditioner, as well as most all styling products, containing emollients (conditioning agents) or film formers, can cause buildup. To eliminate this problem, it is essential to wash your hair with a shampoo that doesn't contain conditioning agents or film formers.

3. Shampoos with film formers and conditioners with film formers were almost always recommended only for those with normal to fine or thin hair. Film formers add a layer over the hair shaft that can add a feeling of thickness, which someone with coarse, thick hair normally would not want.

You Don't Have to Agree

If you're just now reading this section, it is probably after you have picked up this book and quickly looked up the products you are presently using, have used in the past, or are thinking of using in the future. You went to those sections first because my credibility often hinges on whether you agree with my assessments of the products you are using. However, be aware that you need not agree with all my reviews to obtain benefit from this book. As you read my comments, you may indeed find yourself disagreeing with me. That is perfectly understandable and as it should be, because the criteria you use to evaluate cosmetics may differ from mine. Or, for any one of a dozen reasons (personal preference, different expectations, actual usage—once a week versus twice a day, for example), a product I dislike may work well for you. Or just the opposite can be true: you may hate a product I love. What I cannot account for is how millions of women will feel about a particular product or the nuances in usage or specific preferences.

What I present in the following pages are merely guidelines, based on my extensive research and experience about what works and what doesn't. If you decide to follow any of my suggestions, be aware that my recommendations are not a guarantee, but a suggestion as to how to narrow down the endless options the hair-care industry sells and how to approach their relentless, deceptive marketing language more realistically. It is my earnest desire to help you chose from this very crowded field so you can make the best choices possible—but the final choice is up to you.

Hair Note: For all the reviews that follow, it is assumed that chemically treated hair is not automatically a hair type. If you have your hair permed or dyed, whatever hair "type" it is, how normal, dry, or damaged it is depends on the type of chemical process you have done, how often you have it done, how much you keep your hair out of the sun, and what type of hair you started out with. Chemically treated hair is not automatically either dry or damaged, so make your selections based on how your hair feels and behaves, not by this arbitrary "hair type" assumption. **For the most part, I took for granted that damaged, chemically treated, or dyed hair had the exact same needs as dry or extremely dry hair.**

Adorn

Adorn has been around forever—well, almost forever. These hairsprays aren't the fanciest on the market, but for hairspray they work just fine. Their reputation for "helmet hair" is not true. Believe it or not, they do brush through and leave just about the same amount of stiffness and stickiness as other firm-hold hairsprays do. Keep in mind that the entire hair-care industry is using the exact same "film-forming" ingredients.

For more information about Adorn call (800) 872-7202 or visit its Web site at www.gillette.com.

☺ **Hairspray for Long Lasting, Touchable Hold, Extra Hold (Aerosol) Scented and Unscented** *($2.92 for 7.5 ounces)* contains mostly alcohol, propellant, film former, and fragrance. It provides a light to medium hold that can easily be brushed through. The unscented version contains a masking fragrance.

☺ **Hairspray for Long Lasting, Touchable Hold, Frequent Use No Build Up (Aerosol)** *($2.92 for 7.5 ounces)* is almost identical to the one above. The claim of no buildup is impossible; the very nature of all hairstyling products is that they grab on and hold on to hair. If they didn't, they wouldn't work.

African Pride

African Pride claims it has "discovered the secret to fabulous looking hair! Our recipes contain the finest herbs and oils for hair that's soft, shiny and full of body." That sounds better than it ends up being. The oils and emollients in its products are the same ones that show up in lots of products for African American hair, including Vaseline, lanolin, mineral oil, castor oil, and plant oils, but none of that makes its products different from the rest. What those ingredients do more often than not is make hair greasy. There are other options to make hair feel softer and smoother without greasing it out, but the African Pride line has only one or two examples of that newer technology, namely, using silicone instead of a preponderance of plant oils, lanolin, and Vaseline.

The "African herbal liquid complex" in these products is about as far removed from Africa as you can get. It is simply tea water made of hemp, nettle, rosemary, burdock, birch, rose hips, carrageenan, coltsfoot, wild cherry bark, dandelion, *Sambucus nigra* (black elder), horsetail, and coneflower. Even if these plants were harvested in Africa, that wouldn't automatically make them better for curly, kinky hair. My concern about a long list of plant extracts is the risk they pose of an allergic or sensitizing skin reaction. If you have problems with an itchy scalp, that may be the source of the itch.

At best, most of these conditioning product formulations are fairly dated. They create a greasy-looking shine to hair and can be a problem on the scalp (by clogging pores and cutting off healthy growth). That's not the best for damaged hair, dry scalp, or thin hair growth.

African Pride also sells some snake oil in the form of Vitamagic Miracle Hair Vitamins with "healthier hair growth guaranteed." While a healthy diet can make a difference in hair growth, there are no secret nutrients to do this. Vitamins cannot change the genetic structure of hair.

For more information about African Pride, call (800) 223-2339 or check out its Web site at www.african-pride.com.

☺ **Shampoo and Conditioner 2-in-1 Formula** *($3.99 for 12 ounces)* contains tea water, detergent cleansing agents, lather agents, thickeners, conditioning agents, fragrance, and preservatives. This is an extremely standard but very good shampoo with minimal conditioning agents, so if you have dry hair you will still need a conditioner. The tea water sounds good but offers no benefit for the hair or scalp.

☺ **African Miracle Hair & Scalp Spray** *($5.49 for 12 ounces)* contains mostly tea water, slip agent, glycerin, conditioning agents, thickeners, detangling agent, fragrance, and preservatives. This is a good lightweight conditioner for normal to slightly dry hair. There is nothing miraculous about any of it.

☹ **Castor Oil & Mink Oil Conditioner** *($3.99 for 5.5 ounces)* contains mostly Vaseline, plant oils, mink oil, shea butter, lanolin, thickeners, plant extracts, and fragrance. This is greasy kid stuff that can be hard to wash out of hair. The mink oil and plant extracts in here do not offer any added benefit for the hair.

☹ **Dream Kids Miracle Creme** *($5.99 for 4 ounces)* contains mostly tea water, plant oils, Vaseline, wax, lanolin, thickeners, silicone, preservatives, and fragrance. This conditioner can make hair look greasy and it is difficult to wash out.

☺ **Instant Oil Moisturizing Hair Lotion** *($5.49 for 12 ounces)* contains mostly tea water, mineral oil, thickeners, detangling agent, silicone, fragrance, preservatives, and coloring agents. This is slightly less greasy, but only minimally so; other than that it is a good mineral oil–based conditioner for extremely dry hair.

☺ **Leave-in Conditioner** *($3.99 for 12 ounces)* contains mostly tea water, aloe, detangling agents, silicone, conditioning agents, fragrance, and preservatives. This is a very good lightweight conditioner that would be best for someone with normal to slightly dry hair.

☺ **Wonder Weave Moisturizing Styling Gel** *($3.99 for 8.5 ounces)* contains mostly tea water, slip agent, thickener, glycerin, film former, preservatives, coloring agents, and fragrance. This very lightweight styling gel can provide minimal hold and control along with minimal stiffness or sticky feel.

☺ **Braid Sheen Spray** *($3.99 for 12 ounces)* contains mostly tea water, slip agent, silicone, thickeners, preservative, conditioning agents, and fragrance. This lightweight silicone spray can definitely add shine to hair or braids.

☺ **Braid Sheen Spray Extra Conditioning Formula** *($4.99 for 8 ounces)* contains mostly tea water, slip agent, glycerin, silicone, conditioning agent, detangling agent, fragrance, and preservatives. This is a good lightweight spray that can add shine and some softness to hair or braids.

☺ **Wonder Weave Intensive Shine Glosser** *($3.99 for 2 ounces)* is a standard silicone spray that can add shine to hair.

☺ **Hair, Scalp & Skin Oil** *($3.99 for 8 ounces)* contains mostly plant oils, castor oil, plant extracts, wax, and fragrance. This is greasy stuff and not much different from taking olive oil from your pantry to apply to your skin or hair. It can be helpful for extremely dry hair.

☺ **Magical GRO Magical Herbal Recipe** *($4.99 for 5.5 ounces)* contains mostly Vaseline, plant oils, castor oil, plant extracts, lanolin, thickeners, and fragrance. This won't help hair grow in the least; if anything, it's hard to wash out of hair and can clog the hair follicle. If left on the ends of hair, it can be good for dry hair but be careful and use it sparingly—this stuff can be greasy. This product and the next two, Magical GRO and the Miracle Creme, can't do a thing to stop breakage from hair relaxers or hot styling tools.

☺ **Magical GRO Magical Oil Recipe** *($3.99 for 5.5 ounces)* is almost identical to the one above and the same comments apply.

☺ **Magical GRO Maximum Herbal Strength** *($4.99 for 5.5 ounces)* is almost identical to the two above and the same comments apply.

☺ **Miracle Creme** *($3.99 for 5.5 ounces)* is almost identical to the three above and the same comments apply.

☺ **Miracle Sheen Oil Sheen & Conditioning Spray** *($2.99 for 12.5 ounces)* contains mostly mineral oil, propellant, alcohol, plant extracts, and fragrance. This is a good but greasy way to evenly spray oil over the hair and can help very dry hair.

☺ **Wonder Weave Conditioning Sheen Spray** *($3.49 for 2 ounces)* contains mostly plant oils, castor oil, emollient, plant extracts, vitamins, coloring agents, and fragrance. This is a good way to evenly spray oil over the hair, but it is "oily" and can eventually build up and look greasy, so be careful.

AllWays Natural by African Pride

☺ **Neutralizing Conditioning Shampoo with Color Action** *($3.99 for 12 ounces)* contains mostly tea water, detergent cleansing agents, lather agents, minimal conditioning and detangling agents, fragrance, preservatives, and coloring agent. This is a very good, gentle shampoo for most all hair types. It won't clean heavy conditioning agents out of the hair, so it is best only if you are using minimal styling or nongreasy products. It also contains minimal conditioning agents, which would not cause a problem with buildup.

☺ **Shampoo Moisturizing Formula** *($3.19 for 12 ounces)* contains mostly tea water, detergent cleansing agents, lather agent, thickeners, plant oil, vitamin, conditioning agents, detangling agent, slip agent, and preservatives. This is a good, minimally conditioning shampoo that can be good for most hair types.

☺ **100% Natural Indian Hemp Herbal Hair and Scalp Treatment Conditioner** *($4.79 for 4 ounces)* contains mostly Vaseline, plant oils, lanolin, wax, plant extract, preservatives, and vitamins. This is greasy stuff and the gentle shampoos in this line won't wash this amount of Vaseline and lanolin away. It can be good for ends of very dry hair, but keep this away from the scalp. Hemp serves no purpose for hair.

☺ **100% Natural Indian Hemp Super Lite Herbal Hair and Scalp Treatment Conditioner** *($3.09 for 4 ounces)* is similar to the version above and the same basic comments apply.

☺ **Castor Oil Conditioning Hair Dress** *($2.29 for 5.5 ounces)* contains mostly Vaseline, castor oil, lanolin, plant extracts, emollients, preservative, and fragrance. This is greasy kid stuff and best used minimally on ends of extremely dry hair only.

☺ **Conditioner Moisturizing Formula** *($3.99 for 12 ounces)* contains mostly plant extracts, plant oils, slip agent, thickeners, lanolin, film former, and preservatives. This can be very greasy and is best used on the ends of extremely dry hair and only minimally.

☺ **Indian Hemp Conditioning Hair Dress** *($3.99 for 5.5 ounces)* contains mostly Vaseline, lanolin, plant oils, wax, emollient, preservative, and fragrance and is best used on the ends of extremely dry hair and only minimally.

☹ **IsoGRO, Menthol & Chamomile, to Condition Dry Hair and Scalp** *($3.79 for 5.5 ounces)* contains menthol, which can be an irritant and drying agent for the scalp.

☺ **Super GRO Conditioning Hair Dress** *($3.49 for 5.5 ounces)* contains mostly Vaseline, wax, plant oils, plant extracts, vitamins, preservatives, and fragrance. This very greasy conditioner can easily build up on hair and is best used on extremely dry ends only. It is also exceptionally difficult to wash out of hair.

☺ **Super Lite Indian Hemp Conditioning Hair Dress** *($3.99 for 5.5 ounces)* isn't light in the least—it is virtually identical to the one above except for the inclusion of lanolin.

☺ **Super Lite Super GRO Conditioning Hair Dress** *($3.99 for 5.5 ounces)* is almost identical to the ones above and the same comments apply.

☺ **911 Heat Protector Heat Styling Protection** *($3.29 for 8 ounces)* contains mostly water, detangling agent/film former, vitamins, more film former, slip agent, silicones, glycerin, plant extracts, fragrance, and preservatives. This is a good, light-weight styling spray that would work well to add minimal hold with minimal stickiness and stiffness, though it can't protect from heat damage. Nothing can stop a curling iron or blow dryer radiating heat at over 200 degrees Fahrenheit from causing damage to hair, or skin for that matter. It would be great for wavy or curly hair that isn't overly dry.

☺ **911 Leave-in Conditioner, Extra Dry Formula** *($4.59 for 16 ounces)* is supposed to repair damage; it can't. But it is a good lightweight leave-in conditioner for normal to slightly dry, thin, or fine hair. It contains mostly water, detangling agent/film former, vitamins, conditioning agents, silicone, plant extracts, preservatives, and fragrance. This is a good conditioner for normal to slightly dry hair but it can leave a somewhat stiff feel on hair. This formula would not be good for extremely damaged hair.

☺ **911 Leave-in Conditioner, Feather Light Creme Formula, Extra Dry** *($3.19 for 18 ounces)* contains mostly tea water, Vaseline, wax, thickeners, vitamins, silicone, detangling agents, fragrance, and preservatives. For extremely dry hair this product could work well, though the petrolatum can leave the hair feeling fairly greasy.

☺ **911 Leave-in Creme Conditioner, Original Formula** *($3.19 for 8 ounces)* is similar to the Feather Light version above and the same comments apply.

☺ **911 Leave-in Hair Conditioner, Original Formula** *($3.62 for 8 ounces)* contains mostly water, detangling agent/film former, conditioning agents, detangling agent, silicone, plant extracts, preservatives, and fragrance.

☺ **911 Leave-in Hair Treatment** *($4.39 for 16 ounces)* is almost identical to the one above, except for the addition of lanolin, which makes it better for drier hair.

☺ **911 Leave-in Hair Treatment, Extra Dry Formula** *($4.39 for 16 ounces)* isn't best for extra-dry hair, at least not in comparison to the one above. Other than that it is a good leave-in conditioner for normal to slightly dry, thin, or fine hair.

☺ **Instant Oil Moisturizer Leave-in Conditioner** *($4.19 for 12 ounces)* doesn't contain as much oil as the name implies. It contains mostly tea water, thickeners, glycerin, plant oils, slip agent, and preservatives. It would be good for very dry, coarse hair.

☺ **911 Styling Spritz Extra Firm Hold** *($2.71 for 8 ounces)* contains mostly alcohol, film formers, plant extracts, silicone oil, and fragrance. This is a good, standard, light- to medium-hold hairspray that can add some amount of shine to hair and give a combable hold with minimal stiffness or sticky feel. Don't worry about the alcohol; it evaporates before it can dry the hair.

☺ **911 Super Spritz** *($2.71 for 8 ounces)* is similar to the Extra Firm Hold version above only with more hold. It can have more of a stiff and sticky feel.

☺ **Break No More Creme Hair Dressing** *($3.39 for 4 ounces)* contains plant extracts, Vaseline, thickeners, and preservatives. Vaseline can't stop hair breakage but it can add a greasy feel to hair and be difficult to wash out. This is best when used only on extremely dry ends of hair and then only minimally.

African Royale

African Royale is a line of hair-care products aimed at African Americans. The line says its "Gelatin Rich Oils (G.R.O.) plus 14 herbs condition and pamper your hair so that it looks and smells its best. Like the Egyptian Kings and Queens whose attendants knew the herbal secrets of beauty, treat your hair to a Royale treatment." That we have any idea what ancient Egyptians used on their hair is a stretch of history, and what is known is more like mythology than anything else. These extremely standard products contain mineral oil, castor oil, standard detergent cleansing agents, silicone, and a plethora of other ingredients no one knew about until recent times.

Several of the African Royale products claim to "soothe the itching often associated with braids, weaves, and extensions." The itching associated with braids is generally due to the tightness and weight placed on the hair follicle and scalp from the weave or extension, as well as less frequent washing. The products don't contain ingredients that can reduce such itching—if anything, the long list of plant extracts can be sensitizing for many skin and scalp types.

Despite the exotic claims, there are some good products to be found here that work for dry hair and for those who wear braids or have extensions.

For more information about African Royale call (800) 241-6151.

☺ **BRX Braid & Extensions Spray on Shampoo** *($3.99 for 12 ounces)* is a very good, gentle shampoo (more like baby shampoo) with minimal film-forming agents and fragrance. It includes a rather long list of plant extracts ranging from elm bark to yarrow that have no effect on hair.

☺ **Soft As Me Herbal Shampoo** *($3.49 for 8 ounces)* is a standard detergent-based cleanser, slightly more potent than the one above. It contains minimal styling agents and conditioners, so it should clean well without buildup. It does contain fragrance and coloring agents, as well as the same long list of plant extracts as the one above. If you're the allergic type, these could be a problem and they serve no purpose for scalp or hair.

☹ **Castor G.R.O. Gelatin Rich Oils** *($3.99 for 6 ounces)* is greasy stuff that contains mostly Vaseline, plant oils, castor oil, thickener, vitamins, silicone, plant extracts, and fragrance. This would be good for extremely dry hair but it contains walnut shell pieces that can leave bits on the hair and scalp.

☺ **Daily Doctor Leave-in Conditioner** *($3.49 for 12 ounces)* is a good lightweight, leave-in conditioner for normal to slightly dry hair. It contains mostly water, glycerin, soothing agent, silicone, emollient, fragrance, and preservatives. The same long list of plant extracts that sound interesting are here again, but serve no purpose for hair.

☺ **Extra Light Creme of Ginseng** *($3.49 for 6 ounces)* contains mostly water, mineral oil, detangling agent, castor oil, slip agent, silicone, preservatives, and fragrance. This isn't light, and it can be greasy. It could be good for the ends of extremely dry hair, but be careful about buildup or using too much. Ginseng brings no benefit to hair.

☺ **Extra Light Super G.R.O. with Ginseng** *($5.19 for 6 ounces)* is a conditioner with nothing light about it. It contains mostly Vaseline, plant oils, castor oil, thickener, vitamins, silicone, plant extracts, and fragrance. It can be good for extremely dry hair but it can also be greasy. There is nothing in this formula that will "G.R.O" hair.

☺ **Maximum Strength Super G.R.O.** *($5.19 for 6 ounces)* is similar to the Extra Light versions and the same comments apply.

☹ **Super G.R.O. Gelatin Rich Oils** *($3.99 for 6 ounces)* contains mostly Vaseline, plant oils, thickener, vitamins, silicone, plant extracts, coloring agents, and fragrance. This would be good for extremely dry hair but it contains walnut shell pieces that can leave bits on the hair and scalp.

☹ **Mink Oil Gel for Hair and Scalp** *($3.49 for 6 ounces)* is a greasy mix of water, glycerin, slip agent, mink oil, lanolin, mineral oil, silicone, protein, thickener, plant extracts, preservatives, and fragrance. It would be good for extremely dry ends of hair, but this gunk (it isn't really a gel) has pieces of walnut shell in it that can flake off of the hair and leave bits on the scalp.

☺ **M.O.M. Miracle Oil Moisturizer** *($3.59 for 8 ounces)* contains mostly water, plant oils, castor oil, detangling agents, thickeners, mineral oil, plant extracts, preservatives, and fragrance. This can leave a greasy film over the hair, but it definitely can help prevent dryness.

☺ **Royale Mist Natural Spray for Hair & Scalp** *($3.99 for 12 ounces)* contains mostly water, glycerin, slip agents, detangling agents, thickeners, mineral oil, plant oil, plant extracts, preservatives, and fragrance. This very lightweight spray adds a little bit of detangling agents and some oil for normal to dry hair.

☺ **BRX Braid and Extensions Sheen Spray** *($3.49 for 12 ounces)* contains mostly water, slip agents, detangling/film-forming agents, protein, silicone, plant extracts, preservatives, and fragrance. This is supposed to reduce itching, but there are no ingredients in here that can do that. Other than that, it is a good lightweight spray to add a little bit of shine that won't appear greasy.

☺ **Diamond Drops** *($3.99 for 2 ounces)* contains mostly silicones, plant oil, plant extracts, and fragrance. Now this product can add shine without grease and also make hair feel like silk. It is a standard silicone serum for dry hair.

☺ **Hot Six Oil** *($3.79 for 8 ounces)* contains mostly plant oils, castor oil, vitamins, silicone, plant extracts, and fragrance. This is just oil, and inexpensive at that, but it can leave a greasy buildup on the hair and be difficult to wash out. It can be good for extremely dry hair when used minimally.

Alberto

Alberto has been around for decades and is one of the least expensive groups of hair-care products you'll find at the drugstore. There are many urban myths about this line that hairstylists love to tell their clients. I've heard everything from "Alberto eats hair" to "it can perm hair if you leave it on long enough!" None of that is true. What is true is that the Alberto shampoos are fairly drying and the conditioning treatments are fairly standard, with little to no silicone, emollients, or extensive conditioning agents. That makes them more suitable for normal to slightly dry hair—and that's about it. It definitely isn't for everyone, but it is one of the most popular lines at the drugstore.

For more information on Alberto, call (708) 450-3000, (800) 333-6666 or visit its Web site at www.alberto-culver.com.

☹ **Balsam & Protein Shampoo, Conditions and Enhances Shine** *($0.99 for 15 ounces)* uses sodium lauryl sulfate as the main detergent cleansing agent, which can be too drying for the hair and too irritating for the scalp. It also contains balsam, which can leave a stiff resin on the hair that easily builds up and leaves hair limp and sticky.

☹ **Clarifying Formula Shampoo** *($0.99 for 15 ounces)* uses sodium lauryl sulfate as the main detergent cleansing agent, and is not recommended.

☹ **Extra Body Shampoo, Maximum Fullness with Collagen** *($0.99 for 15 ounces)* uses sodium lauryl sulfate as the main detergent cleansing agent, and is not recommended.

☹ **Fresh Cleansing Shampoo Fresh Apple with Pectin** *($0.99 for 15 ounces)* uses sodium lauryl sulfate as the main detergent cleansing agent, and is not recommended.

☹ **Henna Shampoo, Enhances Shine** *($0.99 for 15 ounces)* uses sodium lauryl sulfate as the main detergent cleansing agent, and is not recommended.

☹ **Jojoba Shampoo, Revives Overworked Hair** *($0.99 for 15 ounces)* uses sodium lauryl sulfate as the main detergent cleansing agent, and is not recommended.

☹ **Moisturizing Shampoo, Moisture-Rich with Aloe** *($0.99 for 15 ounces)* uses sodium lauryl sulfate as the main detergent cleansing agent, and is not recommended.

☹ **Naturals Shampoo, Fresh Botanicals (wild thyme, balsam, jojoba)** *($1.49 for 15 ounces)* uses sodium lauryl sulfate as the main detergent cleansing agent, and is not recommended.

☹ **Naturals Shampoo, Fruitsation (melon, wild berry, wheat germ extract)** *($0.99 for 15 ounces)* uses sodium lauryl sulfate as the main detergent cleansing agent, and is not recommended.

☹ **Naturals Shampoo, Vanilla Blossom (vanilla, honeysuckle, chamomile)** *($0.99 for 15 ounces)* uses sodium lauryl sulfate as the main detergent cleansing agent, and is not recommended.

☹ **Normal Shampoo, Gentle Every Day Cleansing** *($0.99 for 15 ounces)* uses sodium lauryl sulfate as the main detergent cleansing agent, and is not recommended.

☹ **Pear Mango Passion Herbal Shampoo, Dry, Color-Treated or Permed, Aloe and Passion Flower Extracts** *($0.99 for 15 ounces)* uses sodium lauryl sulfate as the main detergent cleansing agent, and is not recommended.

☹ **Split Ends Treatment Shampoo, Protects and Reduces Breakage** *($0.99 for 15 ounces)* uses sodium lauryl sulfate as the main detergent cleansing agent, and is not recommended.

☹ **Strawberry 'n Creme Shampoo, Essence of Wild Strawberry** *($1.49 for 15 ounces)* uses sodium lauryl sulfate as the main detergent cleansing agent, and is not recommended.

☹ **Sun Kissed Raspberry Herbal Shampoo, Normal, Juniper and Chamomile Extracts** *($0.99 for 15 ounces)* uses sodium lauryl sulfate as the main detergent cleansing agent, and is not recommended.

☹ **VO Fine Thickening Shampoo, Dry, Color Treated, Permed** *($3.09 for 13 ounces)* uses sodium lauryl sulfate as the main detergent cleansing agent, and is not recommended.

☹ **VO Fine Thickening Shampoo, Regular** *($3.09 for 13 ounces)* uses sodium lauryl sulfate as the main detergent cleansing agent, and is not recommended.

☹ **Balsam & Protein Conditioner, Conditions and Enhances Shine** *($0.99 for 15 ounces)* contains balsam, which can easily build up on hair making it stiff and sticky.

☺ **Clarifying Formula Conditioner, Daily Light Conditioning** *($0.99 for 15 ounces)* contains mostly water, thickener, detangling agent, fragrance, preservatives, minimal conditioning agent, and coloring agents. This is an OK but exceptionally standard conditioner that will add some amount of combability to normal hair that is normal to fine or thin.

☺ **Extra Body Conditioner, Maximum Fullness with Collagen** *($0.99 for 15 ounces)* is similar to the Clarifying one above except with the addition of a small amount of conditioner, vitamins, and plant oil. It can be better for hair that is slightly dry as well as normal to fine or thin.

☺ **Extra Body Permed/Color Treated Conditioner, Maximum Fullness** *($1.49 for 15 ounces)* is almost identical to the one above and the same review applies.

☹ **Hair Therapy Fortifying Leave-in Conditioner** *($2.99 for 8 ounces)* contains TEA-lauryl ether as the third ingredient, which can be drying and irritating to the scalp.

☺ **Hair Therapy Revitalizing Daily Conditioner** *($2.59 for 8 ounces)* contains mostly water, thickeners, detangling agents, glycerin, silicones, film former, preservatives, fragrance, and coloring agents. This doesn't penetrate deeply but it is a good lightweight conditioner for normal to slightly dry, fine, thin hair.

☺ **Henna Conditioner, Enhances Shine** *($0.99 for 15 ounces)* contains mostly water, thickeners, detangling agent, henna, vitamins, plant oil, fragrance, preservatives, and coloring agent. Henna can build up on hair and make it feel dry and brittle. However, for occasional use it can be a good conditioner for someone with normal to slightly dry, thin, fine hair.

☺ **Jojoba Conditioner, Revives Overworked Hair** *($0.99 for 15 ounces)* contains mostly water, thickeners, detangling agent, plant oil, glycerin, vitamins, conditioning agent, preservatives, and coloring agent. This basic but good conditioner would work well for normal to slightly dry hair.

☺ **Moisturizing Conditioner, Moisture and Softness** *($0.99 for 15 ounces)* is similar to the Jojoba Conditioner above and the same comments apply.

☺ **Naturals Conditioner, Fruitsation (melon, wild berry, wheat germ extract)** *($0.99 for 15 ounces)* includes fruit extracts that are completely useless for hair, but other than that it contains mostly water, thickeners, detangling agent, plant oils, fragrance, and preservatives. This is a good, basic conditioner for someone with normal to slightly dry hair.

☺ **Naturals Conditioner, Tropical Dreams (awapuhi, papaya, aloe)** *($1.49 for 15 ounces)* features plant extracts that are useless for hair, but other than that it is a good but extremely standard conditioner for someone with normal hair that needs help with combing. It contains mostly water, thickeners, detangling agent, fragrance, and preservatives.

☺ **Naturals Conditioner, Vanilla Blossom (vanilla, honeysuckle, chamomile)** *($0.99 for 15 ounces)*, except for the change in unnecessary plant extracts, is almost identical to the one above except for the addition of some corn oil, which makes it a little better for normal to slightly dry hair.

☺ **Normal Conditioner, Superb Manageability** *($0.99 for 15 ounces)* is virtually identical to the Vanilla Blossom version above and the same comments apply.

☺ **Pear Mango Passion Herbal Conditioner, Dry, Color-Treated or Permed, Aloe and Passion Flower Extracts** *($0.99 for 15 ounces)* is virtually identical to the Vanilla Blossom version above and the same comments apply.

☺ **Sun Kissed Raspberry Herbal Conditioner, Normal, Juniper and Chamomile Extracts** *($0.99 for 15 ounces)* is virtually identical to the Vanilla Blossom version above and the same comments apply.

☺ **Normal Daily Light Conditioning Conditioner** *($0.99 for 13 ounces)* is a good but extremely standard and basic conditioner for someone with normal hair that needs help with combing. It contains mostly water, thickeners, detangling agent, fragrance, and preservatives.

☺ **Salon Formula Conditioner** *($1.49 for 15 ounces)* is virtually identical to the Normal Daily Light above and the same comments apply.

☺ **Split Ends Treatment Conditioner** *($0.99 for 15 ounces)* is almost identical to the Normal Daily Light above and the same comments apply. This conditioner is useless for split ends or damaged hair of any kind.

☺ **Strawberry 'n Creme Conditioner, Essence of Wild Strawberry** *($1.49 for 15 ounces)* is almost identical to the Normal Daily Light above and the same comments apply.

☺ **VO Fine Thickening Conditioner, Dry, Color Treated, Permed** *($3.09 for 13 ounces)* contains mostly water, thickeners, detangling agents, film formers, silicones, conditioning agents, water-binding agents, plant extracts, slip agent, fragrance, and preservatives. The amount of film formers in this conditioner would be a problem for dry or extremely dry hair, making it feel stiff or brittle. It would be a far better for someone with dry hair that is normal to fine or for thin hair to help it feel thicker.

☺ **VO Fine Thickening Conditioner, Regular** *($3.09 for 13 ounces)* is almost identical to the one above and the same comments apply.

☺ **Conditioning Hairdressing, Extra Body for Fine Hair** *($2.99 for 1.5 ounces)* contains mostly mineral oil, water, Vaseline, thickeners, lanolin, waxes, fragrance, preservatives, and coloring agents. This is fairly greasy and heavy but can work well to smooth dry ends of very damaged hair. It definitely adds shine, but this much grease and wax is a problem for fine hair.

☺ **Conditioning Hairdressing, Gray, White & Silver Blonde Hair** *($2.99 for 1.5 ounces)* contains mostly mineral oil, Vaseline, lanolin, thickeners, fragrance, and coloring agents. Talk about greasy kid stuff! This can be good for very extremely dry ends of hair, but it is difficult to wash out and can easily build up on hair. Other than the violet color, there is nothing about this product that makes it suitable for gray hair.

☺ **Conditioning Hairdressing, Normal/Dry Hair** *($2.99 for 1.5 ounces)* is identical to the one above for gray hair and the same basic comments apply.

☺ **Conditioning Hairdressing, Unscented** *($2.99 for 1.5 ounces)* is identical to the one above and it even contains fragrance despite the name. Unscented simply refers to a masking fragrance as opposed to one that adds a distinctive aroma.

☺ **Hot Creme One Minute Intensive Hair Treatment Hydrating with Vitamin E** *($2.99 for two 0.50-ounce tubes)* is neither intensive or all that hydrating. It contains mostly water, thickeners, detangling agents, silicones, film former, preservatives, and fragrance. This is a fairly standard conditioner for normal to slightly dry hair that is normal to fine or thin in thickness.

☺ **Hot Oil Aromatherapy Hair Treatment, Chamomile & Ylang Ylang** *($2.99 for two 0.50-ounce tubes)* contains mostly water, detangling agent, plant extracts, thickeners, water-binding agents, film former, preservatives, fragrances, and coloring agents. There are no oils in this "hot oil" treatment. Other than that, it is a good, standard conditioner for normal to slightly dry hair that is normal to fine or thin in thickness.

☺ **Hot Oil Hair Treatment, Moisturizing, for Permed or Color Treated Hair** *($2.99 for two 0.50-ounce tubes)* is identical to the Hot Oil Treatments above and the same comments apply.

☺ **Hot Oil Hair Treatment, Strengthening** *($2.99 for two 0.50-ounce tubes)* is identical to the Hot Oil Treatments above and the same comments apply.

☺ **Hot Oil Shower Works Hair Treatment, Moisturizing** *($4.66 for 2 ounces)* is identical to the Hot Oil Treatments above, only you get more of this one, but the same comments apply.

☺ **Hot Oil Treatment, Split Ends Control** *($2.99 for two 0.50-ounce tubes)* is identical to the Hot Oil Treatments above and the same comments apply.

☹ **Hot Oil Aromatherapy Hair Treatment, Eucalyptus & Juniper Berry** *($2.99 for two 0.50-ounce tubes)* contains eucalyptus, which can be a scalp irritant. If that doesn't bother you, the same comments apply as to the Hot Oil Treatments, above.

☺ **Alcohol-Free Styling Gel, Extra Control** *($2.07 for 8 ounces)* is a standard styling gel using film formers, conditioning agent, thickeners, fragrance, preservatives, and coloring agents. It has a soft, pliable hold that brushes through easily with minimal stickiness or stiffness.

☺ **Hairdressing Gel for Men, Extra Hold** *($2.39 for 4.5 ounces)* is a standard gel with film formers, fragrance, and coloring agents. It does provide minimal to very soft hold and does brush through easily.

☺ **Alcohol-Free Styling Mousse, Conditioning Extra Hold** *($2.29 for 7 ounces)* is a standard mousse with several film formers, detangling agents, silicones, fragrance, water-binding agents, conditioning agents, and coloring agents. The amount of water-binding agents is negligible, though, so this is an OK soft-hold mousse, with minimal stiff or sticky feel.

☺ **Alcohol-Free Styling Mousse, Extra Body Extra Hold** *($2.59 for 7 ounces)* is similar to the Conditioning one above and the same comments apply.

☺ **Moisturizing Styling Mousse, Extra Control** *($2.69 for 8 ounces)* is similar to the Conditioning one above, though this one has a slightly stiffer, slightly sticky hold, but this a minor difference.

☺ **Finishing Spritz, Firm Hold** *($1.99 for 10 ounces)* is a standard hairspray that has a more soft than firm hold. It has minimal to no stiff or sticky feel and is easy to comb through hair. The distinctive hairspray smell may not be to everyone's liking, but it does fade quickly.

☺ **Hair Spray Hard to Hold** *($2.99 for 8.5 ounces)* is an aerosol hairspray that definitely has a light hold and that easily brushes through hair.

☺ **Hair Spray Hard to Hold, Conditioning** *($1.99 for 8.5 ounces)* is identical to the Hard to Hold one above and the same comments apply. In case you were wondering, there is nothing conditioning about this formula.

☺ **Hair Spray Hard to Hold, Extra Body** *($1.99 for 8.5 ounces)* is almost identical to the Hard to Hold version above and the same comments apply.

☺ **Hair Spray Hard to Hold, Extra Body (Non-Aerosol)** *($1.99 for 10 ounces)* is almost identical to the Hard to Hold one above, only in a nonaerosol version. This one also contains silicone, which can add shine to hair.

☺ **Hair Spray Hard to Hold, Unscented (Non-Aerosol)** *($1.99 for 10 ounces)* is almost identical to the ones above and the same comments apply. This product does have masking fragrance.

☺ **Hair Spray Hard to Hold, Silver** *($1.99 for 8.5 ounces)* is similar to the aerosol Hard to Hold versions above. There is nothing about this product that makes it better for silver hair.

☺ **Hair Spray Hard to Hold, Super** *($1.99 for 8.5 ounces)* is similar to the aerosol Hard to Hold ones above and the same comments apply.

☺ **Hair Spray Hard to Hold, Unscented (Aerosol)** *($1.99 for 8.5 ounces)* is identical to the aerosol Hard to Hold ones above and this one still contains fragrance in the form of a masking scent.

☺ **Naturals Non-Aerosol Hair Spray, Fruitsation (melon, wild berry, wheat germ extract), Super Hold** *($1.99 for 10 ounces)* is similar to the Hard to Hold nonaerosol versions above, only with the addition of plant extracts that have no benefit for hair. This one can have a slighter stiffer finish than the others.

☺ **Naturals Non-Aerosol Hair Spray, Vanilla Blossom (vanilla, honeysuckle, chamomile), Super Hold** *($1.99 for 10 ounces)* is identical to the one above, only with a change of fragrance.

American Crew

American Crew is a line of hair-care products aimed at men. The dramatic packaging, straightforward names, and woodland-fresh aroma are far more attractive to men, who would otherwise eschew products with floral, cinnamon, or sweet fragrances despite their promises of repairing damaged hair. Is there anything unique to make these products better for men? Not in the least, except for the smell, which is more "woodland" than floral. There are some good products to consider for all hair types, but it doesn't take a "man's" line to fit the hair needs of a guy.

For more information on American Crew, call (303) 292 4850, (800) 598-CREW or visit its Web site at www.americancrew.com.

☹ **Anti-Dandruff Shampoo, Formulated for Problem Scalps** *($9.50 for 6.76 ounces)* is a shampoo with several problems. First, as a dandruff shampoo, it doesn't contain any antidandruff ingredients, plus it also contains several skin irritants including menthol and spearmint, which can cause more itching and dryness. Menthol and spearmint make the scalp tingle, but that has no effect on the microbes causing the dandruff. Finally, the detergent cleansing agent is sodium lauryl sulfate, which can also be a scalp irritant and drying to the hair.

☺ **Daily Moisturizing Shampoo for Normal to Dry Hair & Scalp** *($5.95 for 8 ounces)* contains mostly water, detergent cleansing agents, lather agent, plant extracts, plant oil, detangling agents/film formers, silicone, preservatives, and fragrance. The film formers can build up and make hair feel stiff and look heavy. This would be an option for occasional use for someone with slightly dry hair that is thin or fine.

☹ **Daily Shampoo for Normal to Oily Hair & Scalp** *($5.95 for 8 ounces)* is similar to the Moisturizing Shampoo above, only with conditioning agents that are a problem for an oily scalp and hair, plus it also contains menthol—which, other than adding tingling, serves no purpose and is more of a scalp irritant than anything else.

☹ **Daily Conditioner for Hair & Scalp** *($7.95 for 8 ounces)* contains menthol and peppermint oil, which can be too irritating and drying for the scalp.

☹ **Leave-in Conditioner for Hair and Scalp** *($7.95 for 8.45 ounces)* contains several ingredients that can make scalp itchy and dry, including eucalyptus, peppermint, orange, and clove.

☺ **Styling Gel Light Hold** *($8.50 for 8.45 ounces)* is a standard styling spray with film formers, silicones, slip agent, conditioning agent, plant extracts, fragrance, and preservatives. It has a light hold with a slight sticky feel.

☺ **Spray Gel Medium Hold** *($8.50 for 8.45 ounces)* is similar to the Light Hold below and the same comments apply.

☺ **Styling Gel Firm Hold** *($9.50 for 8.45 ounces)* is similar to the Light Hold below, though this one has more of a stiff, sticky feel.

☺ **Fiber Pliable Molding Creme** *($13.50 for 3.53 ounces)* is a standard waxy pomade that can work well for slicking back the hair. It contains mostly water, lanolin, film former, thickeners, castor oil, fragrance, preservatives, and coloring agents. It can feel slightly stiff and greasy, so use it minimally to prevent a heavy feel.

☺ **Grooming Cream for Hold and Shine** *($12.50 for 3.53 ounces)* contains mostly thickeners, lanolin, castor oil, plant oils, more lanolin, water-binding agents, preservatives, and fragrance. It is similar to the Molding Creme above, though with slightly less hold. It is thick, heavy stuff, so use it minimally to create a slicked-back look for hair.

☺ **Texture Creme for Control and Shine** *($10 for 4 ounces)* contains mostly water, slip agent, detangling agents/film formers, lanolin oil, plant extracts, plant oils, water-binding agents, castor oil, preservatives, and fragrance. It's similar to the Grooming Cream above only in more of a lotion form. This is another product to help slick back hair, though it is far less thick and heavy than the Molding Creme and Grooming Cream.

☺ **Pomade for Hold & Shine** *($12.50 for 4 ounces)* contains mostly water, castor oil, thickeners, detangling agents/film formers, plant extracts, preservatives, and fragrance. It's just a different variation on the theme of "grease" in a gel form to create a slicked-back look with medium hold. It can have a sticky, heavy feel, so use it sparingly.

☺ **Grooming Spray** *($9 for 8.45 ounces)* is a standard nonaerosol hairspray that has a light hold and minimal to no stiff feel on hair, and it easily brushes through. Don't worry about the alcohol; it evaporates before it has a chance to be drying on the hair.

☺ **Thickening Lotion for Thicker Fuller Hair** *($10.50 for 4.2 ounces)* contains mostly water, film formers, conditioning agents, thickeners, glycerin, plant oils, fragrance, and preservatives. It does contains a small amount of eucalyptus, so you will want to keep this away from the scalp. Other than that, this gel/lotion can coat the hair and give it a slight sticky feel as well. For holding a slick look, it is an option.

Apple Pectin

It's a strange thing to base an entire line of hair-care products on apple pectin. Pectin serves no real function for hair or scalp. Outside of being derived from apples, it is little more than a standard thickening agent in hair-care products. I imagine to the consumer it sounds clean and healthy, but its purpose strictly utilitarian and more of a marketing gimmick than anything else. Some of the products in this lineup are worth considering but, of course, some are worth ignoring.

For more information on Apple Pectin, call (800) 444-0699.

☹ **Moisturizing Shampoo** *($4.99 for 15.5 ounces)* uses TEA-lauryl sulfate as the primary detergent cleansing agent, which is too drying for the scalp and hair, and is not recommended.

☺ **Naturals Irish Moss & Wild Cherry Bark Shampoo** *($4.99 for 16 ounces)* is a standard detergent-based shampoo that would nicely clean normal to slightly dry hair that has normal to fine or thin thickness. The plant extracts serve no purpose. It contains mostly water, cleansing agent, lather agent, plant extracts, detangling agent/ film former, fragrance, preservatives, and coloring agents.

☹ **Naturals Rosemary & Grapefruit Shampoo** *($4.99 for 16 ounces)* contains grapefruit extract, which can be irritating and drying for the scalp.

☺ **Naturals Witch Hazel & Honeysuckle Shampoo** *($4.99 for 16 ounces)* is a standard shampoo that contains mostly water, detergent cleansing agent, lather agent, plant extracts, preservatives, fragrance, and coloring agents. It would be a good standard shampoo for most hair types. There doesn't appear to be enough witch hazel in this product to be a problem for the scalp.

☺ **Plus Shampoo/Conditioner System in One** *($5.49 for 15.5 ounces)* is a standard shampoo that uses silicone and a handful of conditioning and detangling agents. It would work well as a two-in-one, but that only works for those who prefer their hair to be flat, or who have normal and/or short hair.

☺ **Shampoo Concentrate** *($4.99 for 15.5 ounces)* is a very good, basic shampoo with no conditioning additives. The little bit of pectin in here has little function. This can work well for all hair types. It does contain fragrance and coloring agents.

☺ **Creme Conditioner** *($4.99 for 15.5 ounces)* contains mostly water, detangling agent, thickeners, conditioning agents, silicone, preservatives, and fragrance. This is a good standard conditioner for someone with normal to slightly dry hair.

☺ **Deep Moisturizing Treatment for Dry/Damaged Hair** *($3.99 for 4 ounces)* contains mostly water, detangling agent, thickeners, conditioning agents, plant oil, silicone, preservatives, fragrance, and coloring agents. This isn't all that deep of a conditioner, but it would be good for someone with normal to slightly dry hair that is wavy and thick.

☺ **Naturals Hops, Apricot & Almonds Conditioner** *($4.99 for 16 ounces)* contains mostly water, thickeners, detangling agents, slip agent, plant extracts, preservatives, fragrance, and coloring agents. There are no hops in this product and the apricot and almond extracts are useless. Still, it's a good basic conditioner for normal to slightly dry hair.

☺ **Naturals Sunflower, Honey & Hibiscus Conditioner** *($4.99 for 16 ounces)* is identical to the Naturals Hops one above, only this one contains a minimal amount of mineral oil, which makes it slightly better for drier hair.

☺ **Naturals Orange Flower & Clove Styling Gel** *($4.49 for 8 ounces)* contains mostly water, film former, plant extracts, slip agent, thickener, preservatives, fragrance, and coloring agents. This lightweight-hold gel is easily brushed through and has little to no sticky or stiff feel.

☺ **Scentsates Apple Raspberry Spray Gel Medium Hold** *($4.49 for 8 ounces)* contains mostly water, film former, thickeners, plant extracts, conditioning agent, silicone, preservatives, fragrance, and coloring agents. It has a good medium hold with minimal sticky or stiff feel.

☺ **Naturals Chamomile & Sage Mousse** *($4.49 for 8 ounces)* is a standard mousse with light to minimal hold. It contains slip agent, detangling agents/film formers, silicone, conditioning agents, plant extracts, preservatives, and fragrance.

☺ **Ultra Hold Styling Mousse** *($4.99 for 8 ounces)* doesn't hold hair all that well, but is a good mousse, similar to the Naturals version above, only with more film formers.

☺ **Scentsates Apple Peach Styling Cream** *($4.99 for 4 ounces)* contains mostly water, silicones, film former, thickeners, plant extracts, preservatives, and fragrance. This is a good option for straightening hair, but use it minimally—it can easily make hair heavy and stiff.

☺ **Naturals Raspberry Leaves & Vitamin E Hair Spray** *($4.49 for 11 ounces)* is a standard aerosol hairspray, with film former, silicone, conditioning agent, and fragrance. It can give a good soft hold with shine from the silicone.

☺ **Naturals Rose Hips & Lemon Grass Spritz** *($3.99 for 8 ounces)* contains mostly alcohol, film formers, water, slip agent, plant extracts, silicone, coloring agents, and fragrance. This hairspray provides a firm, almost stiff hold. The alcohol isn't a problem for hair; it would evaporate before it would have any drying effect.

☺ **Ultra Hold Spritz** *($3.69 for 8 ounces)* contains mostly alcohol, film former, water, more alcohol, and fragrance. This does have a firm, almost stiff hold. The alcohol isn't a problem for hair; it would evaporate before it would have any drying effect.

Aqua Net

Whenever I think of hairspray, I think of Aqua Net. I remember it from when I was very young, and even today the container hasn't changed one bit. Aqua Net was the long-standing creator of helmet hair—but don't expect that effect anymore. Each one of these products has good hold and brushes through easily with minimal stiff or sticky feel. The formulations for these hairsprays are standard ones and the same for every line, from the most expensive hairsprays to the least expensive. Don't ignore this one just because it sounds dated; it can still work for some limited hairstyles.

For more information on Aqua Net, call (800) 626-7283.

☺ **1 All-Purpose All Day All Over Hold, Fresh Fragrance and Unscented** *($0.97 for 7 ounces)* is a good, light-hold aerosol hairspray. It can leave minimal to no stiff or sticky feel on the hair. It does contain alcohol, but it would evaporate before it would be a problem for hair.

☺ **2 Super Hold All Day All Over Hold, Fresh Fragrance and Unscented** *($0.97 for 7 ounces)* has a slightly stiffer feel than the 1 All Day above but the same basic comments apply.

☺ **3 Extra Super Hold All Day All Over Hold, Fresh Fragrance and Unscented** *($0.97 for 7 ounces)* is similar to the 2 Super Hold above and the same comments apply.

☺ **4 Ultimate Hold All Day All Over Hold, Fresh Fragrance and Unscented** *($0.97 for 7 ounces)* is similar to the 2 Super Hold above and the same comments apply.

ARTec

ARTec was one of the first hair-care lines around that added coloring agents to its shampoos and conditioners for the purpose of helping extend the life of hair color between hair dyes or to just add a wee bit of color to undyed hair. Though each product is named in a way that leads you to believe the coloring additives are natural, nothing could be further from the truth. The plant extracts aren't what's helping add color to the hair shaft—rather, it is the very unnatural dye agents such as basic brown #17, basic blue #99, basic red #104, hc blue #2, hc red #3, d&c red #33, and fd&c blue #1 that are helping out the hair. Those ingredients aren't bad for hair, but companies don't advertise their "unnatural" ingredients hoping the consumer won't notice and the companies can maintain their fake "natural" image.

The one negative about shampoos with coloring agents is that the color tends to wash out as you rinse. To allow the color to penetrate better, some women leave it on the hair longer, which can make hair dry and brittle so it's not the best option. Instead, the conditioners in this group of products are a better source of adding color. You can leave them on longer (which helps penetration under and around the cuticle and also helps add softness) because the longer you leave a conditioner on the hair, the more effective it can be.

For more information about ARTec, call (800) 323-6817.

☺ **$$$ Blue Orchid Color Enhancing Shampoo** *($20 for 16 ounces)* is a standard color-enhancing shampoo with detergent cleansing agents, lather agents, several conditioning agents, preservatives, fragrance, and dye agents. With overuse, this can leave a brittle, dry feeling on hair and it's probably not best for someone with extremely dry or coarse hair. It can add a hint of color.

☺ **$$$ Cherry Bark Color Enhancing Shampoo** *($20 for 16 ounces)* is similar to the one above and the same comments apply.

© **$$$ Coco Bean Color Enhancing Shampoo** *($20 for 16 ounces)* is similar to the ones above and the same comments apply.

© **$$$ Lemon Flower Color Enhancing Shampoo** *($20 for 16 ounces)* is similar to the ones above and the same comments apply.

© **$$$ Orange Marigold Color Enhancing Shampoo** *($20 for 16 ounces)* is similar to the ones above and the same comments apply.

© **$$$ Red Clover Color Enhancing Shampoo** *($20 for 16 ounces)* is similar to the ones above and the same comments apply.

© **$$$ Sunflower Color Enhancing Shampoo** *($20 for 16 ounces)* is similar to the ones above and the same comments apply.

© **$$$ Walnut Color Enhancing Shampoo** *($20 for 16 ounces)* is similar to the ones above and the same comments apply.

☹ **Kiwi Natural Enhancing Shampoo** *($20 for 16 ounces)* has sodium C14-16 olefin sulfonate as its main cleansing agent, which can be too drying for all hair and scalp types. It does contain plant oils that can reduce some of the drying effect, but why use a shampoo that fights itself?

☹ **White Violet Color Enhancing Shampoo** *($20 for 16 ounces)* has sodium lauryl sulfate as its main cleansing ingredient, which can be too drying for all hair and scalp types.

© **$$$ Blue Orchid Color Moisturizer** *($23 for 16 ounces)* contains mostly water, detangling agents, thickeners, preservatives, fragrance, and coloring agents. There aren't many conditioning properties in here, so it is really basically best for someone with normal to slightly dry hair of any thickness who wants to add a hint of color. Just don't expect any real coverage.

© **$$$ Cherry Bark Color Moisturizer** *($23 for 16 ounces)* is similar to the one above and the same comments apply.

© **$$$ Coco Bean Color Moisturizer** *($23 for 16 ounces)* is similar to the one above and the same comments apply.

© **$$$ Lemon Flower Color Moisturizer** *($23 for 16 ounces)* is similar to the one above and the same comments apply.

© **$$$ Orange Marigold Color Moisturizer** *($23 for 16 ounces)* is similar to the one above and the same comments apply.

© **$$$ Red Clover Color Moisturizer** *($23 for 16 ounces)* is similar to the one above and the same comments apply.

© **$$$ Sunflower Color Moisturizer** *($23 for 16 ounces)* is similar to the one above and the same comments apply.

© **$$$ Walnut Color Moisturizer** *($23 for 16 ounces)* is similar to the one above and the same comments apply.

© **$$$ White Violet Color Moisturizer** *($23 for 16 ounces)* is similar to the one above and the same comments apply.

☺ **Kiwi Coloreflector Weightless Conditioner** *($23 for 16 ounces)* is meant to hold or seal your color in. It can't do that. This is similar to the ones above, minus the coloring agents, but with a welcome addition of conditioning agents and silicones. This would be fine for dry hair of any thickness.

☺ **Kiwi Leave-in Bodifying Detangler** *($10 for 8.4 ounces)* contains mostly water, plant extracts, plant oil (fragrance), more plant extracts, detangling agents/film former, silicones, conditioning agents, more film former, more plant oil, preservatives, and fragrance. This is a good leave-in conditioner for someone with normal to dry and fine, thin hair. The film formers can build up, leaving hair feeling brittle and dry. It does contain superoxide dismutase, which is a good antioxidant, but it delivers no benefit for hair because it has little to no ability to cling to the cuticle.

☺ **Moisture PAC Salon Hydrating Treatment** *($20 for 14 ounces)* is a good conditioner. The almond meal isn't the best for hair as it can chip away at the cuticle.

Texture Line by ARTec

☺ **Smoothing Shampoo** *($9.40 for 12 ounces)* is a standard shampoo with plant extracts, conditioning agents, fragrance (in the form of essential oils), film former, plant oil, preservatives, and fragrance. This would be a good shampoo for someone with normal to dry hair that was also fine or thin. There is nothing in this product that can smooth hair any better than other shampoos with conditioning agents and film former.

☺ **Volume Shampoo** *($9.40 for 12 ounces)* is almost identical to the one above and the same comments apply. The film-forming ingredient can add some coating to the hair shaft and make it feel slightly thicker.

☺ **Smoothing Conditioner** *($10.46 for 8 ounces)* is an extremely standard conditioner for dry, coarse hair that contains mostly water, plant extracts, thickeners, conditioning agents, detangling agent, fragrance (in the form of essential oils), plant oils, silicones, preservatives, and fragrance.

☺ **Volume Conditioner** *($9.98 for 8 ounces)* contains mostly water, plant extracts, thickeners, detangling agent, fragrance (as essential oils), preservatives, and fragrance. This won't add much volume but it is a good lightweight conditioner for normal to slightly dry hair that has normal to fine or thin thickness.

☺ **Texture Gel** *($10.46 for 8 ounces)* is a standard styling gel that contains conditioning agents, film former, slip agent, plant oil, silicone, thickeners, preservatives, and fragrance. This is a good, lightweight gel with a soft hold that is easily brushed through for styling; it can have a slight sticky feel. The plant extracts in here have no effect on hair. It does contain tea tree oil, which can be a scalp irritant.

☺ **Volume Gel** *($10.46 for 8 ounces)* is almost identical to the Texture Gel above. It doesn't add any more volume to the hair than any other gel, but it does work well for styling. It also contains tea tree oil, which can be a scalp irritant.

☺ **Aeromousse (Aerosol)** *($12.96 for 10 ounces)* is a mousse dispensed in a spray form. I'm not sure that improves the traditional kind of mousse—if anything, this can get all over the place until you learn how to control the dispensing. It contains mostly alcohol, propellant, film former, plant extracts, conditioning agents, silicone, thickeners, preservatives, and fragrance. It has a medium hold with a somewhat sticky feel. It does contain tea tree oil, which can be a scalp irritant.

☺ **Texture Mousse** *($11.96 for 8.5 ounces)* contains mostly water, film former, foaming agent, plant extracts, conditioning agents, thickener, more film former, detangling agent, preservatives, and fragrance. This is a nonpropellant mousse dispensed in an aerated container. It has a medium hold and a slight sticky feel on the hair, but does keep hair in place well. It also contains tea tree oil, which can be a scalp irritant.

☺ **$$$ Shine & Frizz Repair** *($12 for 2 ounces)* is a standard silicone serum that also contains alcohol, emollients, and fragrant oils. It is a great silicone product, though overpriced.

☺ **Smoothing Serum** *($12.56 for 8 ounces)* contains mostly water, detangling agent, film former, plant extracts, conditioning agents, plant oils, thickeners, slip agents, fragrant oils, preservatives, fragrance, and coloring agents. This is a good light-hold gel that can help smooth out frizzies. It can have a slight greasy, sticky feel, so use it sparingly.

☺ **Texture Creme** *($15.70 for 8.4 ounces)* contains mostly water, plant extracts, fragrant oils, conditioning agents, film former, thickeners, plant oil, preservatives, and fragrance. This lotion has a soft hold, but the creamy part can feel heavy on hair. It can help straighten stubborn hair but use it minimally to prevent buildup and a thick, heavy feel. It takes only a drop of this when styling curly hair straight.

☺ **Texture Shine** *($12.56 for 2.64 ounces)* contains mostly water, castor oils, lanolin, detangling agents, film former, slip agent, preservatives, and fragrance. It's a thick gel, with a greasy feel that contains sparkles. It can definitely help straighten hair when styling, but it can also leave a greasy, sticky, heavy feel on hair, so use sparingly. Going for the shine part is up to you.

☺ **Texture Freeze (Non-Aerosol)** *($8.36 for 8 ounces)* contains mostly alcohol, water, film former, silicones, thickeners, plant extracts, conditioning agents, fragrant oils, slip agent, and fragrance. It has a good medium hold and a slight stiff feel, though it is easy to comb through.

☺ **Texture Shine Spray (Non-Aerosol)** *($12.56 for 4 ounces)* contains mostly alcohol, silicones, emollients, plant extracts, conditioning agent, film former, and fragrance. This is mostly silicone, which does add shine to hair and acts as a minimal styling agent for light hold.

☺ **Texture Spray (Aerosol)** *($9.76 for 10 ounces)* is a standard aerosol hairspray that has a good medium hold and a slight stiff feel, though it is easy to comb through.

☺ **Texture Spray Firm (Aerosol)** *($9.76 for 10 ounces)* is similar to the Texture Spray above, only with slightly more hold. It does have a minimal amount of silicone and conditioning agents for shine.

Aubrey Organics

An interesting item in *The Rose Sheet* for March 15, 1999, mentioned that Aubrey Organics was "in violation of catalog mislabeling and Good Manufacturing Practices. . . . [The] FDA investigators also determined several Aubrey products . . . bear labeling that cause them to be drugs and, therefore, are not in compliance with . . . topical . . . [guidelines]." And, separate from this citation from the FDA, there are other problems with many of Aubrey's claims.

If there is any such thing as a true believer in "natural" products, Aubrey Hampton is indeed one. His books, *Natural Organic Hair and Skin Care* (Organica Press) and *What's in Your Cosmetics* (Odonian Press), articulately express his convictions. Foremost is his philosophic position regarding his products: "I make my natural shampoos, conditioners, soaps, and so forth the way my mother taught me almost 50 years ago—without chemicals, using herbs known to be beneficial to the hair and skin." While I'm sure Hampton's mother was a wonderful woman, what she didn't know about hair care could fill several books. It's nice to think Mom knew it all, but I wouldn't make a hair-care decision based on such fanciful, romantic thinking. Further, an Aubrey product may start out organic, but by the time it's formulated to clean, condition, or style hair, it isn't organic anymore. After all, when was the last time you saw a shampoo or hairspray growing from the ground?

Hampton also lauds his position on animal testing, yet a few of his hair-care products contain lanolin, which is an animal by-product. Given Aubrey's excessive claims about plants, this is a stark contradiction.

He also states that he knows his products are "safe to use because they contain ingredients that have been used for hundreds, sometimes thousands, of years by people all over the world. That's the best track record, don't you think?" Well, I don't think so in the least. First, there are many ingredients ranging from panthenol to mucopolysaccharides, PABA (paraminobenzoic acid), and many others, in these products that weren't available until very recent times. I am also skeptical that Aubrey is providing a complete ingredient listing. None of his ingredient labels include standard preservatives, which, given these formulations, means these products would run a high risk of contamination from mold and bacteria, and that would be exceedingly risky for the eyes and skin. His ingredient labels do list vitamins C, A, and E as the preservatives, but these have their own stability problems and deteriorate quickly with exposure to air. Second, given the consistency and feel of the products, particularly the conditioners and styling products, I simply don't believe the ingredient listing. I do my reviews assuming the ingredient list is accurate, and with an educated guess on how much of each ingredient they probably do contain, given the vast number of published hair-care formulations I've studied.

Another Hampton phobia, shared by many other "natural" eccentrics in the world, is petrochemicals. He states, "Petrochemicals, [which] are infinitely cheaper and much more convenient for mass manufacturers to use . . . [make] our hair and skin suffer as a result. What's worse, the long-term effects of these harsh chemicals on both the body and the environment are still unknown. . . . "

Suggesting that all petrochemical derivatives are harsh and all plant derivatives are good is as uninformed as thinking that eating any plant you encounter in the wild won't kill you because it is natural. Plus, all this ignores the fact that petrochemicals have a decidedly natural source: they come from decomposed plant and animal life and have a decidedly organic base!

If you are one of the myriad "natural" hair-care seekers out there, this line won't hurt your pocketbook. Of course, I question what it can really do for hair, but that final decision is up to you. For more information on Aubrey products, call (813) 877-4186, (800) AUBREY H, or visit its Web site at www.aubrey-organics.com.

☺ **Blue Camomile Shampoo** *($8.50 for 8 ounces)* uses coconut oil soap as the detergent cleansing agent, which can be extremely drying to the hair. It does contain some conditioning agents and emollient, but that means this is a shampoo that has to fight itself.

☺ **Blue Green Algae Hair Rescue Vegetal Protein Shampoo** *($10 for 8 ounces)* uses coconut oil soap as the detergent cleansing agent, which can be extremely drying to hair. It does contain some plant oil and protein, but that won't undo the drying effect of the soap. Blue-green algae serves no purpose for hair care.

☹ **Calaguala Fern & Cade Tar Scalp Treatment Shampoo** *($9.65 for 8 ounces)* uses coconut and corn oil soap as the detergent cleansing agents, which can be drying to hair. It also contains juniper resin, which can coat the hair and make it feel brittle and stiff, and lemon oil, which can be an irritant for the scalp.

☹ **Camomile Luxurious Herbal Shampoo** *($13.90 for 16 ounces)* uses coconut oil soap as the detergent cleansing agent, and adds some conditioning agents and plant extract. The soap can be drying to the hair and scalp.

☹ **Egyptian Henna Shampoo** *($7.75 for 8 ounces)* uses coconut oil soap as the detergent cleansing agent, which can be drying to hair and scalp. It does contain conditioning agents, which is nice, but that won't undo the overall drying effects. It also contains henna, which can eventually build up on hair, leaving a brittle, dry feel.

☹ **Green Tea Hair Treatment Shampoo** *($9 for 8 ounces)* uses coconut oil soap as the detergent cleansing agent, which can be drying to hair. The plant extracts serve no purpose for the hair.

☹ **Honeysuckle Rose Conditioning Shampoo** *($7.45 for 8 ounces)* contains coconut oil soap as the detergent cleansing agent, which can be drying to hair. It also contains some protein as a conditioning agent, but that won't undo the drying effect of the soap. The oils in this product are added for fragrance, not as conditioning agents.

☹ **Island Naturals Island Butter Shampoo** *($7.56 for 8 ounces)* uses coconut oil soap as the detergent cleansing agent, which can be drying to hair. It also contains some emollients and conditioning agents. These can add a heavy feeling to hair and won't undo the drying effect of the soap.

☹ **J.A.Y. (Jojoba/Aloe/Yucca) Desert Herb Shampoo** *($20.20 for 16 ounces)* uses coconut oil soap as the detergent cleansing agent, which can be drying to hair. The plant extracts serve no purpose for the hair.

☹ **Mandarin Magic Gingko Leaf & Earth Smoke Shampoo** *($7.45 for 8 ounces)* uses coconut oil soap as the detergent cleansing agent, which can be drying to hair. The plant extracts serve no purpose for the hair.

☹ **Primrose & Lavender Herbal Shampoo** *($6.95 for 8 ounces)* uses coconut oil soap as the detergent cleansing agent, which can be drying to hair. The plant extracts and fragrant oils serve no purpose for the hair. There is conditioning agent in here, but it won't undo the drying effect of the shampoo.

☹ **Rosa Mosqueta Rose Hip Herbal Shampoo** *($8.50 for 8 ounces)* uses coconut oil soap as the detergent cleansing agent, which can be drying to hair. The plant extracts and fragrant oils serve no purpose for the hair.

☹ **Polynatural 60/80 Shampoo** *($8.50 for 8 ounces)* is similar to the Herbal Shampoo above and the same comments apply.

☹ **QBHL Quillaya Bark Hair Lather** *($7.20 for 8 ounces)* is similar to the Herbal Shampoo above and the same comments apply. This one also contains balsam, a resin that can build up on hair and make it feel brittle and dry.

☹ **Saponin A. A. C. Herbal Root Shampoo** *($9.95 for 8 ounces)* uses coconut oil soap as the detergent cleansing agent, which can be drying to hair. There is conditioning agent in here, but it won't undo the drying effect of the shampoo. Saponin refers to plant components that produce lather.

☹ **Selenium Blue Shampoo** *($8.50 for 8 ounces)* uses coconut oil soap as the detergent cleansing agent, which can be drying to hair. There are conditioning agents and plant oil in here, but they won't undo the drying effect of the shampoo. Selenium can be a good antioxidant for skin, but exactly how that benefits hair no one knows for sure. Plus, even if it could have an effect, it wouldn't hold under shampooing and rinsing.

☹ **Swimmers Shampoo** *($13.55 for 16 ounces)* is similar to many of the above formulations; what makes it better for swimming is anyone's guess.

☹ **White Camellia & Jasmine Conditioning Shampoo** *($8.15 for 8 ounces)* is similar to the ones above and the same basic comments apply.

☺ **Blue Green Algae Hair Rescue Vegetal Protein Cream Rinse** *($12 for 8 ounces)* contains mostly emollients, water, aloe, and fragrance. It can be a good conditioner for dry hair, though the plant extracts are useless for hair.

☺ **Calaguala Fern & Cade Tar Hair Thickener and Conditioner** *($9.95 for 8 ounces)* uses two forms of plant gums along with a plant resin to coat the hair. There are also some conditioning agents, but only minimal amounts. This definitely can add thickness to the hair, but it can also build up to a stiff, brittle feel.

☹ **GPB (Glycogen Protein Balancer) Hair Conditioner and Nutrient** *($16.85 for 16 ounces)* contains mostly emollients, conditioning agent, plant extracts, and balsam. This can be good for normal to dry hair, though the balsam can build up and make hair feel brittle and stiff.

☺ **Green Tea Herbal Cream Rinse** *($9.65 for 8 ounces)* contains mostly emollients, aloe, thickener, plant oil, and plant extracts. This can be a good emollient conditioner for dry and coarse hair. The plant extracts serve no purpose for hair.

☺ **Honeysuckle Rose Hair & Scalp Conditioner** *($8.75 for 4 ounces)* is similar to the Herbal Cream Rinse above, only this one has more fragrant oils. The same basic comments apply.

☺ **Island Naturals Island Spice Cream Rinse** *($7.75 for 8 ounces)* is similar to the Herbal Cream Rinse above, only this one contains more emollients, which makes it good for dry or extremely dry coarse, thick hair.

☹ **Jojoba & Aloe Hair Rejuvenator & Conditioner** *($12.85 for 4 ounces)* is mostly jojoba oil and emollient. It can leave hair feeling greasy.

☺ **Mandarin Magic Gingko Leaf & Ginseng Root Hair Moisturizing Jelly** *($10.55 for 8 ounces)* contains mostly water, conditioning agent and plant extract. The "jelly" part is the plant gum extract, which can leave a coating on the hair that has minimal hold with a slight sticky feel. That can definitely help shape hair.

☺ **Polynatural 60/80 Conditioner** *($9 for 8 ounces)* contains mostly emollients, plant extracts, and plant oil. This would be good for dry, coarse hair.

☺ **Rosa Mosqueta Rose Hips Conditioning Hair Cream** *($9.35 for 4 ounces)* is similar to the 60/80 version above and the same comments apply.

☺ **Swimmers Conditioner** *($8.15 for 8 ounces)* delivers nothing that can benefit a swimmer's hair problems. It is similar to the conditioning hair cream above and the same basic comments apply. This one does contain PABA, a sunscreen known for being a skin irritant, but there isn't enough in here to have any sun protection value.

☹ **Rosemary & Sage Hair & Scalp Rinse** *($7.45 for 8 ounces)* contains water, witch hazel, plant extracts, and minimal conditioning agents. The witch hazel would be rinsed off before it could be irritating or drying for the scalp. This is an exceptionally lightweight conditioner for normal hair to help make it easier to comb.

☺ **White Camellia Shine Conditioner Spray** *($6.95 for 4 ounces)* uses two forms of plant gum to form a coating over the hair, along with some conditioning agents. For building fullness, this leave-in conditioner is an option for normal to slightly dry hair that is fine or thin.

☺ **Biotin Hair Repair** *($14.80 for 4 ounces)* is a good, lightweight conditioner for normal to slightly dry hair; it contains amino acids, plant oil, and water-binding agent. Biotin can't repair hair.

☺ **Blue Green Algae Hair Rescue Conditioning Mask** *($13.50 for 4 ounces)* contains emollients, aloe, and plant extracts. This can be good for dry hair.

☹ **Egyptian Henna Hair Rinse** *($8.15 for 8 ounces)* includes henna, which can easily build up on hair, leaving it feeling brittle and stiff and also give it a strange orange/red color. But for some hair types, if used intermittently, it can coat the hair and create a feeling of thickness. This product does contain peppermint oil, which can cause irritation and dryness and be a problem for the scalp.

☹ **$$$ Jojoba Oil** *($15.35 for 0.36 ounce)* is merely 100% jojoba oil, which you can buy at any health food store for a fraction of the price. Used on the hair, it can leave a greasy residue.

☹ **$$$ Rosa Mosqueta Rose Hip Seed Oil** *($15.35 for 0.36 ounce)* is pure rose-hip oil. If you think this will feed dead hair, think again. It is just plant oil, and that's nice, but the jojoba oil from your cabinet, mentioned above, would do just as well for very dry, coarse or thick hair.

☹ **$$$ White Camellia Oil** *($15.35 for 0.36 ounce)* is pure plant oil; what special function this has for hair other than to leave a greasy, nice-smelling scent is anyone's guess.

☺ **B-5 Design Gel** *($10.55 for 8 ounces)* uses plant gum as the film-forming agent. It has minimal hold but can help when styling; it also leaves no stiff or sticky feel on hair.

☺ **Chestnut Brown Natural Body Highlighter Mousse** *($7.75 for 8 ounces)* is just a gel with some coloring agents; the amount of color is so faint it won't affect your own hair color much, if at all. It is similar to the Design Gel above and the same comments about hold and styling apply.

☺ **Golden Camomile Natural Body Highlighter Mousse** *($7.75 for 8 ounces)* is similar to the one above and the same comments apply.

☺ **Soft Black Natural Body Highlighter Mousse** *($7.75 for 8 ounces)* is similar to the one above and the same comments apply.

☺ **Natural Missst Hairspray** *($6.35 for 4 ounces)* contains alcohol, conditioning agent, gum, aloe vera, and plant oil. It has soft hold and minimal to no stiff or sticky feel.

☺ **Primrose Tangle-Go/Lusterizing Spray** *($6.95 for 4 ounces)* contains mostly water, witch hazel, fragrance, lanolin, and conditioning agent. This can be good to add shine and to smooth frizzies for dry hair. The witch hazel would evaporate before it had a chance to be drying to the hair or scalp.

Aura

Aura is a line of inexpensive hair-care products found in some drugstores and beauty supply houses such as Sally's. These products are supposed to be based on botanicals and aromatherapy. Like many hair-care product lines, there is definitely fragrance in these. Some plant extracts are also thrown in for show, but they serve no purpose for hair. All of the standard, nonbotanical ingredients are in these products too, and they *can* make a difference on the hair. There are some good options here to consider for your hair. For more information about Aura, call (800) 444-0699.

☺ **Black Malva Shampoo for All Shades of Black Hair** *($5.25 for 16 ounces)* contains mostly tea water, detergent cleansing agent, lather agent, thickeners, minimal conditioning agent, plant oil, preservatives, fragrance, and coloring agents. This is a good standard shampoo for most hair types. The amount of hair color in here is not much, but it can add a bit of color.

☺ **Blue Malva Shampoo for Blonde, Bleached and Light Shades of Hair** *($5.49 for 16 ounces)* is similar to the one above and the same comments apply.

☺ **Camomile Shampoo for Medium-to-Blonde Shades of Hair** *($4.99 for 16 ounces)* is similar to the ones above and the same comments apply. This version does have some plant extracts that might cause scalp irritation, such as orange peel, clove, turmeric, and grapefruit seed.

☹ **Clove Shampoo for Brunettes and Medium-to-Dark Shades of Hair** *($4.99 for 20 ounces)* contains several ingredients that can be problematic for the scalp, including clove, sage, peppermint, and grapefruit seed. If you tend not to have an itchy scalp, this product will help you have one.

☺ **Madder Root Shampoo for All Shades of Red Hair** *($4.99 for 16 ounces)* has some problematic ingredients for the scalp, but other than that, this one is identical to the ones above and the same comments apply.

☺ **Pure Organic Shampoo Enriched Cleansing for All Hair Types** *($4.99 for 16 ounces)* may be pure but it isn't purely organic. It does contain several plant oils—some fragrant and some just plain conditioning ones—but the rest of the ingredients are standard detergent cleansing agents, lather agents, castor oil, conditioning agents, silicone, detangling agent/film former, vitamins, preservatives, and fragrance. This is also not for all hair types—the conditioning agents in here make it appropriate for dry or coarse hair.

☺ **Cherry Almond Bark Revitalizing Conditioner for Dry, Damaged Hair** *($6.99 for 8.75 ounces)* contains mostly water, thickeners, silicone, conditioning agents, plant oils, fragrance, and preservatives. This is a good conditioner for dry or extremely dry hair that is coarse or thick.

☹ **Rosemary Mint Rinse for Hair and Scalp** *($4.99 for 20 ounces)* contains peppermint and menthol, which can cause irritation and dryness for the scalp, and it is not recommended.

☺ **Elixir Leave-on Conditioner for Hair Rejuvenation** *($4.69 for 8 ounces)* won't rejuvenate hair in the least, but it is a good, standard, leave-in conditioner for normal to dry hair that is normal to fine or thin. It contains mostly water, detangling agent, thickeners, slip agent, fragrance, silicones, film former, preservatives, and plant extracts. This product does contain a tiny amount of peppermint, so keep it away from the scalp.

☺ **Jojoba Hot Oil Treatment, Heat Activated Conditioning that Helps Repair and Revitalize Hair** *($1.59 for 1 ounce)* contains mostly water, film former, thickeners, preservatives, plant oil, fragrance, and coloring agents. This is a very lightweight leave-in conditioner that would work for normal hair that is fine or thin to normal. It contains a tiny amount of mint, so keep it away from the scalp.

☺ **Flax Seed Aloe Sculpting Gel** *($5.49 for 8 ounces)* is a standard gel containing mostly water, film formers, thickeners, detangling agent, preservatives, and fragrance. It gives a soft, combable hold.

☺ **Flax Seed Aloe Spray-on Gel** *($5.39 for 8 ounces)* contains mostly water, alcohol, film formers, fragrance, slip agents, and preservatives. This is a standard styling gel with medium hold. It can leave a slightly stiff and sticky feel on the hair. The alcohol in this product would evaporate before it had a chance to dry the hair.

☺ **Lemongrass Mousse Alcohol-Free Formula** *($4.99 for 9 ounces)* is a standard mousse that contains mostly water, propellant, film former, detangling agent, plant oil, preservatives, and fragrance. It has a soft hold with minimal to no stiff or sticky feel.

☺ **Lavender Ultra-Firm Freezing Spray** *($4.99 for 7 ounces)* contains mostly alcohol, propellant, film formers, conditioning agent, and fragrance. This is a good, standard, very firm-hold hairspray. It can leave a stiff, sticky feel behind on hair. The alcohol in this product, as is true for most spray-type products, would evaporate before it had a chance to dry the hair.

☺ **Witch Hazel Hair Spray (Non-Aerosol)** *($4.69 for 8 ounces)* is similar to the one above only in nonaerosol form. The same comments apply. The witch hazel and alcohol are not a problem for the hair, as they evaporate quickly in spray form.

☺ **Witch Hazel Super Shaping Hair Spray (Aerosol)** *($5.99 for 10 ounces)* is similar to the one above, only in aerosol form. The same comments apply.

Aussie

Like many small companies, this previously family-owned business grew to be a sizable concern and has been bought up, in this case by Bristol-Meyers Squibb. So far that hasn't changed much, but it only happened recently, near the end of 1999. It is yet to be seen what Squibb has in mind for this seemingly friendly, down-under, reasonably priced hair-care line. Is there anything really Australian about this line other than the birthplace of its originators? An occasional plant extract like kangaroo paw flower, Queensland macadamia nut oil, or eucalyptus extract shows up, but other than having cute, engaging names, these ingredients deliver no benefit for hair. All the other ingredients are the same ones used throughout the hair-care industry, with some problematic ingredients that you should watch out for.

For more information on Aussie products, call (800) 947-2656, (800) 363-0731, ext. 3077, or in Canada call (514) 333-3077. You can also visit its Web site at www.bms.com.

☹ **All Over Hair & Body Shampoo Moisturizing** *($2.98 for 12 ounces)* has sodium lauryl sulfate as one of its main detergent cleansing agents, which can be too drying for the hair and irritating for the skin; it is not recommended.

☺ **All Over Hair & Body Shampoo Refreshing** *($2.98 for 12 ounces)* is a standard shampoo that contains mostly water, detergent cleansing agents, silicone, detangling agent, preservatives, fragrance, and coloring agents.

☹ **Citrifier Shampoo for Dull, Lifeless Hair** *($3.59 for 16 ounces)* contains sodium lauryl sulfate as one of its main detergent cleansing agents, and it also contains peppermint, grapefruit, and eucalyptus, which can be too drying for the hair and irritating for the skin; it is not recommended.

☹ **Color Mate Shampoo** *($3.59 for 16 ounces)* contains sodium lauryl sulfate as one of its main detergent cleansing agents, which can be too drying for the hair and irritating for the skin; it is not recommended. The claim that it will help permed or color-treated hair doesn't hold up with the drying detergent cleansing agents in here.

☹ **Intermissions Color Enhancing Shampoo Amber Dawn** *($3.59 for 10 ounces)* is similar to the version above and the same comments apply.

☹ **Intermissions Color Enhancing Shampoo Fiery Sunset** *($3.59 for 10 ounces)* is similar to the version above and the same comments apply.

☹ **Intermissions Color Enhancing Shampoo Warm Sky** *($3.59 for 10 ounces)* is similar to the version above and the same comments apply.

☹ **Intermissions Color Enhancing Shampoo Moonlight Reflections** *($3.59 for 10 ounces)* contains sodium lauryl sulfate as one of its main detergent cleansing agents, which can be too drying for the hair and irritating for the skin; it is not recommended.

☺ **Intermissions Color Enhancing Shampoo Magenta Sky** *($3.59 for 10 ounces)* contains mostly water, detergent cleansing agents, film former, plant extracts, preservatives, fragrance, and coloring agents. This can add some highlights to the hair but not a lot. It is a gentle shampoo though the film-forming agent can cause an eventual buildup.

☹ **Mango Smoothy Shampoo for Coarse, Unruly Hair** *($2.98 for 16 ounces)* contains sodium lauryl sulfate as one of its main detergent cleansing agents, which can be too drying for the hair and irritating for the skin; it is not recommended.

☹ **Mega Shampoo for Everyday Cleansing** *($3.99 for 16 ounces)* contains sodium lauryl sulfate as one of its main detergent cleansing agents, which can be too drying for the hair and irritating for the skin; it is not recommended.

☹ **Moist Shampoo for Dry/Damaged Hair** *($3.99 for 16 ounces)* contains sodium lauryl sulfate as one of its main detergent cleansing agents, which can be too drying for the hair and irritating for the skin; it is not recommended.

☹ **Real Volume Shampoo for Fine to Normal Hair** *($3.59 for 16 ounces)* contains sodium lauryl sulfate as one of its main detergent cleansing agents, which can be too drying for the hair and irritating for the skin; it is not recommended.

☹ **Skip a Step Shampoo Cleanser/Conditioner Duo***($3.59 for 16 ounces)* contains sodium lauryl sulfate as one of its main detergent cleansing agents, which can be too drying for the hair and irritating for the skin; it is not recommended.

☺ **3 Minute Miracle Reconstructor Deep Conditioning for Damaged Hair** *($6.39 for 16 ounces)* contains mostly water, thickeners, conditioning agents, plant extracts, detangling agents, more thickeners, fragrance, preservatives, plant oils, silicone, and coloring agents. This is nothing even close to a miracle, nor is it all that deep. But it is a good conditioner for normal to dry hair that is also wavy and slightly coarse.

☹ **Curing Muddy Revitalizer for Fine to Normal Hair** *($5.44 for 12 ounces)* includes clay, which is drying for hair, so using it on the hair serves no purpose. This product also contains eucalyptus oil, which can be a scalp irritant.

☺ **DewPlex Leave-in Conditioner & Styler in One** *($5.99 for 8 ounces)* contains mostly water, film former, silicones, plant extracts, detangling agents, more film former, and fragrance. Because this one contains more styling agents than conditioners, it is only appropriate for normal hair that is normal to fine or thin. It can build up a sticky, stiff feel on the hair.

☺ **Hair Insurance Leave-in Conditioner Vitamin Enriched** *($3.99 for 8 ounces)* contains mostly water, silicones, vitamins, minerals, detangling agents, film former, emollients, preservatives, and fragrance. This is a good leave-in conditioner for dry or extremely dry or slightly coarse hair.

☺ **Hair Salad Conditioner for Fine, Flyaway Hair** *($3.59 for 12 ounces)* contains mostly water, slip agent, detangling agents/film formers, thickeners, plant extracts (including peppermint, which can irritate the scalp), fragrance, and preservatives. This is a standard conditioner for normal to slightly dry hair that is fine or thin. The film former can build up and feel heavy or stiff. The plant extracts sound interesting but provide no benefit for hair.

☺ **Instant Daily Conditioner for Daily Conditioning, High Protein Conditioner** *($5.39 for 12 ounces)* contains mostly water, mineral oil, thickeners, conditioning agents, fragrance, slip agent, and preservatives. This is a good, standard conditioner for dry to extremely dry hair that is coarse or thick. It has minimal protein and more mineral oil, which is fine, but it can leave a slight greasy feel on the hair.

☺ **Real Volume Leave-in Volumizer** *($5.99 for 8 ounces)* is a standard, leave-in conditioner that works best for normal hair that is fine or thin to normal. It contains mostly water, detangling agents/film formers, conditioning agents, vitamins, silicone, plant extracts, preservatives, and fragrance. The film formers can coat hair and make it feel somewhat thicker, but only ever so slightly.

☺ **Slip Detangler** *($3.99 for 12 ounces)* contains mostly water, thickener, detangling agents, plant extracts, silicone, slip agent, preservatives, and fragrance. For normal or slightly dry hair that just needs help with combing through after washing, this is a great leave-in conditioner.

☺ **Gelloteen Smoothing Gel** *($2.89 for 8 ounces)* is a standard styling gel that contains water, film formers, plant extracts, thickeners, preservatives, and fragrance. This can give good, light hold with no stiff or sticky feel.

☺ **MiraCurls Curls & Curves** *($2.83 for 8 ounces)* contains mostly water, alcohol, film formers, conditioning agents, slip agents, silicone, and fragrance. It is a standard styling spray with soft, light hold and minimal to no stiff or sticky feel. It works well for any styling need whether it's for smoothing or lightly holding curls place.

☺ **Natural Gel** *($2.83 for 7 ounces)* contains mostly water, film former, plant extracts, thickeners, silicone, detangling agent, and fragrance. This standard gel provides light hold with minimal to no stiff or sticky feel. It can be brushed through without feeling sticky.

☺ **Spray Gel** *($2.83 for 12 ounces)* contains mostly water, film formers, silicone, conditioning agent, preservatives, and fragrance. There are several plant extracts in here that can be problematic for the scalp, so be careful and avoid that area. Other than that, this is a standard, light-hold styling spray with minimal to no stiff or sticky feel.

☺ **Styling Gel** *($3.89 for 8 ounces)* contains mostly water, film formers, plant extracts, thickeners, detangling agent, silicone, preservatives, castor oil, and fragrance. It's a standard gel with medium hold and minimal stiff or sticky feel that easily brushes through.

☺ **Maximum Hold Mousse** *($2.83 for 6.5 ounces)* contains mostly water, conditioning agent, propellant, film formers, plant extracts, preservatives, and fragrance.

This isn't maximum hold, but it is a good light-hold mousse that can be brushed through with minimal to no sticky or stiff feel.

☺ **12-Hour Humidity Spray** *($2.83 for 12 ounces)* is just a hairspray and has no special properties to keep humidity out of hair. It contains mostly alcohol, water, film former, plant extracts, conditioning agent, silicone, slip agent, and fragrance. It is a good medium-hold hairspray that can leave a slight stiff feel on hair but it is easy to brush through. The alcohol would evaporate before it could have a drying effect on hair.

☺ **AirDo Flexible Hold Professional Styling Mist Aerosol** *($2.97 for 7 ounces)* contains mostly alcohol, propellant, film former, conditioning agents, slip agents, plant extracts, plant oil, water, and fragrance. This basic aerosol hairspray has a light hold with minimal to no stiff or sticky feel. Don't worry about the alcohol in here; as in all styling products, it would evaporate before it could have a drying effect on hair.

☺ **AirDo Flexible Hold Professional Styling Mist Non-Aerosol (Unscented and Scented)** *($2.97 for 8 ounces)* is similar to the AirDo Aerosol version above and the same comments apply. The unscented version contains a masking fragrance.

☺ **Instant Freeze Aerosol** *($2.83 for 7 ounces)* is a standard aerosol hair spray with light hold and minimal to no stiff or sticky feel on hair. It contains mostly alcohol, propellant, film former, water, conditioning agents, slip agent, silicone, and fragrance.

☺ **Instant Freeze Non-Aerosol** *($3.59 for 8 ounces)* is similar to the one above, only in nonaerosol form and the same comments apply.

☺ **Mega Styling Spray, Aerosol** *($2.78 for 14 ounces)* is similar to the aerosol Instant Freeze above and the same comments apply.

☺ **Mega Styling Spray, Non-Aerosol** *($2.83 for 12 ounces)* is similar to the Instant Freeze nonaerosol above and the same comments apply.

☺ **Sprunch Spray Non-Aerosol (Scented and Unscented)** *($3.59 for 12 ounces)* is similar to the Instant Freeze nonaerosol above and the same comments apply.

☺ **TwinFixx Spray Gel and Hairspray in One** *($5.29 for 12 ounces)* contains mostly alcohol, water, film former, silicone, detangling agent, plant extracts, fragrance, and slip agent. This standard light-hold hairspray can be used for styling or as a hairspray with minimal to no stiff or sticky feel.

☺ **Gloss** *($5.44 for 2.02 ounces)* is a good, standard silicone fluid with a small amount of plant oil added to the mix that can add a silky feel and shine to hair.

☹ **Instant Shine, Shine Treatment** *($4.59 for 15 capsules)* is identical to the Gloss above only in capsule form, which is a waste of money. There is nothing about silicone or plant oil that needs to be encapsulated, other than to create a more scientific or medical look to an ordinary product.

☺ **Instant Mend Split End Treatment** *($4.59 for 15 capsules)* is similar to the one above only with some water-binding agents. Water-binding agents are nice, but they don't have any effect on split ends.

Aveda

Aveda makes a fuss about other hair-care products, saying "Would you moisturize with petroleum? Enjoy the sweet smell of methyl-octine-carbonate?" and so on. Other than the fact that no one in the world of hair care or skin care uses any petroleum (meaning gasoline, as the name implies) in their products, how wonderful do ingredients like sodium methylcocoyltaurate, cocamidopropyl betaine, polyquaternium 10, or lauramide DEA sound? Yet these very unnatural ingredients, among dozens and dozens of others, fill out every Aveda product. Only Aveda can rationalize the use of ingredients such as formaldehyde-releasing diazolidinyl urea (a major preservative in most all of its hair products) as having a natural source. But then again, I guess formaldehyde can be considered natural.

Aveda's claim that "what you put on your body should be as healthy and natural as what you'd put into it" is at best disingenuous because no one is going to eat these products. "That's why we use plant-derived ingredients, organically grown whenever possible," it says, yet how does it explain the extensive list of non-plant-derived ingredients in its formulations? It can't. Throwing in some plants and exotic claims can indeed fool lots of consumers, but not once they catch on to this pervasive marketing game of selling unnatural products under the guise of being all natural.

Separate from the bogus natural claims, Aveda does have some great hair-care options. The prices are high for what you get, but for the most part the performance is reliable.

For more information about Aveda, call (888) 288-0006, (800) 328-0849, or visit its Web site at www.aveda.com. Aveda is now owned by the Estee Lauder company.

☺ **Shampure, Above and Beyond Shampoo** *($9.84 for 8.4 ounces)* is similar to many of the Aveda shampoos, only this one contains more conditioning agents and plant oils. It contains mostly tea, detergent cleansing agents, lather agent, conditioning agents, castor oil, silicones, detangling agents, vitamins, and preservatives. This would be good for someone with very dry and coarse hair.

☺ **Hair Detoxifier** *($9 for 8.45 ounces)* is a standard detergent-based shampoo that does contain a chelating agent, sodium gluconate, which can help remove mineral salts from the hair.

☺ **Madder Root Pure Plant Shampoo** *($6.50 for 8 ounces)* is a shampoo that's as natural as the computer I work on! It contains mostly tea, detergent cleansing agents, lather agent, conditioning agents, film former, fragrance, thickeners, silicone, and preservatives. It is a good standard shampoo for most hair types, with minimal conditioning agents. It can cause buildup with continued use.

☺ **$$$ Cherry/Almond Bark, Reconstructive Hair Conditioner** *($21.50 for 7.9 ounces)* is supposed to be "nature's purest conditioning," but there is nothing natural about stearalkonium chloride or peg 12 distearate. It also can't reconstruct damaged hair. However, it is a good basic conditioner for normal to dry hair. It contains mostly tea, thickeners, detangling agent, plant oil, slip agent, conditioning agent, fragrant plant oils, and preservatives.

☺ **$$$ Curessence Intensive Repair Treatment for Damaged Hair** *($25.44 for 18.4 ounces)* can't repair hair, though it is a good conditioner for dry or extremely dry hair that is coarse or thick. It contains mostly tea, thickeners, detangling agent, silicones, conditioning agents, fragrances, film former, and preservatives. It also contains peppermint, which can cause scalp irritation. This is best used only on the length of hair.

☺ **$$$ Deep-Penetrating Hair Revitalizer, Intensive Hair Conditioner** *($23.88 for 7.9 ounces)* is similar to the Curessence above and the same comments apply.

☺ **Rosemary/Mint Equalizer, Hair Conditioning Rinse** *($8.40 for 8.45 ounces)* contains mostly tea, detangling agent/film former, thickeners, vinegar, fragrance (plant extracts), plant oil, conditioning agents, and preservatives. This is a good conditioner for normal to dry hair that iss normal to fine or thin. The peppermint in here can be a problem, causing irritation and dryness, so keep it off the scalp.

☺ **Elixir Daily Leave-on Hair Conditioner** *($9.60 for 8.45 ounces)* contains mostly tea, detangling agents, thickeners, silicone, more thickeners, glycerin, fragrance (plant extracts), conditioning agents, and preservatives. This is a very good leave-in conditioner for normal to dry hair that is normal to fine or thin. It doesn't contain film former so it doesn't give a stiff feel. It does contain peppermint, which can be an irritant for the scalp.

☺ **Styling Curessence Hair Renewal for Strength and Control** *($14 for 8.4 ounces)* contains mostly tea, detangling agents/film formers, conditioning agents, fragrance, and preservatives. This leave-in conditioner/styling spray is a good option for normal hair that is normal to fine or thin. It can easily build up on hair.

☺ **Volumizing Tonic for All Hair Types** *($10.50 for 3.7 ounces)* is more of a leave-in conditioner than a styling spray. It has slight hold and can make hair feel thicker. It is actually quite similar to the Volumizing Finisher below and the same basic comments apply.

☺ **Volumizing Finisher** *($12.60 for 3.7 ounces)* contains mostly alcohol, tea, film former, conditioning agents, and fragrance. This is a standard hairspray with a soft hold and minimal stiff or sticky feel.

☺ **Scalp Remedy Anti-Dandruff Styling Tonic** *($12.60 for 3.7 ounces)* contains zinc pyrithione, which is the same active ingredient to fight dandruff that Head

& Shoulders contains. Despite the higher price for this one, the benefit of being able to apply the active ingredient in a lotion form that can stay on the scalp overnight is helpful in comparison to shampoo, where the ingredient is rinsed out.

☺ **Flax Seed/Aloe Strong Hold Spray On Styling Gel** *($10 for 8.45 ounces)* contains mostly alcohol, tea, film formers, slip agent, fragrance, and silicone. This standard styling gel has a medium hold with minimal stiff or sticky feel.

☺ **Phomollient** *($13.20 for 7 ounces)* contains mostly tea, thickeners, film formers, fragrance, and water-binding agents. This styling product is dispersed in a foam, so the closed system requires no preservatives—at least as far as Aveda is concerned. It is a good standard styling foam, similar to a mousse. It has a soft hold that is easily brushed through with minimal sticky feel.

☺ **Self Control Hair Styling Stick** *($18.60 for 2.5 ounces)* contains mostly tea, thickeners, film former, fragrance, and preservatives. This stick-form pomade works well on stubborn frizzies. It can feel slightly sticky, stiff, and heavy, so use it sparingly.

☺ **Air-O-Sol Witch Hazel Hair Spray (Aerosol)** *($21 for 14.75 ounces)* contains mostly alcohol, silicone, conditioning agent, plant oils, and film former. The alcohol in here is not witch hazel, but it evaporates before it could have a drying effect on the hair. Other than that, this is a standard hairspray that has a soft to medium hold and minimal stiff or sticky feel.

☹ **Confixor Conditioning Fixative** *($16 for 8.4 ounces)* contains mostly tea, thickeners, film formers, alcohol, slip agent, silicone, conditioning agents, detangling agent, fragrance, and preservatives. It's a standard, lightweight styling gel for most normal, fine, thin hair for a soft hold. This product does contain peppermint, a skin irritant, so keep it away from the scalp. Though I generally don't comment on fragrance, because that preference is so individual, this product struck me as having the oddest smell, which I just can't describe but it caused me to wince.

☺ **Firmata Firm Hold Hair Spray** *($12.50 for 8.4 ounces)* contains mostly alcohol, tea, film former, silicone, fragrance, conditioning agents, and plant oil. It is a good, standard, firm-hold hairspray. It has a somewhat stiff, sticky feel. The alcohol evaporates before it has a chance to have a drying effect on the hair.

☺ **Witch Hazel Medium Hold Hair Spray (Aerosol)** *($9 for 8.45 ounces)* contains mostly alcohol, film former, silicone, fragrance, conditioning agent, plant oil, and more film former. The alcohol in here is not witch hazel, but it doesn't have a drying effect on the hair; it evaporates before it could. Other than that, this is a standard hairspray that gives medium to firm hold with a slight stiff feel.

☺ **Black Malva Shampoo** *($6 for 8.45 ounces)* is a standard detergent-based shampoo that contains mostly tea, detergent cleansing agents, lather agent, conditioning agents, detangling agent/film former, water-binding agents, silicone, thickeners, preservatives, and coloring agents. It also has a small amount of color additives to enhance brown hair. It works well for most hair types.

☺ **Blue Malva Shampoo** *($6 for 8.45 ounces)* is almost identical to the Black Malva and the same comments apply.

☺ **Camomile Shampoo** *($6 for 8.45 ounces)* is almost identical to the Black Malva one above and the same comments apply.

☺ **Clove Shampoo** *($6 for 8.45 ounces)* is almost identical to the Black Malva one above and the same comments apply.

☺ **Annatto Color Conditioner** *($19.20 for 7.9 ounces)* contains mostly tea, thickeners, silicones, detangling agent, plant extracts, conditioning agents, preservatives, and coloring agents. There is annatto in here, but also some standard, unnatural dye agents that help this conditioner impart a tiny amount of color to hair. This is a very good conditioner for dry hair of any thickness.

☺ **Bixa Color Conditioner** *($19.20 for 7.9 ounces)* is similar to the Annatto Color Conditioner above and the same comments apply.

☺ **Black Malva Color Conditioner** *($19.20 for 7.9 ounces)* is similar to the Annatto Color Conditioner above and the same comments apply.

☺ **Blue Malva Color Conditioner** *($19.20 for 7.9 ounces)* is similar to the Annatto Color Conditioner above and the same comments apply.

☺ **Chamomile Color Conditioner** *($19.20 for 7.9 ounces)* is similar to the Annatto Color Conditioner above and the same comments apply.

☺ **Clove Color Conditioner** *($19.20 for 7.9 ounces)* is similar to the Annatto Color Conditioner above and the same comments apply.

☺ **$$$ Madder Root Color Conditioner** *($19.20 for 7.9 ounces)* is similar to the Annatto Color Conditioner above and the same comments apply.

Pure-Fume by Aveda

☺ **Pure-Fume Brilliant Shampoo for Treated, Dry, or Textured Hair** *($10 for 8 ounces)* is a simple, basic shampoo that contains mostly tea, detergent cleansing agent, lather agent, plant extracts (fragrance), detangling agent/film former, and preservatives. This is a great shampoo for all hair types.

☺ **Pure-Fume Brilliant Conditioner for Treated, Dry, or Textured Hair** *($18 for 7.9 ounces)* contains mostly tea, detangling agents, thickeners, plant oil, silicone, plant oil, plant extracts (fragrance), emollient, and preservatives. This would be a very good conditioner for dry, extremely dry, coarse, or thick hair.

☺ **Pure-Fume Brilliant Forming Gel** *($10.50 for 4 ounces)* contains mostly tea, film former, conditioning agents, thickeners, fragrance, and preservatives. It is a thick gel, with a light to medium hold and minimal stiff or sticky feel. It can help when making stubborn hair stay smooth.

☺ **Pure-Fume Brilliant Retexturing Gel** *($15 for 7.9 ounces)* is similar to the Forming Gel above and the same comments apply.

☺ **$$$ Pure-Fume Brilliant Anti-Humectant Pomade** (*$14 for 2 ounces*) is a standard, rather greasy pomade that contains mostly thickeners, castor oil, silicones, fragrance, plant oil, and preservatives. With no film formers, this pomade is strictly a styling "wax," so it would not add any stiffness or hold to the hair but would control frizzies. Appropriate for coarse, dry hair, it can feel heavy and sticky, so use it sparingly.

☺ **$$$ Pure-Fume Brilliant Humectant Pomade** (*$12.60 for 2 ounces*) is a relatively greasy gel with minimal hold. It has no stiff or sticky feel so it can be helpful for smoothing stubborn curls and frizzies, but it can feel heavy and have a slight sticky feel, so it is best used minimally.

☺ **$$$ Pure-Fume Brilliant Thermal Styling Creme** (*$14 for 8 ounces*) is a thick cream-type styling product that can leave hair feeling thick and heavy, so be careful how much you use. It is great for straightening away frizzies, but just use it minimally. It contains mostly tea, film former, silicones, thickeners, castor oil, plant oil, fragrance, and preservatives.

☺ **$$$ Pure-Fume Brilliant Emollient for Hair** (*$14 for 3 ounces*) is a standard silicone liquid with fragrance and plant oil. It works as well as any—silicone is silicone—so the price is hardly warranted, given the availability of far less expensive versions.

☺ **$$$ Pure-Fume Brilliant Spray On for Hair** (*$14 for 3 ounces*) is a spray-on silicone, with alcohol, plant oils, and fragrant oils. It works great for dry, coarse hair but is overpriced given the standard formulation.

All Sensitive by Aveda

☺ **All Sensitive Shampoo** (*$9.50 for 5.7 ounces*) contains mostly tea water, detergent cleansing agents, conditioning agents, silicone, preservatives, fragrant oil, and preservatives. This is a good but standard shampoo with conditioning agents. It can work well for dry, extremely dry, coarse, or thick hair. There are some plant extracts in here known for having anti-irritant properties, but they would be washed away before they had much of a chance to have an effect.

☺ **All Sensitive Conditioner** (*$9.50 for 5.5 ounces*) does contain plant extracts known for being anti-irritants, but it also contains a few that can be irritants, particularly those that have strong fragrances. Perhaps they balance each other out. Other than that, this is a good basic conditioner for dry or extremely dry hair that is coarse or thick; it contains mostly tea, detangling agents, conditioning agents, plant oil, thickeners, silicone, and preservatives.

☺ **All Sensitive Styling Gel** (*$12 for 5.7 ounces*) contains the same extracts as the products above and the same comments apply. Other than that, it contains mostly film former, glycerin, castor oil, silicone, more film formers, thickener, fragrance (plant oil), and preservatives. This is a standard gel with medium hold. It can have a sticky, heavy feel for some hair types.

Avon Hair Care

Avon's hair products aren't exciting, but they are good, basic formulations with great prices. For more information on Avon, call (302) 453-7460, (800) 367-AVON, in Canada call (800) 265-AVON, or visit its Web site at www.avon.com.

☹ **Techniques Tri-Nutriv Formula Brightening Shampoo for Gray or Blond Hair** *($4.99 for 11 ounces)* uses TEA-lauryl sulfate as one of the primary detergent cleansing agents, which is too drying for all hair types and a potential scalp and skin irritant; plus the blue tint in here has minimal effect on hair color.

☺ **Techniques Tri-Nutriv Formula Controlling Dandruff Shampoo Plus Conditioner in One** *($4.99 for 11 ounces)* is a standard zinc pyrithione–based dandruff shampoo that contains standard detergent cleansing agents, lather agents, silicone, fragrance, preservatives, and detangling agent. It is a good option for a dandruff shampoo, but the conditioning agent isn't enough for someone with dry or extremely dry hair that is coarse or thick.

☺ **Techniques Tri-Nutriv Formula Fortifying Shampoo Plus Conditioner in One** *($3.99 for 11 ounces)* contains mostly water, detergent cleansing agents, conditioning agents, lather agent, fragrance, silicone, and preservatives. This is a good basic shampoo with minimal conditioning agents. It can work well for all hair types but can build up on hair with repeated use.

☺ **Techniques Tri-Nutriv Formula Hydrating Shampoo for Dry/Damaged Hair** *($3.99 for 11 ounces)* contains mostly water, detergent cleansing agents, lather agents, fragrance, silicone, conditioning agents, and preservatives. This is a good basic shampoo with minimal conditioning agents. It can work well for all hair types but can build up on hair.

☺ **Techniques Tri-Nutriv Formula Restructuring Shampoo for Permed/ Color Treated Hair** *($3.99 for 11 ounces)* is similar the one above, only this one includes minimal film-forming agents, which can leave a slight stiff feel on hair. This is best for someone with normal to fine hair looking to add some volume.

☺ **Techniques Tri-Nutriv Formula Volumizing Shampoo for Fine/Thin Hair** *($3.99 for 11 ounces)* is similar to the Restructuring Shampoo above and the same comments apply.

☺ **Techniques Tri-Nutriv Formula Replenishing Shampoo for Normal Hair** *($3.99 for 11 ounces)* is a great basic shampoo with minimal conditioning agents. It would work well for all hair types with minimal to no risk of buildup.

☺ **Techniques Tri-Nutriv Formula Hydrating Conditioner for Dry/Damaged Hair** *($3.99 for 11 ounces)* contains mostly water, thickeners, fragrance, conditioning agents, slip agent, plant oil, silicone, lanolin oil, and preservatives. This is a very good emollient conditioner for dry or extremely dry hair that is coarse or thick.

☺ **Techniques Tri-Nutriv Formula Replenishing Conditioner for Normal Hair** *($3.99 for 11 ounces)* contains mostly water, thickeners, fragrance, preservatives, slip agents, detangling agents, and conditioning agents. This is an exceptionally light conditioner that would be fine for normal hair that needed help with comb-through.

☻ **Techniques Tri-Nutriv Formula Restructuring Conditioner for Permed/Color Treated Hair** *($3.99 for 11 ounces)* is actually quite similar to the one above for normal hair, only this one contains silicone. That's helpful for normal to slightly dry hair, but it isn't conditioning enough for coarse or extremely dry hair.

☺ **Techniques Tri-Nutriv Formula Volumizing Conditioner for Fine/Thin Hair** *($3.99 for 11 ounces)* contains mostly water, thickeners, detangling agents, fragrance, conditioning agent, preservatives, film former, and slip agents. This is a good, standard conditioner that would work well for fine, thin hair.

☺ **Techniques Tri-Nutriv Formula Leave-in Treatment for Lightweight Conditioning** *($5.99 for 11 ounces)* contains mostly water, silicones, slip agents, preservatives, detangling agent/film former, and conditioning agents. This is mostly a silicone spray that is great for dry, coarse hair as a leave-in conditioner with minimal to no stiff feel.

☺ **Techniques Tri-Nutriv Formula Hot Oil Treatment for Hair** *($5.99 for two 1-ounce tubes)* doesn't contain any oil, but it does contain water, detangling agent, fragrance, thickener, conditioning agents, film former, preservatives, and coloring agents. It is a good lightweight conditioner, but it isn't an improvement over any of the other conditioners in the Avon range of conditioners.

☺ **Techniques Tri-Nutriv Formula Sculpting Gel for Shape & Control** *($3.99 for 6 ounces)* is a standard styling gel that contains mostly water, alcohol, film former, more alcohol, slip agents, thickener, silicone, fragrance, conditioning agents, and preservatives. This is a lot of alcohol, even for a styling product, but it shouldn't prove drying in the long run. Other than that, it has a soft hold with minimal to no stiffness, which makes it good for styling most hair types.

☺ **Techniques Tri-Nutriv Formula Spray Gel for Ultimate Control** *($3.99 for 7.6 ounces)* contains mostly water, alcohol, film former, conditioning agent, castor oil, preservatives, silicone, and coloring agents. This is just a styling spray that has light hold and minimal to no stiff or sticky feel.

☺ **Techniques Tri-Nutriv Formula Styling Mousse for Volume and Control** *($3.99 for 6 ounces)* is a standard mousse that contains mostly water, propellant, film former, thickeners, fragrance, silicone, preservatives, detangling agents, and conditioning agents. The minimal conditioning agents in here have little effect on hair, but this is a good basic mousse for light hold with minimal stiff or sticky feel.

☺ **Techniques Tri-Nutriv Formula Hair Volumizer** *($5.99 for 7.6 ounces)* contains mostly water, alcohol, slip agent, conditioning agents, film formers, fragrance, and coloring agents. This is a good leave-in gel/lotion that can add a slight layer of film former over the hair, which can make the hair feel thicker. It has minimal to no stiff or sticky feel.

☺ **Techniques Tri-Nutriv Formula Finishing Hair Spray for Natural Hold and Control** *($3.99 for 11 ounces)* contains mostly alcohol, water, film formers, conditioning agents, fragrance, and silicone. This is a good light-hold hairspray with minimal to no stiff or sticky feel.

☺ **Techniques Tri-Nutriv Formula Hair Spray for Extra Hold and All-Over Control Aerosol** *($3.99 for 8 ounces)* is similar to the Natural Hold above, only this one is in aerosol form. The same basic comments apply.

☺ **Techniques Tri-Nutriv Formula Mega Hold Styling Spritz** *($3.99 for 7.6 ounces)* contains mostly, alcohol, water, film formers, conditioning agent, castor oil, fragrance, silicones, and coloring agents. This is a good light-hold hairspray (not a "mega"-hold type). It brushes through easily with minimal to no stiff or sticky feel.

☺ **Techniques Tri-Nutriv Formula Dry End Serum** *($5.99 for 1 ounce)* is a standard silicone spray. It works great for dry, coarse hair!

☺ **$$$ Techniques Tri-Nutriv Formula Frizz Treatment Capsules** *($5.99 for 18 capsules, 0.58 ounce total)* is almost identical to the one above, only for twice the price, plus there is no reason to encapsulate silicone except to make it look more like a real "treatment" for hair.

☺ **Techniques Tri-Nutriv Formula Heat Guard Blow Dry Treatment for Hair** *($5.99 for 6.7 ounces)* is a very lightweight silicone spray that works more like a leave-in conditioner than anything else. It can help normal to slightly dry hair of any thickness. It has no hold but provides some smoothing.

☹ **Techniques Tri-Nutriv Formula Hair Treatment Mask** *($5.99 for 8.4 ounces)* contains both clay and alcohol, which are suspect in a product meant to be moisturizing, as clay and alcohol can rob moisture from hair. There's no reason to ever put anything like this on the hair.

☹ **Techniques Tri-Nutriv Formula Hair Freshness Spray** *($4.99 for 4.2 ounces)* is just a spray mist of cologne, more like air freshener than something you would want to spray on your hair.

Back to Basics

Available at most drugstores, this large line has some great inexpensive options to consider. For more information on Back to Basics, call (760) 918-3600 or (800) 456-9322.

☺ **Aloe Vera Daily Shampoo for All Hair Types** *($5.95 for 10 ounces)* is a standard, detergent-based shampoo that contains mostly tea, detergent cleansing agents, lather agents, thickeners, conditioning agents, silicone, vitamins, slip agents, preservatives, fragrance, and coloring agents. Despite the name, the conditioning agents make it inappropriate for all hair types—it's a good shampoo for only normal to dry hair.

☺ **Beer Shampoo Black Cherry Stout for Dry, Damaged Hair** *($7.95 for 10 ounces)* contains mostly tea, detergent cleansing agents, lather agent, conditioning agents, detangling agent, detangling agent/film former, plant oil, preservatives, fragrance, and coloring agents. This is a good shampoo for dry hair that is normal to fine or thin. The minimal amount of hops in here is useless for hair and the beer packaging is cute but meaningless for hair.

☺ **Beer Shampoo Honey Wheat Pilsner for All Hair Types** *($7.95 for 10 ounces)* contains mostly tea, detergent cleansing agents, lather agent, conditioning agents, detangling agent, film formers, preservatives, fragrance, and coloring agents. This is appropriate only for someone with normal hair that is fine or thin to normal. The film-forming agents can make hair feel thicker but can also build up and feel stiff. The minimal amount of hops in here is useless for hair. Is anyone falling for this beer gimmick? How did beer ever obtain the status of having benefit for hair when it doesn't?

☺ **Beer Shampoo Peach Amber Ale for Volumizing Fine Hair** *($7.95 for 10 ounces)* contains mostly tea, detergent cleansing agents, lather agent, conditioning agents, detangling agent, film former, preservatives, fragrance, and coloring agents. This is a good shampoo for someone with normal hair that is normal to fine or thin. The beer publicity stunt is silly—the minimal amount of hops in here is useless for hair.

☺ **Honey Hydrating Shampoo, for Overworked Hair** *($6.95 for 12 ounces)* contains mostly tea, detergent cleansing agents, lather agent, conditioning agents, silicone, detangling agents/film formers, plant oil, vitamins, preservatives, fragrance, and coloring agents. This is a good shampoo for someone with dry to extremely dry hair that is normal to fine or thin.

☺ **Milk Shampoo** *($7.95 for 12 ounces)* is almost identical to the Honey Hydrating Shampoo above and the same comments apply.

☺ **Raspberry Almond Intensive Shampoo** *($7.95 for 12 ounces)* is similar to the Honey Hydrating Shampoo above, only with more plant oil, and that makes it better for coarser hair types.

☺ **Sunflower Moisture Infusing Shampoo, for All Hair Types** *($6.95 for 12 ounces)* contains mostly water, detergent cleansing agents, lather agent, conditioning agents, thickeners, film former, vitamins, preservatives, fragrance, and coloring agents. This doesn't contain much moisture, but it is a good shampoo for someone with normal to fine and thin hair. The film former can build up with repeated use.

☺ **White Grapefruit Clarifying Shampoo** *($7.95 for 12 ounces)* uses TEA dodecyl benzensulfonate as one of the main detergent cleansing agents. It can strip hair color (dyed or natural) and be drying to the hair and scalp.

☺ **Wild Berry Volumizing Shampoo, for All Hair Types** *($7.50 for 12 ounces)* is just a standard shampoo with conditioning agents. This isn't all that volumizing, but it is a good basic shampoo for most hair types. It's not an option for oily hair and scalp.

☺ **Beer Conditioner Oat Bran Lager for All Hair Types** *($7.95 for 10 ounces)* contains mostly tea, thickeners, slip agent, detangling agents, conditioning agents, plant oil, preservatives, and fragrance. This is a good basic conditioner for normal to dry hair.

☺ **Honey Hydrating Conditioner for Overworked Hair** *($8.95 for 12 ounces)* contains mostly water, thickeners, slip agent, detangling agents, plant oil, plant extracts, conditioning agents, silicones, preservatives, and fragrance. This is a good conditioner for dry to extremely dry hair that is coarse or thick.

☺ **Milk Conditioner** *($8.95 for 12 ounces)* is similar to the Honey Hydrating Conditioner above and the same basic comments apply.

☹ **Mint Leaf Daily Conditioner for All Hair Types** *($6.95 for 12 ounces)* does contain mint and peppermint, which can be a problem for the scalp and definitely serve no purpose for the hair.

☺ **Raspberry Almond Intensive Conditioner** *($8.95 for 12 ounces)* contains mostly tea, detangling agents, plant oils, conditioners, silicone, vitamins, thickeners, preservatives, and fragrance. This is a very good conditioner for dry or extremely dry hair that is coarse or thick. The vitamins can't help the hair or scalp.

☺ **Sunflower Detangling and Conditioning Spray** *($6.95 for 8 ounces)* contains mostly tea, detangling agent, water-binding agent, conditioning agents, vitamins, slip agents, and preservatives. This is a very good leave-in conditioner for all hair types except coarse and extremely dry hair.

☺ **Sunflower Moisture Infusing Conditioner for All Hair Types** *($7.95 for 12 ounces)* is similar to the Detangling version above and the same basic comments apply.

☺ **Wild Berry Volumizing Conditioner for All Hair Types** *($8.95 for 12 ounces)* is similar to the Sunflower Detangling conditioner above, only with a tiny amount of silicone and film former. That can work to give the feel of thicker hair.

☺ **Vanilla Bean Forming Gel** *($8.50 for 12 ounces)* is a standard styling gel that contains mostly tea, film formers, conditioning agents, vitamins, thickeners, silicone, preservatives, and fragrance. This would work well for a light to medium hold with minimal stiff or sticky feel.

☺ **Wild Berry Firm Holding Styling Gel** *($8.95 for 8.5 ounces)* is almost identical to the one above and the same comments apply.

☺ **Sunflower Sculpting Lotion** *($3.95 for 4 ounces)* contains mostly tea, film former, thickeners, conditioning agents, plant oil, silicone, vitamins, castor oil, preservatives, and fragrance. This would work well as a straightening product or to keep stubborn curls and frizzies under control. It can have a slight stiff, sticky feel, but it easily brushes through hair.

☺ **Sunflower Texturizing Creme** *($9.98 for 4 ounces)* is similar to the version above, only with no stiff or sticky feel. It can feel heavy and weight hair down, though, so use it minimally.

☺ **Sunflower Whipped Creme Mousse** *($8.95 for 8 ounces)* is a standard mousse containing tea, propellant, film former, slip agent, preservatives, silicone, conditioner, plant oil, and fragrance. This is a good, light-hold mousse with minimal stiff or sticky feel.

☺ **Chamomile Sculpting and Volumizing Spray** *($6.95 for 8 ounces)* contains mostly tea, alcohol, film former, vitamins, conditioning agents, slip agent, and fragrance. It has a light to medium hold, and like all film-forming products can add a feel of thickness to the hair. It can also have a slight stiff, sticky feel.

☺ **Comfrey Natural Hold Finishing Spray** *($6.95 for 8 ounces)* contains mostly tea, alcohol, film former, conditioning agents, silicone, vitamins, slip agent, and fragrance. This is a standard hairspray with light hold and minimal to no stiff feel on hair.

☺ **Sunflower Firm Hold Hair Spray** *($9.95 for 10 ounces)* doesn't have firm hold; rather, it is similar to the Comfrey Natural version above, only in an aerosol.

☺ **Witch Hazel Firm Hold Hair Spray** *($7.95 for 8 ounces)* is similar to the Comfrey Natural version above, only in a nonaerosol version.

Basic Texture by Back to Basics

☺ **Be Thick Thickening Shampoo** *($7.95 for 12 ounces)* contains mostly water, detergent cleansing agents, lather agent, plant oils, conditioning agents, film former, preservatives, and fragrance. For dry hair that is thin or fine, this shampoo would work well, but it can easily build up, making hair limp.

☺ **Get Curly Curl Enhancing Shampoo** *($7.95 for 12 ounces)* contains mostly water, detergent cleansing agent, plant oils, emollient, silicone, detangling agents/ film formers, lather agent, thickeners, preservatives, and fragrance. If you don't have curls this won't help, but for a little bit of hold for dry, coarse, curly hair, this works, though it can also leave a stiff feel over hair.

☺ **So Straight Smoothing & Anti-Frizz Shampoo** *($7.95 for 12 ounces)* is similar to Get Curly above, only this one has more plant oil. That can be better for dry, coarse hair. It won't make it straight, but it can help make things somewhat smoother.

☺ **Be Thick Thickening Conditioning Rinse** *($8.95 for 12 ounces)* contains mostly water, plant oils, thickeners, detangling agents, film former, vitamins, preservatives, and fragrance. This would work well for dry hair that is normal to fine or thin.

☺ **Get Curly Curl Enhancing Conditioner** *($8.95 for 12 ounces)* is similar to the Be Thick version above, only this one includes castor oil, which can add a bit of thickness for normal to dry hair that is fine or thin. It can have a slightly sticky feel to hair and also build up with repeated use.

☺ **So Straight Smoothing Anti-Frizz Conditioner** *($8.95 for 12 ounces)* contains mostly water, thickener, detangling agent, slip agent, plant oils, thickeners, silicones, vitamins, preservatives, and fragrance. This is a good emollient conditioner for dry or extremely dry hair that is coarse or thick.

☺ **Be Thick Thickening & Texturizing Spray Gel** *($8.95 for 8.5 ounces)* is a standard gel that contains alcohol, water, film former, plant oils, vitamins, and fragrance. This is a good gel with light to medium hold and minimal stiff or sticky feel. It can be too heavy for someone with fine or thin hair. The alcohol would evaporate before it would be a problem for the hair.

☺ **Get Curly Curl Enhancing Gel** *($9.95 for 6.8 ounces)* is a standard lightweight gel for a light hold; there is nothing in here that will stimulate the hair to go curly. It contains mostly water, slip agents, plant oils, silicone, thickeners, film former, vitamins, preservatives, and fragrance.

☺ **Get Control Volumizing Mousse** *($8.95 for 8.5 ounces)* is a standard mousse with a tricky dispensing system that tends to spew the foam out, so be careful when you first use it. It contains mostly water, propellant, film former, slip agents, silicone, vitamins, plant oil, and fragrance. It gives light to medium hold and would work well for most hair types, though it does have a somewhat sticky feel.

☺ **So Straight Anti-Frizz Straightening Balm** *($9.95 for 6.8 ounces)* contains mostly water, thickeners, detangling agent/film former, plant oils, conditioning agents, vitamins, silicones, preservatives, and fragrance. This isn't a balm at all, but a styling gel with no hold—just a slick, waxy feel that works great to smooth frizzies and curls with no stiff or sticky feel. It can build up on hair, so use it sparingly.

☺ **Be Thick Thickening Hair Creme** *($9.95 for 6.8 ounces)* contains mostly water, film formers, thickeners, plant oils, conditioning agents, vitamins, silicones, more film formers, preservatives, and fragrance. It is definitely an emollient thickening cream that can help straighten hair, but it can also be heavy and thick so use it sparingly. It is best for coarse, dry hair.

☺ **Get Control Maximum Hold Hair Spray** *($9.95 for 11.5 ounces)* contains mostly alcohol, propellant, film former, silicone, conditioning agent, vitamins, more silicone, more conditioning agents, and fragrance. This is a standard hairspray with medium to firm hold and a somewhat stiff, sticky feel, though it can brush through.

Bain de Terre

Bain de Terre means "bath of the earth." As evocative as that sounds, there's very little about the earth in these products. The tiny amounts of plant extracts are at the end of the ingredient listings and so are barely present. All of the main ingredients comprising more than 99 percent of the products' contents are the same standard detergent cleansing agents, lather agents, film formers, detangling agents, and preservatives that show up in all hair-care products. For more information on Bain de Terre, call (800) 242-WAVE or in Canada (800) 626-3684.

☺ **Aloe Bath Moisturizing Shampoo** *($8.95 for 16.9 ounces)* contains mostly water, detergent cleansing agent, lather agent, plant oils, slip agents, detangling agent/film former, castor oil, conditioning agents, preservatives, fragrance, and coloring agents. It's a good shampoo for dry, coarse hair.

☺ **Alpine Mist Dandruff Shampoo** *($6.50 for 8.5 ounces)* is a standard zinc pyrithione–based dandruff shampoo. It would work well for all hair types with dandruff.

☻ **Botanical Boost Volumizing Wash** *($7 for 10.2 ounces)* contains mostly water, detergent cleansing agent, lather agent, thickeners, fragrance, detangling agents, film former, conditioning agents, preservatives, plant extracts, and coloring agents. Like all volumizing shampoos, this one uses a film former to coat the hair. It works well enough, but can cause buildup.

☹ **Green Meadow Daily Shampoo** *($7.95 for 16.9 ounces)* contains both sodium C14-16 olefin sulfonate and sodium lauryl sulfate as the main detergent cleansing agents, which is a double whammy for dryness and potential scalp irritation.

☺ **Recovery Complex Repairative Shampoo** *($10 for 16.9 ounces)* contains mostly water, detergent cleansing agents, lather agent, thickeners, fragrant oils, conditioning agents, film former, preservatives, fragrance, and coloring agents. This won't repair anything, but it is a good basic shampoo for normal to dry hair that is normal to fine or thin. It can cause buildup with repeated use.

☺ **Botanical Boost Fortifying Conditioner** *($8 for 10.2 ounces)* isn't all that botanical. It contains mostly water, thickener, silicones, detangling agents, thickeners, preservatives, fragrance, plant extracts, and coloring agents. This is a good conditioner for dry or extremely dry hair that is coarse or thick.

☺ **Herbal Conditioning Seal** *($5.95 for 8 ounces)* contains mostly water, conditioning agent, silicone, detangling agent, film former, plant extracts, preservatives, fragrance, and coloring agents. It is a good conditioner for dry or extremely dry hair that is coarse or thick.

☺ **Marithyme Moisture-Rich Conditioner** *($7.50 for 5 ounces)* contains mostly water, silicone, thickeners, detangling agents, conditioning agents, preservatives, fragrance, and coloring agents. It is a good standard conditioner for dry or extremely dry hair that is coarse or thick.

☹ **Recovery Complex Intensive Treatment Conditioner** *($18.95 for 4 ounces)* contains clay and that's intensely drying for the hair.

☺ **$$$ Recovery Complex Spa Therapy** *($22 for 4 ounces)* is a standard silicone serum with fragrant oils and a tiny amount of film former. That can add shine and combability, but the price is absurd for this ordinary silicone spray.

☺ **White Clover Daily Detangling Conditioner** *($8.95 for 16.9 ounces)* contains mostly water, thickener, detangling agent, silicone, plant extracts, fragrance, slip agent, and preservatives. This is a great, simple, standard leave-in conditioner. It would do just what the name implies, and can work for all hair types who want a little more help with combability.

☺ **Herbal Reconstructing Pac** *($8.50 for 4 ounces)* won't reconstruct one hair on your head, but it is a good conditioner for normal to dry hair that is normal to fine or thin. It contains mostly water, thickener, detangling agents/film former, plant extracts, silicones, fragrance, and preservatives.

☺ **Beezwax Styling Stick** *($8.95 for 1.9 ounces)* contains mostly thickening agents, silicone, Vaseline, fragrance, and preservatives. This is a basic, waxy pomade that can help control frizzies. It would add weight without stiffness but it can look heavy and greasy, so use sparingly.

☺ **Botanical Boost Uplifting Root Foam** *($8.95 for 8 ounces)* has a directional nozzle that, if used as intended, would deposit too much foam in one area. Just use it as a regular mousse and it should work fine. It contains mostly water, propellant, film formers, conditioning agents, plant extracts, detangling agents, silicone, preservatives, and fragrance. This would work as well as any mousse for a light to medium hold and slightly sticky feel that can easily be brushed through.

☺ **Herbal Styling Mousse** *($6.95 for 6.5 ounces)* is similar to the Botanical Boost Uplifting Root Foam above and the same comments apply.

☺ **Botanical Boost Volumizing Mist** *($8.50 for 8 ounces)* is a standard aerosol spray that contains mostly alcohol, propellant, film former, silicone, plant extract, and fragrance. It isn't any more volumizing than any other light-hold hairspray with minimal to no stiff feel.

☺ **Botanical Boost Volumizing Elixir** *($7.95 for 7.6 ounces)* is similar to the one above and the same basic comments apply.

☺ **Currant Expressions Sculpting Texturizer** *($19.95 for 14.5 ounces)* is a standard styling gel with medium to firm hold that can feel somewhat sticky. It contains mostly water, film formers, thickener, plant extracts, castor oil, conditioning agents, silicone, preservatives, and fragrance.

☹ **Flax Seed Styling Gel** *($7.50 for 5 ounces)* contains mostly water, film former, slip agents, thickeners, plant extracts, preservatives, fragrance, and coloring agents. It has medium hold with a sticky feel.

☺ **Finishing Mist** *($6.95 for 13 ounces)* is a standard aerosol hairspray with medium to firm hold and a slightly stiff feel that does brush through. It contains mostly alcohol, propellant, film formers, fragrant oil, plant extracts, and fragrance.

☺ **Finishing Spritz** *($6.95 for 8 ounces)* is similar to the Finishing Mist above, only this one is nonaerosol.

☺ **Goldenseal Shaping Spray** *($6.95 for 7.6 ounces)* is similar to the Finishing Spritz above and the same comments apply.

☹ **Mint Balm Spray Stylizer Spray Gel** *($7.50 for 7.6 ounces)* is similar to the Flax Seed Styling Gel above, only in spray form.

☺ **Red Clover Shaping Spray** *($8.95 for 13 ounces)* is almost identical to the Finishing Mist above and the same comments apply.

☹ **Super Hold Flax Seed Hair Spray** *($8.50 for 13 ounces)* is similar to the Flax Seed Styling Gel above, only in spray form.

Beauty Without Cruelty (BWC)

Many companies proudly boast that they do not test their products on animals. However, it isn't always clear whether the products contain animal-derived ingredients or whether individual ingredients were ever tested on animals. Some companies, including The Body Shop, have a self-imposed five-year "grandfather clause," which means they use ingredients previously tested on animals as long as the testing took place five years before the date the raw ingredient was purchased. Beauty Without Cruelty is one of the few companies with a strict, rigorously defined position concerning animal testing. Its products are not tested on animals, none of its products contain animal by-products, and not one of the ingredients it uses has been tested on animals since 1965. In this regard, the ethics of this company are admirable.

Of course, the company makes elaborate claims about the benefits of their plant extracts, though these have no real effect on hair or scalp. The other ingredients are the same that are present in all hair-care products and they work well. Beauty Without Cruelty products are typically distributed in health food stores and sometimes in drugstores. For more information on Beauty Without Cruelty, call (707) 769-5120, (800) 227-5120, or visit its Web site at www.avalonproducts.net.

☺ **Daily Benefits Shampoo, Benefits All Hair Types** *($6.95 for 16 ounces)* contains mostly tea, detergent cleansing agents, lather agents, conditioning agents, fragrance, and preservatives. This is a good standard shampoo for most hair types. The amount of conditioning agent in here is fairly minimal, so it shouldn't be a problem for oily scalps.

☺ **Moisture Plus Shampoo, Benefits Dry/Treated Hair** *($6.95 for 16 ounces)* contains mostly tea, detergent cleansing agents, slip agent, conditioning agents, plant oils, thickeners, fragrant oils, and preservatives. This is a good shampoo for dry or extremely dry hair that is coarse or thick.

☺ **Daily Benefits Conditioner, Benefits All Hair Types** *($6.95 for 16 ounces)* contains mostly tea, thickeners, conditioning agents, fragrant oils, and preservatives. It is a good basic conditioner for someone with normal to slightly dry hair.

☺ **Moisture Plus Conditioner, Benefits Dry/Treated Hair** *($6.95 for 16 ounces)* contains mostly tea, thickeners, conditioning agents, fragrant oils, and preservatives. This is a good conditioner for someone with normal to dry hair.

☺ **Revitalize Leave-in Conditioner, Benefits Dry/Treated Hair** *($6.95 for 8.5 ounces)* contains mostly tea, thickener, conditioning agents, plant oil, and preservatives. This is a good conditioner for someone with normal to dry hair.

☺ **Volume Plus Spray Gel** *($6.95 for 8.5 ounces)* is a standard spray gel that contains mostly tea, film former, conditioning agent, castor oil, thickeners, and preservatives. It would give a good light to medium hold with a slight sticky feel.

☺ **Natural Hold Hair Spray** *($6.95 for 8.5 ounces)* is a standard nonaerosol hairspray that contains mostly alcohol, plant extracts, film former, conditioning agents, and silicone. It works well for a light to medium hold with minimal to no stiff feel.

BioSilk

Farouk Shami is the owner of BioSilk. His Farouk Systems products are supposed to be free of harsh chemicals. His BioSilk Liquid Gel Color, BioGlitz Creme Color 2100, and BioSilk Perms and AlphaSilk Texturizing (for hair straightening) are hardly free of harsh chemicals. That doesn't makes them bad, it just makes the claim misleading. These products are the same as all hair-coloring and perming products on the market. Being ammonia-free doesn't mean there aren't a lot of other ingredients available that can raise the pH of a product.

According to the company, "Farouk Systems' mission statement has always been and still is: Environment, Education, and Ethics," but some educational elements seem to be left out. For example, several of the shampoos contain TEA-lauryl sulfate and sodium C14-16 olefin sulfonate, both well known for being drying and irritating detergent cleansing agents. Other products contain mint and menthol, which can irritate and dry out the scalp (watch out if you tend to have an itchy scalp) and serve no purpose for skin or hair. A few of the products also make claims about containing alpha and beta hydroxy acids. While those can have benefit for the face to help exfoliate the skin, they can also denature the hair shaft, and so are problematic ingredients in hair-care products. Thankfully, none of the products actually contain the right pH or the right form of AHA or BHA to cause exfoliation, but the information is still misleading. So much for education.

For more information on BioSilk, call (281) 876-2000, (800) 237-9175, or visit its Web site at www.farouk.com.

☹ **Equinox Shampoo** *($7.78 for 10 ounces)* uses TEA-lauryl sulfate as the main cleansing agent and is not recommended.

☹ **Hydrating Shampoo** *($8.88 for 10 ounces)* uses TEA-lauryl sulfate as the main ingredient and is not recommended. It also contains balm mint, which can cause irritation on the scalp.

☹ **Shampoo Out** *($7.78 for 10 ounces)* uses sodium C14-16 olefin sulfonate as the main ingredient and is not recommended. It also contains mint extract, which can cause an itchy, dried-out scalp.

☹ **Volumizing Shampoo** *($7.78 for 10 ounces)* uses TEA-lauryl sulfate as the main ingredient, and is not recommended.

☺ **Conditioner Moisturizer** *($8 for 10 ounces)* contains mostly rose water, thickeners, detangling agent, conditioning agents, plant oil, silicones, vitamin, preservatives, plant extracts, fragrance, and coloring agents. This is a good conditioner for normal to dry hair of any thickness.

☺ **Fruit Cocktail Reconstructing Treatment** *($11 for 10 ounces)* contains mostly water, detangling agent, silicone, thickener, plant oil, silicone, conditioning agents, vitamins, plant extracts, preservatives, coloring agents, and fragrance. This is a very good conditioner for dry or extremely dry hair that is thick or coarse.

☹ **Hydrating Conditioner Rehydrating Treatment** *($8 for 10 ounces)* contains peppermint and mint, and these can be a problem for the scalp.

☺ **Pre Plus Volumizing Detangler** *($4 for 10 ounces)* contains mostly rose water, thickeners, detangling agents, conditioner, plant extracts, coloring agents, preservatives, and fragrance. This is a good, extremely standard detangling spray. It won't add volume to the hair, and be sure to keep it off the scalp, because the mint in here can cause irritation.

☺ **Sealer Plus Finishing Rinse** *($8.80 for 10 ounces)* contains mostly rose water, detangling agent, slip agent, conditioning agent, plant oil, plant extracts, vitamins, silicone, preservatives, fragrance, and coloring agents. It is a good but standard lightweight conditioner for normal to slightly dry hair.

☺ **Silk Filler Leave-in Repairative Treatment** *($11 for 10 ounces)* contains mostly rose water, detangling agent, conditioning agents, slip agent, preservatives, plant extracts, preservatives, and fragrance. It is a good standard leave-in conditioner for normal to slightly dry hair.

☺ **Tone & Shine Color Enhancing Conditioner for Normal and Chemically Treated Hair, Black Orchid for Black and Brunette Hair** *($9.90 for 10 ounces)* contains mostly water, thickeners, detangling agents, mineral oil, plant oils, silicone, conditioning agents, vitamins, preservatives, fragrance, and coloring agents. This is a good conditioner for dry, coarse, thick hair. It can be too emollient for someone with fine or thin hair. The coloring agents do add a hint of color.

☺ **Tone & Shine Color Enhancing Conditioner for Normal and Chemically Treated Hair, Coffee Bean for Brown Hair** *($9.90 for 10 ounces)* is identical to the one above, only with different coloring agents, and the same comments apply.

☺ **Tone & Shine Color Enhancing Conditioner for Normal and Chemically Treated Hair, Dark Chocolate for Brown Hair** *($9.90 for 10 ounces)* is virtually identical to the one above, only with different coloring agents.

☺ **Tone & Shine Color Enhancing Conditioner for Normal and Chemically Treated Hair, Mahogany Red for Brown and Red Hair** *($9.90 for 10 ounces)* is virtually identical to the one above, only with different coloring agents.

☺ **Tone & Shine Color Enhancing Conditioner for Normal and Chemically Treated Hair, Marigold for Brown and Red Hair** *($9.90 for 10 ounces)* is virtually identical to the one above, only with different coloring agents.

☺ **Tone & Shine Color Enhancing Conditioner for Normal and Chemically Treated Hair, Platinum Blonde for Beige and Silver Hair** *($9.90 for 10 ounces)* is virtually identical to the one above, only with different coloring agents.

☺ **Tone & Shine Color Enhancing Conditioner for Normal and Chemically Treated Hair, Red Auburn for Brown and Red Hair** *($9.90 for 10 ounces)* is virtually identical to the one above, only with different coloring agents.

☺ **Tone & Shine Color Enhancing Conditioner for Normal and Chemically Treated Hair, Silver Minx for Gray and White Hair** *($9.90 for 10 ounces)* is virtually identical to the one above, only with different coloring agents.

☺ **Tone & Shine Color Enhancing Conditioner for Normal and Chemically Treated Hair, Summer Blonde for Blonde Hair** *($9.90 for 10 ounces)* is virtually identical to the one above, only with different coloring agents.

☺ **Glazing Gel Medium Hold** *($8 for 10 ounces)* is a standard gel containing mostly rose water, film formers, thickeners, conditioning agent, preservatives, fragrance, and coloring agents. This is a good basic gel for light hold with minimal to no stiff or sticky feel.

☺ **Rock Hard Gelee Hard Hold Gel** *($10 for 4 ounces)* is similar to the Glazing Gel above and the same basic comments apply, which means there is nothing "rock hard" about this gel in the least.

☺ **Silk Mousse Medium Hold** *($9 for 10 ounces)* is a standard mousse with a light hold and minimal stiff or sticky feel. It contains mostly water, propellant, film former, conditioning agents, plant extracts, preservatives, fragrance, and silicone. It does contain some amount of mint so it would best not to apply this on the scalp.

☺ **Molding Silk Designing Paste** *($10 for 4 ounces)* is a thick cream with film formers that can help straighten hair and smooth frizzies. It is also heavy and can be sticky so use it sparingly. It contains mostly water, thickeners, film former, detangling agent, silicones, preservatives, coloring agents, and fragrance.

☺ **Silk Pomade Designing Finish** *($10 for 4 ounces)* contains mostly rose water, film former, mineral oil, thickeners, preservatives, and fragrance. This is a good soft-hold gel-like pomade. It will smooth out stubborn frizzies, but it can leave a heavy, greasy feel on hair, so use it sparingly.

☺ **Finishing Spray Natural Hold (Aerosol)** *($10.80 for 10 ounces)* is a standard aerosol hairspray that contains mostly alcohol, propellant, film formers, conditioning agents, silicone, and fragrance. It has a light brushable hold with minimal to no stiff feel on hair.

☺ **Finishing Spray Firm Hold (Aerosol)** *($10.80 for 10 ounces)* is similar to the Natural Hold version below only with slightly more hold (but not much), and the same basic review applies.

☺ **Spray Spritz Firm Hold Styling Spray (Non-Aerosol)** *($8.80 for 10 ounces)* is a firm-hold nonaerosol spray similar to the aerosol versions above and the same basic comments apply.

☺ **$$$ Shine On Brilliant Finish** *($19.50 for 5 ounces)* is a standard silicone serum with a small amount of conditioning agents and fragrance. It would work well, but the price is a burn given the basic formulation.

☺ **$$$ Silk Therapy** *($40 for 4 ounces)* is almost identical to the one above and the same comments apply.

☺ **Silk Polish Shining Paste** *($10 for 4 ounces)* contains mostly Vaseline, mineral oil, plant oils, thickeners, preservatives, and fragrance. This is greasy kid stuff but would work well over extremely dry ends to control frizzies.

☹ **Silk Strate Temporary Straightener** *($5 for 5 ounces)* is a standard gel with no hold, which also means no stiffness and minimal to no sticky feel. It can help with styling curly hair straight but not more than any other gel. It contains mostly rose water, detangling agent, thickeners, conditioning agents, preservatives, plant extracts, and fragrance.

The Body Shop

The Body Shop's hair-care distinction is that it was one of the first ones out of the gate to popularize the myth around natural ingredients. It goes without saying (because by the end of this book you will have heard it more times than you care to hear) that none of these products are natural in the least. The little bits of plant extracts and the natural-sounding names thrown in for show won't help your hair.

There are some good products to consider, but if you were hoping for a truly natural hair-care line, there isn't one!

For more information on The Body Shop, call (800) BODYSHOP or in Canada (800) 387-4592. You can also visit its Web site at www.usa.the-body-shop.com.

☺ **Banana Shampoo for Normal to Dry Hair** *($9.50 for 16.9 ounces)* contains mostly water, detergent cleansing agent, lather agents, thickeners, slip agent, fragrance, preservatives, and coloring agents. The banana serves no purpose in this product other than as a thickening agent. This is just a standard shampoo that would work well for most hair types.

☺ **Brazil Nut Rich Shampoo for Dry, Damaged & Chemically Treated Hair** *($9.50 for 16.9 ounces)* contains mostly water, detergent cleansing agent, lather agent, silicone, film former, preservatives, thickeners, fragrance, and coloring agents. The film former in here makes this a problem for adding stiffness to extremely dry hair that already has a stiff feel, but it could work well for dry hair that is normal to fine or thin.

☺ **Chamomile Shampoo for Dry or Blonde Hair** *($9.50 for 16.9 ounces)* is a good standard shampoo with minimal conditioning agents. It would work well for all hair types. It contains mostly water, detergent cleansing agent, thickener, detangling agent, fragrance, preservatives, and coloring agents.

☺ **Seaweed & Peony Shampoo for Normal Hair** *($9.50 for 16.9 ounces)* is similar to the Chamomile Shampoo above and the same comments apply.

☹ **Ice Blue Shampoo for Oily Hair** *($5.50 for 8.4 ounces)* contains menthol and peppermint oil, which can be irritating and drying for the scalp.

☺ **Tangerine Beer Shampoo for Normal Hair** *($6 for 5 ounces)* does contain beer, but that serves no purpose for hair. This is basically just a shampoo with a strong detergent cleansing agent and thickeners. It would work well for all hair types, especially for getting rid of styling product buildup.

☺ **Amlika Leave-in Conditioner All Hair Types** *($10.50 for 16.9 ounces)* is a good, extremely basic conditioner for normal to slightly dry hair. It contains mostly water, thickener, slip agent, detangling agent, silicone, preservatives, and fragrance. While this product does contain a sunscreen, it isn't enough to protect hair from the sun.

☺ **Banana Conditioner for Normal to Dry Hair** *($10.50 for 16.9 ounces)* is only minimally a conditioner, and more of a detangling product for normal hair, not dry hair. It contains mostly water, thickener, detangling agent, slip agent, conditioning agent, preservatives, fragrance, and coloring agents.

☺ **Brazil Nut Damage Care Conditioner for Dry, Damaged & Chemically Treated Hair** *($10.50 for 16.9 ounces)* is a good but exceptionally basic conditioner for normal to slightly dry hair that is normal to fine or thin. It contains mostly water, thickeners, plant oil, detangling agent, fragrance, and preservatives.

☺ **Brazil Nut Conditioner, Dry, Damaged & Chemically Treated Hair Extra Rich and Moisturizing** *($10.50 for 16.9 ounces)* is almost identical to the one below and the same comments apply.

☹ **Ice Blue Revitalizing Conditioner for Oily Hair** *($6 for 8.4 ounces)* contains menthol and peppermint oil, which can be irritants for the skin and scalp.

☺ **Intensive Treatment for Normal to Dry, Damaged & Chemically Treated** *($8 for 5 ounces)* is a good conditioner for dry to extremely dry hair that is thick or coarse. It contains mostly water, thickener, detangling agent, silicone, more thickeners, plant oils, preservatives, and conditioning agent.

☹ **Intensive Treatment for Normal to Oily Hair** *($8 for 5 ounces)* isn't intensive in the least, but it does contain menthol, which can irritate and dry out the scalp. That doesn't help absorb oil at all.

☺ **Light Conditioner for Normal to Oily Hair** *($4.50 for 5 ounces)* is a good conditioner for normal to slightly dry hair—there is never a reason to apply conditioner to oily hair. It contains mostly water, thickener, silicone, plant extract, preservatives, detangling agents, fragrance, and coloring agents.

☺ **Seaweed & Peony Strengthening Conditioner Normal Hair** *($6 for 8.4 ounces)* is similar to the Light Conditioner above and the same comments apply.

☺ **Coconut Oil Hair Shine** *($5.45 for 1.7 ounces)* contains mostly thickeners, plant oils, lanolin, fragrance, and preservatives. Packaged to look like shoe polish, this is just a standard pomade that can help in controlling frizzies and stubborn curls. It has no hold, which means no chance of stiffness, but it can feel greasy and thick on hair so apply it minimally.

☺ **Define & No Frizz Cream Texturizer, with Rose Hips Oil & Ginseng** *($7.95 for 5.3 ounces)* is mostly water, silicones, thickeners, plant oils, film former, fragrance, and preservatives. It can smooth out frizzies and stubborn curls with minimal hold and no stiffness, but it can feel fairly greasy and heavy, so use it sparingly.

☺ **Slick** *($6.95 for 5.3 ounces)* is a gel with plant oil and film former along with fragrance and preservatives. It can slick hair back but it can feel greasy too, so use it sparingly.

☺ **Styling Gel Medium Hold, with Wheat Protein** *($5.95 for 5.1 ounces)* is a standard, light-hold styling gel containing mostly water, film former, thickeners, conditioning agent, preservatives, and fragrance. It has minimal to no stiff or sticky feel.

Bumble and Bumble

This line was originally created by Michael Gordon, owner of the Bumble and Bumble salon that opened in New York City in 1977. It's one of the many lines that has a hair designer behind the scenes. The claim for all these designer-established lines is, Who should know better about hair care than a hair designer? While I implicitly trust a talented hair designer with the cutting and styling of hair, creating hair-care formulations is an entirely different subject. You might love the way an interior designer can help you decorate your home, but you wouldn't necessarily want that same interior designer building your furniture.

Bumble and Bumble's claim is "while our products have never been tested on animals, they are thoroughly tested on models until we are sure they can style [for] the pages of *Vogue*, and satisfy our widely varied clientele." That's an enticing idea, but there are lots of product lines that can make the same claim. The bottom line is that these formulations don't differ from a wide range of other products on the market, and using them won't make your hair look like the models in *Vogue* (unless you have great hair and a designer who helps with your daily hairdo). What counts is how the formulations work for you every day, not just for a designer who has the leisure to work and rework a model's hair until he gets it right.

For more information on Bumble and Bumble, call (800) 7-BUMBLE or visit its Web site at www.bumbleandbumble.com.

☺ **Clarifying Shampoo** *($9 for 8 ounces)* is a good basic shampoo with no conditioning agents, and that makes it great for all hair types.

☹ **Gentle Shampoo** *($12 for 8 ounces)* has sodium C14-16 olefin sulfonate as one of its main detergent cleansing agents, and that isn't gentle; it is drying and hard on hair. There are also strong film-formers in this shampoo that can make hair feel stiff.

☺ **Seaweed Shampoo** *($9 for 8 ounces)* is a standard shampoo with no conditioning agents, and that makes it great for all hair types. It contains mostly water, detergent cleansing agent, lather agent, thickeners, preservatives, fragrance, and coloring agents.

☺ **Thickening Shampoo** *($11 for 8 ounces)* contains mostly water, detergent cleansing agent, lather agent, film former, conditioning agents, thickeners, preservatives, and fragrance. The film former can make hair feel slightly thicker so this would work well for someone with normal to fine thin and slightly dry hair.

☹ **Tonic Shampoo** *($12.20 for 8 ounces)* contains several ingredients, including peppermint and menthol, that can be a problem for the scalp.

☺ **Deep Conditioner** *($15.20 for 5 ounces)* is an exceptionally standard but good conditioner, though it isn't all that deep, for normal to dry hair that is normal to fine or thin. It contains mostly water, thickeners, detangling agents, plant oil, plant extracts, conditioning agents, silicone, preservatives, and fragrance.

☺ **Leave in Conditioner** *($12.40 for 8 ounces)* is a good, basic leave-in conditioner with no film former, so it won't feel stiff. It would work well for normal to slightly dry hair that is fine or thin. It contains mostly water, thickener, conditioning agents, preservatives, and fragrance.

☺ **Seaweed Conditioner** *($9.20 for 8 ounces)* features seaweed, though that won't help hair in the least. This is an ordinary detangling agent for normal to slightly dry hair that is normal to fine or thin. It contains mostly water, thickeners, detangling agents, preservatives, fragrance, and coloring agents.

☺ **Prep** *($10 for 8 ounces)* is a standard leave-in conditioner that would work well for normal to dry hair of any thickness. It contains mostly water, silicone, detangling agents, thickeners, plant extracts, vitamins, conditioning agents, slip agent, preservatives, and fragrance.

☺ **Grooming Creme** *($19 for 5 ounces)* contains mostly water, Vaseline, thickeners, plant oils, castor oil, silicone, preservatives, and fragrance. This is a good, fairly greasy styling cream for smoothing out stubborn frizzies or curls or taming coarse hair. It can feel heavy, so use it sparingly.

☺ **Styling Creme** *($17 for 8 ounces)* contains mostly water, film formers, thickeners, silicone, detangling agent, preservatives, and fragrance. This standard styling cream has a light hold and can help when styling curly hair straight. It can have a slight stiff, sticky feel.

☺ **Styling Wax** *($10.40 for 1.25 ounces)* is basically just wax, castor oil, and silicone. It is a standard thick pomade in a shoe-polish-type container. It can have a slight sticky and rather heavy feel, so use it sparingly. It does provide slick control when styling curly or frizzy hair straight. The claim that this wax washes out easily isn't true; products like this are all tricky to get out of the hair.

☺ **Brilliantine** *($12.40 for 2 ounces)* contains mostly water, thickeners, castor oils, preservatives, and coloring agents. It is similar to the Styling Wax below only in cream form, with a slight sticky feel on the hair.

☺ **Thickening Spray** *($15.20 for 8 ounces)* contains mostly alcohol, water, film formers, conditioning agents, and fragrance. As is true with any styling gel in a spray form, it can coat hair and make it feel thicker, and can also have a slight sticky feel.

☺ **Hairspray** *($9.20 for 8 ounces)* is a standard nonaerosol hair spray that contains mostly alcohol, water, film former, silicone, fragrance, and coloring agent. It gives a light hold and has minimal to no stiff or sticky feel on hair.

☺ **Holding Spray** *($9.20 for 8 ounces)* is similar to the Hairspray above and the same comments apply, only this one has a firmer hold.

☺ **$$$ Defrizz** *($18.40 for 4 ounces)* is an exceptionally overpriced, standard silicone serum. There are identical versions at the drugstore for a quarter of the cost.

☺ **$$$ BB Straight** *($18.40 for 5 ounces)* is similar to the Defrizz below only this one is in gel form; the same basic comments apply. This works as well as any silicone serum when used with the right styling tools, but the price is just silly.

☺ **Gloss** *($11.20 for 4 ounces)* contains mostly alcohol, thickeners, silicone, conditioning agents, and fragrance. It's similar to the Defrizz and BB Straight above only in spray form, meaning it has less silicone so is better for a lighter application.

☹ **Sun Spray** *($20.40 for 4 ounces)* does contain sunscreen, but without an SPF number you have no idea how much protection you are getting or how long it will last. It could be an SPF 2. Plus, the sunscreen's effectiveness easily brushes away.

☹ **Tonic** *($13.20 for 8 ounces)* contains several problematic ingredients, including peppermint and menthol, for the scalp, and it is not recommended.

Citre Shine

Citre Shine is a drugstore hair-care line owned by Advanced Research Laboratories (ARL), which also makes the Thicker Fuller Hair line available at drugstores. ARL would like you to believe that its products "naturally create shine through the inclusion of exotic citrus fruits. The secret to achieving the product's superior shine enhancing properties is a specially patented purification process of the extracts. Combined with low molecular weight keratin and wheat amino acids, these extracts penetrate the hair shaft to increase the hair's ability to reflect and refract light. . . in other words, to shine." Wow! What a shame citrus in any form can't do any of that. The conditioning agents are useful and do help smooth hair, which indeed makes it look shinier, but they aren't unique to Citre Shine. If this technology is so wonderful, what is truly curious is why it isn't it being used in the Thicker, Fuller Hair hair-care line owned by ARL. That line makes claims for superior shine too. Whatever the answer is, it turns out that the citrus mixture in the Citre Shine products can be irritating and drying for the scalp. If you tend to have an itchy scalp, these can make matters worse. For more information on Citre Shine, call (714) 556-1028, (800) 966-6960, or visit its Web site at www.citreshine.com.

☹ **Moisturizing Shampoo for Dry or Damaged Hair** *($3.99 for 16 ounces)* contains several problematic ingredients for the scalp and hair, including sodium lauryl sulfate, grapefruit, citrumelo, tangelo, tangerine, satsuma, and pummelo extracts.

☹ **Perm Color Treated Shampoo for Chemically Treated Hair** *($3.99 for 16 ounces)* is similar to the Moisturizing Shampoo above and is not recommended.

☹ **Revitalizing Shampoo for All Hair Types** *($3.99 for 16 ounces)* is similar to the Moisturizing Shampoo above and is not recommended.

☺ **Volumizing Shampoo for Fine to Normal Hair** *($3.42 for 16 ounces)* contains mostly citrus water, detergent cleansing agent, lather agent, film former, preservatives, and fragrance. If you don't have problems with the citrus, this can be a good basic shampoo for normal to fine thin hair. The film former can cause buildup.

☺ **Instant Conditioner for All Hair Types** *($3.42 for 16 ounces)* contains mostly citrus water, thickeners, detangling agents, silicone, preservatives, and fragrance. The citrus can be a problem, but this could be a good lightweight conditioner for normal to dry hair.

☺ **Instant Repair Miracle Creme Conditioner for Dry or Damaged Hair** *($3.99 for 5 ounces)* contains mostly citrus water, silicones, thickeners, film former, conditioning agents, preservatives, and fragrance. It's a good emollient conditioner for dry, coarse hair, but it doesn't repair anything.

☺ **Perm Color Treated Conditioner for Chemically Treated Hair** *($3.99 for 16 ounces)* contains mostly citrus water, conditioning agent, detangling agent, silicone, thickener, preservatives, and fragrance. There is nothing special about this product for permed hair, but it can be good for normal to dry hair that is normal to fine or thin.

☺ **Reconstructing Conditioner for Dry or Damaged Hair** *($3.99 for 16 ounces)* doesn't include anything that will restructure hair, but it is a good standard conditioner for normal to dry hair that is normal to fine or thin. It contains mostly citrus water, thickeners, detangling agents, conditioning agents, preservatives, and fragrance.

☺ **Volumizing Conditioner for Fine to Normal Hair** *($3.42 for 16 ounces)* contains mostly tea, thickeners, lots of silicones, detangling agents, conditioning agents, preservatives, and fragrance. With this much silicone, this conditioner is only suitable for dry hair that is thick to coarse.

☺ **Leave-in Volumizing Treatment Conditioner for Normal to Fine/Limp Hair** *($3.42 for 12 ounces)* contains mostly citrus water, conditioning agents, silicone, detangling agents, film former, preservatives, and fragrance. It is a good leave-in conditioner for normal to dry hair of any thickness.

☺ **Self-Heating Hot Oil Treatment for Dry or Damaged Hair** *($3.42 for three 1-ounce treatments)* is just a standard conditioner, identical to the ones above, which makes it good for normal to dry hair of any thickness. Warming up any conditioner and leaving it on the hair for longer periods of time can help it penetrate better, but that doesn't require a separate product. This one contains mostly citrus water, conditioning agents, thickener, detangling agents, fragrance, and coloring agents. By the way, it doesn't contain any oil.

☺ **Vitamin C Citrus Hot Oil** *($3.99 for three 1-ounce treatments)* is almost identical to the one above and the same comments apply.

☺ **Style & Shine Gel, Clear Shine** *($3.42 for 12 ounces)* contains mostly water, film former, citrus extracts, thickeners, silicone, conditioning agents, preservatives, and fragrance. It is a standard, light-hold gel that has minimal to no stiff or sticky feel.

☺ **Style & Shine Gel, Extra Body** *($3.42 for 12 ounces)* is similar to the Clear Shine version above, only this one has slightly more hold; for the most part the same comments apply.

☺ **Style & Shine Gel, Frizz Control** *($3.42 for 12 ounces)* is identical to the Clear Shine version above and the same comments apply.

☺ **Style & Shine Gel, Mega Hold** *($2.99 for 16 ounces)* is identical to the one above and the same comments apply.

☺ **Style & Shine Gel, Super Hold** *($3.42 for 12 ounces)* is identical to the one above and the same comments apply.

☺ **Super-Hold Styling Mousse Styler, for Wet or Dry Application** *($3.42 for 8 ounces)* contains mostly citrus water, conditioning agents, detangling agents/ film formers, propellant, silicones, fragrance, and preservatives. This is a light-hold mousse with minimal stiff or sticky feel.

☺ **Volumizing Mousse** *($3.42 for 8.5 ounces)* is similar to the Super-Hold version above and the same comments apply. This version contains something called Therm-shield, a mixture of plant oils and a conditioning agent. It is good for adding shine, but it can't protect the hair from heat any more than it could protect your skin or scalp.

☺ **Styler Glossing Wax** *($4.29 for 1.4 ounces)* is as good a pomade as any for straightening or smoothing stubborn ends, and can also have a heavy feel, so it use sparingly. It contains mostly Vaseline, thickeners, mineral oil, plant oil, preservatives, and fragrance. Without film formers it has minimal hold but no stiff feel.

☺ **Styler Texture Style Potion** *($3.42 for 5 ounces)* contains mostly citrus water, film formers, thickeners, silicones, plant oils, detangling agent, preservatives, and fragrance. It is a standard gel with a soft, brushable hold.

☺ **Straightening Balm** *($3.42 for 3.3 ounces)* is a gel that is basically just silicone, thickeners, and film former. This can help straighten hair and smooth frizzies with minimal to no stiff or sticky feel. It can have a heavy feel, so use it sparingly.

☺ **Shine Miracle Anti-Frizz Polisher for All Hair Types** *($5.91 for 4 ounces)* is one of the original silicone serums and it is great for making the hair feel silky soft and look shiny, especially if you don't mind the citrus fragrance.

☺ **Shine Miracle Laminator: An Extraordinary Shine Treatment for All Hair Types** *($3.42 for 1 ounce)* is identical to the one above and the same comments apply.

☺ **Shine Mist Spray Laminator for All Hair Types** *($3.42 for 3 ounces)* is similar to the Miracle Laminator above, only this one is in spray form and has a lighter feel on hair.

☺ **Shine Miracle Volumizing Polisher for Normal to Fine Hair** *($4.29 for 5 ounces)* is a silicone gel with a light hold. It can be too heavy or easily build up for normal to fine hair, but it can be good for styling curly hair straight and smoothing frizzies when used minimally.

☺ **Volumizing Shine Miracle Hair Polisher for Normal to Fine Hair** *($5.91 for 4 ounces)* is identical to the Miracle Volumizing version above and the exact same comments apply. It's just Citre Shine using the same formula with two different marketing angles.

☺ **Mega-Hold Finishing Spray Styler, for Dry Application (Non-Aerosol)** *($3.42 for 12 ounces)* is a standard hairspray that contains mostly alcohol, citrus water, conditioning agents, film formers, silicone, and fragrance. It has a medium to firm hold and a somewhat stiff, sticky feel.

☺ **Mega-Hold Finishing Spray Styler, Professional Hair Spray (Aerosol)** *($3.42 for 10 ounces)* is similar to the Dry Application above, only in aerosol form.

☺ **Shaping Hair Spray** *($3.42 for 8 ounces)* is a standard aerosol spray with film formers and some conditioning agents. It works as well as any for light hold and minimal to no stiff or sticky feel.

☺ **Ultra-Hold Design Spritz Styler for Wet or Dry Application** *($3.27 for 12 ounces)* is a standard but good styling spray that can help smooth hair during styling with minimal to no stiff or sticky feel. It contains mostly alcohol, citrus water, conditioning agents, film former, and silicone.

Clairol

Clairol is one of the largest hair-care companies around, with a major presence at both the salon and drugstore. Better known for its drugstore selections, Clairol has many product lines under its belt. Herbal Essence, Daily Defense, and Frizz Control are the current favorites, and when you count hair dyes, Clairol takes up a lot of space on the drugstore shelves. Clairol's hair-dye products are by far some of the best around, but its other hair-care products for the most part aren't anywhere near as interesting.

In my newsletter, *Cosmetics Counter Update,* I gave the entire Daily Defense line an unhappy face because I felt the whole premise of the line was misleading. The advertising for these products leads you to believe that the ingredients can protect the hair from the sun and pollution, when neither is possible. All of the ingredients in Daily Defense are completely standard and basic (and thoroughly boring) shampoo and conditioning ingredients. The minute amount of sunscreen agents that are added would be rinsed down the drain in use, leaving the hair exposed to any and all damage the environment had to offer.

Frizz Control is a small group of products that work as well as any, but Herbal Essence is just a highly fragranced product line with minimal herbs of any kind.

For more information on Clairol, call (800) 223-5800 or visit its Web site at www.clairol.com.

Frizz Control by Clairol

☹ **Hydrating Shampoo** *($3.78 for 12 ounces)* uses sodium lauryl sulfate as one of the main detergent cleansing agents, and that can be drying for the hair and scalp.

☺ **Taming Conditioner** *($3.78 for 12 ounces)* contains mostly water, thickeners, detangling agents, plant oils, fragrance, slip agents, conditioning agents, and preservatives. This is a good emollient conditioner for dry or extremely dry hair that is coarse or thick.

☺ **Taming Balm** *($3.78 for 2 ounces)* contains mostly water, thickeners, plant extracts, water-binding agent, fragrance, slip agent, film former, and preservatives. This is a lightweight balm that has minimal conditioning agent and a tiny amount of film former. It could work well for styling fine, thin hair.

☺ **Restructurizing Mousse** *($2.99 for 8 ounces)* is a standard mousse that contains mostly water, propellant, film former, conditioning agents, silicone, fragrance, and preservatives. It is a good light- to medium-hold mousse that brushes through easily with minimal sticky or stiff feel. It doesn't mend split ends in the least.

☺ **Defrizz Refresher & Shiner** *($3.78 for 5 ounces)* is a standard aerosol silicone spray with film former. It provides light hold and shine with no stiff or sticky feel.

☺ **High Gloss Hair Serum** *($4.79 for 2 ounces)* is a very good, standard silicone serum, and it works great for dry, coarse hair.

Herbal Essences by Clairol

☹ **Anti-Dandruff Shampoo for All Hair Types** *($2.78 for 12 ounces)* uses sodium lauryl sulfate as the main detergent cleansing agent, which can be drying for the hair and scalp. That won't help dandruff but it can make flaking worse.

☹ **Shampoo, Clarifying for Normal to Oily Hair** *($3.48 for 12 ounces)* uses sodium lauryl sulfate as one of its main detergent cleansing agents, which can be drying for the hair and scalp.

☹ **Shampoo, Extra Body for Fine/Limp Hair** *($3.48 for 12 ounces)* is similar to the Clarifying version above and is therefore not recommended.

☹ **Shampoo, Moisture-Balancing for Normal Hair** *($3.48 for 12 ounces)* is similar to the Clarifying version above and is therefore not recommended.

☹ **Shampoo, Replenishes Colored/Permed/Dry/Damaged Hair** *($3.48 for 12 ounces)* is similar to the Clarifying version above and is therefore not recommended (it would be particularly a problem for extremely dry hair).

☺ **Conditioner, Clean-Rinsing for Normal to Oily Hair** *($3.48 for 12 ounces)* contains mostly water, thickeners, detangling agent, conditioning agent, fragrance, preservatives, and coloring agents. It would be good for normal to dry hair that is either normal to fine or thin in thickness.

☺ **Conditioner, Intensive Conditioning Balm for Dry/Damaged/Over-stressed Hair** *($3.48 for 10.2 ounces)* is similar to the Clean-Rinsing one above and the same comments apply. This would not have enough conditioning agents or emollients for extremely dry hair.

☺ **Conditioner, Protects Colored/Permed/Dry/Damaged Hair** *($3.48 for 12 ounces)* is similar to the Clean-Rinsing conditioner above and the same comments apply.

☺ **Conditioner, Light Conditioning for Fine/Limp Hair** *($3.48 for 12 ounces)* contains mostly water, thickeners, detangling agent, conditioning agent, film former, fragrance, preservatives, and coloring agents. It would be good for normal to slightly dry, fine or thin hair to help make it feel fuller.

☺ **Conditioner, Moisturizing for Normal Hair** *($3.48 for 12 ounces)* is similar to the Light Conditioning one above, but without the film former. It would still be good, but without film former it doesn't impart much fullness. Still, it doesn't cause buildup either.

☺ **Leave-in Conditioner, Lightweight Formula for All Hair Types** *($3.48 for 10.2 ounces)* isn't all that lightweight. It contains mostly water, silicone, film former, conditioning agent, castor oil, detangling agent, slip agents, fragrance, and preservatives. It would be good for dry hair that is normal to fine or thin, but can have a slight sticky feel.

☺ **Conditioner, Dry Scalp for Use with Anti-Dandruff Shampoo** *($2.78 for 12 ounces)* is similar to the Leave-in Conditioner below and contains nothing that would fight dandruff, so just use it on your hair; there is no reason to apply these ingredients to an oily scalp.

☺ **Spray Gel, Extra Hold for Targeted Control** *($3.48 for 8.5 ounces)* contains mostly water, film former, plant extracts, conditioning agents, fragrance, castor oil, slip agents, preservatives, detangling agent, and coloring agent. This is a good light to medium hold styling spray that can have a slight sticky feel.

☺ **Styling Gel, Extra Hold for Shape & Control** *($3.48 for 8.5 ounces)* contains mostly water, film formers, thickener, plant extract, conditioning agents, silicone, fragrance, preservatives, and coloring agents. It's a good light- to medium-hold gel that brushes through easily without a stiff after-feel.

☺ **Styling Mousse, Extra Hold, for Volume and Manageability** *($3.12 for 8 ounces)* is a standard mousse that contains mostly water, propellant, film formers, conditioning agents, silicone, thickeners, fragrance, and preservatives. It is a good medium-hold mousse that brushes through easily without a stiff after-feel.

☺ **Styling Mousse, Maximum Hold, for Volume and Manageability** *($3.11 for 8 ounces)* is almost identical to the Extra Hold version above and the same comments apply.

☺ **Hairspray, Extra Hold, for All-Over Control (Aerosol)** *($3.48 for 8 ounces)* is a standard aerosol hairspray with light- to medium-hold and minimal to no stiff feel. It contains mostly alcohol, water, propellant, film former, silicones, fragrance, and slip agents.

☺ **Hairspray, Extra Hold, for Lasting Control (Non-Aerosol)** *($3.48 for 8.5 ounces)* is similar to the All-Over Control above, only with a slightly firmer hold and in nonaerosol form; the same basic comments apply.

☺ **Hairspray, Maximum Hold, for All-Over Control (Aerosol)** *($3.11 for 8 ounces)* is a standard aerosol hairspray with medium to firm hold and a somewhat stiff feel. It contains mostly alcohol, water, propellant, film formers, silicones, conditioning agents, fragrance, and slip agents.

☺ **Hairspray, Maximum Hold, for Lasting Control (Non-Aerosol)** *($3.11 for 8.5 ounces)* is similar to the Maximum Hold above, only in nonaerosol form, and the same basic comments apply.

☺ **Styling Spritz, Maximum Hold, for Ultimate Control** *($3.48 for 8.5 ounces)* is almost identical to the two Maximum Hold hairsprays above and the same comments apply.

Daily Defense by Clairol

☹ **Shampoo Defense 1 for Fine Hair** *($3.48 for 13.5 ounces)* uses sodium lauryl sulfate as one of its main detergent cleansing agents, which can be drying for the hair and scalp. That won't help dandruff, but it can make flaking worse.

☹ **Shampoo Defense 2 for Normal Hair** *($3.48 for 13.5 ounces)* uses sodium lauryl sulfate as one of its main detergent cleansing agents, which can be drying for the hair and scalp.

☹ **Shampoo Defense 3 for Color-Treated/Permed Hair** *($3.48 for 13.5 ounces)* uses sodium lauryl sulfate as one of its main detergent cleansing agents, which can be drying for the hair and scalp.

☹ **Shampoo Defense 4 for Dry/Damaged Hair** *($3.48 for 13.5 ounces)* uses sodium lauryl sulfate as one of its main detergent cleansing agents, which can be drying for the hair and scalp.

☺ **Conditioner Defense 1 for Fine Hair** *($3.48 for 13.5 ounces)* contains mostly water, thickeners, detangling agent, conditioning agents, fragrance, and preservatives. It is a good, lightweight conditioner for normal to slightly dry hair of any thickness except coarse. There is nothing in this product that can protect hair from environmental damage of any kind, and the claims about sun protection are bogus.

☺ **Conditioner Defense 2 for Normal Hair** *($3.48 for 13.5 ounces)* is almost identical to the one above and the same comments apply.

☺ **Conditioner Defense 3 for Color-Treated/Permed Hair** *($3.48 for 13.5 ounces)* is almost identical to the one above and the same comments apply.

☺ **Conditioner Defense 4 for Dry/Damaged Hair** *($3.48 for 13.5 ounces)* is almost identical to the one above, only with a small amount of silicone added. That does make it better for slightly drier hair but not dry or damaged hair.

☺ **Intensive Conditioner, Extra Defense for Damaged/Overstressed Hair** *($3.29 for 10.2 ounces)* is similar to the Defense 4 above, only with slightly more conditioning agents and silicone. That does make it better for dry, coarse hair, but it is hardly intensive.

☺ **Fortifying Leave-in Conditioning Spray** *($3.48 for 10.2 ounces)* is basically a silicone spray with conditioning agents and film formers that would be very good to use to add a feeling of thickness to dry hair that is fine or thin, though it can have a slight stiff, sticky feel on hair.

☺ **Gel, Extra Hold for Styling Control** *($3.18 for 7 ounces)* contains mostly water, film formers, thickeners, conditioning agents, castor oil, silicones, fragrance, slip agents, preservatives, and coloring agents. This is a standard gel with light to medium hold that has minimal to no stiff or sticky feel.

☺ **Spray Gel, Extra Hold for Styling Versatility** *($3.18 for 8 ounces)* is similar to the Extra Hold Gel above and the same comments apply.

☺ **Mousse, Extra Hold for Body and Volume** *($3.18 for 8 ounces)* is a standard mousse that contains mostly water, propellant, film formers, conditioning agents, vitamins, silicones, castor oil, fragrance, and preservatives. This is a good light- to medium-hold mousse with minimal stiff feel.

☺ **Hairspray, Extra Hold for Lasting Control (Aerosol)** *($3.18 for 8 ounces)* is a standard aerosol hairspray that has medium hold and a slightly stiff feel. It contains mostly alcohol, water, propellant, film former, conditioning agents, silicone, castor oil, and fragrance.

☺ **Non-Aerosol Hairspray, Extra Hold for Lasting Control** *($3.18 for 8 ounces)* is similar to the aerosol Extra Hold above only, in nonaerosol form, and the same comments apply.

☺ **Hairspray, Maximum Hold, for Lasting Control (Non-Aerosol)** *($2.99 for 8.5 ounces)* is similar to the Extra Hold version above and the same comments apply.

Conditions 3-in-1 by Clairol

☺ **Shampoo Plus, Clean and Light, Shampoo/Sheer Conditioner/Protectant** *($1.75 for 12 ounces)* contains mostly water, detergent cleansing agents, foaming agents, detangling agents, silicone, fragrance, preservatives, and coloring agents. This is a good standard shampoo with conditioning agents that can be good for someone with dry hair of any thickness. It can build up on hair.

☹ **Shampoo Plus, Dry Hair, Shampoo/Sheer Conditioner/Protectant** *($1.75 for 12 ounces)* uses sodium lauryl sulfate as one of the main detergent cleansing agents, which can be drying for the hair and scalp.

☹ **Shampoo Plus, Extra Body, Shampoo/Sheer Conditioner/Protectant** *($1.75 for 12 ounces)* uses sodium lauryl sulfate as one of the main detergent cleansing agents, which can be drying for the hair and scalp.

☹ **Shampoo Plus, Normal Hair, Shampoo/Sheer Conditioner/Protectant** *($1.75 for 12 ounces)* uses sodium lauryl sulfate as one of the main detergent cleansing agents, which can be drying for the hair and scalp.

☹ **Shampoo Plus, Permed/Color Treated Hair, Shampoo/Sheer Conditioner/Protectant** *($1.75 for 12 ounces)* uses sodium lauryl sulfate as one of the main detergent cleansing agents, which can be drying for the hair and scalp.

☺ **Detangler Plus** *($1.75 for 8 ounces)* contains mostly water, silicones, fragrance, film former, more fragrance, detangling agent, slip agents, and preservatives. This is a good leave-in conditioner for normal to slightly dry hair that is fine or thin. It can have a slight sticky feel, but it can also make fine or thin hair feel thicker.

☺ **Protein Enriched Beauty Pack Treatment, Extra Body Formula** *($5.62 for 4 ounces)* contains mostly water, conditioning agents, thickeners, detangling agent, fragrance, and preservatives. This is a good basic conditioner for dry hair of any thickness except coarse.

☺ **Gel, Extra Hold** *($1.75 for 4 ounces)* contains mostly water, film formers, conditioning agents, silicone, fragrance, and preservatives. It has a light to medium hold and minimal stiff or sticky feel.

☺ **Gel, Maximum Hold** *($1.75 for 4 ounces)* is similar to the Extra Hold version above, only with medium hold and a slight sticky feel.

☺ **Gel, Moisturizing** *($1.75 for 4 ounces)* isn't that much more moisturizing than the two above. It has a light to medium hold and minimal stiff or sticky feel.

☺ **Gel, Natural Hold** *($1.75 for 4 ounces)* is similar to the Extra Hold version above and the same comments apply.

☺ **Spray Gel, Extra Hold** *($1.75 for 4 ounces)* contains mostly water, film formers, conditioning agents, silicone, fragrance, and preservatives. It has a light hold and minimal stiff or sticky feel.

☺ **Spray Gel, Maximum Hold** *($1.75 for 4 ounces)* is similar to the Extra Hold version above, only with medium hold and a slight sticky feel.

☺ **Spray Gel, Ultra Control** *($1.89 for 8 ounces)* contains mostly water, film formers, detangling agent, conditioning agent, castor oil, and preservatives. This does have slightly more hold than the other two spray gels above, though it also has a slightly sticky feel.

☺ **Mousse, Extra Hold** *($1.75 for 6 ounces)*. The similarity between all of the following mousses is rather shocking. They are all standard, containing mostly water, propellant, film former, conditioning agent, fragrance, silicone, and preservatives. Each one has a light to medium hold with a slight sticky feel, though they do brush through easily.

☺ **Mousse, Maximum Hold** *($1.89 for 6 ounces)* is similar to the Extra Hold version above with a medium to firm but still flexible hold.

☺ **Mousse, Moisturizing** *($1.75 for 6 ounces)* is almost identical to the Extra Hold version above and the same comments apply.

☺ **Mousse, Natural Hold** *($1.75 for 6 ounces)* is almost identical to the Extra Hold version above and the same comments apply.

☺ **Hairspray, Extra Hold (Aerosol—Scented and Unscented)** *($1.75 for 7 ounces)* is a standard aerosol hairspray containing mostly alcohol, water, propellant, film former, silicone, and fragrance. This is a good light-hold hairspray with minimal to no stiff or sticky feel, and it brushes through easily.

☺ **Hairspray, Extra Hold (Non-Aerosol—Scented and Unscented)** *($1.75 for 8 ounces)* is similar to the version above, only this one is nonaerosol.

☺ **Hairspray, Maximum Hold (Aerosol—Scented and Unscented)** *($1.75 for 7 ounces)* is a standard aerosol hairspray containing mostly alcohol, water, propellant, film former, silicone, and fragrance. This is a good light to medium hold hairspray with minimal to no stiff or sticky feel. It brushes through easily.

☺ **Hairspray, Maximum Hold (Non-Aerosol—Scented and Unscented)** *($1.75 for 8 ounces)* is similar to the one above, only this one is nonaerosol.

☺ **Hairspray, Natural Hold (Aerosol—Scented and Unscented)** *($1.75 for 7 ounces)* is a standard aerosol hairspray containing mostly alcohol, water, propellant, film former, silicone, and fragrance. This is a good light-hold hairspray with minimal to no stiff or sticky feel.

☺ **Sculpting Spritz** *($1.75 for 8 ounces)* is similar to the Maximum Hold nonaerosol hairspray above and the same comments apply.

☺ **Curl Refresher** *($1.75 for 8 ounces)* contains mostly water, conditioning agents, fragrance, and preservatives. This is more of a leave-in conditioner than anything else. It has a soft feel and minimal to no holding power. That can work great for wetting hair and adding a slight sheen, without adding a stiff or sticky feel.

Complements by Clairol
(available in beauty supply stores)

☺ **Color-Enhancing Shampoo with Sunscreen and Conditioner, Ash Blonde** *($4.99 for 8 ounces)* contains mostly water, detergent cleansing agent, lather agent, detangling agent, thickeners, film former, fragrance, preservatives, and coloring agents.

This is a good gentle shampoo with temporary coloring agents added. It works as well as any, though this detergent cleansing formula is more gentle than most, and that would help keep the color in and prevent dryness. Though it can add a feel of thickness, the film former can cause buildup, plus, without an SPF, sunscreen in hair-care products are useless.

☺ **Color-Enhancing Shampoo with Sunscreen and Conditioner, Ash Brown** *($4.99 for 8 ounces)* is almost identical to the one above and the same comments apply.

☺ **Color-Enhancing Shampoo with Sunscreen and Conditioner, Golden Blonde** *($4.99 for 8 ounces)* is almost identical to the one above and the same comments apply.

☺ **Color-Enhancing Shampoo with Sunscreen and Conditioner, Natural Blonde** *($4.99 for 8 ounces)* is almost identical to the one above and the same comments apply.

☺ **Color-Enhancing Shampoo with Sunscreen and Conditioner, Red-Copper** *($4.99 for 8 ounces)* is almost identical to the one above and the same comments apply.

☺ **Color-Enhancing Shampoo with Sunscreen and Conditioner, Red Plum** *($4.99 for 8 ounces)* is almost identical to the one above and the same comments apply.

Final Net by Clairol

Some lines are eternal, and Final Net seems to be one of them. It doesn't quite deserve its reputation as a way to create helmet hair because there are some good hairsprays here for medium to firm hold, and it does brush through. All of the formulations are aerosol.

☺ **All-Day Hold Hairspray, Extra Hold, Light Scent** *($2.59 for 12 ounces)* has medium to firm hold with a slight stiff, sticky feel. It contains mostly water, film formers, conditioning agent, silicone, fragrance, and preservatives.

☺ **Hold That Moves Hairspray, Extra Hold, Scented and Unscented** *($2.59 for 12 ounces)* is similar to the one above and the same comments apply.

☺ **Hold That Moves Hairspray, Regular Hold, Scented and Unscented** *($2.59 for 12 ounces)* is similar to the one above and the same comments apply.

☺ **Hold That Moves Hairspray, Ultimate Hold, Scented and Unscented** *($2.59 for 12 ounces)* is similar to the one above, only this one does have a firmer hold and a somewhat stiff, sticky feel.

Clinique

There is every reason to buy makeup or skin care from Clinique, at least within reason, because some of those products are exceptional. Its hair-care products, on the other hand, are incredibly average and ordinary. There's really very little reason to buy hair care from Clinique. For more information on Clinique, call (212) 572-3800, or visit its Web site at www.clinique.com.

☺ **Daily Wash Shampoo** *($10 for 6 ounces)* contains mostly water, detergent cleansing agent, thickeners, lather agent, plant extracts, preservatives, and coloring agents. This is a good standard shampoo with no conditioning agents. It would work great for all hair types.

☹ **Extra Benefits Shampoo** *($10 for 6 ounces)* contains TEA-lauryl sulfate as the main detergent cleansing agent, which is too drying for the hair and irritating for the scalp.

☺ **Extra Benefits Conditioner** *($10 for 4 ounces)* contains mostly water, thickeners, plant extracts, detangling agents, preservatives, and coloring agents. This is a good lightweight conditioner for normal to slightly dry hair that is normal to fine or thin.

☺ **Hair Shaper Gel Alcohol-Free** *($10 for 4 ounces)* contains mostly water, slip agent, thickeners, film former, preservatives, and coloring agents. This is a good lightweight gel with a soft, combable hold.

☺ **Serious-Hold Hairspray Unscented** *($10 for 6 ounces)* is a good light- to medium-hold standard hairspray with a slight stiff, sticky feel. It contains mostly alcohol, water, film former, and silicone.

☺ **Non-Aerosol Hairspray Unscented** *($10 for 8 ounces)* is similar to the Serious-Hold above and the same comments apply.

Dark & Lovely

Dark & Lovely is a line of hair-care products designed for African-American women. Like the styling products in most all hair-care lines marketed to African American women, the ones here are loaded with Vaseline, lanolin, plant oils, and mineral oil. That makes them greasy, thick, and heavy. It's also a dated way of dealing with the problems of making tightly curled hair straight. There are far better options, ranging from pomades to styling balms and waxes. The shampoos and conditioners are fairly standard, with no special features related to the problems of fine, fragile, or relaxed hair. If anything, in order to wash these same styling products out of the hair, the line's shampoos won't be of much help. For more information on Dark & Lovely, call (800) 442-4643.

☺ **3-in-1 Plus Detangling/Conditioning Shampoo** *($2.49 for 16 ounces)* contains mostly water, detergent cleansing agents, lather agent, thickener, conditioning agent, detangling agents, film former, preservative, and coloring agents. This is a good shampoo with conditioning agents for dry hair, but the film former can leave a stiff feel on fragile hair, which makes it best for fine or thin hair.

☺ **Beautiful Beginnings Vitamin E & Aloe Conditioning Shampoo Plus Detangler** *($2.19 for 8 ounces)* is similar to the 3-in-1 version above and the same comments apply.

The Reviews C

☺ **Color Care Shampoo** *($2.29 for 8 ounces)* is similar to the 3-in-1 version above and the same comments apply.

☹ **Color Signal Neutralizing Deep Conditioning & Decalcifying Shampoo** *($3.89 for 16 ounces)* contains nothing that's particularly "decalcifying." It is just the same basic shampoo as those above with a few more conditioning agents added. It would work well for dry hair but it could also cause buildup with repeated use.

☺ **24-Hr. Therapy Moisture & Shine Replenisher** *($4.99 for 8 ounces)* contains mostly water, mineral oil, Vaseline, lanolin, thickeners, silicones, castor oil, plant oils, vitamins, slip agents, preservatives, and fragrance. This is definitely moisturizing, but it can also be extremely greasy, can build up on hair, and can be difficult to wash out—so use it sparingly.

☺ **Beautiful Beginnings Vitamin E & Aloe Leave-in Conditioner Plus Detangler** *($2.59 for 8 ounces)* contains mostly water, slip agents, conditioning agents, detangling agents/film formers, preservatives, coloring agents, and fragrance. This is a good leave-in conditioner for dry hair that is normal to fine or thin. The film formers can leave a slight stiff feel on hair.

☺ **Beautiful Beginnings Vitamin E & Aloe Natural Oil Moisturizer Plus Detangler** *($3.59 for 8 ounces)* contains mostly water, mineral oil, slip agent, silicone, thickeners, detangling agents, conditioning agents, plant oils, vitamins, preservatives, coloring agents, and fragrance. This is a good leave-in conditioner for very dry, coarse hair. The mineral oil and plant oils can be heavy for fine or thin hair.

☺ **Ultra Cholesterol Super Moisturizing & Conditioning Treatment** *($2.49 for 15 ounces)* contains mostly water, thickeners, lanolin, detangling agents, conditioning agents, plant oils, vitamins, coloring agents, preservatives, and fragrance. This doesn't strengthen or repair as the label claims, but it is a very good, albeit heavy, conditioner for very dry, coarse hair.

☺ **Vitamin E & Oil Scalp Conditioner and Hair Dress** *($3.19 for 4 ounces)* contains mostly Vaseline, mineral oil, thickeners, lanolin, plant oils, vitamins, preservatives, and fragrance. It's fairly greasy and heavy and can easily build up, but it can help smooth hair when used minimally. It would take a very good clarifying shampoo to get it out of the hair.

☺ **Ultra Cholesterol Plus Super Moisturizing/Conditioning Treatment** *($2.49 for 15 ounces)* contains mostly thickeners, lanolin, detangling agent, conditioning agents, plant oils, vitamins, coloring agent, preservatives, and fragrance. The lanolin makes this fairly heavy, but it can help smooth coarse, dry hair when used minimally. It would take a very good clarifying shampoo to get it out of the hair.

☺ **Color Care Conditioner** *($2.29 for 8 ounces)* contains mostly water, silicone, thickeners, detangling agent/film former, conditioning agents, preservatives, and fragrance. It is a good lightweight conditioner for dry hair that is normal to fine or thin. There is nothing about it, though, that is better for color-treated hair.

☺ **Corrective Leave-in Condition Therapy** *($4.29 for 8 ounces)* is basically mineral oil, coloring agents, and fragrance. That can be good for extremely dry hair, and also greasy. If used minimally it can be an option for dry, coarse hair.

☺ **Deep Penetrating Conditioner for Relaxed and Color-Treated Hair** *($1.19 for 0.75 ounce)* contains mostly water, slip agent, thickeners, conditioning agent, detangling agent, silicone, mink oil, fragrance, lanolin, plant oil, vitamins, and preservatives. This isn't all that deep, or even related to chemically treated hair, at least not any more than any other conditioner. It is a good conditioner for dry, coarse hair.

☺ **Pro Therapy Protein Intensive Conditioner** *($2.99 for 16 ounces)* contains mostly water, thickeners, detangling agent, silicone, slip agent, plant oils, vitamins, conditioning agents, preservatives, and fragrance. This is a good conditioner for dry, coarse hair.

☺ **Restore & Repair Reconstructive Hair Therapy** *($2.59 for 4 ounces).* Not one ingredient in this product, or any hair product for that matter, can repair or reconstruct hair. However, like all the conditioning products in this line, this is while fairly greasy, it is still an option when used minimally over extremely dry, coarse hair. It contains mostly mineral oil, water, petrolatum, lanolin, thickeners, silicone, detangling agent/film former, conditioning agents, castor oil, plant oils, vitamins, coloring agents, preservatives, and fragrance. The film former and castor oil in here can leave a stiff sticky feel on hair.

☺ **Rich & Natural Hair Dress Conditioner** *($2.79 for 4 ounces)* is similar to the Restore & Repair version above and the same comments apply.

☺ **Conditioning Setting Lotion for Relaxed & Color-Treated Hair** *($2.79 for 8 ounces)* is a standard styling spray that contains mostly water, film formers, conditioning agents, fragrance, detangling agents, and preservatives. It has a soft hold and minimal to no stiff, sticky feel.

☺ **Conditioning Set & Wrap All-Day Hold** *($2.79 for 8 ounces)* is similar to the Setting Lotion above only with slightly more hold and a slightly sticky feel.

☺ **Silky Set Conditioning Set & Wrap Lotion All-Day Hold** *($3.69 for 8 ounces)* is similar to the Setting Lotion above and the same comments apply.

☺ **Quick Styling Regular Hold Gel** *($2.29 for ounces)* contains mostly water, conditioning agents, plant extract, thickener, coloring agents, film former, and fragrance. This is a very soft-hold gel that would work for light-hold combable styling.

☺ **Quick Styling Super Hold Gel** *($2.29 for 4.5 ounces)* is almost identical to the Regular Hold Gel above and the same comments apply.

☹ **Healthy Shine Super Conditioning Oil Sheen Spray** *($4.99 for 14 ounces)* is basically just an aerosol spray of mineral oil. This can be fairly greasy stuff. It contains mostly mineral oil, emollient, lanolin oil, plant oils, vitamins, fragrance, and propellant. This may not be the shine you want on hair that is already loaded up with the conditioners from this line, but it can add shine.

☺ **The Restorer Super Strengthening Hot Oil** *($4.99 for 8 ounces)* is mostly plant oils, slip agent, preservatives, and fragrance. This is fine, but these oils can't strengthen. There is little difference between this and applying olive oil from your cupboard on hair. It can be greasy, but it is also good for extremely dry hair.

☺ **Quik Freeze Super Shine Spritz** *($3.49 for 8 ounces)* is a standard hairspray, with alcohol, water, film former, slip agents, silicones, and fragrance. It has a light to medium hold and minimal to no stiff feel.

Denorex

Denorex is one of the classic options for fighting dandruff. It offers a small range of products that use either zinc pyrithione or coal tar. Unfortunately, most of the formulations are disappointing because of the addition of ingredients that generate a tingle, such as menthol, which can cause more drying and flaking, or alcohol, which can cause dryness and irritation. Neither menthol nor alcohol have any effect on the cause of dandruff. There are better options for fighting dandruff than these.

For more information on Denorex, call (800) 322-3129, or in Canada (201) 660-5500. You can also visit its Web site at www.ahp.com.

☹ **Advanced Formula Dandruff Shampoo** *($7.88 for 8 ounces)* is a standard zinc pyrithione–based shampoo, though this version also contains menthol, which can cause problems for the scalp. It also has minimal detergent cleansing agents, so it isn't the best at cleaning hair.

☹ **Medicated Shampoo and Conditioner** *($7.32 for 8 ounces)* is a standard coal tar–based shampoo, but this one also contains alcohol and menthol and a small amount of TEA-lauryl sulfate, all of which can add up to a drier, more flaky scalp.

☹ **Medicated Shampoo, Mountain Fresh Scent** *($7.32 for 8 ounces)* is identical to the one above and the same comments apply.

☹ **Vitamin Enriched Extra Strength Medicated Shampoo and Conditioner** *($9.39 for 8 ounces)* is identical to the one above and the same comments apply.

Dep

This is the original styling-gel group of products, and for cost effectiveness and performance it's still hard to beat. For more information on Dep, call (310) 604-0777, (800) 326-2855, or visit its Web site at www.dep.com.

☺ **Alcohol-Free Spray Gel Extra Super Control** *($2.99 for 8 ounces)* is just film former and thickening agents with some fragrance, coloring agents, and preservatives, of course! It works as well as any spray gel, with a light hold and minimal to no stiff or sticky feel.

☺ **Level 2 Water-Based Gel Extra Shine with Light Control** *($2.99 for 12 ounces)* is similar to the one above except in traditional gel form, and it works great for light hold and minimal to no stiff or sticky feel.

☺ **Level 3 Shine Gel Natural Hold** *($1.99 for 4 ounces)* is similar to the Level 2 above, only with silicone. That doesn't change the performance, so except for adding a bit of extra shine, the same basic review above applies.

☺ **Level 4 Water-Based Gel Super Control with Moisturizers** *($2.99 for 12 ounces)* is similar to the Level 2 above and the same basic comments apply.

☺ **Level 4 Shine Gel Natural Hold Non-Sticky** *($2.99 for 12 ounces)* is indeed a light-hold gel with no stiff or sticky feel, similar to the Level 2 above, and the same basic comments apply.

☺ **Level 5 Volumizing Gel Flexible Hold** *($2.99 for 12 ounces)* is almost identical to the Level 4 above only, with slightly more hold (but only slightly); otherwise the same comments apply.

☺ **Level 5 Water-Based Gel Extra Super Control** *($2.40 for 12 ounces)* is almost identical to the Level 5 Volumizing Gel above and the same comments apply.

☺ **Level 6 Moisturizing Gel Extra Hold** *($2.40 for 12 ounces)* is almost identical to the Level 5 above, only with more hold and a slightly stiffer, more sticky feel.

☺ **Level 6 Volumizing Spray Gel Extra Hold** *($2.40 for 8 ounces)* is almost identical to the Level 6 above, only in spray form, and the same comments apply.

☺ **Level 7 Shaping Gel Extra Super Hold** *($2.99 for 12 ounces)* is similar to the Level 6 above and the same comments apply.

☺ **Level 8 Texturizing Gel Ultimate Hold** *($2.99 for 12 ounces)* is similar to the Level 6 above and the same comments apply; in other words, this does not deliver "ultimate" hold.

☺ **Level 7 Finishing Hairspray Extra Super Hold** *($3.19 for 8 ounces)* has a medium to firm hold and a slightly stiff feel.

☺ **Level 5 Straightening Cream Flexible Hold** *($3.19 for 5 ounces)* is more of a gel than a cream, and contains mostly water, thickeners, detangling agent, silicones, film formers, conditioning agents, fragrance, and preservatives. The hold is light and extremely flexible, with no stiff or sticky feel. It can be helpful when styling hair straight.

Fabao 101

In the world of hair-growth snake-oil treatments, perhaps none fits the bill better than Fabao 101. This hair tonic is widely advertised by various retailers on the Internet but—what a shock—does not have FDA approval as a treatment for hair loss of any kind.

The Reviews F

Doctors Zhuang-Guang Zhao and Yoshikata Inaba of Tokyo created this product, and their success has received mention in both the *New York Times* and *Newsweek*. They haven't successfully grown much, if any, hair, but the scale of their marketing escapades is substantial.

One study does exist for this product. It was published in the *Journal of Clinical Epidemiology*, vol. 44, no. 4/5, 1991, pages 439–47. Basically this study was a randomized, double-blind trial using 396 males with androgenetic alopecia (male-pattern baldness). The men took the Chinese herb Dabao for six months and the effects were evaluated by counting the number of hairs per unit area, by asking for the subjective opinion of the users, and by semiquantitative analysis of before-and-after photographs of the scalp.

The researchers reported that "Comparing Dabao and placebo groups after six months there was an increase in the observed amount of hair; average 133 and 109 hairs respectively per a 5 cm^2 marked area (a difference of 24 hairs between the groups). Subjective responses from the men in the trial suggested 42% of the Dabao users and 37% in placebo users reported positive results (a 5% difference)." Is 5 percent statistically significant to warrant a success? Not from my point of view. Plus, these men were taking the Dabao as a supplement, which Fabao isn't; it's a topical product, applied to the surface of the skin.

The claim the doctors who make this stuff are sticking to is that Fabao 101 unclogs pores and improves the quality of the blood supply to hair follicles, thereby encouraging hair growth. Unfortunately, that theory of hair regrowth is not proven. According to a paper by Richard L. De Villez, MD, associate professor, Division of Dermatology, University of Texas Health Science Center, San Antonio, Texas, "Many attempts have been made to stimulate hair growth . . . by increasing blood flow by massage methods and by topical administration of vasodilators. . . . Much like the association of hair growth to the enervation of the follicle, the relationship of vascularization to hair growth has not been completely resolved. It is generally thought that vascularization by itself does not stimulate follicular activity but that the active follicle determines its own blood supply from the dermal vascular plexus." The conclusions you draw are up to you.

For more information about Fabao 101, call (888) 919-4247, in Canada (888) 919-HAIR (both numbers toll-free), or visit its Web site at www.fabao.com.

The following Fabao tonics are available: **101D Formula** *($69.95 for 2 ounces)* recommended for people in the early stage of hair loss; **101F Formula** *($79.95 for 2 ounces)* for people in the late-stage of hair loss, recommended for oily scalp; **101G Formula** *($79.95 for 2 ounces)* for people in the late-stage of hair loss, recommended for normal or dry scalp; and **101 Shampoo** *($8.95 for 6.6 ounces).*

Finesse

Finesse is owned by Helene Curtis. For more information on Finesse, call (800) 621-2013.

☺ **Bodifying Shampoo for Fine or Thin Hair** *($2.58 for 15 ounces)* contains mostly water, detergent cleansing agent, lather agent, thickener, silicone, conditioning agent, detangling agent/film former, fragrance, preservatives, and coloring agents. This is a good basic shampoo for someone with dry hair that is normal to fine or thin in thickness.

☺ **Enhancing Shampoo for Normal, Healthy Hair** *($2.58 for 15 ounces)* is similar to the one above and the same comments apply.

☹ **Moisturizing Shampoo for Dry or Coarse Hair** *($2.58 for 15 ounces)* uses sodium lauryl sulfate as the main detergent cleansing agent and that isn't moisturizing for hair or scalp, it's drying and potentially irritating.

☺ **Revitalizing Shampoo for Permed, Color-Treated or Overstyled Hair** *($2.58 for 15 ounces)* contains mostly water, detergent cleansing agents, lather agent, silicone, slip agent, thickener, detangling agent, conditioning agent, fragrance, and preservatives. This is a good basic shampoo for someone with normal to dry hair of any thickness.

☺ **Plus Shampoo Plus Conditioner Enhancing for Normal Hair** *($2.58 for 15 ounces)* is almost identical to the one above and the same comments apply.

☺ **Plus Shampoo Plus Conditioner Moisturizing for Dry or Coarse Hair** *($2.58 for 15 ounces)* is almost identical to the Revitalizing Shampoo above and the same comments apply.

☺ **Bodifying Conditioner for Fine or Thin Hair** *($2.58 for 15 ounces)* contains mostly water, thickener, silicone, detangling agent, conditioning agents, fragrance, more thickeners, and preservatives. This is a good conditioner for dry, damaged, and coarse hair.

☺ **Deep Fortifying Conditioner for Weak or Damaged Hair** *($3.49 for 15 ounces)* is almost identical to the one above and the same comments apply.

☺ **Moisturizing Conditioner for Dry or Coarse Hair** *($2.58 for 15 ounces)* is almost identical to the one above and the same comments apply.

☺ **Revitalizing Conditioner for Permed, Colored or Overstyled Hair** *($2.58 for 15 ounces)* is almost identical to the one above and the same comments apply.

☺ **Enhancing Conditioner for Normal, Healthy Hair** *($2.58 for 15 ounces)* is similar to the one above only with slightly less silicone and more detangling agent. It would work well for normal to slightly dry hair of any thickness.

☺ **Light Conditioning Spray for All Hair Types** *($2.58 for 10.5 ounces)* contains mostly water, conditioning agents, detangling agents, fragrance, preservatives,

The Reviews F

and silicone. This is a good, lightweight, leave-in conditioner for normal to slightly dry hair of any thickness.

☺ **Touchables Mousse Extra Control Alcohol Free** *($2.08 for 7 ounces)* is a standard mousse that contains mostly water, propellant, film formers, fragrance, silicones, and preservatives. It has a good light to medium hold with minimal to stiff or sticky feel.

☺ **Touchables Mousse Moisturizing, Alcohol Free** *($2.08 for 7 ounces)* is similar to the one above and the same comments apply.

☺ **Touchables Volumizing Foamer** *($2.08 for 7 ounces)* is similar to the mousse above, only in an aerated dispensing container that creates the foam; the same basic comments apply.

☺ **Touchables Hairspray Extra Hold, Aerosol** (Scented and Unscented) *($2.08 for 7 ounces)* is a standard aerosol hairspray that contains mostly alcohol, propellant, water, film former, conditioning agent, fragrance, and silicones. This gives a light to medium hold with a slight stiff feel. It does brush easily through hair.

☺ **Touchables Hair Spray Extra Hold, Non-Aerosol** *($2.08 for 8.5 ounces)* is similar to the one above, only in nonaerosol form and the same comments apply.

☺ **Touchables Hairspray Maximum Hold, Aerosol** *($2.08 for 7 ounces)* is similar to the aerosol version above, only with definitely more hold.

☺ **Touchables Hairspray Maximum Hold, Non-Aerosol** *($2.08 for 8.5 ounces)* similar to the one above, only in nonaerosol form.

☺ **Touchables Shaping Spray Dual Usage for Wet or Dry Hair** *($2.08 for 7 ounces)* is better as a hairspray for light hold than it is as a styling spray. It has light hold and a minimally stiff, sticky feel.

Focus 21

Focus 21 has a vast range of products showcased at the drugstore, including SeaPlasma, Enviro-Tek Antioxidant, Hair Toys, and Splash. The variety of claims made for each group is astounding—every imaginable plant that grows on the ground or in the ocean is supposed to be good for hair. It always amazes me that all hair-care lines carry on at length about their botanical content, which rarely makes up more than 1 to 2 percent of the product, but never mention the less exotic ingredients that comprise well over 99 percent of the actual formulation. Conditioning agents, whether they come from the sea, land, or air or are synthetically derived, all perform beautifully. The hair can't tell the difference; it's dead. What counts is how the product coats the hair, how it reflects shine, and whether it can build up on the hair—not where it came from.

For more information on Focus 21, call (800) 832-2887 or visit its Web site at www.focus21.com.

☺ **Hair Toys Shampoo** *($3.82 for 8 ounces)* contains mostly water, detergent cleansing agents, lather agent, thickeners, conditioning agent, preservatives, and fragrance. This is a good basic shampoo with minimal conditioning agents that would work well for all hair types with no risk of buildup.

☺ **Jojoba Sebum Emulsifier Shampoo** *($2.29 for 8 ounces)* contains mostly water, detergent cleansing agent, conditioning agents, thickeners, plant oil, lather agent, fragrance, and preservatives. This is a good shampoo for dry hair of any thickness.

☹ **Normal to Dry Hair Shampoo, Herbal Enhanced** *($2.69 for 8 ounces)* has sodium lauryl sulfate as the main detergent cleansing agent, which can be too drying for all hair types and scalps.

☺ **Hair Remoisturizing Treatment** *($3.29 for 4 ounces)* contains mostly water, detangling agent, thickeners, water-binding agent, conditioning agents, film former, preservatives, fragrance, and coloring agents. This is a good conditioner for dry hair that is normal to fine or thin in thickness.

☺ **Hair Toys Moisturizing Spray** *($5.62 for 8 ounces)* is a good leave-in conditioner for dry, damaged, or coarse hair. It contains mostly water, detangling agent, silicone, water-binding agents, preservatives, slip agents, and fragrance.

☺ **Reconditioning Formula** *($3.29 for 8 ounces)* contains mostly water, conditioning agents, detangling agent, thickeners, water-binding agents, plant oil, preservatives, fragrance, and coloring agents. This is a very good conditioner for dry, damaged, and coarse hair.

☺ **$$$ Liposheen Hair Restorer** *($16.79 for 4 ounces)* is a standard silicone serum with silicone and a little alcohol. It works great to add a silky-soft feel and shine to hair but the price is uncalled-for—there are far less expensive versions that have the exact same formulation, if not better.

☺ **Hair Toys Gel** *($3.82 for 8 ounces)* contains mostly water, detangling agent/ film former, thickeners, conditioning agents, preservatives, and fragrance. This is a good, standard, light-hold gel with minimal to no stiff or sticky feeling.

☺ **Panasea Gel** *($10.90 for 4 ounces)* can't repair one hair on your head, so ignore the misleading claims on the label (or any product label that makes this kind of claim). This gel has a medium hold with a somewhat sticky feel. It contains mostly water, thickeners, conditioning agents, menthol, fragrance, and coloring agents. The tiny amount of menthol is probably not a problem, but it's best to keep this gel off the scalp just in case.

☺ **Hair Candy Designing Mousse, Extra Body** *($3.99 for 8 ounces)* is a standard mousse with a cute name. It contains mostly water, alcohol, film formers, propellant, slip agents, silicone, and fragrance. It has light to medium hold with a slight sticky feel. This doesn't add any more body than any other mousse does.

☺ **Thikk Protective Hair Thickener** *($3.46 for 4 ounces)* includes a sunscreen ingredient, although that can't protect hair, but otherwise this is a good standard gel that contains mostly water, conditioning agents, detangling agent, preservatives, fragrance, and coloring agents. It would be good for normal to slightly dry hair that is normal to fine or thin—just don't count on hair becoming all that "thikk." It has minimal to no stiff or sticky feel. It can add a slight feel of thickness to hair, but no more than any other light-hold gel.

☺ **Art Form Sculpting Spray (Non-Aerosol)** *($3.99 for 8 ounces)* contains mostly alcohol, water, film formers, slip agents, and fragrance. This is a standard styling spray with light hold and minimal to no stiff or sticky feel. It can help when styling hair.

☺ **Changes Flexible Hold Hair Spray (Non-Aerosol)** *($3.49 for 12 ounces)* is a standard hairspray that has light to medium hold and minimal to no stiff or sticky feel. It contains mostly alcohol, water, film formers, slip agents, and fragrance.

☺ **Changes Medium to Firm Hold Hair Spray (Non-Aerosol)** *($3.19 for 8 ounces)* is almost identical to the Sculpting Spray above and the same comments apply.

☺ **Illusions Design and Finishing Hair Spray, Medium Hold (Aerosol)** *($4.51 for 10 ounces)* is a good standard hairspray with light to medium hold and minimal to no stiff feel, and it can easily be brushed through. It contains mostly alcohol, propellant, water, film formers, slip agents, silicone, and fragrance.

☹ **Oxy Lock** *($17.64 for 16 ounces)* contains mostly water, thickener, detangling agent, conditioning agent, and preservatives. This overpriced leave-in conditioner is an option for minimally dry hair, but the price could make your hair stiff!

Enviro-Tek by Focus 21

Enviro-Tek Anti-Bacterial is supposed to kill germs, suppress dandruff, and leave hair strong, as well as being "a must for highly polluted environments." Yet the claims about antioxidants and preventing dandruff just don't hold up in the wash. Even if the antioxidants used here did something (and they are just standard vitamins that show up in hundreds of products), they would be rinsed down the drain before they had a chance to have an effect. But don't worry, the entire marketing campaign about antioxidants is all theory, with no proof that they have any valid benefit for skin or scalp. The antibacterial agent in the shampoo is triclosan, which can have some effect against bacteria—but dandruff isn't a bacteria issue, it's a yeast issue, and triclosan isn't known to be effective against yeast.

☺ **Enviro-Tek Antioxidant Shampoo** *($5.58 for 12 ounces)* is just a standard shampoo that contains mostly water, detergent cleansing agent, lather agent, slip agent, plant extracts, conditioning agent, vitamins, preservatives, and fragrance. The plant extracts in here can be irritating for the scalp and the triclosan won't affect dandruff. The antioxidants are nice but they won't do anything noticeable for the scalp or hair; even if they could, in a shampoo they would just be washed away.

☺ **Enviro-Tek Antioxidant Moisturizing Spray** *($5.51 for 12 ounces)* contains mostly water, detangling agent, silicone, slip agents, conditioning agents, preservatives, vitamins, and fragrance. This is a good but exceptionally lightweight leave-in conditioner for normal to slightly dry hair of any thickness. The triclosan in here won't affect dandruff and the antioxidants are nice but won't do anything noticeable for the scalp or hair.

☺ **Enviro-Tek Antioxidant Reconstructor Conditioner** *($6.04 for 12 ounces)* contains mostly water, detangling agent, slip agents, thickeners, plant oil, conditioning agents, preservatives, vitamins, and fragrance. This is a good conditioner for normal to dry hair of any thickness. The triclosan in here won't affect dandruff and the antioxidants are nice but won't do anything noticeable for the scalp or hair. And that bit about reconstructing hair? It isn't true.

☺ **Enviro-Tek Antioxidant Leave-in Conditioner Spray** *($6.14 for 12 ounces)* contains mostly water, detangling agent, thickeners, plant oil, vitamins, preservatives, and fragrance. This is a good lightweight conditioner for normal to slightly dry hair of any thickness. The triclosan in here won't affect dandruff and the antioxidants are nice but won't do anything noticeable for the scalp or hair.

☹ **Enviro-Tek Antioxidant Spray Gel** *($5.51 for 12 ounces)* is a standard gel with medium hold and a slight sticky-stiff feel. It contains mostly alcohol, film formers, plant extract, silicone, slip agent, fragrance, and vitamins.

☺ **Enviro-Tek Antioxidant Styling Spray** *($6.25 for 12 ounces)* contains mostly water, film formers, silicone, plant extracts, vitamins, slip agents, and fragrance. It's a good, basic, lightweight styling spray with soft hold and minimal to no stiff or sticky feel.

SeaPlasma by Focus 21

☺ **SeaPlasma Shampoo** *($3.99 for 12 ounces)* contains mostly water, detergent cleansing agents, lather agent, conditioning agent, thickeners, preservatives, fragrance, and coloring agents. This is a good basic shampoo for all hair types. The minimal conditioning agent in here won't build up on hair.

☺ **SeaPlasma All Purpose Skin and Hair Moisturizer** *($6.29 for 16 ounces)* contains mostly water, detangling agent, silicone, slip agent, water-binding agents, preservative, and fragrance. This is a good, but extremely lightweight, leave-in conditioner for normal to slightly dry hair to help with combing only. There isn't a reason in the world to apply this product to the skin—why would the skin need a detangling agent?

The Reviews F

☺ **SeaPlasma Intensified Hair Booster Plus** *($3.29 for 8 ounces)* contains mostly water, thickeners, detangling agents, water-binding agents, film former, preservatives, fragrance, and coloring agents. This is a good leave-in conditioner that can help make fine or thin, slightly dry hair feel thicker.

☺ **SeaPlasma Designing Gel** *($3.99 for 12 ounces)* contains mostly water, alcohol, film former, water-binding agents, thickener, preservatives, fragrance, and coloring agents. This standard gel has minimal to light hold with minimal to no stiff or sticky feel.

☺ **SeaPlasma Moisture Mousse** *($5.44 for 8 ounces)* isn't a mousse, just a very liquidy gel that has a light hold with a slight sticky feel, though it brushes through easily. It contains mostly water, film formers, silicone, slip agents, and preservatives.

Splash by Focus 21

☹ **Splash Shampoo** *($3.99 for 12 ounces)* contains sodium lauryl sulfate as the main detergent cleansing agent, which is drying for both the scalp and hair. It also contains ammonium xylene sulfate, which can be extremely drying for hair and scalp as well.

☺ **Splash Detangler** *($5.99 for 12 ounces)* contains mostly water, detangling agents, slip agents, plant extracts, preservatives, and fragrance. This is a good but exceptionally light detangling leave-in conditioner for normal hair that needs help with comb-through after washing.

☺ **Splash Leave-in Conditioner Spray** *($3.99 for 12 ounces)* is almost identical to the one above only with plant oil. That makes it better for someone with normal to dry hair of any thickness.

☺ **Splash Sculpting Gel Extra Firm** *($8.39 for 16 ounces)* contains mostly water, alcohol, film former, thickeners, and fragrance. This simple, standard gel works well for medium hold with a slight sticky feel, though it does brush through easily.

☺ **Splash Sculpting Gel Firm Alcohol Free** *($2.97 for 12 ounces)* contains mostly water, film former, thickeners, preservatives, and fragrance. It's almost identical to the version above, only without alcohol, and the basic performance is the same.

☺ **Fashion Splash Design and Finishing Hair Spray, Extra Firm Hold (Aerosol)** *($6.99 for 9.5 ounces)* is a standard aerosol hairspray with medium hold that has a slight stiff feel, though it easily brushes through. It contains mostly water, propellant, film formers, silicones, preservatives, conditioning agent, and fragrance.

☺ **Splash Finishing Spray** *($2.97 for 12 ounces)* is almost identical to the aerosol version above, only this one is in nonaerosol form. The hold and feel are the same.

☺ **Splash Flexible Hold Spray** *($2.97 for 12 ounces)* is almost identical to the one above, with the same hold and feel.

BIO2 Tanicals by Focus 21

☹ **Luxurious Mango Shampoo** *($7.95for 12 ounces)* uses ammonium xylene sulfate as its detergent cleansing agent, which can be drying for the hair and drying and irritating for the scalp.

☺ **Moistrex Moisturizing Hair Conditioner** *($8.50for 12 ounces)* is an exceptionally standard conditioner for normal to slightly dry hair that is normal to fine or thin. It contains mostly water, detangling agent, thickeners, plant extracts, preservatives, and fragrance.

☺ **Hair & Skin Leave On Moisturizing Mist, Mango Tahitian** *($5.71 for 12 ounces)* is a leave-in conditioner that should be used only on hair and not skin. It is best for normal hair to help with combing, and that's about it; it's a very lightweight, almost do-nothing conditioner. It contains mostly water, detangling agent, silicone, slip agents, plant extracts, preservatives, and fragrance.

☺ **Spray Gel Plus Shine, Mango** *($9.20 for 12 ounces)* is a standard gel that contains mostly water, film formers, plant extracts, silicone, and fragrance. It has a light hold and minimal to no stiff or sticky feel and brushes through easily.

☺ **Thermal Shine Super Shine Texturizing Volumizing Sculpting Lotion** *($10 for 12 ounces)* contains mostly water, thickeners, film formers, silicone, conditioning agents, slip agents, fragrance, preservatives, and plant extracts. This is a styling liquid that should come in a spray container; as it is, this liquid spills through your fingers before you can get it on your hair. It has light to medium hold and a slight sticky, stiff feel.

☺ **Flash Freeze Plus Design and Finishing Hair Spray, Extra Firm Hold (Aerosol)** *($10.90 for 10 ounces)* contains mostly alcohol, propellant, film formers, silicones, preservatives, and fragrance. This is a standard, medium- to firm-hold aerosol hairspray that has a slight stiff feel but lets you easily brush through hair.

☺ **Flash Freeze Plus Shine Mango Design and Finishing Hair Spray, Extra Firm Hold (Non-Aerosol)** *($9.70 for 12 ounces)* is a very simple hairspray, with alcohol, film former, fragrance, and plant extracts. It works much like the one above.

Folligen
(also see Tricomin)

Folligen is sold by Skin Biology Incorporated as a product for regrowing hair. As is true for many non-FDA-approved products for hair regrowth, this one has quite a history. Folligen is about copper peptides and a Dr. Loren Pickart, who graduated with a degree in biochemistry from the University of California at San Francisco in 1973. At the time, Pickart's thesis was on copper peptides and how they helped skin healing. How does this relate to hair growth? Pickart continued his work on copper peptides with his new company, ProCyte, when some of the peptides he was working on stimulated hair growth in the mice that were being used for research in skin healing.

Does Pickart have rigorous studies proving copper peptides work for hair re-growth? By his own admission, the answer is no. All the information on hair regrowth with copper peptides is anecdotal. Yet ProCyte decided to start marketing Tricomin anyway.

Is there science behind any of this? The way the theory goes, testosterone can play a major part in hair loss by shrinking the blood supply to the hair follicle and making it inactive. However there are lots of men with low levels of testosterone who have full heads of thick hair. These men must have an abnormally thriving blood supply to the hair follicle! The thinking about copper peptides is that they stimulate the growth of the blood supply, which reinvigorates the hair follicle. The follicle then ignores any alternative message from the reduced testosterone.

If you want to believe that's science, which is what lots of hair-regrowth compa-nies would like you to believe, then this line is an option. But where does Folligen come into play? Folligen was later developed and is being sold by Pickart after he left ProCyte and Tricomin behind and started a new company called Skin Biology.

Do Tricomin and Folligen work the same? Not surprisingly, Pickart feels Folligen is better because, as the inventor of both, he says the form of copper peptides in Folligen is the next generation. "The primary difference between the two is that Tricomin is a single peptide that holds copper, Folligen uses a mixture of peptides that will bind the copper. Tricomin uses alanine/histidine/lysine polypeptide copper HCl and Folligen uses hydrolyzed soy protein and copper sulfate." Is that a difference your hair follicles will notice? There is no way to know because there are no studies showing the way, just lots of products for sale promising to grow hair on your head.

For more information about Folligen, call Skin Biology at (800) 405-1912 or visit its Web sites at www.skinbio.com or www.folligen.com.

The following products are available: **Folligen Lotion** *($17.95 for 2 ounces)*; **Folligen Cream** *($17.95 for 2 ounces)*; and **Folligen Solution Therapy Spray** *($31.95 for 8 ounces)*.

Framesi Biogenol

Framesi is a line of hair-care products carefully aimed at women who color their hair, perhaps in response to the fact that, as Framesi sees it, "by the year 2000, sev-enty-five percent or more clients will be using color. The market is turning to color." I agree, the market is turning to color, but the question remains, Do these products provide any extra benefit for chemically treated hair? Framesi feels that its Biogenol Color Care System is for "Color clients [who] require shampoos, conditioners and styling products formulated to the highest professional performance level, and with special ingredients to enhance, and not diminish, the beauty of their color." That sounds great, but not only are the ingredients in these products quite standard, some of them are also problematic; for example, some of the shampoos contain sodium lauryl sulfate, a fairly drying detergent cleansing agent. Most everything else is just standard shampoos, conditioners, and styling products. Some of the products do contain a good antioxidant—superoxide dismutase—but it doesn't hold up well under washing and rinsing, so it's useless in shampoos and conditioners. It can be interesting in leave-on products (for the scalp it's a good moisturizing agent), but there is no information about the effectiveness of any antioxidants on the hair, and that's about it.

For more information on Framesi Biogenol, call (416) 252-9591, (800) 245-6323, or visit itsWeb site at www.styl.com.

☺ **Clarifying Shampoo** *($5.99 for 8 ounces)* contains mostly water, detergent cleansing agents, lather agent, conditioning agent, preservatives, and fragrance. This is a very good, standard shampoo with an insignificant amount of conditioning agents, and that makes it great for all hair types.

☹ **Nourishing Shampoo** *($5.95 for 8 ounces)* contains TEA-lauryl sulfate as the main detergent cleansing agent, which is drying for both the scalp and hair.

☹ **Replenishing Shampoo** *($5.95 for 8 ounces)* contains TEA-lauryl sulfate as the main detergent cleansing agent, which is drying for both the scalp and hair.

☺ **Ultra Body Shampoo** *($5.95 for 8 ounces)* contains mostly water, detergent cleansing agents, film former, lather agent, thickeners, silicone, conditioning agents, antioxidant, more silicone, more conditioning agents, more thickeners, fragrance, and preservatives. This is a good shampoo for dry hair that is normal to fine or thin, though it can cause buildup in a few washings.

☺ **Bathe Moisturizing Shampoo** *($3.96 for 4 ounces)* contains mostly water, detergent cleansing agents, lather agent, antioxidant, detangling agents, film former, conditioning agents, fragrance, and preservatives. This is a good shampoo for dry hair of any thickness, although the film former can cause buildup.

☺ **Moisture Rinse** *($6.95 for 8 ounces)* contains mostly water, thickener, detangling agents, film former, more thickeners, antioxidant, conditioning agents, silicone, preservatives, and fragrance. This is a good lightweight conditioner for normal to dry hair that is normal to fine or thin.

☺ **Reconditioner for Dry, Damaged Hair** *($8.50 for 5 ounces)* contains mostly water, thickener, detangling agents, more thickeners, antioxidant, conditioning agents, preservatives, fragrance, and coloring agents. This is a good lightweight conditioner for normal to dry hair regardless of hair thickness.

☺ **Ultra Deep Conditioner** *($16.96 for 8 ounces)* contains mostly water, thickeners, detangling agents, antioxidant, conditioning agents, slip agent, silicone, fragrance, and preservatives. This isn't all that deep of a conditioner but it is a good lightweight conditioner for normal to dry hair of any thickness.

☹ **Leave-in Conditioner** *($9.95 for 10 ounces)* contains mostly water, thickener, detangling agents, film former, antioxidant, conditioning agents, silicone, castor oil, preservatives, and fragrance. This can have a sticky, stiff feel but can work for someone with normal to fine or thin hair to give a feel of thickness.

☺ **Biogenol Color Care System Ultra-Deep Masque Deep Conditioner** *($11.95 for 4 ounces)* is an emollient conditioner for dry hair that is coarse or thick. It contains mostly water, thickeners, detangling agents, conditioning agents, slip agent, silicone, fragrance, and preservatives.

☺ **$$$ Shine In Prep-It Style Start** *($19.98 for 4 ounces)* contains mostly water, slip agent, film formers, conditioning agents, silicone, antioxidant, fragrance, and preservatives. This is just a liquidy gel with light hold and a slight sticky feel. It is supposed to be a "prep" to allow other styling products to work better. If the other styling products can't work well, there is something wrong with them; it shouldn't require another product. By itself, this styling product is just fine.

☺ **Shine In Polishing Spray** *($9.50 for 2 ounces)* contains mostly alcohol, slip agents, silicone, castor oil, conditioning agents, antioxidant, and fragrance. It is basically a silicone spray that can add shine and a silky feel to hair, and this one can add a teeny amount of hold too.

☺ **Shine In Polishing Stick** *($16 for 2.5 ounces)* is a gel version of the Polishing Cream above and the same basic comments apply.

☺ **Shine In Polishing Cream** *($16 for 5 ounces)* is just an overpriced greasy styling cream that would work well to smooth frizzies and stubborn curls. It can have a greasy feel so use it sparingly. It contains mostly water, thickeners, castor oils, more thickeners, conditioning agents, antioxidant, fragrance, and preservatives. It can leave a sticky feel behind on the hair. There are similar products for far less.

☺ **Biogenol Color Care System Spray Gel Firm Hold** *($8.99 for 10 ounces)* is a spray gel that has light to medium hold and a slight stiff, sticky feel. It contains mostly water, film formers, antioxidant, conditioning agents, silicone, slip agents, fragrance, and preservatives.

☺ **Biogenol Color Care System Bodifying Foam Strong Hold** *($9.96 for 9 ounces)* is a standard mousse with medium hold and a slight sticky, stiff feel. It contains mostly water, film formers, propellant, antioxidant, conditioning agents, slip agents, fragrance, and preservatives.

☺ **Biogenol Color Care System Forming Glaze Strong Hold** *($6.49 for 8 ounces)* contains mostly water, detangling agents/film formers, antioxidant, thickeners, conditioning agents, slip agents, fragrance, and preservatives. This is a light- to medium-hold gel with minimal stiff or sticky feel.

☺ **Biogenol Color Care System Bodifying Spray** *($8.96 for 10 ounces)* is a standard light-hold styling spray with minimal to no stiff or sticky feel. It contains mostly water, detangling agents/film formers, conditioning agents, antioxidants, silicone, slip agents, preservatives, and fragrance.

☺ **Biogenol Color Care System Design Spray Strong Hold (Aerosol)** *($9.90 for 10 ounces)* is a standard but good aerosol hairspray with medium hold and a somewhat stiff feel that can be brushed through easily. It contains mostly alcohol, water, film formers, conditioning agents, silicone, and fragrance.

☺ **Biogenol Color Care System Finishing Spray Firm Hold (Non-Aerosol)** *($8.90 for 10 ounces)* is almost identical to the aerosol version above and the same comments apply.

☺ **Shine In Take Hold (Aerosol)** *($8.49 for 10 ounces)* is almost identical to the Design Spray Aerosol version above and the same comments apply.

☺ **Biogenol Color Care System One Tip Slip Ends Repair and Shiner** *($9.90 for 2 ounces)* contains mostly water, alcohol, propellant, film formers, silicones, conditioning agents, fragrance, and preservatives. This is an aerosol silicone spray with some minimal hold. It works well to smooth frizzies and help styling, along with delivering the benefits of silicone and adding a silky feel and shine to hair, but it can't repair anything.

☺ **Biogenol Brash Hard Gel** *($5.99 for 5 ounces)* contains mostly water, film formers, thickener, antioxidant, silicone, conditioning agents, more film former, castor oil, fragrance, and preservatives. This isn't all that hard; rather, it is a good medium-hold gel with a slight stiff, sticky feel that easily brushes through.

☺ **Biogenol Definition Conditioning Cream Gel** *($15.99 for 8 ounces)* contains mostly water, film formers, thickeners, antioxidant, conditioning agents, fragrance, and preservatives. It isn't a cream but a rather standard gel with medium hold and a somewhat stiff, sticky feel.

☺ **Biogenol Dew Humectant Pomade** *($12.99 for 2 ounces)* contains mostly water, castor oil, thickeners, more castor oil, detangling agents, silicone, fragrance, and preservatives. It is a gel-like pomade that can be fairly heavy and greasy, so use sparingly. It can definitely control coarse, frizzy hair and stubborn curls. It has no film formers so there is minimal hold but also no stiff feel on hair.

☺ **Biogenol Pro-Form Thermal Setting Lotion** *($8.99 for 10 ounces)* contains mostly water, alcohol, film former, conditioning agents, silicone, antioxidant, fragrance, and preservatives. There is nothing special about this for setting purposes, but it is a good lightweight-hold styling spray for all hair types.

☺ **Biogenol Hold 10 Extra Strong Hold** *($9.99 for 10 ounces)* is a standard aerosol hairspray that contains mostly alcohol, propellant, film formers, slip agents, and fragrance. It has a medium hold with a slight stiff, sticky feel.

☺ **Biogenol Myste Finishing Spray** *($8.99 for 10 ounces)* is similar to the Hold 10 version above, only in nonaerosol form.

☺ **Biogenol Snapp Curl Rejuvenator** *($8.99 for 10 ounces)* contains mostly water, film formers, conditioning agents, silicones, detangling agents, thickener, and preservatives. It can be either a leave-in conditioner or a styling spray; either way it has a soft hold and no stiff or sticky feel. It can help with any styling need for most all hair types, it all depends on the styling tools used.

☺ **Biogenol Stop-Frizz Anti-Humectant** *($12.99 for 2 ounces)* is a standard no hold styling cream that contains mostly water, thickeners, silicones, detangling agent, antioxidant, fragrance, and preservatives. This is a good styling cream for smoothing stubborn frizzies and straightening curls, with no stiff or sticky feel. However, it can feel heavy and greasy, so use sparingly.

Freeman

For all the discussion of naturalness and the very fruity-herbal-looking packaging the Freeman products are dressed up in, it turns out that this line is overflowing with synthetic ingredients and is owned by the very unnatural-sounding Dial Corporation. That isn't good or bad, just an interesting marketing perspective. There are several lines under the Freeman header, including Aromatherapy, Beautiful Hair, Botanicals, Papaya Provita/Silk, Salon Textures, Big Thick Hair, Super Straight Hair, Real Shiny Hair, and, if you can take one more, Sparkling Silver Hair. Rather than going into each marketing claim, I'll let the individual product reviews stand as description enough. Just keep in mind that fragrance and plants can't affect the hair, though they can negatively impact the scalp by irritation.

For more information on Freeman, call (800) FREEMAN, or visit its Web site at www.freemancosmetics.com.

Aromatherapy by Freeman

☺ **Aromatherapy Calming 2-in-1 Shampoo Cleansing Plus Conditioning for Normal to Dry Hair** *($4.11 for 16 ounces)* contains mostly water, detergent cleansing agent, lather agent, silicone, thickeners, fragrance, conditioning agent, plant extracts, detangling agent, preservatives, and coloring agents. This is a good standard shampoo with silicone that can work for normal to dry hair but not coarse or thick hair. It can also build up and make hair look flat, a risk with all two-in-one products.

☺ **Aromatherapy Calming Shampoo for Normal to Dry Hair** *($4.11 for 16 ounces)* contains mostly water, detergent cleansing agents, lather agents, fragrance, conditioning agent, film former, plant extracts, preservatives, and coloring agents. This is an exceptionally ordinary shampoo with almost nonexistent conditioning agents. That makes it good for most hair types, though the small amount of film former can be better for thin or fine hair.

☺ **Aromatherapy Energizing 2-in-1 Shampoo** *($4.11 for 16 ounces)* contains mostly water, detergent cleansing agent, lather agent, silicone, thickeners, plant extracts, conditioning agents, detangling agent, preservatives, fragrance, and coloring agents. This is a good standard shampoo with silicone that can work for normal to dry hair but not coarse or thick hair. The film former makes it better for fine or thin hair though it can also build up and make hair look flat.

☺ **Aromatherapy Energizing Shampoo** *($4.11 for 16 ounces)* contains mostly water, detergent cleansing agent, lather agent, thickeners, plant extracts, conditioning agents, detangling agent/film former, castor oil, preservatives, and coloring agents. It's a standard shampoo that can work for normal to dry hair but not coarse or thick hair. The film former and castor oil can make fine or thin hair feel thicker, though they can also build up and make hair look flat.

☺ **Aromatherapy Calming Conditioner for Normal to Dry Hair** *($4.11 for 16 ounces)* contains mostly water, thickener, detangling agents, fragrance, plant extracts, conditioning agents, silicone, and preservatives. The tiny amount of conditioning agents in here make it inappropriate for dry hair, though it can work well for normal to slightly dry hair of most any thickness.

☺ **Aromatherapy Energizing Conditioner for Normal to Dry Hair** *($4.11 for 16 ounces)* is almost identical to the Calming version above and the same comments apply.

Beautiful Hair by Freeman

☹ **Beautiful Hair Botanicals Apple, Pear & Peach Amazing Body Volumizing Shampoo** *($3.49 for 16 ounces)* contains balsam, which can dry out hair, as well as clove, which can be irritating to the scalp. It also contains some quantity of sodium lauryl sulfate, which can also be drying, and that's too many potential problems for one product.

☹ **Beautiful Hair Citrus Pure Deep Shine Revitalizing Shampoo** *($2.85 for 16 ounces)* is similar to the one above, only with lemon and lime, and they can be problems for the scalp too.

☺ **Beautiful Hair Hawaiian Ginger Supremely Silk Texturizing Shampoo** *($2.88 for 16 ounces)* doesn't contain sodium lauryl sulfate, but it does contain several plant extracts that could be irritating to the scalp. Other than that, it could be a good shampoo for dry hair of any thickness; it contains mostly water, detergent cleansing agent, lather agent, plant extracts, slip agent, plant oil, detangling agent, thickeners, preservatives, fragrance, and coloring agents.

☺ **Beautiful Hair Wild Cherry Extra Humectant Moisturizing Shampoo** *($2.88 for 16 ounces)* contains mostly water, detergent cleansing agents, lather agent, plant oil, conditioning agents, film former, slip agent, preservatives, fragrance, and coloring agents. There is sodium lauryl sulfate in this product, but probably not enough to be a problem. It can be a good shampoo for dry hair.

☺ **Beautiful Hair Hawaiian Ginger Supremely Silk Texturizing Conditioner** *($3.49 for 16 ounces)* contains mostly water, detangling agents, plant extracts, plant oil, conditioning agents, slip agent, preservatives, and fragrance. It's a good standard conditioner for normal to dry hair that isn't coarse or thick.

☺ **Beautiful Hair Kiwi Fruit Ultra Therapy Treatment Conditioner** *($2.88 for 16 ounces)* contains mostly water, thickeners, detangling agents, plant extracts, conditioning agent, plant oil, preservatives, fragrance, and coloring agents. This isn't "ultra" in the least, though it is a good lightweight conditioner for normal to slightly dry hair of any thickness to help with combing.

☺ **Beautiful Hair Botanicals Kiwi Fruit No Frizz Styling Gel Ultimate Hold** *($3.49 for 8.5 ounces)* contains mostly water, alcohol, film formers, plant extract, conditioning agent, slip agents, thickener, fragrance, and coloring agents. This is a standard spray gel with light hold and minimal to no stiff or sticky feel that can be brushed through easily.

☺ **Beautiful Hair Botanicals Wild Cherry Shaping Shine Gel** *($2.99 for 8.5 ounces)* is similar to the No Frizz version above, only with medium hold.

☺ **Beautiful Hair Botanicals Hawaiian Ginger Conditioning Freeze Spritzer Maximum Hold** *($3.49 for 8.5 ounces)* is a standard hairspray that contains mostly alcohol, water, film former, conditioning agent, plant extract, silicone, fragrance, and coloring agent. This is a good light- to medium-hold hairspray with minimal stiff or sticky feel.

☺ **Beautiful Hair Botanicals Apple, Pear, and Peach Shaping Curl Control** *($2.48 for 8.5 ounces)* contains mostly water, film former, slip agent, silicone, preservatives, fragrance, and coloring agents. It is a soft- to light-hold styling spray with minimal to no stiff or sticky feel. It can help form any style, whether curly or straight.

Botanicals by Freeman

☹ **Apple Nectar Shampoo for Fine or Thin Hair** *($3.49 for 16 ounces)* contains sodium lauryl sulfate as one of the main detergent cleansing agents, which is drying for both the scalp and hair.

☹ **Citrus Clarifying Shampoo** *($2.85 for 16 ounces)* contains sodium lauryl sulfate as one of the main detergent cleansing agents, which is drying for both the scalp and hair.

☺ **Hawaiian Ginger Shampoo Ultra Body and Shine** *($3.49 for 16 ounces)* contains mostly water, detergent cleansing agent, lather agent, detangling agent, plant oil, preservatives, fragrance, and coloring agents. This is a good shampoo for normal to slightly dry hair of any thickness.

☺ **Kiwi Fruit Therapy Shampoo for Dry or Damaged Hair** *($3.49 for 16 ounces)* contains mostly water, detergent cleansing agent, lather agent, conditioning agent, plant extracts, film former, slip agent, preservatives, fragrance, and coloring agents. This is a good shampoo for normal to slightly dry hair that is fine or thin. The film former can add a feel of thickness though it can feel stiff on dry, coarse hair.

☹ **Apple Nectar Conditioner Thickening Formula** *($3.49 for 16 ounces)* contains balsam, which can build up on hair and feel stiff. Other than that, it is a very standard conditioner for normal to slightly dry hair that is normal to fine or thin in thickness. It contains mostly water, thickeners, detangling agent, plant extracts, conditioning agents, preservatives, and fragrance.

☺ **Cherry Humectant Conditioner for Dry or Damaged Hair** *($3.49 for 16 ounces)* contains mostly water, thickeners, detangling agent, conditioning agent, plant extracts, plant oil, preservatives, and fragrance. This is a good conditioner for dry, coarse, or damaged hair of any thickness.

☺ **Hair Rescue Conditioner** *($3.49 for 8 ounces)* contains mostly water, thickeners, castor oil, detangling agent, conditioning agent, plant extracts, plant oil, preservatives, fragrance, and coloring agents. This is a good conditioner for dry, coarse hair to gain control, though it can also have a slight sticky, stiff feel.

☺ **Hawaiian Mango Conditioner for Normal Hair** *($2.99 for 16 ounces)* contains mostly water, thickeners, slip agent, detangling agent, plant extracts, conditioning agents, preservatives, fragrance, and coloring agents. It is a good lightweight conditioner for normal to slightly dry hair of any thickness but coarse.

☺ **Instant Infusion Treatment, Sunflower Oil, Gardenia and Pennyroyal** *($3.49 for 16 ounces)* contains mostly water, slip agent, detangling agents, film former, silicones, conditioning agents, plant oil, plant extracts, preservatives, and fragrance. This is a very good leave-in conditioner for dry, damaged hair of any thickness.

☺ **Shaping Styling Gel Mega Hold Limeflower, Pineapple and Nettle** *($2.85 for 8.5 ounces)* contains mostly water, alcohol, film formers, plant extracts, conditioning agent, slip agent, thickener, fragrance, and coloring agents. This standard gel has medium hold with a somewhat sticky feel, though it can brush through.

☺ **Shaping Styling Gel Mega Hold Factor 30** *($2.85 for 8.5 ounces)* is similar to the one above only with medium to firm hold.

☺ **Freeze Spritzer Mega Hold, Prescription for Maximum Hold, Honeysuckle, Marigold and Wild Chamomile** *($2.48 for 8 ounces)* is a standard hairspray with light to medium hold and minimal stiff or sticky feel that can easily be brushed through. It contains mostly water, alcohol, water, film former, plant extracts, silicone, conditioning agent, and fragrance.

☺ **Peach Kernel, Butter Rose and Kola Nut Shaping Curl Control** *($2.48 for 8.5 ounces)* contains mostly water, film former, slip agent, silicone, conditioning agent, plant extracts, preservatives, fragrance, and coloring agents. This is a standard styling spray that can provide medium hold for any style, not just holding curls, and it has a slight sticky, stiff feel.

☺ **Split-End Mender** *($1.99 for 5 ounces)* won't mends end of any kind, but it is a good leave-in conditioner for dry, damaged, and thick, coarse hair. It contains mostly water, thickener, detangling agent, slip agent, conditioning agents, emollient, plant extracts, mineral oil, and preservatives.

☺ **Hair Thickening Serum** *($3.99 for 4 ounces)* is a lightweight styling serum that has minimal hold but can add some control and a feel of thickness to hair with minimal to no stiff or sticky feel. It contains mostly water, glycerin, detangling agent/film former, slip agents, plant extracts, conditioning agents, thickeners, castor oil, preservatives, and fragrance.

☺ **Botanical Hair Thickening Spritz** *($3.99 for 6 ounces)* is a light- to medium-hold styling spray/gel that has a slight stiff, sticky feel. It can help when styling hair and can add a feel of thickness—but this is more about styling hair than thickening it. It contains mostly water, glycerin, detangling agent/film former, slip agents, plant extracts, conditioning agents, thickeners, castor oil, preservatives, and fragrance.

Papaya Provita by Freeman

☺ **Papaya Provita Miracle Shampoo for Ultra Body** *($2.99 for 16 ounces)* contains mostly water, detergent cleansing agent, lather agent, conditioning agent, plant extracts, slip agents, plant oil, film former, preservatives, fragrance, and coloring agents. This is a good shampoo for dry hair that is fine or thin. The film former can add a feel of thickness, though it can feel stiff on dry, coarse hair.

☹ **Papaya Provita Moist Shampoo for Colored or Permed Hair** *($1.99 for 16 ounces)* has sodium C14-16 olefin sulfonate as the main detergent cleansing agent, which makes it too drying for all hair types, and especially for chemically treated hair.

☺ **Papaya Provita Shampoo plus Conditioner in One for Normal to Dry Hair** *($1.99 for 16 ounces)* is a standard, silicone-based two-in-one shampoo. It would work as well as any for normal to dry hair but it can easily cause buildup with repeated use.

☺ **Papaya Silk Miracle Shampoo with Ginseng, Extra Nourishing Formula for Normal Hair** *($1.99 for 16 ounces)* contains mostly water, detergent cleansing agent, lather agents, plant extracts, conditioning agents, thickeners, film former, slip agent, preservatives, coloring agents, and fragrance. This is a good shampoo for someone with dry hair that is normal to fine or thin in thickness. The film former can eventually cause buildup.

☺ **Papaya Silk 1-Minute Miracle Treatment Conditioner with Ginseng, Ultra Body** *($2.39 for 16 ounces)* contains mostly water, thickener, detangling agents, plant extracts, conditioning agent, preservatives, and fragrance. This is a lightweight conditioner that is best used as a detangler for normal to slightly dry hair of any thickness.

☺ **Papaya Provita Styling Gel Hold Factor 30** *($3.39 for 13.5 ounces)* contains mostly water, film formers, slip agent, conditioning agents, thickeners, preservatives, fragrance, and coloring agents. This is a good medium-hold styling gel with a somewhat sticky feel, though it can be brushed through.

☹ **Papaya Silk Miracle Hold Anti-Frizz Sculpting Gel Mega Hold Factor 25** *($2.85 for 13.5 ounces)* is almost identical to the Hold Factor 30 above and the same comments apply.

☺ **Papaya Silk Miracle Control Ultra Spritzer with Ginseng Maximum Hold & Ultimate Control** *($1.99 for 10.1 ounces)* contains mostly alcohol, water, film former, plant extracts, conditioning agent, silicone, slip agent, and fragrance. There is nothing miraculous about this, it's simply a standard hairspray with light to medium hold and a slight stiff or sticky feel.

☺ **Papaya Provita Sculpting Spritzer for Touchable Hold** *($1.99 for 10.1 ounces)* is almost identical to the Maximum Hold above and the same comments apply.

☺ **Papaya Silk Miracle Anti-Frizz Curling Spray with Ginseng** *($1.99 for 10.1 ounces)* is a soft- to light-hold styling spray with minimal to no stiff or sticky feel. It can help lightlyform any style, whether curly or straight.

Salon Textures by Freeman

☹ **Salon Textures Moisturizing Aire Shampoo** *($3.99 for 16 ounces)* contains orange, lemon, mandarin, grapefruit, and lime extracts, which can be scalp irritants.

☺ **Salon Textures Volumizing Aire Shampoo** *($4.99 for 16.9 ounces)* contains mostly water, detergent cleansing agent, lather agent, slip agent, thickener, conditioning agent, plant oil, plant extracts, preservatives, fragrance, and coloring agents. There is nothing about this that will make hair thick, but it is a good shampoo for dry and coarse hair.

☺ **Salon Textures Daily Aire Conditioner** *($3.99 for 7 ounces)* contains mostly water, thickener, detangling agent, conditioning agents, silicone, preservatives, fragrance, and coloring agents. It is a good conditioner for dry, damaged, and thick or coarse hair.

☺ **Salon Textures Intense Aire Conditioner** *($3.99 for 5.3 ounces)* is similar to the Daily Aire above, only without silicone, and that makes it better for slightly dry hair of any thickness.

☺ **Salon Textures Leave-in Aire Conditioner** *($3.99 for 5.3 ounces)* contains mostly water, slip agent, thickeners, film formers, conditioning agent, detangling agent, plant oils, silicone, preservatives, fragrance, and coloring agents. This is a very good leave-in conditioner for dry hair that is fine, or for thin hair to make it feel fuller. The film former can cause buildup.

☺ **Salon Textures Volumizing Aire Mousse** *($4.99 for 8 ounces)* is a standard mousse that contains mostly water, film former, alcohol, propellant, conditioning agents, silicone, detangling agent, and fragrance. It has a light to medium hold with minimal stiff or sticky feel.

☺ **Salon Textures Easy Hold Aire Spritzer** *($4.99 for 8 ounces)* contains mostly alcohol, water, film former, conditioning agents, plant extracts, slip agents, silicone, fragrance, and coloring agents. This hairspray gives a medium to firm hold with a stiff, sticky feel.

☺ **Salon Textures Shaping Aire Hair Spray** *($4.99 for 8 ounces)* contains mostly alcohol, film formers, propellant, conditioning agent, slip agents, and fragrance. This aerosol hairspray has a light hold with minimal to no stiff or sticky feel that easily brushes through.

☺ **Salon Textures Zero Alcohol Aire Hair Spray** *($4.99 for 8 ounces)*. Alcohol in styling products isn't a problem for hair, but for some consumers, alcohol-free may be an important factor. This one contains mostly water, film formers, conditioning agents, silicone, preservatives, fragrance, and coloring agents. It has a light hold with minimal stiff or sticky feel, but it isn't as weightless as the label claims.

Big Thick Hair by Freeman

☹ **Big Thick Hair Shampoo** *($3.42 for 12 ounces)* contains sodium lauryl sulfate as one of the main detergent cleansing agents, which is drying for both the scalp and hair. It also contains menthol, which can be irritating to the scalp.

☺ **Big Thick Hair Conditioner** *($3.42 for 12 ounces)* contains mostly water, thickener, detangling agents, conditioning agent, plant extracts, slip agent, preservatives, fragrance, and coloring agents. This won't help make thin hair thick, but it is a good conditioner for normal to slightly dry hair of any thickness. It does contains balm mint and menthol, which can be a problem for the scalp, so keep it away from that area.

☹ **Big Thick Hair Serum Original Formula, Mint & Rosemary** *($3.29 for 4 ounces)* contains mostly water, slip agent, film former, conditioning agents, plant extracts, thickeners, castor oil, preservatives, fragrance, and coloring agents. This can help make normal to dry hair feel thicker, but the film former can cause buildup. It also contains balm mint detangling agents, which can be irritating for the scalp, so keep it away from that area.

☺ **Big Thick Hair Spritzer** *($2.74 for 6 ounces)* is a standard hairspray that contains mostly alcohol, water, film former, conditioning agent, slip agents, silicone, fragrance, and coloring agents. This has a medium hold with minimal stiff or sticky feel and can easily be brushed through. The mint in here can be a problem for the skin so keep this off the scalp.

Super Straight Hair by Freeman

☺ **Super Straight Hair Shampoo, Honeydew & Lilac** *($3.42 for 12 ounces)* doesn't contain anything that will straighten hair. This one is just shampoo with conditioning agents, which is fine for dry hair, and that's about it.

☺ **Super Straight Hair Conditioner, Honeydew & Lilac** *($3.42 for 12 ounces)* is just a lightweight conditioner for normal to slightly dry hair of any thickness. It contains mostly water thickeners, detangling agents, silicone, and a tiny amount of emollients. This is just fine, but it absolutely won't help make anything straight.

☹ **Super Straight Hair Straightening Spray, Honeydew & Lilac** *($3.42 for 10 ounces)* is just fragrant water with a slight sticky feel. It can minimally help in smoothing out curls and frizzies with a tiny bit of hold, and the stickiness does brush through. There are far better products for styling hair straight than this one.

☺ **Super Straight Hair Straightening Balm, Honeydew & Lilac** *($3.69 for 5.3 ounces)* isn't a balm at all, but a creamy lotion that can help straighten stubborn curls and frizzies. It contains mostly water, thickeners, silicones, conditioning agent, film formers, detangling agent, castor oil, preservatives, fragrance, and coloring agents. It can have a heavy, slightly stiff, sticky feel, so use it minimally.

Real Shiny Hair by Freeman

☹ **Real Shiny Hair Shampoo Original Formula, Orange and Lemon** *($3.42 for 12 ounces)* contains sodium lauryl sulfate as the main detergent cleansing agent, which is drying for both the scalp and hair; the orange and lemon are also irritating for the scalp.

☺ **Real Shiny Hair Conditioner, Orange & Lemon** *($3.42 for 12 ounces)* can be a problem for the scalp because of the orange and lemon, but if you keep this on only the hair it shouldn't be a problem. It contains mostly water, thickeners, detangling agents, conditioning agents, preservatives, fragrance, and coloring agents. There is nothing about this product that will add shine, but it is a good conditioner for normal to dry hair that is normal to fine or thin.

☹ **Real Shiny Hair Original Formula Glossing Spray, Orange & Lemon** *($3.29 for 2 ounces)* is a standard silicone spray that can help hair look shiny and feel silky. This one does contain lemon and orange extract, so keep it off the scalp.

☺ **Real Shiny Hair Spritzer** *($2.74 for 6 ounces)* is a standard hairspray with medium hold and a slight stiff, sticky feel, though it does brush through. It contains mostly alcohol, water, film former, plant extracts, conditioning agent, slip agent, silicone, fragrance, and coloring agents.

Sparkling Silver Hair by Freeman

☺ **Sparkling Silver Hair Shampoo for Gray or Blond Hair, Violet & Gardenia** *($3.29 for 12 ounces)* contains mostly water, detergent cleansing agents, lather agents, thickeners, conditioning agent, plant extracts, slip agent, preservatives, fragrance, and coloring agents. There is nothing about this shampoo special for silver hair other than the violet-looking coloring agents. This is a good basic shampoo with insignificant conditioning ingredients that would work for most all hair types.

Frizz-Ease
(see John Frieda)

Fudge

The only information Fudge seems to want you to know about its expertise in hair care is that it is an "Australian thing." I guess the original Aussie hair-care line available at drugstores made the concept of Australian-made hair-care products popular. While there's nothing about the ingredients here that is unique to Australia, these are some good products to consider regardless of their origin. What is absolutely unique about Fudge is its product names. Marketing goes a long way to sell ordinary formulations, but Fudge takes it to a whole new contemporary level. It must only take a name to convince a consumer to waste money on otherwise standard products such as Skrewd Gives Hair That Unexpected Twist Heat Responsive (which is nothing more than a styling gel), or Erekt Cold Turkey for Curly Hair (which is merely a silicone serum).

What Fudge really has to offer is an intriguing range of styling products that can make hair conform to any imaginable shape. Many of its styling products take the meaning of waxing hair literally. For more information on Fudge, call their Australian number (61) 2997 54122 or visit its entertaining but completely uninformative Web site at www.fudge.com.

☺ **The Shampoo for Normal to Dry Hair** *($8 for 10.1 ounces)* contains mostly water, detergent cleansing agent, lather agents, thickeners, conditioning agents, preservatives, and fragrance. As the name implies, this is a good shampoo for normal to dry hair that is fine, thin, or normal in thickness.

☺ **Oomf Shampoo** *($8 for 10.1 ounces)* contains mostly water, detergent cleansing agent, lather agents, thickeners, conditioning agents, silicone, detangling agent/film former, slip agent, preservatives, fragrance, and more preservatives. This would be a good shampoo for normal to dry hair that is normal to fine or thin. The film former can make hair feel thicker but it can cause buildup too.

☺ **$$$ 1 Shot** *($5.50 for 0.88 ounce)* contains mostly water, thickeners, silicones, detangling agent, film former, slip agent, preservatives, fragrance, and coloring agents. This is a very overpriced, very standard, silicone-based conditioner for someone with dry, coarse, or damaged hair.

☺ **The Conditioner** *($8 for 10.14 ounces)* is similar to the one above, only the price is less absurd; the same performance comments apply.

☺ **Dynamite Hair Rebuilder** *($16 for 5.2 ounces)* won't rebuild hair, but it is a good conditioner for dry or damaged hair that is also coarse or thick. It contains mostly water, thickeners, detangling agents, plant oil, silicone, more plant oil, conditioning agent, preservatives, and fragrance.

☺ **Oomf Conditioner Extra Gutz for Fine Limp Hair** *($12 for 6.76 ounces)* contains mostly water, thickeners, silicones, conditioning agent, detangling agent, slip agents, preservatives, and fragrance. This is great for dry, damaged, coarse hair, though it would be too emollient for fine or limp hair.

☺ **$$$ Erekt Cold Turkey for Curly Hair** *($17 for 4 ounces)* is an overpriced silicone-based styling gel. It contains mostly silicones, slip agent, film former, preservatives, coloring agents, and fragrance. It works as well as any silicone serum with a tiny bit of hold to help with styling curly, coarse hair straight, but it isn't a "nonchemical hair straightener"—it requires styling tools to have any effect. It has a minimal sticky feel.

☺ **Hair Gum Hair Controller Hold Factor 1** *($14 for 5.2 ounces)* contains mostly water, film formers, thickeners, preservatives, and fragrance. This is just a standard gel with a clever name. It has a light to medium hold and a slight stiff sticky feel.

☺ **Oomf Booster Styling Muscle for Fine Limp Hair** *($12 for 6.76 ounces)* contains mostly water, film formers, silicone, conditioning agents, plant extracts, plant oil, slip agent, thickeners, preservatives, and fragrance. This is a rather liquidy styling gel that has a light hold and minimal to no stiff or sticky feel. There is nothing about this gel that's better for fine hair; it can work well for all hair types.

☺ **$$$ Skrewd Gives Hair That Unexpected Twist Heat Responsive** *($17 for 4.2 ounces)* is a great name for an average, extremely overpriced styling gel. It contains mostly water, film formers, thickeners, silicone, preservatives, and fragrance. This is a good light- to medium-hold styling gel with minimal stiff or sticky feel, but that's it, which makes the price ludicrous for what you get.

☺ **$$$ Pump Up** *($20 for 7.1 ounces)* is just mousse that dispenses in a gel form that turns foamy. It's an interesting delivery for a basic light to medium hold with a slight sticky feel. It contains mostly water, propellant, film formers, slip agents, conditioning agents, preservatives, and fragrance.

☺ **Hair Licorice Hold Factor 5** *($14 for 3.5 ounces)* contains mostly water, mineral oil, silicones, thickeners, film former, lanolin, castor oil, licorice, and preservatives. This doesn't smell like or act like licorice. It's a rather strange-textured creamy gel with minimal hold, though the grease can help smooth frizzies and curls. It has no stiff or sticky feel but it can have a heavy wax finish, so use it minimally.

☺ **Hair Putty Hold Factor 3** *($14 for 3.5 ounces)* contains mostly water, film formers, thickeners, silicones, carnauba wax, clay, conditioning agent, preservatives, and fragrance. This is just a standard pomade that has a heavy hold on hair. It can have a sticky feel and is best when used minimally to smooth stubborn frizzies and curls.

☹ **Hair Shaper Firm Hold Factor 2** *($14 for 3.5 ounces)* contains mostly water, alcohol, lanolin, Vaseline, thickener, film formers, mineral oil, carnauba wax, castor oil, preservatives, and fragrance. This delivers a gummy, heavy hold, with a slight sticky feel. It can work to smooth and hold stubborn hair but it easily builds up on hair and weighs it down.

☺ **Hair Varnish Hold Factor 4** *($14 for 3.17 ounces)* contains mostly Vaseline, thickeners, castor oil, carnauba wax, preservative, and fragrance. This standard pomade is just like applying greasy wax to the hair (after all, carnauba wax is the same wax used in car wax). When used minimally it can help smooth stubborn frizzies and curls. It can have a slight sticky feel as well as a heavy wax texture, so use it minimally.

☺ **Hair Cement the Exceptional Finishing Spray** *($9 for 10.01 ounces)* contains mostly alcohol, film formers, water, conditioning agents, and fragrance. This isn't cement, it's just a good light- to medium-hold hairspray with minimal to no stiff or sticky feel that easily brushes through.

☺ **Head Polish Silicone Shine** *($14 for 1.4 ounces)* contains mostly slip agent, water, silicones, film former, conditioning agents, alcohol, preservatives, and fragrance. This is a good silicone gel with a light hold and minimal sticky feel to straighten out coarse, dry, or damaged hair.

Garden Botanika Hair Care

Garden Botanika has been having a hard time of it. In 1999 Garden Botanika closed 95 stores and laid off 1,200 employees after filing Chapter 11 in a Seattle bankruptcy court on April 20. In the long run, Garden Botanika is just one of several cosmetics companies that have done their own versions (read, knock-offs) of The Body Shop—an all-purpose cosmetic boutique with a mix of environmentalism and infusions of plants. What all these types of stores offer is an intimate shopping atmosphere, low-key salespeople, reasonable prices, and all the vegetable, botanical, herb, fruit, and random plant extracts you could ask for. Do you need all those plants on your hair? No, but the other less exotic-sounding ingredients in the products are all standard to the hair-care industry and they work well.

For more information on Garden Botanika, call (425) 881-9603, (800) 968-7842, or visit its Web site at www.gardenbotanika.com.

☺ **Botanika Cleanse Black Cherry Color Enhancing Shampoo Adds Deep, Rich Auburn Tones** *($12.50 for 12 ounces)* contains mostly water, detergent cleansing agents, lather agent, conditioning agent, detangling agent/film former, dye agents, more conditioning agents, plant extracts, fragrance, and preservatives. This is a good color-enhancing shampoo. It works best for normal to dry hair that is normal to fine or thin. The film former can make thin hair feel thicker but it can also cause buildup with repeated use.

☺ **Botanika Cleanse Cattail Color Enhancing Shampoo Enriches Warm Brown Tones** *($12.50 for 12 ounces)* is similar to the one above and the same basic comments apply.

☺ **Botanika Cleanse Dandelion Color Enhancing Shampoo Brightens Blonde Hair** *($12.50 for 12 ounces)* is similar to the ones above and the same basic comments apply.

☺ **Botanika Cleanse Marigold Color Enhancing Shampoo Adds Golden Highlights** *($12.50 for 12 ounces)* is similar to the ones above and the same basic comments apply.

☺ **Botanika Cleanse Poppy Color Enhancing Shampoo Adds Warm, Red Highlights** *($12.50 for 12 ounces)* similar to the ones above and the same basic comments apply.

☺ **Chamomile Moisture & Shine Shampoo** *($8 for 12 ounces)* contains mostly water, detergent cleansing agents, lather agents, plant extract, conditioning agents, fragrance, detangling agent/film former, and preservatives. This is a very good shampoo for dry, coarse hair. The minimal amount of film former should not be a problem for most all hair types.

☺ **Tri Wheat Hair Repair Shampoo** *($8.50 for 12 ounces)* is almost identical to the Chamomile version above, and the same comments apply.

☹ **Exhilarating Mint Conditioning Shampoo** *($8.50 for 8 ounces)* definitely contains peppermint, which can be drying and irritating for the scalp.

☺ **Fruit Complex Daily Conditioner** *($9 for 12 ounces)* contains mostly water, thickeners, detangling agent, plant extracts, conditioning agents, more thickeners, fragrance, and preservatives. This is a very good conditioner for normal to dry hair of any thickness except coarse.

The Reviews G

☺ **Kelp & Nettle Leave-in Conditioner** *($9 for 12 ounces)* contains mostly water, conditioning agents, plant extracts, film former, slip agent, preservatives, and fragrance. This is a very good leave-in conditioner for normal to dry hair of any thickness except coarse.

☺ **Panthenol Remoisturizing Conditioner** *($9 for 12 ounces)* contains mostly water, thickeners, detangling agent, conditioning agents, plant oils, preservatives, and fragrance. This is a very good conditioner for dry hair of any thickness.

☹ **Flax-Seed Styling Gel** *($8 for 5 ounces)* is a standard medium-hold gel containing mostly water, film formers, conditioning agents, plant extracts, silicone, thickeners, preservatives, and fragrance. It can have a rather sticky hold.

☺ **Protein Protective Spray Gel** *($9.50 for 12 ounces)* is a standard light-hold spray gel with minimal to no stiff or sticky feel that can easily be brushed through. It contains mostly water, film formers, conditioning agents, plant extracts, silicone, thickeners, preservatives, and fragrance.

☺ **Natural Finishing Spray** *($8.50 for 12 ounces)* is a good standard hairspray for light hold, containing mostly alcohol, film former, water, plant extracts, conditioning agents, silicones, and fragrance. It brushes through easily with minimal stiff or sticky feel.

☹ **Russian Silt Hair Mask** *($8.50 for 5 ounces)* contains silt, which is sort of like clay and sand. Either way it's drying for the hair, and that can only make matters worse.

☹ **Stimulating Peppermint Treatment** *($9.50 for 12 ounces)* contains peppermint oil and menthol, which can be irritating to the scalp.

☹ **Terra Cotta Hair Mud** *($12.50 for 8 ounces)* is a clay mask and there is no reason to apply clay to the hair. Clay is drying and serves no purpose for the hair.

Goldwell

Goldwell has been in the business of hair care for over 50 years. That's a long time. Over the years it has become a mainstay in the world of salon hair-care products. Its education programs are well known among stylists the world over. What then of its hair-care products? As you may already suspect, it has some good products and some disappointments. Goldwell has many lines under its belt, each with its own set of promises.

The Kerasilk line is supposed to be "specifically formulated with hydrolyzed silk proteins to give hair a healthy, vibrant sheen." That's fine, but while silk proteins sound like they can impart a silky shine to your hair, they are no better than any other protein for conditioning hair. Goldwell's Definition line is "specially formulated with alpha hydroxy acids (AHAs) for healthy, shiny hair." Thankfully none of these products contain an active or effective form of AHA. If they did, it would degrade the hair's cuticle. But itsColorance Color 'n Care is an interesting group of hair coloring and styling products for temporary color enhancement.

For more information on Goldwell, call (800) 333-2442 or in Canada (800) 387-4910. You can also visit its Web site at www.goldwellky.com.

☺ **Shampoo 5 Turbocharged Shampoo for Dry and Damaged Hair** *($5.90 for 8.4 ounces)* contains mostly water, detergent cleansing agent, thickener, detangling agent/film former, vitamins, plant extract, conditioning agent, castor oil, preservatives, fragrance, and coloring agents. This is a very good shampoo for dry hair of normal to heavy thickness. The castor oil can weigh down fine or thin hair.

☺ **Care 5 Turbocharged Intensive Conditioner for Dry and Damaged Hair** *($11.90 for 8.4 ounces)* contains mostly water, thickeners, detangling agent, mineral oil, conditioning agents, plant oil, preservatives, castor oil, plant extracts, vitamins, fragrance, and coloring agents. This is a very good conditioner for dry, damaged, coarse, or thick hair.

☺ **Care R Leave In Revitalizer** *($11.90 for 7.6 ounces)* contains mostly water, silicone, slip agents, detangling agent, castor oil, preservatives, and fragrance. This is a very good silicone-based leave-in conditioner for hair that is dry, damaged, and coarse or thick.

Colorance by Goldwell

☺ **Colorance Color 'n Care Conditioning Color Balm (available in Brown, Copper, Gold, Pearl, and Red)** *($11 for 5.2 ounces)* contains mostly water, thickeners, detangling agent, conditioning agent, mineral oil, preservatives, fragrance, and dye agents. This is a good color-enhancing conditioner for most all hair types.

☹ **Colorance Color Styling Gel, Silver** *($10 for 1.8 ounces)* contains mostly water, alcohol, film former, slip agents, thickeners, castor oil, conditioning agent, fragrance, and coloring agents. This standard, light-hold creamy gel imparts a metallic shine that really sticks to hair like a layer of paint. This may not be everyone's idea of adding some "spark" to gray hair.

☹ **Colorance Color Styling Mousse (comes in 14 shades)** *($9.99 for 2.4 ounces)* is a standard light- to medium-hold mousse with no stiff or sticky feel. The color concentration for these mousses imparts almost no color worth mentioning to the hair. For soft styling they're fine, but that's about it. These contain mostly water, alcohol, propellant, film formers, conditioning agent, detangling agent, silicone, preservatives, and coloring agents.

☹ **Colorance Hair Shimmer, Hairspray with a Soft Color Glow, Crystal Rose or Sandy Pearls** *($10 for 2 ounces)* is reminiscent of spray paint, but it is just a sticky, fast-drying, firm-hold hairspray that adds a minute bit of color—though it does add a noticeable shiny finish. This is stiff stuff, and the "glow" may not be worth it, given the texture.

Definition by Goldwell

☹ **Definition Balance & Vitality Shampoo** *($7.90 for 12 ounces)* uses sodium C14-17 alkyl sec sulfonate, a sulfonate that can be drying on the hair and strip hair color.

☺ **Definition Coated & Oily Shampoo** *($7.90 for 12 ounces)* is a good standard shampoo with minimal conditioning agent, so it should work well for all hair types. It contains mostly water, detergent cleansing agent, lather agent, detangling agent/film former, thickener, preservatives, and fragrance.

☺ **Definition Color & Highlights Shampoo** *($7.90 for 12 ounces)* contains mostly water, detergent cleansing agents, lather agent, thickener, fragrance, detangling agent/film former, slip agent, preservatives, and plant extracts. The detergent cleansing agents in here make this a fairly drying shampoo, though it may be OK for someone with very oily hair and scalp. The amount of AHA in here is insignificant.

☺ **Definition Demineralizing Shampoo for Coated and Oily Hair** *($7.95 for 12 ounces)* contains mostly water, detergent cleansing agent, lather agent, thickeners, conditioning agent, plant extracts, slip agents, preservatives, and fragrance. This is a good basic shampoo for all hair types. The amount of conditioning agent is insignificant, so the chance for buildup is minimal.

☺ **Definition Dry & Porous Shampoo** *($7.90 for 12 ounces)* contains mostly water, detergent cleansing agent, lather agent, thickeners, detangling agent/film former, vitamins, plant extract, conditioning agent, castor oil, preservatives, fragrance, and coloring agents. This is a good shampoo for dry to coarse hair of any thickness except fine or thin.

☺ **Definition Permed & Curly Shampoo** *($7.95 for 12 ounces)* contains mostly water, detergent cleansing agent, thickeners, lather agent, plant oil, conditioning agents, AHAs, detangling agent/film former, preservatives, and fragrance. This is a good shampoo for dry to coarse hair of any thickness. The pH of this shampoo is too high (about 5.5) for the AHAs in here to be effective; if it were effective, it could denature the hair shaft. Nothing about this shampoo makes it particularly beneficial or helpful for curly hair.

☺ **Definition Balance & Vitality Conditioner** *($11.95 for 12 ounces)* contains mostly water, thickeners, detangling agents, conditioning agent, AHAs, preservatives, and fragrance. This is a good conditioner for someone with normal to slightly dry hair that is normal to fine or thin.

☺ **Definition Color & Highlights Conditioning Treatment** *($11.95 for 12 ounces)* is almost identical to the Vitality version above and the same comments apply.

☺ **Definition Dry & Porous Conditioner** *($11.90 for 12 ounces)* contains mostly water, thickeners, detangling agents, mineral oil, conditioning agent, plant oil, preservatives, castor oil, vitamins, fragrance, and color agents. This is a good conditioner for someone with dry, coarse hair of any thickness but fine or thin.

☺ **$$$ Definition Dry & Porous Intensive Treatment** *($25.95 for 16 ounces)* contains mostly water, thickeners, castor oil, plant oil, conditioning agents, AHAs, detangling agent, preservatives, and fragrance. This is a very good conditioner for dry, coarse, thick hair.

☺ **Definition Permed & Curly Conditioning Treatment** *($11.90 for 12 ounces)* contains mostly water, thickeners, castor oil, detangling agents, mineral oil, conditioning agents, AHAs, preservatives, and fragrance. This is a very good conditioner for dry, coarse, thick hair.

☹ **Definition Permed & Curly Foam Conditioner** *($11.90 for 9 ounces)* contains mostly water, thickeners, castor oil, detangling agent, preservatives, and fragrance. This is a good conditioner for dry, coarse, thick hair. It can have a slightly stiff feel and can build up with repeated use.

☹ **$$$ Definition Color & Highlights Spray Leave-in Conditioner** *($25.95 for 32 ounces)* contains mostly water, detangling agent, conditioning agent, silicone, AHAs, film formers, castor oil, slip agents, preservatives, and fragrance. This is a good conditioner for normal to dry and thin to thick hair. It can have a slightly stiff, sticky feel on the hair and can easily build up with repeated use.

☹ **Definition Permed & Curly Foam Leave-in Conditioner** *($11.95 for 9 ounces)* contains mostly water, propellant, plant extract, conditioning agents, detangling agents/film formers, silicone, AHAs, slip agents, more silicone, preservatives, and fragrance. The mousse-like application is clever but it doesn't help. This is a good leave-in conditioner for normal to dry hair that ei normal to fine or thin. It can have a stiff feel and can easily build up on hair.

☺ **Definition Finish & Shine Hair Shiner** *($7.50 for 3.6 ounces)* contains mostly propellant, alcohol, silicones, AHAs, slip agent, and fragrance. This is basically just silicone and it does add shine to hair.

☹ **Definition Style & Shine Glaze** *($7.50 for 8 ounces)* contains mostly water, alcohol, film formers, thickeners, castor oil, preservatives, fragrance, and AHAs. This is a standard gel with a medium to firm hold, and it can have a stiff, sticky feel.

☺ **Definition Style & Shine Spray Gel** *($7.90 for 8 ounces)* contains mostly alcohol, water, film formers, thickeners, silicone, fragrance, slip agent, and AHAs. This is a good standard spray gel with a light hold and minimal to no stiff or sticky feel. The AHAs in here are useless for hair, they are just a clever marketing gimmick to make these products sound *au currant.*

☺ **Definition Style & Shine Creative Pomade** *($7.90 for 3.4 ounces)* is more of a gel than a pomade. It contains mostly water, mineral oil, thickeners, slip agents, preservatives, detangling agent, AHAs, and fragrance. It gives minimal hold but a good soft finish to smooth stubborn curls and frizzies, or can work for just an extra-soft hold.

☺ **Definition Finish & Shine Finishing Hairspray (Aerosol)** *($9 for 8 ounces)* is a standard aerosol hairspray that contains mostly propellant, alcohol, water, film formers, silicone, and fragrance. It has a firm hold with a somewhat stiff feel.

☺ **Definition Finish & Shine Finishing Hairspray (Non-Aerosol)** *($9 for 8.5 ounces)* is similar to the aerosol version above and the same comments apply.

Exclusives by Goldwell

☺ **Exclusives Body-Building Shampoo** *($5.90 for 8 ounces)* contains mostly water, detergent cleansing agents, lather agent, thickeners, conditioning agents, fragrance, and preservatives. This basic shampoo with minimal conditioning agents would work well for all hair types.

☺ **Exclusives Color Care Shampoo** *($5.90 for 8 ounces)* contains mostly water, detergent cleansing agents, lather agent, thickeners, fragrance, detangling agent/film former, preservatives, plant extracts conditioning agents, and preservatives. This basic shampoo would work well for normal to slightly dry hair that is normal to fine or thin.

☺ **Exclusives Deep Cleansing Shampoo** *($5.90 for 8 ounces)* contains mostly water, detergent cleansing agents, lather agent, thickeners, detangling agent/film former, fragrance, and preservatives. This shampoo is mostly detergent cleansing agents with minimal film former, so it would work well for all hair types.

☺ **Exclusives Body-Building Conditioner** *($8.50 for 8 ounces)* contains mostly water, thickeners, detangling agent, conditioning agent, and fragrance. This rather ordinary conditioner would work well for normal to slightly dry hair of any thickness.

☺ **Exclusives Color Care Conditioner** *($8.50 for 8 ounces)* contains mostly water, thickeners, castor oil, detangling agents, mineral oil, preservatives, and fragrance. This rather ordinary conditioner would work well for dry hair that is coarse or thick.

☺ **Exclusives Conditioner Moisturizing** *($14 for 16 ounces)* contains mostly water, thickeners, detangling agents, mineral oil, conditioning agents, plant oil, preservatives, castor oil, plant extracts, vitamins, and fragrance. The vitamins and plant extracts are practically nonexistent, but this rather basic conditioner would work well for dry hair that is coarse or thick.

☺ **Exclusives Revitalizing Conditioner Spray** *($11.90 for 8 ounces)* is a very good, lightweight leave-in conditioner for normal to slightly dry hair of any thickness. It contains mostly water, silicone, slip agents, detangling agents, castor oil, preservatives, and fragrance.

☺ **Exclusives Turbo-Hydrating Conditioner** *($9 for 12 ounces)* contains mostly water, thickeners, detangling agents, mineral oil, conditioning agents, plant oil, castor oil, plant extracts, vitamins, preservatives, fragrance, and coloring agents. The vitamins and plant extracts are practically nonexistent, but this rather basic conditioner would work well for dry hair that is coarse or thick.

☺ **Exclusives Designing Body-Building Styling Gel** *($7.90 for 6 ounces)* contains mostly water, film former, thickener, conditioning agent, castor oil, preservatives, and fragrance. This basic gel has a very light hold with minimal stiff or sticky feel.

☺ **Exclusives Body-Building Styling Gel, Alcohol Free** *($7.90 for 6 ounces)* is similar to the Designing Gel above only in spray form.

☺ **Exclusives Designing Gel Polish** *($10 for 2 ounces)* is a thick gel in a jar. It contains mostly water, thickeners, mineral oil, slip agents, silicone, preservatives, detangling agents, and fragrance. It would work well to smooth out curls and frizzies with no stiffness, but use it sparingly to prevent a heavy feel.

☺ **Exclusives Designing Super Shine Spray Gel** *($9.50 for 8 ounces)* contains mostly alcohol, water, film formers, silicone, slip agent, and fragrance. This is a light-to medium-hold spray gel, and it can work to keep hair in place with minimal stiff or sticky feel.

☺ **Exclusives Designing Firm Holding Mousse** *($9.50 for 10.2 ounces)* is a standard light- to medium-hold mousse with minimal stiff, sticky feel. It contains mostly water, alcohol, propellant, film formers, alcohol, silicone, fragrance, thickeners, castor oil, and conditioning agents.

☺ **Exclusives Body-Building Designing Glaze** *($7 for 8 ounces)* contains mostly water, alcohol, film formers, thickeners, conditioning agent, castor oil, preservatives, fragrance, and coloring agents. This standard gel has light hold with no stiff or sticky feel.

☺ **Exclusives Designing Firm Holding Forming Lotion** *($7.90 for 8 ounces)* is almost identical to the Glaze above, only this one has slightly more hold and a very slight sticky feel that easily brushes through.

☺ **Exclusives Finishing Super Firm & Dry Spray** *($9.50 for 8.5 ounces)* is a standard hairspray with medium to firm hold and a somewhat stiff feel. It contains mostly alcohol, water, film formers, silicone, and fragrance.

☺ **Exclusives Finishing Super Firm Spray (Non-Aerosol)** *($7.90 for 8 ounces)* is similar to the Super Firm one above and the same comments apply.

Kerasilk by Goldwell

☺ **Kerasilk Care & Smoothness Conditioning Shampoo for Dry, Damaged, or Curly Hair** *($5.90 for 8 ounces)* contains mostly detergent cleansing agents, thickeners, conditioning agents, detangling agent/film former, preservatives, slip agent, and fragrance. This is a good shampoo for normal to dry hair that is normal to fine or thin.

☺ **Kerasilk Care & Volumizing Shampoo** *($6.50 for 8 ounces)* is similar to the one above and the same comments apply. This one does contain AHAs, but the amount is negligible.

☺ **Kerasilk Care & Gloss Shining Conditioner for All Hair Types** *($9.50 for 5 ounces)* contains mostly water, silicones, alcohol, detangling agents, conditioning agents, plant oil, vitamins, AHA, film former, fragrance, preservative, and coloring agents. It's a good conditioner for dry, thick, or coarse hair.

☺ **Kerasilk Care & Smoothness Conditioning Treatment for Dry, Damaged, or Curly Hair** *($7 for 3.4 ounces)* contains mostly water, thickeners, detangling agent, mineral oil, conditioning agents, preservatives, and fragrance. This is a very good conditioner for dry, coarse, and thick hair. Though I haven't generally warned about product aroma, this one does deserve mentioning because it may knock you over!

☺ **Kerasilk Conditioner** *($7.25 for 3.3 ounces)* is almost identical to the Smoothness version above and the same comments apply.

☺ **Kerasilk Volumizing Leave-in Conditioner** *($8.90 for 6 ounces)* contains mostly water, alcohol, silicone, detangling agents, conditioning agent, film former, AHAs, slip agents, preservatives, fragrance, and coloring agents. The AHAs in here are useless, but this is a good leave-in conditioner for dry to very dry hair of all thicknesses.

Graham Webb

Graham Webb's Classic line uses an ingredient called Thermacore Complex in some of the products. It is nothing more than a blend of panthenol, allantoin (a skin soothing agent, that would be rinsed away in a shampoo and in styling agents wouldn't make it to the scalp), and an ingredient to keep the two mixed together. Primarily this just functions as a standard conditioning agent, no better or worse than those found in hundreds and hundreds of products, although Webb has dubbed it with an impressive name. For more information on Graham Webb, call (760) 918-3600 or (800) 456-9322.

Bodacious by Graham Webb

☺ **Bodacious Moisturizing Shampoo** *($6.95 for 8.5 ounces)* contains mostly water, detergent cleansing agents, lather agent, conditioning agents, film formers, thickeners, silicone, preservative, fragrance, and coloring agent. This is a very good shampoo for dry hair that is fine or thin to make it feel thick. The film formers in here can easily build up with repeated use.

☺ **Bodacious Moisturizing Conditioner Renew & Revitalize** *($9 for 10 ounces)* contains mostly water, detangling agents, thickeners, slip agents, conditioning agents, silicone, preservatives, and fragrance. This is a good basic conditioner for normal to dry hair of any thickness.

☺ **Bodacious Sculpting Foam** *($8.95 for 8 ounces)* is a standard mousse containing mostly water, propellant, film former, preservatives, silicone, and fragrance. It has a medium hold with a somewhat sticky feel.

☹ **Bodacious Hair Creme Define & Design** *($11.95 for 3 ounces)* contains mostly water, film former, thickeners, slip agent, castor oil, conditioning agents, silicones, detangling agents, more slip agents, preservatives, and fragrance. This is a relatively sticky hair gel that looks like Vaseline but has a sticky, stiff feel. It can be good for straightening the most stubborn hair or for a slicked-back look, but basically this is just very heavy sticky stuff.

☺ **Bodacious Finishing Hair Spray** *($6.95 for 10 ounces)* is a standard medium- to firm-hold aerosol hairspray with a slight stiff or sticky feel that does brush through. It contains mostly alcohol, propellant, film former, conditioning agents, silicones, and fragrance.

☺ **Bodacious Silky and Soft Spray Shine** *($8.75 for 4 ounces)* contains mostly alcohol, slip agent, silicones, and fragrance. This is a basic silicone spray and it works as well as any to add shine and a soft feel to hair.

Classic by Graham Webb

☺ **Cleanse Infusion Shampoo for Fine, Thin & Limp Hair** *($9.95 for 8 ounces)* contains mostly water, detergent cleansing agents, lather agent, conditioning agents, vitamins, plant oil, preservatives, fragrance, and coloring agents. This is a good shampoo for all hair types, but it's best for dry hair of any thickness. The amount of conditioning agents in here isn't large, so they shouldn't build up, though they would be a problem for oily hair and scalp.

☺ **Cleanse Thermal Care Shampoo for Dry, Damaged and Chemically Treated Hair** *($8.26 for 8.5 ounces)* is similar to the Infusion version above and the same comments apply.

☺ **Cleanse Stick Straight High Gloss Smoothing Shampoo** *($8 for 8.5 ounces)* contains mostly water, detergent cleansing agents, lather agent, detangling agent/film former, conditioning agents, silicone, thickeners, preservatives, fragrance, and coloring agents. This is a good shampoo for normal to dry hair that's fine or thin. The film former in here can cause buildup.

☹ **Ice Cap Revitalizing & Moisturizing Shampoo** *($8.26 for 8 ounces)* uses TEA-lauryl sulfate as one of the main detergent cleansing agents, which makes it too drying for the hair and too irritating and drying for the scalp. It also contains menthol, another scalp irritant.

☹ **Visibility Shampoo for Deep Cleansing & Purification** *($10.75 for ounces)* uses TEA dodecylbenzenesulfonate as one of its main detergent cleansing agents, which can be drying for hair and scalp.

☺ **24 Karat, Leave-in Conditioner, Reconstructor and Shine** *($10.95 for 8 ounces)* contains mostly water, detangling agent, conditioning agents, silicones, thickeners, castor oil, film formers, slip agents, preservatives, fragrance, and coloring agents. This is a good conditioner for very dry, fine or thin hair. It can easily build up on the hair with repeated use.

☺ **30 Second Sheer Conditioner for Daily Use** *($9.96 for 8.5 ounces)* contains mostly water, thickeners, detangling agent, conditioning agent, silicones, slip agent, preservatives, and fragrance. This is a good conditioner for dry hair of any thickness except coarse.

☺ **Condition Stick Straight High Gloss Smoothing Conditioner** *($8 for 8.5 ounces)* is similar to the one above only with slightly more silicone; it would work best for very dry hair of any thickness.

☹ **Ice Cap Hypothermic Bonding Conditioner** *($9.80 for 8 ounces)* is a lightweight conditioner for normal to slightly dry hair, mostly to help with easier combing. It contains mostly water, thickener, slip agent, detangling agents, preservatives, and fragrance. It does contain menthol, which can be a problem if applied on the scalp.

☺ **Ice Cap Protein Reconstructor Mist** *($11 for 8 ounces)* contains mostly water, thickener, conditioning agents, silicone, film former, slip agents, preservatives, fragrance, and coloring agents. This is a very good leave-in conditioner for dry hair of any thickness except coarse. It does contain menthol, which can be a problem if applied on the scalp.

☺ **The Untangler Leave-in Detangling Spray** *($11 for 8.5 ounces)* contains mostly water, detangling agent, water-binding agent, plant extracts, conditioning agents, slip agents, preservatives, and fragrance. This is a very good leave-in conditioner for normal to slightly dry hair of any thickness except coarse.

☺ **Styling Exothermic Styling Gel** *($9.96 for 8.5 ounces)* contains mostly water, film formers, conditioning agents, vitamins, plant oil, silicone, thickeners, slip agent, preservatives, and fragrance. This is a good standard gel for a light hold with minimal stiff or sticky feel.

☺ **Style Magnitude Mousse for Volume & Condition** *($5.94 for 3 ounces)* contains mostly water, propellant, film former, slip agent, silicone, conditioning agent, and fragrance. This is a good standard mousse with a light hold and minimal to no stiff or sticky feel.

☺ **Hair Wax for Shine & Definition** *($10.50 for 4.5 ounces)* is a standard hair-straightening wax that contains mostly slip agent, thickeners, castor oil, water, conditioning agent, silicone, preservatives, and fragrance. This can have a sticky feel.

☺ **Styling Root Infusion Root Volumizing Serum** *($10 for 4 ounces)* contains mostly water, film formers, thickeners, plant extracts, silicone, conditioning agent, slip agents, preservatives, and fragrance. This is more of a basic styling gel than anything else. It has a light hold and minimal to no stiff or sticky feel and doesn't help volumize any more than any other light-hold gel. The most unique thing is the applicator tip that looks like it will get right to the root of the matter, but it deposits too much in one area so you end up using the gel as you would otherwise, working it through the hair with your fingers.

☺ **Styling VHS Volumizing & Thickening Spray** *($10.96 for 8.5 ounces)* is a good light-hold styling spray that can make hair feel thicker, though the result will depend on the styling far more than this product.

☺ **Styling Voltage High Gloss Sculpting Spray** *($10.96 for 8.5 ounces)* is a styling spray with a firm hold and a somewhat sticky feel. It does brush through, but this one is more for getting hair to stay put.

☺ **Jet Stream** *($7.95 for 8 ounces)* is a standard hairspray that contains mostly alcohol, water, film former, conditioning agents, vitamins, plant oil, silicone, and fragrance. It has a medium to firm hold with minimal stiff or sticky feel.

☺ **Finish Energy Lock Maximum Hold Hair Spray** *($12.04 for 10 ounces)* is a great name for a very standard aerosol hairspray with medium to firm hold and a slight stiff feel that does brush through. It contains mostly alcohol, propellant, film former, silicones, conditioning agent, and fragrance.

☺ **Finish Super Hold & Shine Firm Hold Hair Spray** *($10.96 for 8.5 ounces)* is a standard hairspray with medium to firm hold and with a stiff feel that brushes through easily. It contains mostly alcohol, film former, silicones, conditioning agents, and fragrance.

☺ **Stick Straight Curl Relaxer Straightens & Smoothes** *($13.16 for 6 ounces)* contains mostly water, thickener, slip agent, conditioning agent, preservatives, fragrance, and coloring agents. This is a thick, creamy gel with no real hold, it just places a layer of emollient over the hair to help when smoothing curls or frizzies.

☺ **$$$ Stick Straight High Gloss Shine and Anti-Frizz Serum** *($16 for 2 ounces)* is a standard silicone serum that contains mostly silicone, slip agent, conditioning agent, and fragrance. The price tag is absurd; there are identical versions formulated like this at the drugstore for a fraction of the cost.

Intensives by Graham Webb

☺ **Intensives Super Silk Shampoo Reconstructive Shampoo for Dry, Brittle, & Chemically Treated Hair** *($7.80 for 6 ounces)* contains mostly water, detergent cleansing agent, lather agent, plant oils, conditioning agents, detangling agent/film former, silicone, thickeners, preservatives, and fragrance. It is a good shampoo for very dry, coarse hair.

☹ **Intensives Vivid Color Conditioning Moisturizing Shampoo for Color Treated Hair** *($11 for 10.5 ounces)* uses sodium C14-16 olefin sulfonate as one of the main detergent cleansing agents, which makes it too drying for all hair types but especially for chemically treated hair.

☺ **Intensives Extreme Clean After Shampoo Clarifying Conditioner** *($15 for 12 ounces)* contains mostly water, thickeners, detangling agent, conditioning agent, plant oil, slip agent, preservatives, and fragrance. This is an exceptionally standard conditioner for normal to slightly dry hair of any thickness.

☺ **Intensives Pure Gold Conditioner Intense Moisturizer** *($9.95 for 6 ounces)* contains mostly water, thickeners, castor oil, detangling agents, conditioning agents, plant oils, thickeners, slip agent, preservatives, and fragrance. This is a very good conditioner for dry, coarse hair of any thickness. It can build up on hair with re-peated use.

☹ **Intensives ThermaClay Hair Maximizer Hair Strengthening Conditioner** *($9.95 for 6 ounces)* contains clay as the second ingredient, and that makes this in-credibly drying for hair; clay serves no purpose for the scalp or for the health of the hair shaft.

☺ **Intensives ThermaSilk Therapy Advanced Hair Recovery Treatment** *($4 for 1 ounce)* contains mostly water, pH balancer, thickeners, detangling agent, condi-tioning agents, plant oils, vitamin, silicone, slip agent, preservatives, fragrance, and coloring agents. This is a very good conditioner for dry, coarse, or thick hair. It won't recover or undo any damage.

☺ **Intensives Vivid Color Moisturizing Conditioner** *($11 for 8.5 ounces)* contains mostly water, thickeners, detangling agents, silicone, slip agents, condition-ing agents, more silicone, plant extracts, preservatives, and fragrance. This conditioner claims to protect hair color; it doesn't protect it in the least but it is a good condi-tioner for dry, coarse, and thick hair.

☺ **Intensives Silk Protein Leave In Conditioner and Reconstructor** *($15 for 8.5 ounces)* is similar to the Vivid Color version above and the same comments apply.

☺ **Intensives Power Gel Maximum Hold Styling & Setting Gel** *($13.16 for 8 ounces)* is a standard gel with medium to firm hold and a slight stiff and sticky feel that contains mostly water, film formers, conditioning agents, slip agents, thicken-ers, preservatives, and fragrance.

☺ **Intensives Vivid Color Firm Hold Foaming Gel, Color Locking Foam-ing Gel for Color Treated Hair** *($10.50 for 6 ounces)* won't help keep color in hair but it is a good standard mousse, giving a medium to firm hold that has a slight stiff and sticky feel. It contains mostly water, film formers, propellant, conditioning agent, thickeners, preservatives, castor oil, and fragrance.

☺ **Intensives Making Waves Curl Defining Texturizer** *($13.16 for 8.5 ounces)* contains mostly water, film former, detangling agent, thickener, slip agent, conditioning agents, and fragrance. This is a very good standard gel, almost identical to the Power Hold above, and the same comments apply. There is nothing about this gel better at holding curls than any other styling gel.

☺ **Intensives Total Control Silk Protein Finishing and Styling Hair Spray** *($10.96 for 8 ounces)* is a standard hairspray with medium to firm hold and a slight stiff feel that does brush through. It contains mostly alcohol, water, film formers, conditioning agents, silicone, and fragrance.

☺ **Intensives Visible Control Silk Protein Finishing and Styling Hair Spray** *($10 for 8 ounces)* is similar to the Total Control above and the same comments apply.

☺ **Intensives Vivid Color Hair Spray, Color Locking Protection with Firm Hold for Color Treated Hair** *($12.72 for 10 ounces)* is similar to the Total Control above, only in aerosol form, and the same comments apply. There is nothing in here that can protect hair color.

Montage by Graham Webb

☹ **Montage Hair & Body Shampoo** *($8.80 for 12 ounces).* One of the minerals in this shampoo is copper, but that doesn't make sense—one of the reasons hair turns green when you've been in a swimming pool is because of the copper content in the water. If the ingredient listing is accurate and to be taken seriously, which I always assume it is, this shampoo would be a problem for all hair types. What I suspect is true for the Montage line is that the minerals in these products are included in such trace amounts that they are barely present and that they're there for a marketing angle only. However, I wasn't able to obtain a content breakdown from the company, which means I suggest you err on the safe side and not use the Montage products. If the minerals are there in any significant concentration you would have problems.

☹ **Montage Moisturizing Conditioner** *($11 for 12 ounces)* has copper as one of the minerals in its ingredient list. The comments for the shampoo above apply to this conditioner.

☹ **Montage Hair Gel** *($11 for 6 ounces)* has copper as one of the minerals in its ingredient list. The comments for the shampoo above apply to this gel.

☹ **Montage Thickening Spray Gel** *($10 for 8.5 ounces)* has copper as one of the minerals in its ingredient list. The comments for the shampoo above apply to this spray gel.

☹ **Montage Pomade** *($11 for 2 ounces)* has copper as one of the minerals in its ingredient list. The comments for the shampoo above apply to this pomade.

The Reviews G

⊗ **Montage Texturizing Creme** *($10 for 6 ounces)* has copper as one of the minerals in its ingredient list. The comments for the shampoo above apply to this creme.

⊗ **Montage Hair Spray** *($6.95 for 10 ounces)* has copper as one of the minerals in its ingredient list. The comments for the shampoo above apply to this hairspray.

HairGenesis

Here's another group of hair-care products meant to regenerate hair on a balding head. According to the company, HairGenesis "is a safe, natural formulation designed to combat the effects of . . . male pattern baldness." The brochure for these products explains in scientific-sounding terms that male-pattern baldness is "caused by a series of events within the body. Primary among these events is the metabolic conversion of the male hormone testosterone to dihydrotestosterone or DHT . . . [which] has been shown to bind to receptor sites in the scalp hair follicle (as well as other receptor sites) initiating a chain of events that, in hair genetically programmed to be susceptible to this process, may ultimately result in the loss of hair."

Although that explanation sounds accurate and rather specific (I describe the process in more detail in "Why Does Hair Stop Growing?" in Chapter 2), keep in mind that it is all theory and not fact. For example, this hormonal explanation doesn't explain how transplanted hair can grow beautifully anyplace on the head without being affected by a continuing change in hormonal production. Yet HairGenesis products are supposed to "work(s) by blocking key androgen receptor sites in the hair follicle from damage caused by DHT. Thus the hair follicle is better able to produce a healthier and stronger hair."

As is true with most all non-FDA-approved hair-regrowth products, "results have been reported in as little as two months, a six month period of the use is strongly recommended in order to begin to see real benefits." But that's only after you've spent about $600. That's a lot of money for a theory. Interestingly enough, part of what you get in the initial kit ($199) is minoxidil, the FDA-approved treatment for hair regrowth.

Aside from the minoxidil, the main ingredient in the HairGenesis products is the herb saw palmetto. Saw palmetto has been raised to mythic proportions as a way to naturally grow hair due to its chemical functioning relationship to a drug called Propecia (finasteride). "Yet," according to Kevin J. McElwee, an immunologist and dermatologist involved in the research of hair loss and regrowth, "no scientific research of any kind has been conducted to find [saw palmetto's] true value in treating hair loss." McElwee explains that saw palmetto is used much more widely in treatment of human prostatic hyperplasia, in much the same way finasteride (Propecia) is used to treat benign prostatic hyperplasia (Plosker 1996). Saw palmetto's relationship to finasteride may sound promising but it appears to be nothing more than a dead end. While finasteride itself has been shown to be effective in reducing serum concentrations of dihydrotestosterone, as McElwee notes, "Research shows that saw palmetto does not have an effect on the plasma concentration of testosterone, dihydrotestosterone, or other hormones so systemic production of testosterone is maintained when taking saw palmetto." What saw palmetto may do is inhibit the enzyme 5 alpha reductase, which converts testosterone to DHT, but again that's only theory. Is it worth a try? That's up to you and your hair. For more information on HairGenesis call (800) 736-0729 or visit its Web site at www.hairgenesis.com.

The following HairGenesis kit costs *$199*: **Hair Revitalizing Formulation Softgel caps** *(three bottles, 60 per bottle)*, **Topical Activator Serum with 5% Minoxidil** *(three 2-ounce bottles)*, **Hair Revitalizing Shampoo** *(one 8-ounce bottle)*, and **Hair Revitalizing Conditioner** *(one 8-ounce bottle)*.

Halsa Highlights

Halsa is owned by the Dep Corporation (which also own L.A. Looks). Halsa's Swedish connection is sorely lacking. This small group of products has nothing to do with Sweden in any way, shape, or form. Actually, I have no idea what a Swedish hair-care formula would look like because there are no specialized "Swedish" formulations for hair care or any other kind of beauty care. These are pretty standard products that are actually quite good for many hair types. For more information on Halsa Highlights, call (310) 604-0777 or (800) 326-2855.

☺ **Herbal Swedish Formula Daily Shampoo, Chamomile and Rose Hips** *($2.57 for 20 ounces)* contains mostly water, detergent cleansing agents, thickeners, fragrance, preservatives, and coloring agents. This is a good basic shampoo with negligible conditioning agents, and it would work well for all hair types.

☺ **Herbal Swedish Formula Daily Shampoo, Marigold and Orange Blossom** *($2.57 for 20 ounces)* is identical to the Chamomile version above and the same comments apply.

☹ **Herbal Swedish Formula Daily Shampoo, Mint and Rosemary** *($2.57 for 20 ounces)* contains mint, which won't invigorate the scalp as the label claims, though it will cause irritation and dryness.

☺ **Herbal Swedish Formula Daily Conditioner, Chamomile and Rose Hips** *($2.57 for 20 ounces)* contains mostly water, thickeners, detangling agents, film former, more thickeners, conditioning agent, silicones, plant oil, slip agents, fragrance, preservatives, and coloring agents. This is a very good conditioner for dry, coarse, and thick hair.

☺ **Herbal Swedish Formula Daily Conditioner, Marigold and Orange Blossom** *($2.57 for 20 ounces)* is similar to the Chamomile version above and the same comments apply.

☹ **Herbal Swedish Formula Daily Conditioner, Mint and Rosemary** *($2.57 for 20 ounces)* is similar to the Chamomile version above and the same comments apply. The mint can be an irritant for the scalp.

Hayashi

Hayashi is a line of salon hair care products created by hair designer Sharon Hayashi. For more information on Hayashi, call (818) 716-4716 or (800) 448-9500.

☺ **Daily Shampoo for Frequent Shampooers, Normal to Oily Hair** *($6.90 for 10.6 ounces)* contains mostly water, detergent cleansing agent, lather agent, detangling agents/film formers, conditioning agents, preservatives, coloring agents, and fragrance. This is a very good shampoo for normal to dry hair that is normal to fine or thin, but the film formers and conditioning agents would be a problem for oily hair and scalp.

☺ **Purify Clarifying Shampoo for All Hair Types** *($17.50 for 32.5 ounces)* contains mostly detergent cleansing agents, water, lather agent, water-binding agent, thickener, preservatives, and fragrance. This would be a great standard shampoo with minimal to no conditioning agents. My one concern is the inclusion of sodium sulfite, because it's typically used as a reducing agent in acid perms and can have a lightening effect on hair color.

☺ **Professional Color Shampoo, Amethyst Violet, for White, Pale Blonde, or Highlighted Hair** *($9.50 for 8.4 ounces)* contains mostly water, detergent cleansing agent, lather agent, conditioning agents, plant oil, plant extracts, silicone, detangling agent, preservatives, fragrance, and dye agents. This is a very good color-enhancing shampoo for dry hair of any thickness. There is a tiny amount of lemon extract in this shampoo but it probably isn't enough to be a problem for drying out hair, and lemon can't lighten hair.

☺ **Professional Color Shampoo, Golden Topaz, for Pale, Bright, Medium, Dark Blond, or Highlighted Hair** *($9.50 for 8.4 ounces)* is virtually identical to the version above and the same comments apply.

☺ **Professional Color Shampoo, Red Garnet, for Auburn, Red, Red Brown, or Brown Hair** *($9.50 for 8.4 ounces)* is identical to the version above and the same comments apply.

☺ **Professional Color Shampoo, Ruby Red, for Red, Red Brown, Brown, or Burgundy Hair** *($9.50 for 8.4 ounces)* is identical to the version above and the same comments apply.

☺ **Professional Color Shampoo, Sapphire Blue, for Red Tones, Dark Brown, or Black Hair** *($9.50 for 8.4 ounces)* is identical to the version above and the same comments apply.

☺ **Professional Color Shampoo, Warm Bronze, for Light, Medium, or Dark Brown Hair** *($9.50 for 8.4 ounces)* is identical to the version above and the same comments apply.

☺ **Protect Shampoo Moisturizing Formula for Color Treated Hair** *($7 for 10.6 ounces)* contains mostly water, detergent cleansing agents, lather agent, conditioning agents, silicone, detangling agent/film former, preservatives, fragrance, and coloring agent. This is a good shampoo for normal to dry hair of any thickness, except it can't protect color-treated hair in the least.

☺ **Color Sealing Conditioner Liquid Diamonds** *($10.50 for 8.4 ounces)* contains mostly water, detangling agents, thickeners, conditioning agents, silicones, film formers, plant extracts, slip agent, preservatives, and fragrance. For all its great name, this can't seal in color, but it is a good conditioner for dry hair of any thickness but coarse. The film formers in here can build up on hair.

☺ **Daily Conditioner Detangling Rinse, All Hair Types** *($7.90 for 8.4 ounces)* contains mostly water, detangling agents, thickeners, conditioning agents, fragrant oils, silicone, slip agents, film former, plant extracts, preservatives, and fragrance. This is a very good conditioner for normal to dry hair that is normal to fine or thin in thickness; it wouldn't work well for coarse or extremely dry hair. The minimal amount of film former in here isn't enough to be a problem for buildup.

☺ **Protect Conditioner Moisture Lock for Color Treated Hair** *($7.90 for 8.4 ounces)* contains mostly water, thickeners, detangling agents, film former, conditioning agents, preservatives, and fragrance. This is a very good conditioner for normal to dry hair that is normal to fine or thin; it wouldn't work well for coarse or extremely dry hair. It can't protect color, though the film formers in here can build up on hair.

☺ **No Rinse Leave-in Conditioner for Volume and Shine** *($6 for 8.4 ounces)* is a good, standard, leave-in conditioner for normal to slightly dry hair that is fine or thin. It contains mostly water, detangling agents, film formers, slip agents, conditioning agents, thickeners, silicone, preservatives, and fragrance.

☺ **Moisture Balancer Hair Mask for Healthier Hair** *($19.50 for 16 ounces)* is just a standard conditioner that contains mostly water, thickeners, detangling agent, conditioning agents, vitamins, plant oil, preservatives, coloring agents, and fragrance. This is a very good conditioner for dry hair of any thickness.

☺ **Spaah Skin and Hair Fitness Spray Mist Rehydrante** *($3.80 for 2 ounces)* contains mostly water, thickener, slip agents, water-binding agents, conditioning agents, silicone, detangling agents, preservatives, and fragrance. This is a very good lightweight conditioner for normal hair to help with combing. It does have a small amount of detangling agent in it, which makes no sense for use on skin.

☺ **Spray and Curl Revitalizer for Natural and Permed Hair** *($5.95 for 8.4 ounces)* contains mostly water, film formers, conditioning agents, preservatives, detangling agent, and fragrance. This standard, light-hold styling spray has minimal to no stiff or sticky feel. You can use it to help form curls, but it can be used to create any style depending on the tools you use.

System 911 by Hayashi

☺ **Shampoo Emergency Repair for Dry Damaged Hair** *($6 for 8.4 ounces)* contains mostly water, detergent cleansing agent, lather agent, thickener, conditioning agents, silicone, detangling agent, preservatives, and fragrance. This is a good standard shampoo for most all hair types except oily hair and scalp. The minimal amount of conditioning agents in here shouldn't be a problem for buildup.

☺ **Emergency Pak Reconstructor for Damaged Hair** *($29 for 16 ounces)* contains mostly water, thickeners, conditioning agent, detangling agents, preservatives, fragrance, and coloring agents. This is a standard but good conditioner for dry hair of any thickness.

☺ **Protein Mist Leave-in Conditioner Detangler, Body Building** *($7.90 for 8.4 ounces)* is a standard leave-in conditioner that would work great for dry hair of any thickness except coarse. It contains mostly water, slip agent, detangling agents, conditioning agents, thickeners, film formers, silicone, preservatives, and fragrance.

☺ **Gelplus Fixative Styling Gel with Natural Gums** *($8 for 8.4 ounces)* contains mostly water, slip agents, thickeners, conditioning agent, film former, preservatives, fragrance, and coloring agents. This standard gel has a light hold with minimal stiff or sticky feel.

☺ **Spray Plus Finishing Spray for Damaged Hair** *($8.50 for 8.4 ounces)* is just a standard hairspray that contains mostly alcohol, water, film formers, conditioning agents, and fragrance. There is nothing about this that makes it preferred for damaged hair. It simply has a light to medium hold with a slight stiff feel that easily brushes through.

System Design by Hayashi

☺ **Hi-Gloss Brilliantine** *($7.80 for 2 ounces)* contains mostly water, glycerin, mineral oil, thickeners, lanolin oil, silicone, preservatives, fragrance, and coloring agents. This is a good gel-styled pomade for smoothing and taming frizzies and curls. It can have a greasy finish, so use it sparingly. It also has no film formers, so there is less hold but also no sticky feel on hair.

☺ **$$$ Hi-Shine Polishing Drops** *($11.50 for 1 ounce)* is a standard but extremely overpriced silicone serum. It contains mostly silicone, alcohol, and preservative.

☺ **Spray & Shine Polishing Spray** *($11.50 for 4 ounces)* is a standard silicone spray with some conditioning agents added. It is still just primarily silicone, which is great for dry, coarse hair.

☺ **Instant Replay Gel** *($7.50 for 6 ounces)* contains mostly water, film former, slip agents, conditioning agents, detangling agent/film former, plant extracts, thickeners, castor oil, preservatives, fragrance, and coloring agents. This standard but good styling gel has a light to medium hold and a slight stiff, sticky feel.

☺ **Triple Play Volumizing Mousse Strong Hold** *($9.90 for 7 ounces)* is a standard mousse with medium hold and a somewhat sticky feel. It contains mostly water, film formers, propellant, alcohol, conditioning agent, silicone, more conditioning agent, plant extracts, preservatives, and fragrance.

☺ **Texture Mud Design Adhesive** *($13.90 for 3.5 ounces)* contains mostly water, film formers, thickeners, Vaseline, slip agent, silicone, wax, preservatives, and fragrance. This molding wax has light to medium hold and is thick stuff, but it can help straighten out stubborn curls and smooth down frizzies. Use it sparingly—it can have a thick, waxy feel.

☺ **Freeze-It Working Spray** *($7.90 for 8.4 ounces)* is a standard hairspray that contains alcohol, water, film formers, conditioning agents, silicone, fragrant oil, and fragrance. This has a good light to medium hold with minimal stiff or sticky feel.

☺ **Quikk Fast Dry Working Spray (Aerosol)** *($12.50 for 10.6 ounces)* is similar to the one above only in aerosol form. This does not dry any faster than any other aerosol hairspray.

☺ **Volume + Firm Texture Design Mist** *($7.90 for 8.4 ounces)* is a standard, light- to medium-hold styling spray with a slight sticky, stiff feel that does brush through easily. It contains water, film formers, conditioning agent, plant extracts, and fragrance.

☺ **Uncurl Smoothing Glaze Keeps Hair Straight** *($11.90 for 6.8 ounces)* is a standard liquidy gel with light to medium hold and minimal stiff or sticky feel. It contains mostly water, thickeners, slip agents, film formers, silicone, preservatives, fragrance, and coloring agent. It can help with most any hairstyle, just like any gel, but there's nothing in here special for straightening out hair.

System Hinoki by Hayashi

☺ **Shampoo Volumizing Cleaner for Fine and Thinning Hair** *($6.60 for 8.4 ounces)* contains mostly water, detergent cleansing agent, lather agent, fragrant plant oil, conditioning agents, vitamins, preservatives, coloring agents, and fragrance. This is a very good standard shampoo with minimal conditioning agents that would work for all hair types except oily hair and scalp. The hinoki oil is from a fragrant pine tree. It has some resin properties but not much for holding hair. Mostly it's in here for fragrance and to add a Japanese flair for marketing purposes.

☺ **Conditioner Texturizing Rinse, Normal to Fine Hair** *($7.90 for 8.4 ounces)* contains mostly water, thickeners, castor oil, conditioning agent, vitamins, detangling agent, preservatives, coloring agents, and fragrance. This is a good conditioner for normal to dry hair that is normal to fine or thin. It can have slight sticky feel.

☹ **Hinoki Plus Hair and Scalp Revitalizer for Healthy Hair Growth, Fine and Thinning Hair** *($9.90 for 4 ounces)* contains mostly alcohol, water, glycerin, hinoki oil, conditioning agent, film former, silicone, thickeners, preservatives, and fragrance. There is nothing in this product that can affect hair growth or help the scalp.

☺ **Hair Thickener Leave-in Body Booster for Fine and Thinning Hair** *($9 for 4 ounces)* contains mostly water, thickeners, conditioning agents, silicone, detangling agents, slip agents, film former, preservatives, and fragrance. This is a very good leave-in conditioner for all hair types, though it doesn't add all that much thickness to hair.

☺ **Finishing Spray Control and Shine for Fine and Thinning Hair** *($7.90 for 8.4 ounces)* contains mostly alcohol, water, film formers, hinoki oil, conditioning agent, slip agent, silicone, and fragrance. There is nothing in this hairspray that is especially appropriate for fine or thin hair; it is just a good but extremely standard light- to medium-hold hairspray with a slight stiff feel that easily brushes through.

Head & Shoulders

Head & Shoulders is state of the art when it comes to dandruff shampoos. Almost all of them in this line contain zinc pyrithione, which is a potent antimicrobial agent. If you have dandruff (not dandruff-like conditions, but true dandruff, thought to be caused by a pesky yeast organism), I would recommend starting with one of the Head & Shoulders products to see how it affects your scalp. Two of the Head & Shoulders products use selenium sulfide, the same ingredient in Selsun Blue, and they are also an option. Why not just use zinc pyrithione if that is supposed to be so good for treating dandruff? The answer is that the very nature of any fungus invasion, in or on the human body, is that it is very stubborn. Zinc pyrithione might work for your dandruff (maybe even most dandruff), but definitely not all dandruff. Selenium sulfide is another strong antifungal agent, one I would suggest choosing only if the zinc pyrithione doesn't work. Selenium sulfide can strip hair color.

Head & Shoulders recently expanded its line to include a range of products for different hair types. The same warnings that apply for two-in-one shampoo/

conditioners apply to these dandruff shampoos. If you have an oily scalp, you won't appreciate the conditioning agents (particularly silicone oil), and conditioning agents can build up on fine, limp hair and make it more limp. Depending on your hair type, you may want to apply a separate conditioner (particularly a lightweight leave-in conditioner) if you want to tackle parts of your hair other than the scalp. It is also best, if your scalp doesn't mind, to alternate or rotate a regular shampoo with your dandruff shampoo to reduce the buildup and the drying effect of zinc pyrithione or selenium sulfide. The best products in the following group are the basic Dandruff Shampoo for Fine and Oily Hair and the Dandruff Shampoo for Normal or Dry Hair.

For more information about Head & Shoulders, call (800) 723-9569 or in Canada (800) 668-0151 in Canada. You can also visit the Procter & Gamble Web site at www.pg.com.

☺ **Dandruff Shampoo for Fine or Oily Hair** *($3.39 for 15.2 ounces)* is a standard zinc pyrithione–based dandruff shampoo. It would work well as a place to start the fight against dandruff for all hair types. It does contain a small amount of silicone but it isn't too much for dry hair or to combat the drying effects of the treatment.

☺ **Dandruff Shampoo for Normal Hair** *($3.39 for 15.2 ounces)* is similar to the one above and the same comments apply.

☺ **Dandruff Shampoo Plus Conditioner, 2 in 1, for Fine or Oily Hair** *($3.39 for 15.2 ounces)* is a standard zinc pyrithione–based dandruff shampoo, only with added silicone. That can be somewhat helpful for dry hair, but it would not replace the need for a conditioner. It would work well as a place to start the fight against dandruff for all hair types. There is nothing about this one that makes it more appropriate for fine or oily hair; if anything, the conditioning agent would be a problem for an oily scalp.

☺ **Dry Scalp Dandruff Shampoo Conditioner, 2 in 1, for Normal to Dry Hair** *($3.28 for 15.2 ounces)* is a standard zinc pyrithione–based dandruff shampoo. It would work well as a place to start the fight against dandruff for all hair types. It does contain a small amount of silicone but that isn't much for dry hair or to combat the drying effects of the treatment.

☺ **Dry Scalp Dandruff Shampoo for Normal or Dry Hair** *($4.50 for 25.4 ounces)* is a standard zinc pyrithione–based dandruff shampoo. It would work well as a starting point to fight dandruff for all hair types. It does contain a small amount of silicone but that isn't much for dry hair or combating the drying effects of the treatment.

☺ **Dry Scalp Dandruff Shampoo Plus Conditioner, 2 in 1, for Normal to Dry Hair** *($3.39 for 25.4 ounces)* is a standard zinc pyrithione–based dandruff shampoo. It would work well for all hair types as a starting point to fight dandruff. It does contain a small amount of silicone but that isn't much for dry hair or combating the drying effects of the treatment.

☹ **Intensive Treatment Dandruff and Seborrheic Dermatitis Shampoo for All Hair Types** (*$3.39 for 15.2 ounces*) contains sodium lauryl sulfate as one of the main detergent cleansing agents, which is drying for both the scalp and hair and which doesn't help dandruff in the least. It also contains ammonium xylenesulfonate, which can also be drying and irritating for the hair and scalp.

☺ **Refresh Pyrithione Zinc Dandruff Shampoo for All Hair Types** (*$5.78 for 25.4 ounces*) is a standard zinc pyrithione–based dandruff shampoo. It would work well for all hair types as a place to start the fight against dandruff.

ICE
(see Joico)

Infusium 23

For more information about Infusium 23, call (800) 223-5800 or visit the Clairol Web site at www.clairol.com.

☹ **Professional Pro-Vitamin Shampoo Maximum Body Shampoo** (*$8.81 for 33.8 ounces*) uses sodium lauryl sulfate as one of its main detergent cleansing agents, which makes it too drying for the hair and too irritating and drying for the scalp.

☹ **Shampoo Colored/Permed for Overstressed Hair** (*$5.43 for 16 ounces*) uses sodium lauryl sulfate as one of its main detergent cleansing agents, which makes it too drying for the hair and too irritating and drying for the scalp.

☹ **Shampoo Moisturizing Formula for Normal to Dry Hair** (*$5.99 for 16 ounces*) uses sodium lauryl sulfate as one of its main detergent cleansing agents, which makes it too drying for the hair and too irritating and drying for the scalp.

☺ **Shampoo UV Protection Formula for Damaged Hair** (*$3.44 for 16 ounces*) can't protect the hair from sun damage in the least, but it is a good shampoo for normal to dry hair of any thickness.

☺ **Maximum Body Revitalizing Conditioner for Fine/Thin Hair** (*$5.43 for 16 ounces*) contains mostly water, thickeners, detangling agents, conditioning agents, silicones, water-binding agents, slip agents, film former, fragrance, preservatives, and coloring agents. This is a very good conditioner for dry hair that is anything but fine or thin. The film former is barely present so it isn't a problem for buildup.

☺ **Pro-Vitamin Hair Treatment Maximum Body Treatment for Fine/Thin Hair** (*$5.43 for 16 ounces*) contains mostly water, castor oil, silicones, conditioning agents, detangling agents, slip agents, water-binding agents, thickeners, fragrance, and preservatives. This is a very good conditioner for dry, coarse hair that is anything but fine or thin.

☺ **Pro-Vitamin Hair Treatment Moisturizing Treatment** *($5.43 for 16 ounces)* contains mostly water, film former, conditioning agent, fragrance, detangling agent, thickeners, silicone, preservatives, and fragrance. This is a good conditioner for normal to slightly dry hair that is normal to fine or thin. The film former can make thin hair feel thicker but it can also build up with repeated use.

☺ **Pro-Vitamin Hair Treatment Original Hair Treatment for Damaged/ Unmanageable Hair** *($5.43 for 16 ounces)* contains mostly water, film former, silicone, conditioning agents, fragrance, detangling agent, water-binding agents, thickeners, preservatives, and fragrance. This is a good conditioner for dry hair of any thickness but it can build up with repeated use.

☺ **Re-Vitalizing Conditioner for Normal to Dry Hair** *($5.43 for 16 ounces)* contains mostly water, thickeners, detangling agents, silicones, conditioning agent, water-binding agents, fragrance, film former, and preservatives. This is a very good conditioner for dry hair of any thickness.

☺ **Maximum Body Formula Leave-in Treatment for Fine/Thin Hair** *($4.19 for 8 ounces)* is, just as the name implies, a good leave-in conditioner for normal to slightly dry hair that is normal to fine or thin. It contains mostly water, slip agents, detangling agent/film former, conditioning agents, silicones, fragrance, and preservatives. With repeated use it can build up and have a sticky feel.

☺ **Moisturizing Formula Leave-in Treatment for Normal to Dry Hair** *($3.44 for 8 ounces)* is almost identical to the Maximum Body Formulaversion above and the same comments apply.

☺ **Original Formula Leave-in Treatment for Damaged Hair** *($3.44 for 8 ounces)* is almost identical to the Maximum Body Formula version above and the same comments apply.

☺ **UV Protection Formula Leave-in Treatment for Damaged Hair** *($3.44 for 8 ounces)* is almost identical to the Maximum Body Formula version above and the same comments apply. Without an SPF number, the claim about sun protection is bogus.

☺ **Power Pac Treatment 5 Minute Formula** *($3.44 for 1 ounce)* is just a standard conditioner—and the longer you leave any conditioner in your hair, the better the conditioning. This is a good conditioner for extremely dry, coarse, and thick hair; it contains mostly water, thickeners, detangling agents, silicones, plant oil, conditioning agents, film former, fragrance, lanolin oil, mineral oil, castor oil, and preservatives.

☺ **Hair Treatment Capsules** *($5.43 for 18 0.034-ounce capsules)* is just silicone in a capsule. Putting silicone in a capsule serves no purpose, it just makes a very good product difficult to apply.

☺ **Fortifying Spray Gel Extra Firm Hold Formula** *($3.44 for 8 ounces)* contains mostly water, film formers, detangling agent, fragrance, slip agents, castor oil, and preservatives. This is a good light- to medium-hold spray gel with minimal stiff and sticky feel.

☺ **Fortifying Spray Gel Firm Hold Formula** *($3.44 for 8 ounces)* is almost identical to the Extra Firm spray gel above and the same comments apply.

☺ **Pro-Vitamin Styling Gel Extra Firm Hold Formula** *($3.44 for 4 ounces)* is a standard, medium-hold gel with a slight stiff, sticky feel.

☺ **Pro-Vitamin Styling Gel Firm Hold Formula** *($3.44 for 4 ounces)* is similar to the Extra Firm Hold above, only with a somewhat more stiff and sticky feel.

☺ **Fortifying Mousse Extra Firm Hold Formula** *($3.44 for 6 ounces)* contains mostly water, propellant, film formers, conditioning agents, castor oil, silicone, slip agents, thickeners, fragrance, and preservatives. This is a very good light-hold mousse with minimal to no stiff or sticky feel.

☺ **Fortifying Mousse Firm Hold Formula** *($3.44 for 6 ounces)* is almost identical to the Extra Firm Hold version above and the same comments apply.

☺ **Pro-Vitamin Hair Spray Extra Firm Hold Formula (Non-Aerosol)** *($3.44 for 8 ounces)* is a standard, light- to medium-firm hold hairspray with a stiff, slightly sticky feel, though it can easily be brushed through. It contains mostly alcohol, water, film formers, conditioning agent, silicones, and fragrance.

☺ **Pro-Vitamin Hair Spray Firm Hold Formula (Non-Aerosol)** *($3.44 for 8 ounces)* is almost identical to the one above and the same comments apply.

☺ **Split End Repair, Repair Formula** *($5.43 for 3 ounces)* contains mostly water, detangling agent, film formers, conditioning agents, thickeners, fragrance, and preservatives. This is more a styling serum than anything else. It can't repair split ends, but it can provide light control with minimal stiff or sticky feel on hair.

Ion

For more information about Ion, call (800) 777-5706.

☺ **Anti-Frizz Smoothing Shampoo** *($3.99 for 12 ounces)* contains mostly water, detergent cleansing agents, lather agent, thickeners, conditioning agent, silicone, detangling agents/film formers, fragrance, and preservatives. This can definitely smooth out frizzies, as any conditioning shampoo can, which makes it good for dry hair. Though the film former in here can add a feel of thickness, it can build up and feel heavy, which can be helpful for fine or thin hair.

☹ **Balanced Cleansing Shampoo with Electro-Bond Proteins** *($4.99 for 16 ounces)* uses C14-16 olefin sulfonate as one of its main detergent cleansing agents, which makes it too drying for all hair types.

☹ **Clarifying Shampoo** *($4.99 for 16 ounces)* uses C14-16 olefin sulfonate as one of its main detergent cleansing agents, which makes it too drying for all hair types.

☹ **Moisturizing Shampoo** *($4.99 for 16 ounces)* uses sodium C14-16 olefin sulfonate and TEA dodecylbenzene sulfonate as the main detergent cleansing agents, which makes it too drying for all hair types.

☺ **Anti-Frizz Leave-in Conditioner** *($4.29 for 12 ounces)* contains mostly water, detangling agent, silicone, conditioning agents, slip agents, preservatives, and fragrance. This is a very good leave-in conditioner for dry hair of any thickness.

☺ **Conditioning Miracle Microwavable Treatment Pac** *($1.99 for 1 ounce)* contains mostly water, detangling agent, thickeners, conditioning agents, slip agents, preservatives, plant oil, silicone, and fragrance. This is a good leave-in conditioner for dry hair of any thickness.

☺ **Effective Care Intensive Therapy Treatment** *($3.99 for 4 ounces)* contains mostly water, detangling agents, film former, thickeners, conditioning agents, preservatives, and fragrance. The claim that this very standard, ordinary conditioner "repairs and restructures from the inside out" is bogus, though it is a good conditioner for normal to slightly dry hair of any thickness.

☺ **Finishing Rinse with Electro-Bond Proteins** *($4.99 for 16 ounces)* is a great conditioning rinse for dry hair of any thickness. It contains mostly water, detangling agents, mineral oil, thickeners, conditioning agents, silicone, plant oil, slip agents, preservatives, and fragrance.

☺ **Moisturizing Treatment** *($4.99 for 4 ounces)* is a great conditioner for dry hair of any thickness. It contains mostly water, detangling agents, thickeners, conditioning agents, plant oils, preservatives, fragrance, and coloring agents.

☺ **Reconstructor Treatment** *($8.99 for 16 ounces)* contains mostly water, slip agent, conditioning agents, detangling agents, thickeners, preservatives, and fragrance. This won't reconstruct one hair on your head but it is a good conditioner for normal to dry hair of any thickness but coarse.

☺ **Finishing Detangler** *($4.99 for 16 ounces)* is a very good leave-in conditioner for dry hair of any thickness. It contains mostly water, detangling agent, mineral oil, thickeners, film former, conditioning agents, silicone, plant oil, more thickeners, preservatives, and fragrance.

☺ **Hot 'N' Moist Intensive Hair and Scalp Treatment** *($1.99 for 1 ounce)* is a standard silicone serum with some conditioning agents. Whether warm or cold it helps make hair feel silky.

☺ **Hot Oil Deep Penetrating Treatment** (*$1.69 for 1 ounce*) is a good conditioner for dry hair though it is nothing more than a basic conditioner. It contains mostly plant water, thickeners, detangling agent, conditioning agents, plant oil, film former, silicone, coloring agents, and fragrance.

☺ **Anti-Frizz Gel Styling Mist** (*$3.99 for 11.5 ounces*) is a basic styling spray that gives a light, combable hold; it contains mostly water, film former, slip agent, plant extracts, silicone, thickener, preservatives, and fragrance.

☺ **Anti-Frizz Styling Gelle for Textured and Maximum Hold Styling** (*$4.19 for 6 ounces*) is a basic styling gel with medium hold and a slight sticky feel. It contains mostly water, film former, silicone, slip agent, thickeners, preservatives, and fragrance.

☺ **Styling Glaze Alcohol-Free Sculpting and Designing Lotion** (*$4.29 for 12 ounces*) contains mostly water, film former, slip agents, detangling agents, conditioning agents, preservatives, and fragrance. This is a standard styling liquid that would be far easier to use in a spray form. It pours out and can be messy. It has light to medium hold and minimal stiff, sticky feel.

☺ **Sculpturing & Designing Lotion with Electro-Bond Proteins** (*$3.99 for 8 ounces*) is identical to the Styling Glaze above and the same comments apply.

☺ **Anti-Frizz Liquid Mousse Styling Spray** (*$3.99 for 12 ounces*) isn't a mousse at all but just a styling spray with medium hold and a slight sticky feel. It contains mostly water, film formers, conditioning agents, silicone, slip agents, and preservatives.

☺ **Styling Mousse Alcohol-Free** (*$4.49 for 10 ounces*) is a standard mousse, similar to the Styling Spray mousse above.

☺ **Hydrolac Hair Spray Extra Firm Humidity-Proof Hold** (*$2.99 for 11 ounces*) is a standard aerosol hairspray that has medium to firm hold and a slight stiff feel that can easily be brushed through. It contains mostly water, film formers, conditioning agent, silicones, slip agents, preservatives, and fragrance.

☺ **Long-Lasting Hold Hair Spray with Electro-Bond Proteins** (*$3.99 for 8 ounces*) is similar to the Hydrolac one above, only in nonaerosol form, but the same basic comments apply.

☺ **Styling Spritz Super Hold for Freeze and Shine Styling, Wet or Dry** (*$3.99 for 8 ounces*) is similar to the Hydrolac above only in nonaerosol form, but the same basic comments apply.

☺ **Flexible Hold Finishing Spray** (*$3.99 for 8 ounces*) is similar to the Hydrolac above only in nonaerosol form, but the same basic comments apply.

☺ **Hard-to-Hold Hair Spray** (*$2.99 for 11 ounces*) is similar to the Hydrolac above and the same comments apply.

☺ **Super Hold Spritz with Electro-Bond Proteins** (*$3.99 for 8 ounces*) is similar to the Hydrolac one above, only in nonaerosol form but the same comments apply.

☺ **Shaping Plus Styling Spray Super Hold for Hard to Control Styles** *($4.99 for 10 ounces)* is similar to the Hydrolac above only in nonaerosol form, but the same comments apply.

☺ **Anti-Frizz Alcohol-Free Hair Spray** *($3.99 for 8 ounces)* is similar to the Hydrolac above only in nonaerosol form, but the same comments apply.

☺ **Hard-to-Hold Hair Spray** *($2.99 for 11 ounces)* is similar to the Anti-Frizz Hair Spray above and the same comments apply.

☺ **Anti-Frizz Oil Free Anhydrous Gloss** *($7.99 for 1.8 ounces)* is a pure, standard silicone serum with a little fragrance and works as well as any other silicone serum.

☺ **Anti-Frizz Glossing Mist** *($6.99 for 4 ounces)* is similar to the Gloss above only in spray form.

☺ **$$$ Crystal Clarifying Treatment** *($1.99 for 0.18 ounce)* makes claims about preventing mineral buildup and it takes chelating ingredients to perform that function. This product definitely contains a "chelating" solution. This one is definitely worth a try but the price is steep for regular use.

ISO

For more information about ISO, call (800) ISO HAIR or visit its Web site at www.hairnet.com.

☹ **Aligning Shampoo, Balances and Refreshes** *($6.49 for 10 ounces)* contains ammonium xylenesulfonate as well as a small amount of sodium lauryl sulfate, which makes it too drying for all hair types.

☺ **Purifying Shampoo, Clarifies and Renews** *($6.49 for 10 ounces)* is a good basic shampoo for all hair types; it contains mostly water, detergent cleansing agents, lather agent, fragrance, preservatives, slip agents, thickeners, and coloring agents. It does contain some barely noticeable conditioning agent but not enough to be remotely a concern for buildup.

☹ **Reviving Shampoo, Moisturizing Shampoo** *($6.49 for 10 ounces)* contains ammonium xylenesulfonate, which makes it too drying for all hair types.

☺ **Nourishing Daily Conditioner** *($17.49 for 33.8 ounces)* contains mostly water, thickeners, silicones, detangling agents, preservatives, conditioning agents, and fragrance. This is a good basic conditioner for dry hair of any thickness.

☺ **Recovery Treatment Intensive Moisturizing Conditioner** *($7.49 for 5 ounces)* is similar to the Nourishing version above and the same comments apply.

☺ **Stress Defense Conditioner Leave-in Protection** *($7.49 for 10 ounces)* is similar to the Nourishing version above, only in leave-in form.

☺ **Mistifying Spray Gel, Firm, Weightless Hold** *($8.49 for 9 ounces)* contains mostly water, film formers, slip agent, silicone, thickeners, preservatives, fragrance, and detangling agent. This is a good spray-on gel for a medium holdwith a somewhat stiff sticky feel. It does brush through, but I wouldn't call this "weightless" hold.

☺ **Smoothie Gel, Texture Tamer** *($8 for 5 ounces)* is almost identical to the Spray Gel above, only in regular gel form, but it basically performs the same way.

☺ **Intensifying Gel, Brilliant Hold and Shine** *($8.49 for 5 ounces)* contains mostly water, film formers, thickeners, silicone, detangling agents, slip agents, fragrance, and preservatives. There are a handful of conditioning agents at the end of the ingredient list but they are barely present and don't have an effect. This is a good styling gel for medium hold with minimal stiff or sticky feel.

☺ **Transforming Foam Volumizing Mousse** *($8.49 for 8 ounces)* contains mostly water, alcohol, film former, thickeners, silicone, preservatives, fragrance, conditioning agents, and propellant. This is a good standard mouse with a light to medium hold and a minimal stiff or sticky feel that does brush through.

☺ **Bouncy Creme, Texture Energizer** *($8 for 10.2 ounces)* contains mostly water, slip agent, thickeners, film former, fragrance, conditioning agents, and preservatives. This is a good styling cream for straightening hair with minimal weight or stiffness, but use sparingly—it can build up and feel heavy.

☺ **Defining Lotion, Liquid Texturizer** *($8.49 for 10 ounces)* contains mostly water, detangling agent, film formers, thickeners, silicone, fragrance, preservatives, and conditioning agents. This is a good styling spray with light hold and minimal to no stiff or sticky feel.

☺ **Creative Hair Spray, Flexible Shaping Spray (Aerosol)** *($8.49 for 10 ounces)* is a standard aerosol hairspray with light to medium and a minimal stiff feel that easily brushes through. It contains mostly alcohol, propellant, film formers, fragrance, silicones, detangling agents, and slip agents.

☺ **Enduring Spritz Firm, Lasting Hold** *($8.49 for 10 ounces)* is almost identical to the Creative Hair Spray above, only this one is in nonaerosol form.

☺ **Ultimate Hold Shaping Spray, Firm Extra Hold (Aerosol)** *($10.49 for 10 ounces)* is a standard aerosol hairspray with medium to firm hold and a somewhat stiff feel that does brush through. It contains mostly alcohol, propellant, film formers, fragrance, silicones, detangling agents, and slip agents.

☹ **SportCleanse Daily Shampoo** *($6.49 for 10 ounces)* uses sodium C14-16 olefin sulfonate as one of the main detergent cleansing agents, which makes it too drying for all hair types.

☺ **SportNourish Moisturizing Conditioner** *($7.49 for 10 ounces)* contains mostly water, thickeners, slip agent, detangling agent, more thickeners, conditioning agents, plant oil, preservatives, more detangling agent, fragrance, and coloring agents. It is a good basic conditioner for normal to slightly dry hair of any thickness. It does contain menthol, so keep it off the scalp to avoid irritation.

☺ **SportMist Leave-in Conditioner** *($7.49 for 10 ounces)* contains mostly water, detangling agent, silicones, slip agents, preservatives, vitamins, conditioning agents, fragrance, and coloring agents. This is a very good leave-in conditioner for dry hair of any thickness.

☺ **SportStyler Firm, Flexible Gel** *($8.49 for 5.1 ounces)* is a standard styling gel with light- to medium-hold and minimal stiff or sticky feel that does brush through. It contains mostly water, film former, thickeners, preservatives, fragrance, and coloring agents.

☺ **SportFinish Shaping Spray (Non-Aerosol)** *($8.49 for 10.2 ounces)* contains mostly alcohol, water, film formers, silicone, slip agent, detangling agent, conditioning agent, fragrance, and coloring agents. It is a good medium to firm hold hairspray with a somewhat stiff, sticky feel though it does brush through.

Jason Natural Cosmetics

Next to Kiss My Face on drugstore or health food store shelves is the prolific, reasonably priced Jason Natural Cosmetics line. As the name implies, Jason Natural is about—surprise!—natural ingredients. According to its brochure, "We believe consumers must have a reliable natural alternative to chemically synthesized, technical-grade products, and to that end we are devoted to developing and manufacturing a wide range of personal care and beauty care products that are truly botanical in origin." However, several of the Jason products contain laureth sulfosuccinate, lauramide DEA, cocamidopropyl betaine, and sodium myreth sulfate, among many others. Now, doesn't that sound natural?

Jason also wants you to know that its information dates back to the ancient Egyptians and that much of their "knowledge of the healing power of herbs and their special effects on the skin was gathered into books during medieval times." Is there really anything from ancient Egypt or medieval Europe that would be of interest to us today? After all, they didn't have sunscreens, they didn't have antibiotics, and mostly they didn't live past 40 (the average life expectancy around the year 1900 was 47). While the notion of ancient folklore is romantic, it is nonsense when it comes to the health of your hair or scalp.

Jason also states that its products don't contain offensive chemical ingredients like the lauryl and laureth sulfates, pore-clogging ingredients, and other known irritants. In its brochure it has a big red stamp saying "No Lauryl Sulfate or Laureth Sulfates." But that's simply not true: some of these products absolutely contain those detergent cleansing agents! Jason also states that its products don't contain artificial preservatives when they absolutely do! Phenoxyethylanol, methylparaben, and propylparaben, to name a few of the preservatives listed on the Jason products, are standard industry preservatives. Not that I think any of those are bad—though sodium lauryl sulfate can be drying and irritating for the hair and scalp. If a company states popular misconceptions about what is natural and what isn't, it should at least live up to its own claims. There are good products to consider here, and the prices are more than reasonable, but the company's distortions of fact are just hard to overlook.

One more point: the ingredient listings for these products are immense. They all contain a range of vitamins that show up at the end of the ingredient listing, and so in amounts too trivial to even mention, which is why I'm only mentioning the insignificance of it here instead of repeating the insignificance for hair in each review.

For more information about Jason Natural Cosmetics, call (800) JASON-05 or visit its Web site at www.jason-natural.com.

☺ **Color Enhancing Shampoo for Black Hair** *($6.95 for 12 ounces)* is a standard but very good color-enhancing shampoo with detergent cleansing agents, conditioning agents, thickeners, fragrance, and dye agents (very unnatural coloring agents). The plant extracts in here serve no purpose.

☺ **Color Enhancing Shampoo for Blonde Hair** *($6.95 for 12 ounces)* is similar to the version above and the same comments apply.

☺ **Color Enhancing Shampoo for Brown Hair** *($6.95 for 12 ounces)* is similar to the versions above and the same comments apply.

☺ **Color Enhancing Shampoo for Red Hair** *($6.95 for 12 ounces)* is similar to the versions above and the same comments apply.

☺ **Color Enhancing Shampoo for Silver/Gray Hair** *($7.25 for 12 ounces)* is similar to the versions above and the same comments apply.

☺ **Color Enhancing Shampoo: A Wild Color Enhancing Shampoo, Fuchsia Fun** *($6.95 for 12 ounces)* is similar to the versions above and the same comments apply.

☺ **Color-Treated, Frizzy, Dry Hair Therapy All Natural Damage Control Creme Shampoo** *($11.79 for 16 ounces)* contains mostly plant water, detergent cleansing agents, lather agent, thickeners, plant extracts, silicone, film former, preservatives, and fragrance. This is a good, standard, silicone-based conditioning shampoo for dry hair of any thickness.

☺ **Extra Rich Natural E.F.A. Shampoo, Hair Nourishing Formula for Normal to Dry Hair** *($5.50 for 17.5 ounces)* contains mostly water, detergent cleansing agents, lather agent, thickeners, plant extracts, conditioning agents, water-binding agents, preservatives, and fragrance. This is a good conditioning shampoo for normal to dry hair of any thickness.

☺ **For Kids Only! Extra Mild Shampoo** *($7.50 for 17.5 ounces)* may be for kids, but there's nothing in here that makes this product better for children. It is similar to the Extra Rich above and the same comments apply.

☺ **Forest Essence Conditioning Shampoo** *($7.09 for 17.5 ounces)* contains mostly plant water, detergent cleansing agents, lather agent, thickeners, plant extracts, conditioning agents, water-binding agents, plant oil, preservatives, and fragrance. This is a good conditioning shampoo for normal to dry hair of any thickness.

☺ **Hemp Enriched Shampoo for All Hair Types** *($7.50 for 17.5 ounces)* is similar to the Forest Essence version above and the same comments apply. The hemp seed oil is a good conditioner but it serves no unique or special purpose for hair.

☺ **Natural Aloe Vera 84% Shampoo, Hair Nourishing Formula** *($5.50 for 17.5 ounces)*. All shampoos are about 80 to 90 percent water, and that's true for this one too: it's just 84% plant water. Other than that it is similar to the Forest Essence version above and the same comments apply.

☺ **Natural Apricot Keratin Shampoo** *($2.30 for 17.5 ounces)* is similar to the Forest Essence version above and the same comments apply.

☹ **Natural Biotin Shampoo** *($5.50 for 17.5 ounces)* contains menthol, which can be drying and irritating for the scalp.

☺ **Natural Henna Highlights Shampoo** *($3.10 for 17.5 ounces)* contains henna, which can build up on hair making it feel heavy and stiff. It would be good for occasional use as a basic shampoo with minimal conditioning agents.

☺ **Natural Jojoba Shampoo; UV protection, Extra Body, Super Shine** *($5.50 for 17.5 ounces)* is similar to the Forest Essence version above and the same comments apply. There are no hair care products, this one included, that can protect from sun damage.

☺ **Natural Vitamin A, C & E Shampoo** *($5.50 for 17.5 ounces)* is similar to the Forest Essence version above and the same comments apply.

☺ **Rich Natural Sea Kelp Shampoo, Concentrated Extra Gentle, Super Shine** *($3.10 for 17.5 ounces)* is similar to the Forest Essence version above and the same comments apply.

☺ **Swimmers & Sports Hair and Scalp Reconditioning Shampoo** *($7.09 for 17.5 ounces)* is similar to the Forest Essence version above, though this one does contain silicone and chelating agents that can be helpful to remove minerals from hair.

☹ **Tall Grass Hi-Protein Shampoo** *($7.09 for 17.5 ounces)* contains peppermint, which can be an irritant for the scalp.

☺ **Tea Tree Oil Hair and Scalp Therapy Shampoo** *($5.99 for 17.5 ounces)* is similar to the Forest Essence version above, though this one does contain a tiny amount of tea tree oil. That can be helpful for dandruff.

☺ **Thin-to-Thick Hair and Scalp Therapy, Hair Thickening Shampoo** *($7.59 for 8 ounces)* contains nothing that would be helpful for preventing hair loss or cleaning out follicles. If anything, the thickening agent in here can clog pores. This does contain salicylic acid in a tiny amount, along with AHAs, but the pH is about 4.5 and that isn't low enough for those to work to exfoliate the scalp—which is great, because if it could exfoliate the scalp it could also denature the hair shaft and cause damage to the cuticle.

☺ **Color Sealant Conditioner for All Shades of Hair, Enhances Shine as It Conditions** *($6.69 for 8 ounces)* contains mostly water, thickeners, silicone, plant extracts, conditioning agent, preservatives, and fragrance. This is a good conditioner for dry hair of any thickness.

☺ **Color-Treated Frizzy, Dry Hair Therapy Creme Conditioner** *($9.49 for 8 ounces)* contains mostly water, plant extracts, thickeners, conditioning agents, detangling agents, film former, silicones, fragrance, and preservatives. This is a very good conditioner for very dry hair of any thickness, but it's best for thick or coarse hair.

☺ **Extra Rich Natural E.F.A. Conditioner, Hair Nourishing Formula for Normal to Dry Hair** *($5.50 for 17.5 ounces)* contains mostly water, thickeners, conditioning agents, detangling agents, plant extracts, water-binding agents, plant oil, preservatives, and fragrance. This is a very good conditioner for dry hair of any thickness.

☺ **For Kids Only! Extra Gentle Conditioner** *($7 for 8 ounces)* contains mostly water, plant extract, thickeners, plant oil, conditioning agents, detangling agent, preservatives, and fragrance. There is nothing about this formulation that makes it better for kids, but it is a good conditioner for dry hair of any thickness.

☺ **Forest Essence Vital Conditioner** *($6.69 for 8 ounces)* is similar to the Kids Only version above and the same comments apply.

☺ **Hemp Enriched Conditioner for All Hair Types, Especially Dry/Damaged Hair** *($7 for 8 ounces)* is similar to the Kids Only version above and the same comments apply.

☹ **Henna Hi-Lights Conditioner** *($3.10 for 17.5 ounces)* contains henna, which can build up on hair making it feel heavy and stiff. It would be good for occasional use as a basic lightweight conditioner for normal to slightly dry hair.

☺ **Natural Aloe Vera 84% Conditioner, Hair Nourishing Formula** *($5.50 for 17.5 ounces)* contains mostly plant water, thickeners, conditioning agents, detangling agents, plant extracts, water-binding agents, plant oil, preservatives, and fragrance. This is a very good conditioner for dry hair of any thickness.

☺ **Natural Apricot Keratin Conditioner** *($3.10 for 17.5 ounces)* is similar to the Natural Aloe version above and the same comments apply.

☺ **Natural Biotin Conditioner** *($5.50 for 17.5 ounces)* is similar to the Natural Aloe version above and the same comments apply.

☺ **Natural Jojoba Conditioner** *($5.50 for 17.5 ounces)* is similar to the Natural Aloe version above and the same comments apply.

☺ **Natural Vitamin A, C & E Conditioner** *($5.50 for 17.5 ounces)* is similar to the Natural Aloe version above and the same comments apply.

☺ **Rich Natural Sea Kelp Conditioner; Concentrated Extra Gentle, Super Shine** *($2.30 for 17.5 ounces)* is similar to the Natural Aloe version above and the same comments apply.

☺ **Swimmers & Sports Hair and Scalp Reconditioning Conditioner** *($6.69 for 8 ounces)* is similar to the Natural Aloe version above and the same basic comments apply. This conditioner does contain a chelating agent that can help prevent minerals from bonding to the hair.

☺ **Tall Grass Hi-Protein Conditioner** *($6.69 for 8 ounces)* is similar to the Natural Aloe version above and the same comments apply.

☹ **Tea Tree Oil Hair and Scalp Therapy Conditioner** *($5.99 for 8 ounces)* is similar to the Natural Aloe version above and the same basic comments apply. This one does contain a tiny amount of tea tree oil, which can be helpful for dandruff, but the other conditioning agents in here would be a problem for an oily scalp and oily hair.

☺ **Thin-to-Thick Hair and Scalp Therapy Hair Thickening Conditioner** *($7.59 for 8 ounces)* is similar to the Natural Aloe version above and the same comments apply.

☺ **All Natural Mousse, All Hair Types** *($7.09 for 7 ounces)* is a mousse dispensed in an aerated container instead of with propellant. It has light to medium hold and minimal sticky feel. It contains mostly water, plant extracts, film formers, conditioning agents, silicone, vitamins, thickeners, fragrance, and preservatives.

☺ **Fresh Botanicals Hairspray Super Style Holding Natural Hold Alcohol Free (Non-Aerosol)** *($4.66 for 8 ounces)* is a standard hairspray with a light hold and a slight sticky feel. It contains mostly water, film former, conditioning agents, preservatives, and fragrance.

☺ **All Natural Hi-Shine Plus for Maximum Shine and UV Protection** *($7.09 for 4 ounces)* is a standard silicone spray like many others. It definitely can help add shine and softness to hair. This product has no ability to protect hair from UV damage.

☺ **All Natural Frizz Control, Repairs Damage and Restores Shine for Smooth, Soft Hair** *($7.09 for 2 ounces)* is similar to the Hi-Shine Plus above only in serum form, and the same comments apply.

☹ **Revitalizing Scalp Elixir** *($7.59 for 2 ounces)* won't revitalize anything, but the plant extracts in here, such as mint, clover, and cypress, can be irritating and sensitizing on the scalp.

J. F. Lazartigue

There are no words to convey how overpriced almost every one of the J. F. Lazartigue products is. From my viewpoint, it is the most outrageously priced hair-care line on the market, yet these products contain nothing unique or special for the hair—and I mean *nothing!* Every standard hair-care ingredient in the book is in here, with nary a new twist of an interesting extra touch. Although I would rather not provide space in this book to a long list of overpriced ridiculous products such as **Deep Action Treatment with Carrot Oil** *($52 for 5 ounces)*, **Pre-Shampoo Cream** with **Shea Butter** *($50 for 6 ounces)*, **Liposome Hair Energizer** *($62 for 2.5 ounces)*, or **Milk Shampoo** *($28 for 8 ounces)*, nevertheless I realize it's necessary. Yet to pay even the slightest attention to these products is to encourage a trend in the hair-care industry similar to that in the skin-care world: the more outrageous the price, regardless of the ordinary ingredients, the more women are convinced they are getting a better product. IT ISN'T TRUE. For what they are worth, which, from my point of view isn't a fraction of their price, here are their evaluations.

For more information on J. F. Lazartigue, call (212) 288-2250, (800) 359-9345, or visit its Web site at www.jflazartigue.com.

☹ **Deep Action Treatment with Carrot Oil, Dry Hair Care Pre-Shampoo** *($52 for 5.07 ounces)* contains mostly water, thickeners, detangling agents, plant extract, plant oil, fragrance, and preservatives. All of these ingredients are completely ordinary. You are supposed to believe that carrot extract, and a minuscule amount of carrot extract at that, can restructure the hair. It can't, not even a little. And this is supposed to be used as a prewash, which means you would be washing it right out when you shampoo.

☺ **Nature L Nourishing Repair Treatment Pre-Shampoo for Dry, Brittle Dull Hair** *($9.99 for 5 ounces)* contains mostly water, thickeners, plant oil, film former, preservatives, slip agent, silicone, fragrance, and coloring agents. As a prewash it is useless because you would just be washing it away, but as a lightweight conditioner for normal to dry hair that is normal to fine or thin, it would work great.

☹ **Pre-Shampoo Cream with Shea Butter** *($51 for 6.8 ounces)* contains mostly water, shea butter, detangling agents, thickeners, slip agent, Vaseline, fragrance, preservatives, and carrot extract. Shampoos wash this stuff out of the hair, but even so, $51 for shea butter and Vaseline—I mean, really!

☹ **Propolis Jelly for Oily Scalp, Oily Hair Care Pre-Shampoo** *($36 for 3.4 ounces)* contains mostly water, alcohol, thickeners, slip agent, water-binding agents, plant extracts, conditioning agent, preservatives, and fragrance. This product is supposed to exfoliate the scalp, and it does contain a tiny amount of salicylic acid (BHA), but the amount of BHA is small and the pH of this product isn't low enough for BHA to be effective. That's actually good, because if it could exfoliate the scalp it would exfoliate hair and eat away at the cuticle.

☹ **After Swimming Shampoo (Salt Neutralizer)** *($19 for 5.1 ounces)* uses TEA-lauryl sulfate as one of its main detergent cleansing agents, which makes it too drying for the hair and too irritating and drying for the scalp.

☹ **Anti Dandruff Shampoo** *($25 for 8.4 ounces)* doesn't contain any active anti-dandruff agents, and is not recommended.

☺ **$$$ Cereal Shampoo Volumizing Treatments Shampoo** *($19 for 5.1 ounces)* is as ordinary a shampoo as it gets. This one contains mostly water, detergent cleansing agent, lather agent, conditioning agent, thickeners, preservatives, film formers, and fragrance. Like any other shampoo that includes standard film formers, this can help make the hair feel thick and the conditioning agents are good for dry hair, but the price is bizarre for what you get.

☹ **Deep Cleansing Shampoo with Fruit Acids to Combat Scalp Imbalances for Healthy Scalps** *($17 for 5.07 ounces)* uses TEA-lauryl sulfate as the main detergent cleansing agent, which makes it too drying for the hair and too irritating and drying for the scalp.

☺ **$$$ Essentials for Curly or Frizzy Hair Nourishing Shampoo, Straightened Hair** *($18 for 6.8 ounces)* contains mostly water, detangling agent, detergent cleansing agent, lather agents, conditioning agents, thickeners, film formers, fragrance, coloring agents, and preservatives. This is a good shampoo for normal to dry hair of any thickness.

☹ **Essentials for Curly or Frizzy Hair Treatment Shampoo, Unstraightened Hair** *($18 for 6.8 ounces)* uses TEA-lauryl sulfonate as one of its main detergent cleansing agents, which makes it too drying for the hair and too irritating and drying for the scalp.

☹ **Micro-Pearl Shampoo for Dry Hair, Dry Hair Care Shampoo** *($32 for 6.8 ounces)* uses TEA-lauryl sulfate as one of its main detergent cleansing agents, which makes it too drying for the hair and too irritating and drying for the scalp.

☹ **Micro-Pearl Shampoo for Oily Hair** *($32 for 6.8 ounces)* uses TEA-lauryl sulfate as one of its main detergent cleansing agents, which makes it too drying for the hair and too irritating and drying for the scalp.

☺ **$$$ Milk Shampoo for Dry Hair, Dry Hair Care Shampoo** *($29 for 8.4 ounces)* contains mostly water, detergent cleansing agent, lather agent, detangling agents/film formers, thickeners, fragrance, conditioning agents, and preservatives. This is a good shampoo for normal to dry hair that is fine or thin. This can make hair feel thicker but the film formers can easily build up.

☹ **Orchid Shampoo, Perfumed Hair Care Shampoo** *($22 for 8.4 ounces)* contains several detergent cleansing agents that can be drying for the hair.

☹ **Rapid Drying Shampoo** *($17 for 5.07 ounces)* uses TEA-lauryl sulfate as one of its main detergent cleansing agents, which makes it too drying for the hair and too irritating and drying for the scalp.

☺ **$$$ Shampoo for Frequent Use Combination Hair Care** *($25 for 8.4 ounces)* is a good but absurdly overpriced shampoo for normal to dry hair that is normal to fine or thin in thickness. It contains mostly water, detergent cleansing agent, lather agent, slip agent, detangling agent, fragrance, and preservatives.

☺ **$$$ Treatment Cream Shampoo with Collagen, Dry Hair Care** *($33 for 6.8 ounces)* contains mostly water, detergent cleansing agent, thickeners, detangling agent, lather agent, film former, slip agent, and preservatives. This is a good basic shampoo for normal to slightly dry fine or thin hair.

☺ **$$$ Anti Dandruff Cream Anti Dandruff Treatments After Shampoo** *($28 for 3.4 ounces)* does contain zinc pyrithione, an effective ingredient for fighting dandruff, but you can get the same active ingredient (used in Head & Shoulders—they invented the technology) for a fraction of the cost. The only benefit to having it in a conditioner as opposed to a shampoo is that it can be left on the scalp without irritating detergent cleansing agents being present.

☺ **$$$ Energizing Elixir After Shampoo for All Hair Types** *($21 for 5.1 ounces)* contains mostly slip agents, detangling agents/film formers, fragrance, conditioning agents, and coloring agents. No matter what the name or price, this is a basic leave-in conditioner for normal to slightly dry hair that is fine or thin in thickness.

☺ **$$$ Essentials for Curly or Frizzy Hair Conditioner Detangling and Nourishing** *($18 for 6.8 ounces)* contains mostly water, thickeners, detangling agents, slip agents, conditioning agent, silicone, fragrance, and preservatives. This is a good leave-in conditioner for normal to dry hair of any thickness.

☺ **$$$ Hair-Body Emulsion Volumizing Treatments After-Shampoo Treatment** *($19 for 5.1 ounces)* contains mostly water, thickeners, slip agents, detangling agents, preservatives, and fragrance. The huge list of negligible ingredients that comes after the preservatives looks impressive but doesn't have much, if any, effect on hair. This is a boring conditioner for normal hair to slightly dry hair.

☹ **Protective Hair Cream, Protection 10** *($21 for 2.54 ounces)* has a protection number, but it's bogus: that is not an SPF. This is a styling cream for straightening hair with silicones, film formers, and a tiny amount of film former, and that's it.

☹ **Protective Hair Milk Sun Protection** *($22 for 2.54 ounces)* does not protect from the sun in the least—this is just a good emollient conditioner that contains mostly water, thickeners, mineral oil, fragrance, and preservatives, and the claim about sun protection is a burn.

☺ **$$$ Vita-Cream with Milk Proteins Dry Hair Care After Shampoo Treatment** *($43 for 6.8 ounces)* contains mostly water, thickeners, detangling agents, film former, silicone, fragrance, preservatives, and coloring agents. This is a good conditioner for normal to dry hair of any thickness.

☺ **$$$ Vita-Cream with Milk-Proteins for Fine Hair, Dry Hair Care** *($43 for 6.8 ounces)* is similar to the Dry Hair Care After Shampoo version above and the same comments apply.

☺ **$$$ Volume Hair Conditioner without Rinse, Volumizing Treatments After Shampoo Treatment** *($22 for 2.54 ounces)* contains mostly water, egg extract, silicone, detangling agent, thickeners, conditioning agent, preservatives, and fragrance. Like any conditioner with this much silicone, this one is good for dry hair of any thickness. It doesn't volumize but it can help when styling to smooth hair and frizzies.

☺ **$$$ Especially for Curly or Frizzy Hair Treatment Oil** *($39 for 3.5 ounces)* contains mostly thickeners, plant oils, fragrance, and preservatives. These are the most overpriced plant oils I've ever seen, but they would be good for dry, coarse, and thick hair.

☺ **$$$ Essentials for Curly or Frizzy Hair, Smoothing Shining Balm** *($20 for 5.1 ounces)* contains only Vaseline, coconut and carrot extract, and fragrance. $20 for Vaseline? This kind of cosmetic insanity should be illegal. It isn't a balm, it's more of a greasy pomade that could work to smooth extremely dry frizzies and stubborn curls but it can easily feel and look oily, so use it minimally.

☺ **$$$ Disentangling Instant Silk Protein Spray** *($18 for 3.4 ounces)* contains mostly water, conditioning agent, detangling agents/film formers, silicone, slip agents, preservatives, and fragrance. This is a good, basic (and overpriced) conditioner for normal to slightly dry hair of any thickness. The film formers can build up on hair and leave a slight sticky feel. Silk protein is just a conditioning agent, and not the source of what helps make hair feel silky—that's what the silicone does.

☺ **$$$ Cereal Hair Mask, Volumizing Treatment After Shampoo Treatment** *($26 for 2.54 ounces)* contains mostly thickeners, conditioning agent, preservatives, and fragrance. This is a good but extremely ordinary conditioner for dry hair of any thickness.

☺ **$$$ Hair Volume Tonic, Root Volumizing Treatments After Shampoo Treatment** *($32 for 3.4 ounces)* contains mostly conditioning agent, water, film formers, fragrance, slip agents, preservatives, and silicone. This styling liquid has a minimal to light hold that can add slight thickness to hair, but not very well, and not better than hundreds of other products for a fraction of the price. This one does actually contain a fractional amount of DNA, although that has no effect whatsoever on hair or scalp. Even the notion that you could change your hair's genetic structure is absurd, but the claims that it is worth this offensive price are not funny.

☹ **Intensive Sebum Treatment for Oily Roots** *($51 for 2.54 ounces)* does contains salicylic acid, though the pH isn't low enough for it to be effective. It also contains 2,3-aminopropane sulfonic acid and sodium scymnol sulfonate, which can be drying to the hair and scalp and irritating for the scalp.

☹ **Marine Hair Care Mask** *($28 for 3.4 ounces)*. Under any name, marine sediment is mud or sand, and that can be drying for the hair.

☺ **$$$ Root Volumizer for Hair, Volumizing Treatments After Shampoo Treatment** *($18 for 2.54 ounces)* contains mostly water, slip agent, silicones, film former, conditioning agents, preservative, and fragrance. This is a standard silicone spray with some film former. That can help dry hair feel smoother, softer, and a little thicker, but it is an understatement to mention that there are far better formulations of this type at the drugstore for a fraction of this price.

☺ **$$$ Hair Styling Gel** *($20 for 3.4 ounces)* contains mostly water, alcohol, slip agent, film formers, thickeners, fragrance, preservatives, and coloring agents. This exceptionally standard styling gel has a light hold with minimal to no stiff or sticky feel.

☺ **$$$ Straightening Gel for Curly Hair, Styling Products After Shampoo** *($17 for 3.4 ounces)* is similar to the gel above, only with a lighter hold.

Jheri Redding

Jheri Redding was a hairdresser in the 1930s and created this line back in the 1960s. Today it is owned by the Conair Corporation. The Redding family went on to create a new line of products separate from this one, called Nexxus.

For more information about Jheri Redding, call (800) 326-6247 or visit its Web site at www.conairpro.com.

☺ **Balsam Shampoo for All Hair Types** *($1.90 for 24 ounces)* contains mostly water, detergent cleansing agents, lather agents, conditioning agents, thickeners, fragrance, preservatives, and coloring agents. This is a good shampoo for slightly dry hair that is normal to fine or thin. The balsam can build up and make hair feel stiff and heavy. The conditioning agents are not appropriate for oily hair.

☺ **Citrus Shampoo for All Hair Types** *($1.90 for 24 ounces)* contains mostly water, detergent cleansing agents, lather agents, thickeners, fragrance, preservatives, and coloring agents. This is a good basic shampoo for all hair types with no conditioning agents to weigh hair down or cause buildup.

☺ **Honey Wheatgerm Shampoo for All Hair Types** *($1.90 for 24 ounces)* is identical to the Citrus version above and the same comments apply. The wheatgerm extract in here is useless for hair.

☺ **Strawberry Shampoo for All Hair Types** *($1.90 for 24 ounces)* is identical to the Citrus version above and the same comments apply. The strawberry scent doesn't affect anything unless you're allergic to strawberry.

☺ **Vanilla Shampoo for All Hair Types** *($1.90 for 24 ounces)* is identical to the Citrus version above and the same comments apply. The wheatgerm extract in here is useless for hair.

☺ **Aloe Vera Conditioner for All Hair Types** *($1.90 for 24 ounces)* contains mostly water, thickeners, detangling agents, film formers, fragrance, slip agents, more fragrance, coloring agents, and preservatives. This is a good basic conditioner for normal to slightly dry hair that is fine or thin. It can cause buildup with repeated use.

☺ **Balsam Conditioner for All Hair Types** *($1.90 for 24 ounces)* contains mostly water, thickeners, detangling agents, balsam, conditioning agents, fragrance, slip agents, fragrance, coloring agents, and preservatives. This is a good basic conditioner for normal to dry hair that is normal to fine or thin. It can cause buildup with repeated use.

☺ **Extra Humidicon Humidifying Conditioner** *($5.99 for 8 ounces)* contains mostly water, thickeners, mineral oil, conditioning agents, detangling agents, slip agents, fragrance, coloring agents, and preservatives. This is a good basic conditioner for dry hair of any thickness.

☺ **Repairers Detangler** *($2.79 for 14 ounces)* doesn't repair anything, but it is a good basic conditioner for normal to dry hair that is normal to fine or thin. It contains mostly water, detangling agent/film former, conditioning agent, silicone, fragrance, and preservatives.

☺ **Extra Bio-Body Biotin Leave-in Treatment for Fine, Weak and Thin Hair** *($5.99 for 8 ounces)* doesn't help strengthen hair. Topically biotin is just an OK conditioning agent, nothing special or superior for hair. This is a good basic conditioner for normal to dry hair of any thickness. It contains mostly water, conditioning agent, detangling agent, silicone, slip agents, fragrance, and preservatives.

☺ **Extra Protein Pac for Extremely Damaged Hair** *($0.99 for 1 ounce)* contains mostly water, thickeners, detangling agent, conditioning agent, lanolin oil, plant oil, vitamins, fragrance, coloring agents, and preservatives. This is a good conditioner for very dry hair of any thickness.

☺ **Natural Protein 100% Natural Conditioner** *($8.49 for 15 ounces)* contains mostly water, conditioning agent, thickener, and vinegar. This is a good simple conditioner for normal to slightly dry hair of any thickness.

☺ **Porofill Conditioner Porosity Equalizer** *($2.99 for 16.5 ounces)* contains mostly water, detangling agent, preservatives, and coloring agent. This is a good simple detangling conditioner for normal to slightly dry hair that is normal to fine or thin in thickness.

☺ **3 in 1 Professional Gel** *($1.89 for 16 ounces)* is a standard styling gel that has a light to medium hold and a slight stiff, sticky feel though it does brush through. It contains mostly water, film former, slip agent, thickeners, conditioning agents, silicone, fragrance, preservatives, and coloring agents.

☺ **Alcohol-Free Straightening Gel** *($2.59 for 16 ounces)* is almost identical to the 3 in 1 Gel above and the same comments apply.

☺ **Alcohol-Free Shine Gel** *($2.79 for 20 ounces)* is similar to the 3 in 1 Gel above only with slightly softer hold and slightly less sticky feel.

☺ **Alcohol-Free Volumizing Gel** *($2.59 for 16 ounces)* is similar to the 3 in 1 Gel above and same comments apply.

☺ **Alcohol-Free Frizz Out Gel** *($2.79 for 20 ounces)* is similar to the 3 in 1 Gel above and the same comments apply.

☺ **Alcohol-Free Mega Hold Gel** *($2.79 for 20 ounces)* is similar to the 3 in 1 Gel above and the same basic comments apply.

☺ **Alcohol-Free Styling Gel Firm Hold** *($2.24 for 8 ounces)* is a standard styling gel that has a light to medium hold with minimal stiff or sticky feel. It contains mostly water, film former, slip agent, thickeners, conditioning agents, silicone, fragrance, preservatives, and coloring agents.

☺ **Alcohol-Free Spray Gel** *($2.24 for 14 ounces)* has soft hold and minimal to no stiff or sticky feel. It contains mostly water, film former, slip agent, thickeners, conditioning agents, silicone, fragrance, preservatives, and coloring agents.

☺ **3 in 1 Professional Mousse, Extra Control** *($2.24 for 8 ounces)* contains mostly water, propellant, film formers, detangling agents, slip agents, fragrance, silicone, and preservatives. This is a good standard mousse with a medium hold and a slight sticky feel.

☺ **Alcohol-Free Mousse, Volumizing Ultra Control (Scented and Unscented)** *($2.24 for 8 ounces)* is similar to the 3 in 1 Mousse above only with slightly softer hold and slightly less sticky feel. The unscented version still contains a masking fragrance.

☺ **Design Spritz, Super Hold (Non-Aerosol) Scented and Unscented** *($2.24 for 14 ounces)* is a standard medium-hold hairspray with a slight stiff feel that does brush through. It contains mostly alcohol, water, film former, fragrance, and silicones.

☺ **Glossing Design Spritz, Super Hold (Aerosol)** *($2.24 for 14 ounces)* is similar to the Design Spritz nonaerosol version above and the same comments apply.

☺ **Flexible Hold Hair Spray (Aerosol)** *($2.59 for 10.5 ounces)* is similar to the Design Spritz nonaerosol version above and the same comments apply.

☺ **Flexible Hold Hair Spray (Non-Aerosol) Scented and Unscented** *($2.24 for 12 ounces)* is similar to the Design Spritz nonaerosol version above and the same comments apply.

☺ **Shine Hair Spray, Super Hold (Aerosol) Scented and Unscented** *($2.24 for 10 ounces)* is similar to the Design Spritz nonaerosol version above and the same comments apply.

☺ **Blow-Dry Activated Thickening Spray** *($2.24 for 6 ounces)* contains mostly water, alcohol, detangling agents/film formers, conditioning agents, silicone, fragrance, slip agents, and preservatives. This is a standard soft-hold styling spray with minimal to no stiff or sticky feel. Like any product with film formers, it can add a feel of thickness but that isn't special or activated by heat.

☺ **Blow-Dry Activated Straightening Lotion** *($2.24 for 6 ounces)* contains mostly water, film former, castor oil, conditioning agent, silicones, fragrance, thickeners, and preservatives. As the name implies, this is a good straightening lotion for styling curly hair and frizzies smooth. It has light hold and a slight sticky feel. Use this minimally or it can easily make hair look heavy and flat.

☺ **Curl Energizer Frizz Control** *($2.24 for 14 ounces)* is a light hold styling spray with minimal to no stiff or sticky feel. It can help with any styling need; it's the tools and brushes that will make the difference. It contains mostly water, alcohol, detangling agents/film formers, conditioning agents, fragrance, slip agents, preservatives, and silicone.

☺ **Frizz Out Hair Serum** *($2.53 for 1.5 ounces)* is a standard silicone serum with a little fragrance that works great for adding shine and adding a silky feel to dry hair.

Professional Prescription by Jheri Redding

☹ **Absolute Shampoo for Normal to Fine Hair** *($4.99 for 15 ounces)* uses sodium lauryl sulfate as the main detergent cleansing agent, which makes it too drying for the hair and too irritating and drying for the scalp.

☺ **Biotin Shampoo for Fine, Thin, or Weak Hair** *($4.99 for 15 ounces)* contains mostly water, detergent cleansing agents, lather agents, plant oil, water-binding agents, silicone, fragrance, preservatives, and coloring agents. This product contains DNA and biotin, but those have no effect on hair strength. Biotin is an OK conditioning agent, and it sounds strong, but that isn't the effect it has on hair. This is just a good shampoo for normal to dry hair of any thickness.

☹ **Curative Daily Strengthening Shampoo for Dry, Weak, or Chemically Treated Hair** *($5.49 for 12 ounces)* uses sodium lauryl sulfate as one of its main detergent cleansing agents, which makes it too drying for the hair and too irritating and drying for the scalp.

☹ **Curative Strengthening Shampoo for Fine, Weak, or Chemically Treated Hair** *($5.49 for 12 ounces)* uses sodium lauryl sulfate as one of its main detergent cleansing agents, which makes it too drying for the hair and too irritating and drying for the scalp.

☹ **Tea Tree Deep Cleanse for Normal to Oily Hair** *($5.99 for 15 ounces)* contains mostly water, detergent cleansing agent, lather agent, tea tree oil, conditioning agents, thickeners, film former, silicone, detangling agent, fragrance, slip agent, preservatives, and coloring agents. Tea tree oil is a disinfectant that may be helpful for dandruff, but it has no benefit for oily scalp or hair. The conditioners and silicone in here can be a problem for oily scalp.

☹ **Transpose Shampoo for Dry, Sun-Damaged, or Chemically Treated Hair** *($4.49 for 15 ounces)* uses sodium lauryl sulfate as one of the main detergent cleansing agents, which makes it too drying for the hair and too irritating and drying for the scalp.

☺ **Curative Body Building Conditioner for Fine, Limp Hair** *($5.99 for 12.5 ounces)* contains mostly water, conditioning agents, thickeners, detangling agents, fragrance, silicones, and preservatives. This is a very good basic conditioner for dry hair that is normal to fine or thin.

☺ **Curative Daily Strengthening Conditioner for Fine, Weak, or Chemically Treated Hair** *($5.99 for 12.5 ounces)* is similar to the Body Building version above and the same comments apply.

☺ **Enforce Conditioner for Normal to Slightly Damaged Hair** *($8.49 for 33.8 ounces)* contains mostly water, thickeners, conditioning agents, plant extracts, detangling agents/film formers, fragrance, coloring agents, and more fragrance. This is a good lightweight conditioner for normal to slightly dry hair that is any thickness but coarse.

☺ **Humectin Humidifier for Dry, Dull, Damaged Hair** *($3.99 for 8 ounces)* contains mostly water, thickeners, mineral oil, conditioning agents, detangling agents, preservatives, film formers, fragrance, and coloring agents. This is a good conditioner for dry hair that is thick or coarse.

☺ **Keratin Reconstructor for Severely Damaged Hair** *($8.49 for 33.8 ounces)* contains mostly water, thickeners, conditioning agents, detangling agent, plant oil, film formers, plant extracts, fragrance, and preservatives. This is a good conditioner for normal to dry hair of any thickness. This product does contain RNA and DNA, but the notion that these can affect hair because they have genetic origins is bogus.

☹ **Tea Tree Conditioner for Normal to Oily Hair** *($8.49 for 33.8 ounces)* does contain tea tree oil, which can be a possible option for treating dandruff, but the conditioning agents in here would be a problem for oily scalp. This would be an option for someone with dandruff and dry hair and scalp.

☺ **Biotin Leave-in Treatment for Fine, Thin, Weak Hair** *($4.99 for 8 ounces)* is a good standard leave-in conditioner for normal to dry hair that is fine or of thin to normal thickness. This contains mostly water, conditioners, detangling agent, film former, silicone, slip agents, fragrance, and preservatives. The biotin is an OK conditioning agent, but it is not inherently better for the hair than any other conditioning agents.

☺ **Super Protein Pac for Extremely Damaged Hair, pH Balanced Formula** *($4.99 for 8 ounces)* contains mostly water, thickeners, detangling agent, conditioning agents, lanolin oil, plant oil, fragrance, preservatives, and coloring agents. This is a very good conditioner for very dry, coarse, or thick hair. The vitamins in here have no impact on the hair.

☺ **Hot Oil Treatment for Dry, Brittle, and Dull Hair** *($5.49 for 4 ounces)* contains mostly water, slip agent, film former, conditioning agents, silicone, plant oil, fragrance, and coloring agents. This is a very good conditioner for very dry coarse or thick hair.

☺ **Replenishing Hair Shiner for All Hair Types** *($7.49 for 4 ounces)* is a silicone serum with a tiny amount of conditioning agents. It works well for dry hair of any thickness to add shine and a silky feel. It can't heal cuticles or split ends though.

☺ **Replenishing Mica Spray Polish for Normal, Dry, Damaged, or Chemically Treated Hair** *($4.99 for 4 ounces)* is identical to the Hair Shiner above, only this one is in spray form.

☺ **Gelle Polish for Normal to Dry Hair** *($4.49 for 8 ounces)* is a standard styling lotion with light- to medium-hold that has a good amount of silicone, which helps when smoothing frizzies and styling hair straight. It contains mostly water, film formers, silicones, conditioning agent, thickeners, fragrance, preservatives, and coloring agents.

☺ **Styling Gel for All Hair Types** *($4.49 for 6 ounces)* contains mostly water, film formers, slip agents, thickeners, plant extracts, fragrance, and preservatives. This is a good light to medium gel with minimal stiff or sticky feel.

☺ **Replenishing Polishing Mousse for Normal to Dry Hair** *($4.49 for 9 ounces)* contains mostly water, propellant, film former, plant extracts, conditioning agents, silicones, fragrance, detangling agent, and preservatives. This is a good light to medium hold mousse with minimal sticky feel.

☺ **Styling Spray for All Hair Types** *($4.49 for 8 ounces)* contains mostly alcohol, water, film former, conditioning agent, silicone, and fragrance. This is a good standard hairspray with light to medium hold that can have minimal stiff feel.

☺ **Ultra Hold Hair Spray for All Hair Types** *($2.69 for 11 ounces)* is similar to the Styling Spray above, only with firm hold, and the same comments apply.

☹ **Curative Strengthening Treatment for all Hair Types** *($5.49 for 4.5 ounces)* includes nothing that will strengthen hair. It is just a basic conditioner that contains mostly water, conditioning agents, film former, detangling agents, fragrance, and preservatives. There is no unique or special ingredient that could deliver on the strengthening claim.

Jhirmack

For more information about Jhirmack (owned by Playtex Beauty Care), call (800) 222-0453.

☺ **EFA Moisturizing Shampoo for Dry/Color Treated or Permed Hair** *($3.69 for 20 ounces)* contains mostly water, detergent cleansing agent, lather agent, thickeners, conditioning agents, detangling agent, plant oils, fragrance, preservatives, and coloring agents. This is a good shampoo for very dry hair.

☺ **Gelave Strengthening Shampoo for Normal Hair** *($3.69 for 20 ounces)* contains mostly water, detergent cleansing agent, lather agent, conditioning agents, detangling agent, fragrance, preservatives, and coloring agents. This is a good shampoo for normal to slightly dry hair of any thickness but coarse. The amount of conditioners in here shouldn't cause a problem with buildup.

☹ **Nutri-Body Volumizing Shampoo for Fine, Thin Hair** *($3.69 for 20 ounces)* uses sodium C14-16 olefin sulfonate as one of its main detergent cleansing agents, which makes it too drying for all hair types.

☺ **Shine Shampoo for All Hair Types** *($3.69 for 20 ounces)* contains mostly water, detergent cleansing agent, lather agent, conditioning agents, silicone, fragrance, slip agent, thickeners, preservatives, and coloring agents. This is a good shampoo for normal to dry hair of any thickness but coarse.

☺ **Silver Brightening Shampoo for Gray, Bleached, or Highlighted Hair** *($3.69 for 20 ounces)* includes violet dye agents that can slightly improve the yellow cast of gray hair. Other than that, this is identical to the Gelave shampoo above and the same comments apply.

☺ **EFA Moisturizing Conditioner for Dry, Permed and Color Treated Hair** *($3.69 for 20 ounces)* contains mostly water, thickeners, detangling agents/film formers, conditioning agent, plant oils, fragrance, preservatives, and coloring agents. This is a good conditioner for dry hair that is fine or of thin to normal thickness. It can easily cause buildup with repeated use.

☺ **Nutri-Body Volumizing Conditioner for All Hair Types** *($2.70 for 11 ounces)* is similar to the EFA conditioner above and the same basic comments apply.

☺ **Shine Conditioner for All Hair Types** *($2.70 for 11 ounces)* is similar to the EFA conditioner above and the same basic comments apply.

☺ **Silver Brightening Conditioner for Gray, Bleached, or Highlighted Hair** *($3.69 for 20 ounces)* is similar to the EFA conditioner above and the same basic comments apply.

☺ **Alcohol-Free Sculpting Gel** *($2.99 for 4 ounces)* contains mostly water, slip agent, detangling agents/film formers, conditioning agents, thickener, preservatives, and fragrance. This is a good basic gel with a light hold and minimal to no stiff or sticky feel.

☺ **Spray Styling Gel** *($2.72 for 8.4 ounces)* contains mostly water, film former, slip agent, silicone, thickeners, conditioning agents, more thickener, lanolin oil, preservatives, and fragrance. This is a good styling spray for smoothing stubborn curls or frizzies, with a light to medium hold and a slight stiff or sticky feel that can easily be brushed through.

☺ **Extra Hold Hairspray Level 2 (Non-Aerosol) Scented and Unscented** *($2.99 for 8.4 ounces)* is a standard hairspray with light to medium hold and a slight stiff, sticky feel that does brush through easily. It contains mostly alcohol, water, film former, conditioning agent, silicone, and fragrance.

☺ **Silver Extra Hold Hairspray Level 2 (Aerosol)** *($2.99 for 7 ounces)* contains nothing that makes it better for silver hair. It is similar to the Freeze Quick Level 4 aerosol above and the same comments apply.

☺ **Ultimate Hold Hairspray Level 3 (Non-Aerosol)** *($2.99 for 8.4 ounces)* is a good light to medium hold hairspray with a slight stiff, sticky feel that does allow you to brush through. It contains mostly alcohol, water, film former, conditioning agent, silicone, and fragrance.

☺ **Freeze Quick Drying Hairspray Level 4 (Aerosol)** *($2.99 for 7 ounces)* contains mostly alcohol, propellant, film former, conditioning agent, silicone, slip agents, and fragrance. This is a good medium- to firm-hold hairspray with a slight stiff feel.

☺ **Freeze Quick Drying Hairspray Level 4 (Non-Aerosol)** *($2.99 for 8.4 ounces)* is similar to the Freeze Quick aerosol version above and the same comments apply.

☺ **Styling Spritz, Extra Hold Styling on Dry or Damp Hair** *($2.99 for 8.4 ounces)* is similar to the Extra Hold Level 2 nonaerosol above and the same comments apply. This is far better as a hairspray than as a styling spray. It has a soft hold with minimal stiff or sticky feel.

☺ **HeatCare Styling Protectant** *($2.99 for 7.7 ounces)* contains nothing that can prevent a curling iron or blow dryer at temperatures over 200 degrees Fahrenheit from damaging hair. This is just a good, exceptionally lightweight silicone spray that is more of a leave-in conditioner for normal hair than it is a styling product. It has no hold and no real texture or feel on hair. It contains mostly water, conditioning agent, silicone, thickener, detangling agent, fragrance, preservatives, and coloring agents.

John Frieda

John Frieda is a hair designer who made his mark by being one of the first to introduce women with coarse, frizzy hair to the wonders of smoothing their wild tresses by using pure silicone or heavily silicone-based products. It probably goes without saying that Frieda's Frizz-Ease products never worked remotely as well in real life as they did in the before-and-after pictures that graced the ads for those products, but they did make a significant difference in the feel of the hair and how it looked after styling. An entire line of products grew up around Frizz-Ease, with some of the products worth considering and others definitely not an option.

Frieda's Sheer Blonde is a separate line of shampoos and conditioners aimed at a very specific hair color. Technically, there's no reason to aim a shampoo formula at a hair color. Hair color has nothing to do with hair's texture, dryness, coarseness, thickness, or the amount of damage present, not to mention the fact that hair color has nothing to do with the condition of the scalp! If you consider that a hair product might have color additives that can add a bit of temporary highlighting, that would be of interest, but shampoos can't deposit coloring agents on the hair shaft very well because the detergent cleansing agents in them tend to keep that from happening. Besides, shampoo needs to be geared to hair type not hair color, and all shampoos should be formulated so that they won't strip hair color. And even supposing that there were a shampoo formula that could be beneficial to a specific hair color, the two Sheer Blonde shampoos here contain TEA-lauryl sulfate as the second ingredient, which is just too drying and irritating for the hair and scalp, not to mention being a potential risk for irritation when it comes in contact with the skin. The Sheer Blonde conditioners, on the other hand, are quite suitable for fine, thin, slightly dry hair, and they do have subtle color additives appropriate for the hair colors indicated.

For more information on John Frieda, call (203) 762-1233 or (800) 521-3189.

Sheer Blonde by John Frieda

☹ **Highlight Activating Shampoo for Natural, Color-Treated or Highlighted Blondes, Formulated for Use on Honey to Caramel Blondes** (*$5.83 for 8.45 ounces*) uses TEA-lauryl sulfate as one of the main detergent cleansing agents, which makes it too drying for the hair and too irritating and drying for the scalp.

☹ **Highlight Activating Shampoo for Natural, Color-Treated or Highlighted Blondes, Formulated for Use on Platinum to Champagne Blondes** (*$5.83 for 8.45 ounces*) uses TEA-lauryl sulfate as one of the main detergent cleansing agents, which makes it too drying for the hair and too irritating and drying for the scalp.

☺ **Instant Conditioner and Highlight Enhancer, Formulated for Use on Honey to Caramel Blondes** (*$5.83 for 8.45 ounces*) contains mostly water, thickeners, plant oil, detangling agents, conditioning agent, preservatives, and dye agents. This is a good color-enhancing conditioner for dry hair of any thickness.

☺ **Instant Conditioner and Highlight Enhancer, Formulated for Use on Platinum to Champagne Blondes** (*$5.83 for 8.45 ounces*) is almost identical to the one above and the same comments apply.

☺ **Blonde Ambition Dual Action Mousse for Natural, Color-Treated, or Highlighted Blondes** (*$4.86 for 7.5 ounces*) contains mostly water, film former, alcohol, propellant, silicone, conditioning agent, castor oil, preservatives, fragrance, and coloring agent. This is a good basic mousse with light hold and a slight sticky feel. The purple color is not the best color enhancement for blonde hair other than to tone overtones of brassy yellow.

☺ **Golden Opportunity Glossing and Grooming Creme** (*$5.83 for 4.4 ounces*) contains mostly water, plant oil, slip agents, thickeners, silicone, film former, conditioning agents, detangling agents, preservatives, fragrance, and coloring agents. This is a good hair-straightening cream with a light hold and a slight sticky feel. It brushes through easily. The lavender color this product has can add a hint of shiny blue to lighter hair colors.

☺ **Spun Gold for Natural, Color-Treated, or Highlighted Blondes, Shaping and Highlighting Balm** *($5.49 for 1.2 ounces)* has a great name for what's just a very heavy wax that has sparkles and a tacky, sticky feel. It contains mostly Vaseline, mineral oil, fragrance, and coloring agents. When styling it can help to smooth stubborn frizzies and curls, but the weight and tacky feel aren't the best and as you brush your hair the sparkles can flake off and get all over.

Frizz-Ease by John Frieda

☺ **Corrective Shampoo and Shiner, Conditioning and Glossing Formula** *($4.14 for 12.7 ounces)* contains mostly water, detergent cleansing agents, lather agents, thickeners, silicones, detangling agents/film formers, fragrance, and preservatives. This is a good, silicone-based shampoo that can work well for dry hair; the film formers can add a feel of thickness, but they can also easily build up with repeated use.

☺ **Glistening Creme Conditioner** *($4.50 for 8 ounces)* contains mostly water, thickeners, silicones, detangling agents, conditioning agents, thickeners, plant oil, fragrance, and preservatives. This is a very good conditioner for dry hair that is normal to coarse in thickness.

☺ **Prescription Oils, Hot Oil Treatment, with Natural Oils and Vitamin E** *($4.99 for 1.8 ounces)* contains mostly slip agents, plant oils, lanolin oil, silicone, conditioning agent, and fragrance. These are good oils for dry hair, but the price is absurd given that you can get the same effect from just using some canola oil from your cupboard.

☺ **Hair Serum** *($13.09 for 3 ounces)* is an overpriced standard silicone serum that works great to add shine and a silky feel to hair.

☺ **Instant Touch-up, Serum Spray** *($6.30 for 3 ounces)* contains mostly alcohol, silicones, slip agent, and fragrance. It's similar to the Serum above only in spray form.

☺ **Corrective Styling Gel with Encapsulated Silicone** *($3.14 for 4 ounces)* is an extremely standard gel with medium hold and a slight sticky feel that contains mostly water, film former, thickeners, slip agents, preservatives, fragrance, silicone, coloring agents, and preservatives.

☺ **Corrective Styling Mousse** *($4.14 for 6 ounces)* contains mostly water, propellant, film former, silicone, conditioning agent, castor oil, preservatives, and fragrance. This is a good standard mousse for a medium hold; it has a slight sticky feel.

☺ **Secret Weapon Styling Creme with 24-Hour Conditioning Action** *($4.99 for 4 ounces)* has a great name, though it's only a standard styling lotion. It contains mostly water, plant oil, silicone, slip agents, thickeners, film former, detangling agent, conditioners, preservatives, fragrance, and coloring agents. This is a good hairstyling cream for straightening hair, with light hold and a minimal to slight sticky feel. This can feel heavy so use it minimally.

☺ **Moisture Barrier Hair Spray (Aerosol)** *($3.14 for 10 ounces)* includes only standard hairspray ingredients, and they don't protect against moisture any better than any other hairspray on the market. This is just a good standard aerosol hairspray with a light to medium hold and minimal to no stiff or sticky feel that easily brushes through hair. It contains mostly water, propellant, film former, fragrance, silicones, and conditioning agent.

☺ **Shape and Shine Flexible Hold Hair Spray (Non-Aerosol)** *($4.14 for 10 ounces)* has a finish that is more stiff than it is flexible; it contains mostly alcohol, water, film former, fragrance, silicones, and conditioning agent.

☺ **5-Minute Manager, Blow-Dry Lotion** *($3.14 for 6.7 ounces)* is a standard styling spray that contains mostly water, film former, silicone, fragrance, and preservatives. It can provide light hold with minimal to no stiff or sticky feel. It can help for a light hold when styling hair, but nothing in here will shorten the time it normally takes to style your hair.

Ready to Wear by John Frieda

☺ **Custom Cleansing and Glistening Shampoo, Tailored for Dry/Chemically Treated Hair** *($4.59 for 11 ounces)* contains mostly water, detergent cleansing agents, lather agents, thickeners, silicones, detangling agents/film formers, fragrance, and preservatives. This is a good silicone-based shampoo that can be helpful for dry hair; the film formers can add a feel of thickness, but they can also easily build up with repeated use.

☺ **Custom Cleansing and Thickening Shampoo, Tailored to Thicken and Shine Fine/Limp Hair** *($4.59 for 11 ounces)* contains mostly water, detergent cleansing agents, lather agents, conditioning agent, detangling agent/film former, fragrance, and preservatives. It's a good shampoo for dry hair that is fine or thin. The film former in here can cause buildup.

☺ **Miracle Mend, Deep Penetrating Conditioner** *($4.99 for 4 ounces)* contains mostly water, thickeners, detangling agents, plant oil, silicone, conditioning agents, preservatives, fragrance, and coloring agents. This isn't a miracle in the least, it's just a good basic conditioner for dry hair that is normal to coarse.

☺ **Miraculous Recovery Conditioning Treatment, Professional Strength** *($6.37 for 4 ounces)* is almost identical to the one above and the same comments apply.

☺ **Wear and Tear Repair, Instant Conditioner and Shiner** *($4.59 for 11 ounces)* contains mostly water, thickeners, detangling agents, film former, conditioning agents, silicone, preservatives, and fragrance. This is a good conditioner for normal to dry hair that is fine or thin.

☺ **Quick Coif, Thickening and Conditioning Mousse** *($4.59 for 7.5 ounces)* is an exceptionally standard mousse with light to medium hold and a minimal to slight sticky feel. It contains mostly water, film former, alcohol, propellant, silicone, conditioning agent, castor oil, preservatives, and fragrance.

☺ **Shaping and Glossing Balm** *($4.58 for 0.9 ounce)* comes in a shoe polish–type metal container and the texture is reminiscent of shoe polish. It is Vaseline, mineral oil, fragrance, and coloring agents! It has a very heavy, waxy hold, and a slight tacky feel, but when used minimally it can help smooth out stubborn frizzies and curls.

☺ **Thickening Lotion, Instant Makeover for Fine/Limp Hair** *($6.89 for 4.2 ounces)* contains mostly alcohol, water, film former, thickener, and fragrance. This is a good standard styling spray with a light hold and no stiff or sticky feel. It can help add a layer of film former over the hair and that can make it feel thicker, but so can any lightweight styling spray.

☺ **Modeling Spray, Flexible Hold Spritz (Non-Aerosol)** *($4.59 for 6.7 ounces)* is a good hairspray with light to medium hold and minimal to no stiff or sticky feel, and it brushes through easily. It contains mostly alcohol, water, film former, silicone, conditioning agents, and fragrance.

Johnson & Johnson

Johnson & Johnson's 1967 patent established the mild, nonirritating capacity of the amphoteric group of detergent cleansing agents, of which the primary ingredient is cocamidopropyl betaine, and set a landmark for baby shampoo. Nowadays, Johnson & Johnson's baby shampoos, as well as most baby shampoos on the market, use a combination of detergent cleansing agents to lower irritancy and improve detergent cleansing, but they are still almost always more gentle than adult versions.

What would really make Johnson & Johnson's and all hair-care products for kids more gentle is the elimination of fragrance and coloring agents. While you may assume that special care has been taken to use only ingredients that will be the most gentle to your baby's skin, that assumption is not truly accurate. Think now about the wafting, appealing fragrances emanating from most all baby products; therein lies a major problem, one that makes me leery of using baby products for anyone's skin, let alone a baby's! Products for babies and young children are usually highly fragranced. That delicious, recognizable aroma you could smell a mile away is nothing more than added fragrance and can cause irritation. Moreover, baby products almost always have a pretty yellow or pink tint, which is contrived by coloring agents, another group of problematic skin-care ingredients for sensitive skin. If baby products were really more gentle than what adults put on their skin, they would be fragrance free and contain no coloring agents, but, sadly, few of those exist. (Only one Johnson & Johnson product eliminates fragrance and coloring agents.)

For more information about Johnson & Johnson, call (908) 874-1000, (800) 526-3967, or visit its Web site at www.johnsonandjohnson.com.

☺ **Kids 2-in-1 Shampoo** *($2.99 for 9 ounces)* is a great gentle shampoo that would work great for a child's hair and not bother the eyes all that much. The conditioning agent is silicone and there's a tiny amount of film former, just as in most two-in-one shampoos.

☺ **Kids No More Tangles Shampoo** *($2.99 for 9 ounces)* is identical to the one above and the same comments apply.

☺ **Kids Xtreme Clean Shampoo** *($2.99 for 9 ounces)* has slightly more detergent cleansing agent than the previous two but it is still not an "extreme" detergent cleansing shampoo. The tiny amount of film former in here would not cause a problem for buildup.

☺ **No More Tears Baby Shampoo** *($3.49 for 20 ounces)* is almost identical to the Xtremeone above and the same comments apply.

☺ **No More Tears Baby Shampoo 2-in-1 Detangler** *($3.49 for 20 ounces)* is almost identical to the Xtreme one above and the same comments apply.

☺ **No More Tears Baby Shampoo Moisturizing Formula with Honey and Vitamin E** *($2.89 for 15 ounces)* is almost identical to the Xtreme one above and the same comments apply. The tiny amounts of vitamin E and honey in here have no effect on hair.

☺ **Ultra Sensitive Baby Shampoo** *($2.73 for 6.75 ounces)* isn't that much different from the above products when it comes to detergent cleansing, though it does eliminate fragrance and coloring agents, and that's great.

☺ **Kids No More Bed-Head Spray** *($2.99 for 10 ounces)* is a very good basic detangling spray for dry hair of any thickness; it contains mostly water, detangling agent, silicone, slip agents, fragrance, and preservatives.

☺ **Kids No More Tangles Spray Detangler** *($2.99 for 10 ounces)* is identical to the Bed-Head spray above and the same comments apply.

☺ **No More Tears Baby Gentle Detangler** *($2.49 for 20 ounces)* is similar to the one above, only without the silicone and with the addition of a small amount of film former. This one is OK, but the two above do a better job and provide a softer feel on the hair.

Joico

Joico's claim to hair-care recognition over the years has been something called Triamine Complex. It is nothing more than hydrolyzed human hair keratin protein. Although it sounds like human hair protein should be able to bond better to hair and provide better conditioning, the reality is that once you take hair and get the protein molecules out and then hydrolyze them, the hair is no longer hair, it is just another protein. That makes Triamine Complex a good conditioning agent, but no better than lots of other conditioning agents used in hair-care products.

For more information about Joico, call (800) 44 JOICO or visit its Web site at www.joico.com.

Blue Line by Joico

☺ **Biojoba Treatment Shampoo** *($8.60 for 8.45 ounces)* contains mostly water, detergent cleansing agent, lather agent, thickener, conditioning agent, film former, plant oils, fragrance, and preservatives. This is a good shampoo for dry hair that is fine or thin to help make it feel thicker. The film former can cause buildup.

☺ **Kerapro Conditioning Shampoo for Normal to Dry & Chemically Treated Hair** *($5.40 for 8.45 ounces)* is similar to the Biojoba above and the same comments apply.

☺ **Lavei Extra Body Shampoo for Fine/Limp Oily Hair** *($4.90 for 8.45 ounces)* is similar to the Biojoba above, only with reduced amounts of conditioner and plant oil. The small quantity of conditioning agents in here is still a problem for oily hair. It can be a good shampoo for normal hair that is fine or thin.

☺ **Resolve Deep Cleansing Chelating Shampoo** *($6.30 for 8.45 ounces)* does contain chelating agents and than can help get rid of mineral buildup in the hair. Other than that, it's a good shampoo with a negligible amount of conditioning agents, so it would work well for most hair types.

☺ **Triage Moisture Balancing Shampoo for Normal Hair** *($5.80 for 8.45 ounces)* is similar to the Biojoba above only with slightly more plant oil, which makes this one slightly better for drier hair.

☺ **Volissima Volumizing Shampoo** *($6.95 for 8.45 ounces)* is similar to the Biojoba above, only with silicone instead of plant oil. The same basic comments still apply.

☺ **Lite Instant Detangler and Conditioner** *($5.50 for 8.45 ounces)* contains mostly water, detangling agents, thickeners, castor oil, slip agent, conditioning agents, fragrance, preservatives, and silicone. This is a good conditioner for dry hair but it isn't all that "lite." It can work well for hair that is normal to fine or thin in thickness.

☺ **Moisturizer Moisture Balancer** *($7.25 for 4.4 ounces)* contains mostly water, thickeners, detangling agents, conditioning agents, Vaseline, film former, fragrance, and preservatives. This is a good basic conditioner for dry, coarse, thick hair.

☺ **Phine Conditioning Chelating Treatment** *($6 for 4.4 ounces)* contains mostly water, thickeners, detangling agent, conditioning agent, preservatives, fragrance, and coloring agents. This is a good basic conditioner for normal to slightly dry hair of any thickness but coarse.

☺ **Volissima Volumizing Reconditioner** *($7.95 for 8.45 ounces)* contains mostly water, thickeners, silicones, conditioning agents, detangling agents, film former, slip agents, preservatives, and fragrance. This is a very good conditioner for dry hair of any thickness, though it isn't all that volumizing.

☺ **Altima Protective Leave-in Reconditioner** *($8.60 for 8.45 ounces)* contains mostly water, thickeners, silicone, conditioning agents, plant oil, detangling agents, preservatives, and fragrance. This is a very good leave-in conditioner for dry hair of any thickness but fine or thin. It does contain a tiny amount of tea tree oil, which can be effective for dandruff, but there probably isn't enough in here to serve that purpose. Tea tree oil has no benefit for the hair shaft.

☺ **Integrity Leave-in Reconditioning Treatment** *($8.60 for 8.45 ounces)* contains mostly water, silicones, thickeners, detangling agents, conditioning agents, preservatives, and fragrance. This is a very good leave-in conditioner for dry hair of any thickness but fine or thin.

☺ **H.K.P. Liquid Protein Hair Reconstructor** *($10 for 8.45 ounces)* is a good leave-in conditioner for normal to slightly dry hair. It has no special ability to repair hair or change hair in any fashion, other than temporarily, just like any other conditioner. You have to wonder, if this "reconstructor" worked, why would Joico need to provide all the other products in its line that make the exact same claim?

☺ **K-Pak Deep Penetrating Creme Hair Reconstructor** *($15.95 for 6.6 ounces)* contains mostly water, thickeners, mineral oil, conditioning agents, fragrance, plant oil, and preservatives. This is a good conditioner for dry hair of any thickness but fine or thin. It isn't any more penetrating or reconstructing than any other conditioner.

☺ **Nucleic Pak Moisturizing Creme Hair Reconstructor** *($12.20 for 4.4 ounces)* contains mostly water, thickeners, detangling agent, plant oil, slip agent, conditioning agent, fragrance, preservatives, and coloring agents. This is a good basic conditioner for normal to slightly dry hair of any thickness.

☺ **Shade Endurance Color Sealant with Antioxidants and UVA-UVB Protection** *($7.95 for 8.45 ounces)*. This product cannot protect hair from the sun. Without an SPF number, the claim about any UVA and UVB protection is bogus. This is a good leave-in conditioner for normal to dry hair of any thickness, but that's it.

☺ **JoiGel Styling Gel** *($7.95 for 8.8 ounces)* is a lightweight, almost no-hold styling gel that contains mostly water, thickeners, conditioning agents, fragrance, preservatives, and coloring agents. That can help for smoothing hair with no stiff or sticky feel whatsoever.

☺ **Spray Gel Liquid Styling Gel** *($6.70 for 8.45 ounces)* is a good styling spray with light to medium hold that has minimal to no stiff or sticky feel. It contains mostly water, film formers, conditioning agent, slip agent, silicone, preservatives, and fragrance.

☺ **Volissima Volumizing Gel** *($9.50 for 8.45 ounces)* contains mostly water, film formers, conditioning agents, silicone, fragrance, and preservatives. This is a good medium-hold gel with minimal stiff or sticky feel. It works the same as any gel, which means styling tools are the trick to get the volume.

☺ **Brilliantine Shine Enhancing Pomade** *($8.65 for 2 ounces)* is a standard pomade that contains mostly Vaseline, wax, silicone, plant oils, preservatives, and fragrance. This would do the trick to smooth out stubborn curls and frizzies with no hold and therefore no stiff feel. It could leave a heavy residue, so use it sparingly.

☺ **Perm Endurance Perm Revitalizer and Styling Spray** *($7.25 for 8.45 ounces)* contains mostly water, film formers, conditioning agents, slip agents, silicone, preservatives, and fragrance. This is a good styling spray with a light hold and minimal to no stiff or sticky feel, but there is nothing about it better for perms; it just helps style and hold hair.

☺ **Styling Spray Thermal Designing Spray** *($8.65 for 8.45 ounces)* is a standard hairspray with light to medium hold and minimal to no stiff, sticky feel that contains mostly alcohol, water, film former, conditioning agents, silicone, and fragrance.

☺ **Transformation Styling Spray** *($8.95 for 8.45 ounces)* is a standard hairspray with medium hold and a somewhat stiff, sticky feel that contains mostly alcohol, water, film former, conditioning agents, silicone, and fragrance.

☺ **Travallo Design and Finishing Spray** *($7.95 for 8.45 ounces)* is a lightweight styling spray with a soft hold and minimal to no stiff or sticky feel. It works well for most any styling need requiring soft hold. It contains mostly alcohol, water, film former, conditioning agents, silicone, and fragrance.

☺ **Jojoba Oil** *($12.50 for 2 ounces)* is just very expensive jojoba oil with a small amount of fragrance and preservatives. It would be fine for dry hair. You could gain the same effect for far less money by using canola oil from your kitchen cupboard. There is nothing about jojoba oil that makes it better for hair.

☺ **Transformations Spray Glace** *($14.95 for 4 ounces)* is a lightweight, standard silicone spray that works well to add shine and a silky feel to hair. There are far less expensive versions with the same formulation available at the drugstore.

☺ **Straight Edge Heat-Activated Straightener** *($11.80 for 8.45 ounces)* gets no more activated by heat than any other styling product that helps shape hair when the heat is turned up. This is a thick styling lotion that contains mostly water, silicones, film former, conditioning agents, thickeners, slip agents, preservatives, and fragrance. This can help straighten and style stubborn curls and frizzies with a light hold and minimal stiff or sticky feel, but that's true only if you use it minimally.

☺ **JoiMist Firm Super-Hold Finishing Spray (Aerosol)** *($8.95 for 10.5 ounces)* is a standard aerosol hairspray with medium hold and a slight stiff, sticky feel, though it does brush through easily. It contains mostly alcohol, propellant, film former, conditioning agents, plant oil, silicones, slip agents, and fragrance.

☺ **JoiMist Shaping Spray** *($9.80 for 10.5 ounces)* is similar to the JoiMist above, only with medium hold.

I.C.E. by Joico

☺ **I.C.E. Gel Super Hold Styling Gel** *($7.95 for 8.8 ounces)* is a good standard gel with medium to firm hold that has a somewhat sticky, stiff feel though it can easily be brushed through. It contains mostly water, film formers, thickeners, conditioning agent, slip agent, silicone, preservatives, and fragrance.

☺ **I.C.E. Whip Designing Foam** *($11.95 for 10 ounces)* is a standard mousse with a light to medium hold and a slight stiff, sticky feel that contains mostly water, film formers, propellant, conditioning agents, plant oil, preservatives, and fragrance.

☺ **Forming I.C.E. Styling Creme** *($12.80 for 4.2 ounces)* is a good basic hair-straightening lotion with medium hold and minimal to no stiff or sticky feel for smoothing stubborn curls and frizzies. It contains mostly water, film former, silicones, thickeners, conditioning agents, plant oils, slip agents, preservatives, and fragrance.

☺ **I.C.E. Sculpting Lotion** *($6.60 for 8.45 ounces)* isn't a lotion, but a rather standard gel with light hold and minimal stiff, sticky feel that easily brushes through. It contains mostly water, film formers, conditioning agents, slip agents, and preservatives.

☺ **Thermal I.C.E. Heat-Activated Volumizer** *($7.95 for 8.45 ounces)* does not activate with heat any more than any other styling product that can help shape hair when the heat is turned up high. This is a liquidy styling gel with light to medium hold that can have a slight stiff feel, though it's easily brushed through. It contains mostly water, film formers, conditioning agents, slip agents, silicone, preservatives, and fragrance.

☺ **I.C.E. Mist Super-Hold Finishing Spray** *($3.60 for 2 ounces)* is a standard hairspray with medium to firm hold and a slight stiff, sticky feel.

ICE by Joico

Do not be confused the I.C.E. products above by Joico with these newly packaged versions called ICE, though both are line extensions of Joico. There isn't much to talk about in this newer version except the nice packaging and the strange array of plant extracts, including kelp, caffeine, and horseradish (which burns if you have a drop of styling product on your fingers and you inadvertently touch your eyes). Other than the strange marketing angle, these provide no improvement for hair or scalp. For more information about Ice, call (800) 44-JOICO or visit its Web site at www.joico.com.

☹ **Washer Shampoo Just Add Water** *($8 for 10 ounces)* contains mostly water, detergent cleansing agents, lather agent, conditioning agent, plant extracts, silicone, thickeners, preservatives, fragrance, and coloring agents. This is a good basic shampoo for most all hair types except oily scalp and hair. One word of warning: it does contain horseradish extract, and if this gets in the eyes, ouch!!!

☹ **Hydrater Conditioner Just a Drop** *($10 for 10 ounces)* contains mostly water, detangling agents, conditioning agents, plant extracts, vitamins, silicones, thickeners, slip agents, preservatives, and fragrance. This is a good conditioner for normal to slightly dry hair of any thickness. One word of warning: this does contain horseradish extract, and if it gets in the eyes, ouch!!!

☺ **Controller Gel Full Effect** *($7 for 5 ounces)* is a standard gel with medium hold and a minimal sticky feel that brushes through easily. It contains mostly water, film formers, thickeners, slip agents, silicone, conditioning agents, plant extracts, vitamins, fragrance, and preservatives.

☺ **Amplifier Mousse** *($13 for 8.8 ounces)* is a standard mousse that has a medium to firm hold and a somewhat sticky feel, though it can be brushed through easily. It contains mostly water, film formers, propellant, conditioning agents, silicone, plant extracts, vitamins, slip agents, and fragrance.

☺ **Molder Texture Cream** *($15 for 4.2 ounces)* is a hair-straightening cream that is best used minimally; this is heavy, sticky stuff and works best for smoothing stubborn curls and frizzies. It contains mostly water, film formers, thickeners, Vaseline, silicones, wax, castor oil, conditioning agents, vitamins, plant extracts, preservatives, fragrance, and coloring agent.

☺ **Slicker Defining Lotion Supple Definition** *($8 for 5 ounces)* is a very good silicone lotion with film formers. It can help straighten hair and smooth frizzies, and is far less heavy and greasy than the Texture Cream above.

☺ **Waxer Water Soluble Wax** *($15.50 for 4.2 ounces)* contains mostly thickeners, plant oil, conditioning agent, plant extracts, vitamins, slip agents, fragrance, preservatives, and coloring agent. This is a good, smooth styling wax that has less weight than you would think. It definitely has no stiff or sticky feel and can smooth hair, but the wax (that's what the thickeners are in this product-thick waxes) can get heavy so use it sparingly.

☺ **Finisher Hair Spray Medium Impact (Aerosol)** *($10 for 10.5 ounces)* is a good standard aerosol hairspray with medium hold and a slightly stiff, sticky feel. It contains mostly alcohol, propellant, film formers, silicone, conditioning agents, slip agents, plant extracts, vitamins, and fragrance.

☺ **Fixer Hair Spray High Impact (Non-Aerosol)** *($10 for 10 ounces)* is similar to the aerosol Finisher above and the same comments apply.

Kenra

For more information on Kenra, call (317) 356-6491 or (800) 428-8073.

☹ **Clarifying Shampoo** *($8.50 for 10.1 ounces)* uses TEA-lauryl sulfate as one of its main detergent cleansing agents, which makes it too drying for the hair and too irritating and drying for the scalp.

☺ **Dandruff Shampoo** *($10.95 for 10.1 ounces)* is a standard zinc pyrithione–based shampoo, which makes it identical to Head & Shoulders, only this one is ten times the price.

☹ **Energizing Shampoo** *($8.50 for 10.1 ounces)* contains menthol, which can be an irritant for the scalp.

☹ **Finishing Shampoo** *($7.50 for 10.1 ounces)* uses TEA-lauryl sulfate as the main detergent cleansing agent, which makes it too drying for the hair and too irritating and drying for the scalp.

☹ **Shampoo for Dry Hair** *($7.50 for 10.1 ounces)* uses sodium C14-16 olefin sulfonate as one of the main detergent cleansing agents, which makes it too drying for all hair types but especially for dry hair.

☹ **Volumizing Shampoo** *($7.50 for 10.1 ounces)* uses sodium C14-16 olefin sulfonate as one of the main detergent cleansing agents, which makes it too drying for all hair types.

☹ **Clarifying Treatment Instant Chelating Treatment for Removing Minerals and Excess Build-Up** *($5.50 for 4 ounces)* contains ingredients that are best kept off the scalp, including lemon and grapefruit, but other than that it doesn't contain any chelating type ingredients.

☺ **Energizing Conditioner Revitalizing Treatment for Healthier Hair and Scalp** *($11.50 for 10.1 ounces)* contains menthol, which can be an irritant for the scalp so keep it off that area. For the hair, this is an exceptionally lightweight conditioner for normal hair to help with combing. It contains mostly water, thickener, detangling agent, conditioning agent, slip agent, preservatives, and fragrance.

☺ **Excell Conditioner** *($10.50 for 10.1 ounces)* contains mostly water, thickeners, detangling agents/film formers, plant extracts, and preservatives. It does contain lemon balm and peppermint, which are problems for the scalp, so avoid that area. For the hair this is a basic conditioner for normal to slightly dry fine or thin hair to help make it feel thicker. The film formers can build up on hair.

☺ **Hair Re-Moisturizer** *($10.50 for 10.1 ounces)* contains mostly water, thickeners, detangling agents, conditioning agents, preservatives, fragrance, and coloring agents. This is a good basic conditioner for normal to slightly dry hair that is fine, thin, or normal in thickness.

☺ **Max Conditioner** *($10.50 for 10.1 ounces)* contains mostly water, conditioning agents, thickeners, detangling agent, preservatives, and fragrance. This is a good basic conditioner for normal to dry hair that is fine, thin, or normal in thickness.

☺ **Max Revitalisant Volumizing Protein-Enriched Conditioner** *($24.95 for 33.8 ounces)* is almost identical to the Max Conditioner above and the same comments apply.

☺ **Daily Provision Lightweight Leave-in Conditioner** *($9.95 for 10.1 ounces)* contains mostly plant water, silicone, detangling agent/film former, conditioning agent, slip agents, preservatives, and fragrance. This is a good leave-in conditioner for dry hair that is fine or thin.

☺ **Reflect Shine Alcohol-Free Spray Shine** *($11.95 for 2.2 ounces)* is a standard, though overpriced, silicone spray that can impart a smooth silky feel to the hair.

☺ **Endurance Gel Extra Firm-Hold Styling Fixative 21** *($9.95 for 10.1 ounces)* contains mostly plant water, film formers, thickeners, slip agents, preservatives, and fragrance. This is a medium- to firm-hold gel that can have a slight sticky, stiff feel, though it can easily be brushed through.

☺ **Outcome Extra Gel Firm Hold Styling Fixative 17** *($8.95 for 10.1 ounces)* contains mostly water, film formers, conditioning agent, plant extracts, thickeners, fragrant oils, silicone, and preservatives. This is a good, standard, firm-hold gel that can have a slight stiff, sticky feel on hair.

☺ **Texture-ize Light Hold Texturing Gel 6** *($6.95 for 4.2 ounces)* is similar to the Outcome Extra above, only this version has more silicone and a lighter hold with minimal to no stiff or sticky feel. It can help add a silky feel and soft hold when styling frizzies or smoothing coarse curls. Use it sparingly or it can make hair look and feel greasy.

☺ **Artformation Mousse Firm Hold Bodifying Formula 17** *($9.95 for 8 ounces)* is a standard mousse with light hold and a slight sticky feel. It contains mostly water, film formers, propellant, thickeners, slip agent, silicone, preservatives, and fragrance.

☺ **Empower Spray Gel Medium to Firm Hold Styling Fixative 15** *($8.95 for 10.1 ounces)* is similar to the Artformation Mousse above only this version does have a more medium to firm hold and a slight sticky feel.

☺ **Volume Styling Mousse Medium Hold Conditioning Formula 12** *($9.95 for 8 ounces)* is almost identical to the Artformation version above and the same comments apply.

☺ **Artform Pomade** *($7.95 for 2 ounces)* is a good soft-hold pomade in gel form that has no stiff or sticky feel; it can feel greasy and heavy, though, so use it sparingly. It contains mostly water, thickeners, mineral oil, slip agents, preservatives, and fragrance.

☺ **Molding Creme Firm Hold for Definition, Separation and Control 18** (*$14.95 for 6.95 ounces*) is a styling cream dispensed in an aerosol-like container, which tends to squirt out more product than you need. This firm-hold cream has a definite sticky feel, and can help hold stubborn hair in place, but use it sparingly— this can be heavy and stiff on hair.

☺ **Styling Lotion Light Hold for Texture, Body and Shine 8** (*$13.95 for 8 ounces*) is more of a gel than a lotion, and it has a good light hold with minimal to no stiff and sticky feel. It contains mostly plant water, film formers, silicones, conditioning agents, preservatives, and fragrance.

☺ **Thickening Spray Light Hold for Volume, Body and Shine 4** (*$11.95 for 8 ounces*) is a standard styling spray that contains mostly plant water, film formers, conditioning agent, silicone, fragrance, and preservatives. This has light hold with minimal to no stiff or sticky feel. It can help when styling, but it's the styling process, not this product or any other, that makes hair feel fuller or smoother.

☺ **Capture Glaze Medium Hold Styling Fixative 14** (*$8.95 for 10.1 ounces*) is a standard, light- to medium-hold gel with a slight stiff, sticky feel that contains mostly water, film formers, conditioning agents, plant extracts, silicone, thickeners, preservatives, and fragrance.

☺ **Thermal Styling Spray Firm Hold Heat Activated Styling Spray 19** (*$10.95 for 8.5 ounces*) is a standard styling spray that contains mostly alcohol, water, film formers, plant extracts, silicones, fragrance, and preservatives. This has medium hold with a slight stiff feel. There is nothing in here especially for "thermal" styling.

☺ **Straightening Serum, Smoothing and Conditioning Curl Relaxant** (*$12.95 for 10.1 ounces*) is a light-hold styling gel-like lotion with no stiff or sticky feel. It contains mostly plant water, thickeners, detangling agents, silicones, film former, preservatives, and fragrance. It can help smooth out most hair types and can add thickness to fine or thin hair without weighing it down.

☺ **Root Volumizing Serum Volumizer for Root Lift and Style Support 20** (*$11.95 for 6 ounces*) contains mostly plant water, alcohol, film former, thickeners, and fragrance. The pointed applicator helps aim this gel-like serum at the root, which is clever but not as helpful as it seems. This has light to medium hold and can have a slight stiff, sticky feel. That can help styling, but you might want to apply this just minimally, and the applicator doesn't quite allow that kind of control.

☺ **Artformation Spray Firm Hold Styling and Finishing Spray 18** (*$11.95 for 12 ounces*) is a standard aerosol hairspray with medium to firm hold and a slight stiff, sticky feel that is easy to brush through. It contains mostly alcohol, propellant, film formers, conditioning agents, and fragrance.

☺ **Design Spray Light Hold Styling Spray 9** (*$11.95 for 12 ounces*) is similar to the Artformation Spray above, only with a firm hold and a slight stiff feel.

☺ **Capture Plus Spray Extra Firm Hold Finishing Formula 23** *($8.95 for 10.1 ounces)* is a standard hairspray with light to medium hold and minimal stiff feel that is easily brushed through. It contains mostly alcohol, propellant, film formers, conditioning agents, and fragrance.

☺ **Endurance Fragrance-Free Long-Lasting Styling Spray 21** *($9.95 for 10.1 ounces)* is similar to the Artformation Spray above, only in nonaerosol form, and this one contains silicone, which helps more with shine.

☺ **Volume Spray Super Hold Finishing Spray** *($11 for 12 ounces)* is similar to the Artformation Spray above and the same basic comments apply.

Kiehl's

The Kiehl's line has the reputation of being both natural and an ersatz pharmaceutical at the same time. It is neither. There are some good products here but they are about as natural as your car, and there is no "medical" benefit to any of them. For more information on Kiehl's, call (212) 677-3171 or (800) KIEHLS-1.

☹ **Castille Shampoo** *($11.50 for 8 ounces)* contains mostly detergent cleansing agents, lather agent, thickeners, preservatives, lanolin, and soap. This can be drying for some hair types and there's not enough lanolin in here to correct the potential problems from the detergent cleansing agents.

☹ **Herbal Treatment Shampoo for Problem Hair and Scalp** *($14.50 for 8 ounces)* uses sodium C14-16 olefin sulfonate as one of its main detergent cleansing agents, which makes it too drying for all hair types, but especially for problem hair and scalp.

☹ **Klaus Heidegger's All-Sport Everyday Shampoo** *($10.95 for 8 ounces)* uses sodium C14-16 olefin sulfonate as one of its main detergent cleansing agents, which makes it too drying for all hair types.

☹ **Lecithin Conditioning Shampoo** *($18.50 for 8 ounces)* uses sodium C14-16 olefin sulfonate as one of its main detergent cleansing agents, which makes it too drying for all hair types. It also contains orange oil, lemon oil, and grapefruit oil, all of which can be scalp irritants.

☹ **Protein Concentrate Chamomile Shampoo** *($12.50 for 8 ounces)* uses TEA-lauryl sulfate as one of its main detergent cleansing agents, which makes it too drying for the hair and too irritating and drying for the scalp.

☹ **Protein Concentrate Shampoo for Dry to Normal Hair** *($11.95 for 8 ounces)* uses TEA-lauryl sulfate as one of its main detergent cleansing agents, which makes it too drying for the hair and too irritating and drying for the scalp.

☹ **Protein Concentrate Shampoo for Oily Hair** *($11.95 for 8 ounces)* uses TEA-lauryl sulfate as the main detergent cleansing agent, which makes it too drying for the hair and too irritating and drying for the scalp.

☺ **Tea Tree Oil Shampoo** *($9.50 for 4 ounces)* does contain a small amount of tea tree oil, which can be helpful for dandruff, but not in this amount. Other than that, this is just shampoo with fragrant oils. That can be great for an oily scalp, unless you're allergic to the fragrance.

☺ **Deep Conditioning Protein Pak** *($22.50 for 4 ounces)* contains mostly water, thickeners, slip agents, lanolin oil, conditioning agents, detangling agents, preservatives, plant oils, and fragrance. This is a good emollient conditioner for very dry hair of any thickness.

☺ **Extra-Strength Conditioning Rinse for Dry Hair** *($17.50 for 8 ounces)* contains mostly water, conditioning agents, fragrance, plant oil, and preservatives. This is a good emollient conditioner for normal to dry hair that is normal to coarse in thickness.

☺ **Extra-Strength Conditioning Rinse with Added Coconut** *($10.95 for 4 ounces)* is almost identical to the Extra-Strength version above. This one is slightly more emollient.

☺ **Hair Conditioning & Grooming Aid Formula 133** *($14.95 for 8 ounces)* is a good conditioner for normal to slightly dry hair. It contains mostly water, detangling agent, thickeners, conditioning agent, preservatives, and fragrance.

☺ **Leave-in Hair Conditioner** *($26.50 for 8 ounces)* makes the claim that it can protect the hair from sun damage; that isn't true. It doesn't have an SPF number so it may only be an SPF 2, which is meaningless for protection; also, it doesn't contain UVA protection, only UVB. Other than that, it is a good lightweight conditioner for normal to slightly dry hair of any thickness.

☺ **Panthenol Protein Hair Conditioner** *($14.95 for 8 ounces)* contains mostly water, panthenol, and preservatives. This is one of the most one-note conditioners I've ever seen. It would work well for normal to slightly dry hair of any thickness.

☺ **Extra Strength Styling Gel** *($14.50 for 4 ounces)* is an exceptionally standard styling gel with light hold and a somewhat sticky feel that contains mostly water, slip agent, film formers, conditioning agents, thickeners, and preservatives.

☺ **Creme de la Creme Groom Repairateur with Silk** *($13.50 for 2 ounces)* is an emollient cream (more like a rich moisturizer than a styling product) that could be helpful for smoothing stubborn curls and frizzies. It has no hold, which means no sticky or stiff feel, but it can feel greasy on hair so use it sparingly. It contains mostly water, thickeners, slip agent, conditioning agents, plant oil, preservatives, and fragrant oils.

☺ **Creme with Silk Groom** *($15.50 for 4 ounces)* is almost identical to the Creme de la Creme above and the same comments apply.

☺ **Shine 'N Lite Groom for Dull or Thick Hair** *($10.95 for 4 ounces)* is almost identical to the Creme de la Creme above and the same comments apply.

☺ **"Wet Look" Groom** *($11.50 for 4 ounces)* contains mostly water, slip agent, thickeners, film former, preservatives, lanolin oil, and preservatives. This is a lotion with a gel-like texture that can slick back hair with light hold. It is just a styling lotion that is actually quite similar to the Creme de la Creme above and works about the same only with a light hold and minimal to no stiff or sticky feel.

☺ **Hair Thickening Spray for Dry or Hard-to-Manage Hair (Non-Aerosol)** *($10.95 for 4 ounces)* contains mostly water, alcohol, film formers, fragrance, conditioning agents, and slip agents. This is a minimal-hold styling spray that is more of a leave-in conditioner. It has minimal to no hold and no stiff or sticky feel. It can help when styling hair.

☺ **Panthenol Protein Hair Conditioner Softener & Grooming Aid** *($14.95 for 8 ounces)* contains mostly water, conditioning agent, film former, preservatives, and slip agents. Is almost identical to the Hair Thickening Spray above and the same comments apply.

☺ **Enriched Massage Oil for Scalp** *($14.50 for 4 ounces),* as the name implies, contains oil, and while that's good for a dry scalp, it's no more so than any oil you may have in your kitchen. This one contains mostly plant oil, slip agents, vitamins, fragrant oil, preservatives, and thickeners. Vitamins are good moisturizing ingredients but they aren't going to help grow hair or revitalize the scalp.

☹ **Herbal Toner for the Scalp** *($22.95 for 8 ounces)* contains mostly water, slip agent, plant water, preservatives, and conditioning agent. This is a do-nothing product that is a waste of time for the scalp. These plants have no benefit for skin.

☺ **High-Gloss Conditioning and Styling Oil for Hair** *($19.95 for 1.5 ounces)* contains mostly plant oils, slip agents, plant extracts, preservatives, and fragrant oils. This is not much different from using safflower or peanut oil from your kitchen cupboard. It works for dry hair, but a silicone product would give better performance.

☺ **Lecithin and Coconut Enriched Hair Masque with Panthenol** *($21.50 for 14 ounces)* is just a good conditioner for dry to very dry hair of any thickness. It contains mostly water, thickeners, emollient, plant oils, detangling agent, preservatives, and fragrance.

KMS

KMS is the abbreviation for kinetic molecular systems, which the line says "expresses our commitment to natural chemistry." There isn't an unnatural chemistry, so the comment is bogus, though it gets across the notion of its ingredients being natural. Not surprisingly, KMS products contain the same standard formulations despite the impressive claims on their labels. In fact, as is true for the entire hair-care industry, the repetitiveness of formulations between lines in all price ranges is astounding.

None of this stops cosmetic companies from trying to convince you that their products are all natural. KMS, like Aveda, labels its most synthetic-sounding ingredients with parenthetical explanations that in essence relay the message that you needn't worry, these ingredients really aren't unnatural. It might make the consumer feel better that methylparaben is "food grade" though this is a strong preservative and you wouldn't want to eat it, or that dmdm hydantoin is from a "plant source" when it can be a formaldehyde releaser. Though I find that misleading, what KMS is completely forthcoming about is its ingredients, which are fully listed on its Web site, something no other company is presently doing! Now that really is something new and different. Another interesting note: KMS is also one of the few companies that has a fragrance-free and coloring agent–free line of products. For someone with a sensitive, itchy scalp, that's good news.

KMS has a huge range of products; many of them are redundant and don't offer much other than great names. For more information about KMS, call (800) DIAL KMS or visit its Web site at www.kmshaircare.com.

☺ **Alternative Protein-Enriched for All Hair Types** *($7.50 for 8 ounces)* contains mostly water, detergent cleansing agent, lather agent, conditioning agents, preservatives, and fragrance. This is a good basic shampoo for normal to slightly dry hair. The amount of conditioning agents is minimal so the chance for buildup is greatly reduced.

☺ **Classic Silver for Gray or Blonde Hair** *($6.95 for 8 ounces)* is made with a violet color, and that's the only thing that makes this product look like it would help reduce the yellow overtones of gray hair, but the dyes in here don't cling well to hair. This is just shampoo with some conditioning agents, which makes it good for dry hair. It contains mostly water, detergent cleansing agent, lather agents, conditioning agents, plant oils, preservatives, and dye agents. This product also contains a small amount of sulfur, which I suspect may be intended to help lift brassiness from the hair. On a regular basis that could prove to be drying.

☺ **Cleanse-pHree Shampoo, Gentle Cleansing for Normal, Healthy Hair** *($5.95 for 8 ounces)* contains mostly water, detergent cleansing agent, lather agent, plant oils, silicone, preservatives, coloring agent, and fragrance. This is a good shampoo for dry hair. The oils make it a problem for normal hair.

☺ **CliniDan the Dandruff Solution** *($7.95 for 8 ounces)* is a standard zinc pyrithione–based dandruff shampoo with minimal conditioning. It would work well, but for the money it is not that much different from Head & Shoulders.

☺ **Color Response Shampoo Nutritive Shampoo for Colored or Color-Highlighted Hair** *($6.95 for 8 ounces)* contains nothing that is special or helpful for dyed hair. This basic shampoo contains mostly water, detergent cleansing agent, thickeners, detangling agent, lather agent, silicone, conditioning agents, preservatives, and fragrance. It would work well for normal to dry hair of any thickness.

☺ **Moisturizing Shampoo, Extra Body for Dry, Damaged Hair** *($5.95 for 8 ounces)* contains mostly water, detergent cleansing agent, lather agent, silicone, detangling agent, film formers, conditioning agents, preservatives, coloring agents, and fragrance. It would work well for dry hair that is normal to fine or thin in thickness.

☺ **NEFA Natural Essence Reconstructive Shampoo for Chemically Treated Hair** *($6.50 for 8 ounces)* contains mostly water, detergent cleansing agent, plant oils, lather agent, conditioning agents, detangling agent/film former, silicone, preservatives, coloring agents, and fragrance. This is a good shampoo for dry to very dry hair of any thickness.

☺ **pHirst Active Clarifier Shampoo for All Hair Types** *($7.45 for 8 ounces)* contains mostly water, detergent cleansing agent, lather agent, chelating agent, detangling agent/film former, silicone, preservatives, and fragrance. This is a good shampoo for normal to dry hair that is normal to fine or thin. It contains a chelating agent, which can help prevent minerals from binding to hair.

☺ **Ultra Volume Shampoo, Extra Body for Fine, Lifeless Hair** *($6.50 for 8 ounces)* is a standard shampoo with just water, detergent cleansing agents, lather agent, preservatives, coloring agents, and fragrance. This shampoo does also contain baking soda, which can help with softness and can slightly swell the hair.

☺ **Color Response Color Last Color Protector and Detangling Spray for Colored or Color-Highlighted Hair** *($7.95 for 8 ounces)* doesn't contain anything that will help keep color in the hair. This is just a good leave-in conditioner for normal to dry hair that is normal to fine or thin in thickness. It contains mostly water, slip agents, detangling agent, film former, silicone, antioxidant, and preservatives. The amount of antioxidant in here is negligible and would not have an effect on hair.

☺ **Color Response Detangling Reconstructor, Advanced Reconstructor and Detangler for Colored or Color-Highlighted Hair** *($8.95 for 8.11 ounces)* is similar to the one above and the same basic comments apply.

☹ **Liquid Asset Recovery Treatment, Exclusive Anti-Aging Complex for Dry, Stressed Hair** *($13.95 for 8 ounces)* contains mostly water, conditioning agents, detangling agent/film former, plant oils, sulfur, preservatives, and fragrance. This does contain a tiny amount of sulfur, and my concern is that sulfur can strip hair color with repeated use.

☺ **pHinish Reconstructor, Active Clarifier for All Hair Types** *($6.50 for 4 ounces)* contains mostly water, detangling agent, thickeners, conditioning agent, detangling agent/film former, preservatives, coloring agent, and fragrance. This is a good basic conditioner for normal to slightly dry hair that is normal to fine or thin.

☺ **Prolimin Gold, the Ultimate Reconstructive Treatment** *($4 for 1 ounce)* contains mostly water, detangling agent, thickeners, conditioning agent, plant oils, detangling agent/film former, preservatives, coloring agents, and fragrance. This is a good conditioner for dry hair of any thickness, but it won't reconstruct one hair on your head.

☺ **RePlace Reconstructor, Moisture-Enriched for Dry, Damaged Hair** *($6.95 for 4 ounces)* contains mostly water, plant oil, thickeners, detangling agent, conditioning agents, preservatives, coloring agents, and fragrance. This is a good conditioner for dry to very dry hair that is thick to coarse.

☺ **Strategy Reconstructor, Nutrient-Enriched for Chemically Treated Hair** *($9.95 for 8.11 ounces)* contains mostly water, detangling agent, conditioning agents, plant oils, thickeners, preservatives, and fragrance. This is a good conditioner for dry hair of any thickness.

☺ **Trilogy Leave-in Reconstructor for All Hair Types** *($7.95 for 8 ounces)* contains mostly water, film-former/detangling agents, conditioning agent, silicone, preservatives, and fragrance. This is a good leave-in conditioner for dry hair that is fine or thin, but it won't reconstruct one hair on your head.

☺ **Ultra-Pak Reconstructor, Extra Body for Fine, Lifeless Hair** *($9.95 for 4 ounces)* contains mostly water, thickener, detangling agent, conditioning agents, plant oils, detangling agent/film former, preservatives, and fragrance. This is a good basic conditioner for dry hair of any thickness.

☺ **Conditioning Fixx Spray Gel, Light Hold Gel for Finishing** *($7.45 for 8 ounces)* contains mostly water, film formers, detangling agents, slip agents, preservatives, and fragrance. This is a good spray gel with a light to medium hold and minimal stiff or sticky feel.

☺ **Pomade Molding Gel** *($14.50 for 4.06 ounces)* contains mostly water, castor oil, thickeners, lanolin, slip agents, film former, preservatives, and fragrance. This is a good, greasy pomade that can have light to medium hold and a somewhat sticky feel and it can definitely smooth stubborn frizzies and curls when used sparingly, but be careful—this can feel and look greasy.

☺ **Paste Molding Paste for All Hair Types** *($12.50 for 3.5 ounces)* is similar to the Molding Gel above only in cream form. This is a thick styling cream with medium hold and a heavy, slightly sticky feel. It will smooth out the stubborn curls and frizzies but it can also feel heavy and look greasy, so use it sparingly. It contains mostly water, alcohol, lanolin wax, Vaseline, film formers, more waxes, mineral oil, castor oil, conditioning agent, and fragrance.

☺ **Configure Molding Creme for Shine, Control and Definition** *($14.50 for 4.06 ounces)* is a good styling cream that contains mostly water, thickeners, preservatives, silicone, film former, and fragrance. It has a minimal to light hold, with a slight sticky feel. The same warnings for the Molding Paste and Pomade Molding Gel apply for this one too.

☺ **Spray Gel, Firm Hold Gel for Finishing** *($9.50 for 8 ounces)* contains mostly alcohol, water, film formers, slip agents, silicone, and fragrance. This is a good spray gel with a light to medium hold and minimal stiff or sticky feel.

☺ **Styling & Setting Gel, Maximum Hold Gel for Finishing** *($9.95 for 8.11 ounces)* contains mostly water, film formers, thickeners, slip agents, preservatives, coloring agents, and fragrance. This is a good standard gel with a light to medium hold and minimal stiff or sticky feel.

☺ **ThermaStat Thermal Styling Spray (Non-Aerosol)** *($7.95 for 8 ounces)* is a standard styling spray with a light to medium hold and minimal to no stiff or sticky feel. This is supposed to be special for use with curling irons, but there's not one unique or special ingredient in here that would make this spray better to use for that.

☺ **Sculpturing Lotion Styling Liquid, Light Hold Liquid for Finishing** *($5.95 for 8 ounces)* contains mostly water, film formers, slip agent, thickeners, preservatives, and fragrance. This is a good basic styling liquid with light to medium hold and a slight sticky feel that is easily brushed through.

☺ **Mousse Styling Foam, Medium Hold Foam for Finishing** *($8.45 for 6.17 ounces)* is a standard mousse that contains mostly water, film formers, alcohol, propellant, conditioning agent, detangling agent, silicone, preservatives, and fragrance. It has a good light to medium hold with a slight stiff or sticky feel.

☺ **HairHold Styling Spray, Medium Hold Spray for Finishing (Non-Aerosol)** *($5 for 8 ounces)* is a good standard hairspray with medium hold and a slight stiff feel that does brush through easily. It contains mostly alcohol, water, film formers, conditioning agent, silicone, and fragrance. The redundant hairsprays similar to this are almost shocking. Didn't KMS think anyone would notice they all perform almost identically?

☺ **ProliFixx Finishing Spray, Medium Hold (Aerosol)** *($9.95 for 9.5 ounces)* is similar to the HairHold version above, only this one is in aerosol form.

☺ **ProliMaxx Finishing Spray, Maximum Hold (Aerosol)** *($9.95 for 9.5 ounces)* is similar to the HairHold version above, only this one is in aerosol form.

☺ **ProliForce Finishing Spray, Maximum Hold Spray for Finishing** *($7.95 for 8 ounces)* is similar to the HairHold version above and the same comments apply.

☺ **ProliFree Alcohol-Free Hairspray, Medium Hold Spray for Finishing (Non-Aerosol)** *($7.95 for 8 ounces)* is similar to the HairHold version above and the same comments apply.

☺ **ProliMist Pure Finishing Spray, Soft Hold Spray for Finishing** *($9.95 for 12 ounces)* is similar to the HairHold version above and the same comments apply.

☺ **Shine Complex Glossifier for Finishing** *($11.95 for 2 ounces)* is a standard silicone serum that can add a silky-soft feel and shine to hair.

☺ **Shine Complex Spray Glossifier, Shines, Smooths, Protects for Finishing** *($10.50 for 4.23 ounces)* is similar to the Shine Complex Glossifier for Finishing above, only this one is in spray form.

AMP: Amino-Magnesium-Panthenol by KMS

☺ **Volume Shampoo for All Hair Types** *($6.67 for 8 ounces)* contains mostly water, detergent cleansing agents, lather agent, conditioning agents, preservatives, and fragrance. This is a good shampoo for normal to dry hair of any thickness. It doesn't add volume to hair.

☺ **Volume Reconstructor for All Hair Types** *($8.95 for 8.11 ounces)* contains mostly water, detangling agent, thickener, conditioning agents, detangling agents, film former, silicone, preservatives, and fragrance. This is a very good standard conditioner for normal to dry hair that is normal to fine or thin in thickness.

☺ **Volume Amplifying Spray for All Hair Types** *($9.95 for 8 ounces)* is a standard styling spray with a light hold and minimal to no stiff or sticky feel. It contains mostly alcohol, water, film former, conditioning agents, detangling agents, silicone, and fragrance.

☺ **Volume Styling Foam, Firm Hold for All Hair Types** *($9.50 for 6.17 ounces)* contains mostly water, film formers, alcohol, propellant, conditioning agent, silicone, preservatives, and fragrance. This is a good basic mousse with light to medium hold and minimal stiff or sticky feel.

☺ **Volume Leave-in Thickening Cream for All Hair Types** *($7.95 for 6 ounces)* is a good styling cream with light to medium hold and a slight sticky feel. It doesn't add any more thickness, at least not any more than any other styling cream, but it can help control curls and frizzies. It contains mostly water, thickener, detangling agent, conditioning agents, preservatives, and fragrance.

Flat Out by KMS

☺ **Flat Out Shampoo, Smoothing Shampoo for All Hair Types** *($7.95 for 8.28 ounces)* contains mostly plant water, detergent cleansing agent, lather agent, silicone, detangling agent, film former, conditioning agent, thickeners, preservatives, coloring agent, and fragrance. This is a good basic two-in-one shampoo much like other silicone-based shampoos; it's best for someone with normal to dry hair that is fine or thin. The film former in here can build up with repeated use.

☺ **Flat Out Hair Repair Curl Control Reconstructor for All Hair Types** *($10.50 for 8.11 ounces)* is a good (though silicone-based) conditioner that contains mostly plant water, thickeners, silicones, slip agents, detangling agent/film former, preservatives, coloring agents, and fragrance. It would work great for dry, thick, or coarse hair.

☺ **Flat Out Lite Relaxing Creme, Non-Chemical Curl Relaxer and Defrizzant** *($17.95 for 6 ounces)* contains mostly plant water, silicones, film former, thickeners, preservatives, and fragrance. This is a very good styling cream with minimal hold and minimal stiff or sticky feel that is best for smoothing out stubborn curls or frizzies.

☺ **Flat Out Relaxing Balm, Non-Chemical Curl Relaxer and Defrizzant** *($16.95 for 6 ounces)* is similar to the Relaxing Creme above, only in gel form, and the same basic comments apply.

☺ **Flat Out Stay Smooth Spray, Soft Hold, High Shine Finishing Spray** *($8.95 for 7 ounces)* is a standard hairspray with a light to medium hold and minimal stiff feel; it can be easily brushed through. It contains mostly alcohol, water, film former, conditioning agent, silicone, and fragrance.

☺ **Flat Out Styling Shine Gel** *($8 for 7 ounces)* contains mostly plant water, film formers, thickeners, silicone, slip agent, preservatives, coloring agents, and fragrance. This is a good styling gel for medium to firm hold with minimal stiff or sticky feel.

☺ **Flat Out Weightless Shine Spray** *($9 for 1.5 ounces)* is a standard silicone spray that adds shine and a silky feel to hair.

☺ **Flat Out Shine Serum** *($8 for 1 ounce)* is identical to the Shine Spray above only this one is in serum form.

Curl Up by KMS

☺ **Curl Up Shampoo** *($10 for 8.3 ounces)* contains mostly plant water, detergent cleansing agent, lather agent, conditioning agent, silicone, detangling agent, film former, thickener, coloring agents, preservatives, and fragrance. There is nothing in this shampoo that will help curls, but it is a good basic shampoo for dry hair that is normal to fine or thin.

☺ **Curl Up Curl Prepare** *($9.95 for 8.1 ounces)* contains mostly plant water, thickeners, film formers, silicone, detangling agent, conditioning agents, thickeners, preservatives, coloring agents, and fragrance. This is a good conditioner for normal to dry hair that is normal to fine or thin. It can have a stiff feel.

☺ **Curl Up Curling Balm, Non-Chemical Curl Intensifier** *($12.95 for 5 ounces)* contains mostly plant water, slip agents, thickeners, preservatives, coloring agent, and fragrance. This hair balm provides a soft conditioning effect on hair with no hold or stiffness.

☹ **Curl Up Bounce Back Spray** *($12.95 for 7 ounces)* contains mostly alcohol, plant water, film formers, conditioning agents, slip agents, coloring agents, and fragrance. This is a good basic styling spray that doesn't have any special curling ability although it can provide a medium to firm hold with some stiff and sticky feel.

Puritives by KMS

☺ **Shampoo** *($8.25 for 8.45 ounces)* contains mostly water, detergent cleansing agents, lather agent, detangling agent, film former, and preservatives. This is a good basic shampoo for all hair types. The amount of film former here is so tiny there isn't much concern about buildup.

☺ **Reconstructor** *($8.95 for 8.79 ounces)* won't reconstruct anything, but it is a good basic conditioner for normal to slightly dry hair of any thickness but coarse. It contains mostly water, thickeners, conditioning agents, detangling agent, and preservatives.

☺ **Pure Gel Medium Hold** *($8.95 for 8.79 ounces)* is a standard gel that contains mostly water, film formers, thickeners, silicone, and preservatives. It has light hold and minimal stiff or sticky feel. This product also contains no fragrance.

☺ **Alcohol Free Hairspray Medium Hold** *($10.25 for 8.45 ounces)* is a standard hairspray that contains mostly water, film formers, and silicone. It has a good light hold with minimal to no stiff or sticky feel.

Hair Play by KMS

☺ **Hair Play Configure Creme** *($10 for 4 ounces)* contains mostly thickeners, slip agent, wax, preservatives, silicone, film formers, and fragrance. This light-hold molding cream has minimal stiffness but can feel greasy and heavy, so use it sparingly. It definitely can smooth hair and frizzies.

☺ **Hair Play Defining Pomade** *($10 for 4 ounces)* is a greasy pomade that contains mostly water, castor oil, thickeners, lanolin, film formers, slip agent, preservatives, and fragrance. It can have a slight sticky feel, but it can also smooth and control frizzies and curls.

☺ **Hair Play Molding Paste** *($9 for 3.4 ounces)* contains mostly water, alcohol, waxes, Vaseline, film former, castor oil, conditioning agent, preservatives, and fragrance. This is a heavy, greasy wax that can have a sticky feel, but it can help control stubborn hair and smooth frizzies and curls.

☺ **Hair Play Tacky Gel** *($12 for 4 ounces)* contains mostly water, film former, slip agent, thickeners, conditioning agents, silicone, detangling agent, preservatives, and fragrance. This is a good standard gel with medium hold and a slightly stiff, sticky feel.

Hair Stay by KMS

☺ **Hair Stay Styling Gel** *($12.95 for 8.1 ounces)* contains mostly water, film former, thickeners, preservatives, coloring agents, and fragrance. This is a great name for a standard styling gel that has medium to firm hold.

☺ **Hair Stay Sculpting Lotion** *($10.95 for 8.1 ounces)* contains mostly water, detangling agent, film formers, slip agent, conditioning agent, thickeners, preservatives, and fragrance. This is a good medium-hold styling lotion with minimal stiff or sticky feel.

☺ **Hair Stay Styling Foam** *($14.95 for 8 ounces)* is a standard mousse with medium hold and a slightly stiff feel; it contains mostly water, film former, propellant, silicone, slip agent, thickeners, preservatives, and fragrance.

☺ **Hair Stay Max Hold Spray (Non-Aerosol)** *($12.95 for 8.5 ounces)* is a standard medium-hold hairspray with a slight stiff feel that contains mostly alcohol, water, film formers, silicone, conditioning agents, and fragrance.

☺ **Hair Stay Medium Hold Aerosol** *($12.95 for 9.5 ounces)* is similar to the Max Hold above, only in aerosol form, and the same basic comments apply.

Silker by KMS

☺ **Silker Shampoo** *($8.50 for 12 ounces)* is a standard shampoo that contains mostly water, detergent cleansing agent, lather agent, thickeners, conditioning agent, detangling agent/film former, silicone, preservatives, and fragrance. This is a good shampoo for normal to dry hair of any thickness. The silk amino acids in here are just conditioning agents; their source doesn't have anything to do with their effect on hair.

☺ **Silker Detangler for All Hair Types** *($8.50 for 8.11 ounces)* contains mostly water, thickener, conditioning agents, detangling agent, detangling agent/film former, preservatives, and fragrance. This is a good leave-in conditioner for normal to dry hair that is fine or thin.

☺ **Silk Reconstructor** *($10 for 8.1 ounces)* contains mostly water, thickener, conditioning agents, vitamin E, detangling agent, film former, preservatives, and fragrance. This is a good conditioner for normal to slightly dry hair of any thickness. It won't reconstruct one hair on your head.

☺ **Silker Leave In Treatment** *($9.50 for 8.5 ounces)* contains mostly water, detangling agents, film former, silicones, conditioning agents, thickeners, preservatives, and fragrance. This is a very good leave-in conditioner for dry hair that is fine to thin.

☺ **Silker 2-in-1 Shaping Cream** *($10 for 4 ounces)* contains mostly water, thickeners, lanolin oil, more thickeners, plant oils, conditioning agents, preservatives, and fragrance. This is a good minimal-hold wax for stubborn, coarse, extremely dry hair.

Moisture Replace by KMS

☺ **Moisture Replace Shampoo** *($10 for 12 ounces)* contains mostly water, detergent cleansing agent, lather agent, silicone, detangling agent, film formers, conditioning agent, preservatives, and fragrance. This is a good silicone-based shampoo that can be good for dry hair, although the film formers in here (the secret "moisture replace" ingredients) can easily build up on hair.

☺ **Moisture Replace Constructor** *($10 for 8.1 ounces)* contains mostly water, plant oil, thickeners, detangling agent, conditioning agent, film former, preservatives, coloring agent, and fragrance. This is a good conditioner for dry to very dry hair of any thickness. The film former can easily build up on hair.

☺ **Moisture Replace Deep Therapy** *($8.95 for 3.4 ounces)* contains mostly water, silicones, thickeners, detangling agent, conditioning agent, film former, preservatives, coloring agent, and fragrance. This is a good conditioner for very dry hair that is thick or coarse. The film former can easily build up on hair.

☺ **Moisture Replace 2-in-1 Styling Spray** *($8.95 for 8.5 ounces)* is a good styling spray that gives a light to medium hold with minimal stiffness; it contains mostly water, film formers, slip agent, detangling agent, conditioning agents, preservatives, and fragrance.

Color Vitality Shampoo by KMS

☺ **Color Vitality Shampoo** *($10 for 8.5 ounces)* is a standard shampoo for normal to dry hair of any thickness. This doesn't contain anything to enhance or protect hair color. It contains mostly water, detergent cleansing agent, lather agent, detangling agent, silicone, thickeners, conditioning agent, antioxidant, preservatives, and fragrance.

☺ **Color Vitality Reconstructor** *($10.95 for 8.1 ounces)* contains mostly water, thickeners, conditioning agents, detangling agent, film former, preservatives, and fragrance. This is a good conditioner for normal to dry hair of any thickness, but the antioxidant in here can't help keep color in the hair. There is no evidence that antioxidants have any effect on hair.

☺ **Color Vitality Color Last Treatment** *($12.95 for 8.5 ounces)* contains mostly water, slip agent, detangling agent, film former, silicone, thickeners, preservatives, and fragrance. This is a good, lightweight, leave-in conditioner for normal to slightly dry hair of any thickness.

Healthy Alternative by KMS

☺ **Healthy Alternative Everyday Shampoo** *($10 for 12 ounces)* contains mostly water, detergent cleansing agents, lather agent, plant oils, conditioning agent, preservatives, and fragrance. There is nothing particularly healthy or unique about this group of shampoos, but this is a good basic one for dry hair of any thickness.

☺ **Healthy Alternative Dandruff Shampoo** *($10 for 12 ounces)* is a standard zinc pyrithione–based shampoo with no conditioning agents. It's a very good, basic dandruff treatment without other ingredients to get in the way.

☺ **Healthy Alternative Totally Clean Shampoo** *($10 for 12 ounces)* is a standard shampoo with no conditioning agents, just detergent cleansing agents, coloring agents, and fragrance. This is a great shampoo for all hair types, with no chance of buildup.

☺ **Healthy Alternative Clarifying Shampoo** *($10 for 12 ounces)* is a standard shampoo that does contain some amount of a chelating agent, which can help prevent minerals from binding to the hair. It also contains film former and silicone, and that makes this one better for normal to slightly dry hair.

☺ **Healthy Alternative Clarifying Treatment** *($10 for 8.1 ounces)* is a good leave-in conditioner that is best only for detangling if you have normal hair. It contains mostly water, detangling agent, thickeners, film former, conditioning agent, preservatives, coloring agent, and fragrance.

L.A. Looks

L.A. Looks is a full line of hairstyling products. The L.A. gimmick is cute but don't count on any celebrity styles lurking in these bottles; that takes styling ability, not just product use. For more information on L.A. Looks, call (310) 604-0777, (800) 326-2855, or visit its Web site at www.lalooks.com.

☺ **Gel 2 Mousse, Extra Super Hold & Body** *($2.29 for 7.5 ounces)* is dispensed like a creamy gel and then turns into mousse. Very cool, but it's still just a mousse with medium hold and a somewhat sticky feel, though it does brush through. It contains mostly water, propellant, thickeners, film former, silicones, fragrance, and preservatives.

☺ **Gel 2 Mousse, Mega Hold & Body** *($2.29 for 7.5 ounces)* is virtually identical to the Gel 2 Mousse Extra Super Hold above and the same comments apply.

☺ **Styling Mousse, Extra Super Body** *($2.29 for 7 ounces)* dispenses like a regular foamy mousse, but the feel and performance is identical to the two Gel 2 Mousses above.

☺ **Gel Blast Extra Super Hold Fine Mist Spray Gel (Level 3)** *($1.99 for 8 ounces)* is a standard spray gel that has light to medium hold and a slight stiff, sticky feel. It contains mostly water, film formers, conditioning agent, slip agents, fragrance, silicones, and preservatives.

☺ **Styling Gel, Body Building (Level 2)** *($2.29 for 16 ounces)* is a standard styling gel with a light hold and minimal to no stiff or sticky feel. It contains mostly water, film former, thickeners, silicone, conditioning agents, fragrance, coloring agents, and preservatives.

☺ **Styling Gel, Frizz Control (Level 2)** *($2.29 for 16 ounces)* is a styling gel with just thickeners and conditioning agent and no film formers. This provides a minimal hold but also minimal to no sticky or stiff feel.

☺ **Styling Gel, Shine Enhancing (Level 2)** *($2.29 for 16 ounces)* is almost identical to the Body Building Level 2 above and the same comments apply.

☺ **Styling Gel, Extra Super Hold (Level 3)** *($2.29 for 16 ounces)* is identical to the Body Building version above and the same comments apply.

☺ **Styling Gel, Mega Hold (Level 4)** *($2.29 for 16 ounces)* doesn't have such a mega hold, though it does have good light to medium hold with minimal stiff or sticky feel. It contains mostly water, film former, thickeners, fragrance, conditioning agent, slip agent, preservatives, and coloring agents.

☺ **Styling Gel, Mega Mega Hold (Level 5)** *($2.29 for 16 ounces)* is similar to the Gel Body Building Level 2 above, except this one has somewhat more hold and somewhat more of a sticky feel—but this is hardly the mega mega hold you were expecting.

☺ **Touchable Hold Finishing Spray (Level 2) (Aerosol)** *($2.29 for 7.5 ounces)* is a standard aerosol hairspray that contains mostly alcohol, water, film former, and fragrance. It has good medium hold and minimal stiff or sticky feel and can easily be brushed through. The redundant, almost identical performance of all the hairsprays in this line is just ridiculous.

☺ **Touchable Hold Finishing Spray (Level 2) (Non-Aerosol)** *($2.29 for 7.5 ounces)* is almost identical to the Finishing Spray (Level 2) (Aerosol) above, only in nonaerosol form, but the exact same comments apply.

☺ **Finishing Spritz, Extra Super Hold (Level 3)** *($2.29 for 7.5 ounces)* is almost identical to the Finishing Spray (Level 2) (Aerosol) above, only in nonaerosol form, but the exact same comments apply.

☺ **Style 'N Hold Shaping Spray, Mega Hold (Level 3) (Non-Aerosol)** *($1.99 for 7 ounces)* is almost identical to the Finishing Spray (Level 2) (Aerosol) above only in nonaerosol form, but the exact same comments apply.

☺ **Style 'N Hold Shaping Spray, Ultimate Hold (Level 4) (Non-Aerosol)** *($1.99 for 7 ounces)* is almost identical to the Finishing Spray (Level 2) (Aerosol) above only in nonaerosol form, but the exact same comments apply.

☺ **Ultimate Finishing Spray, Extra Super Hold (Level 3) (Aerosol)** *($1.77 for 7 ounces)* is almost identical to the Finishing Spray (Level 2) (Aerosol) above and the exact same comments apply.

☺ **Ultimate Finishing Spray, Extra Super Hold (Level 3) (Non-Aerosol)** *($2.29 for 7.5 ounces)* is almost identical to the Finishing Spray (Level 2) (Aerosol) above, only in nonaerosol form, but the exact same comments apply.

☺ **Ultimate Finishing Spray, Mega Hold (Level 4) (Aerosol)** *($2.29 for 7.5 ounces)* is almost identical to the Finishing Spray (Level 2) (Aerosol) above and the exact same comments apply.

Lange

It is an understatement to say that Lange is excited about panthenol when it comes to the health of your hair. To read Lange's brochures about its products, you would think it was the fountain of youth for hair. It makes grand claims about what the right amount of panthenol can do for your hair, including everything from re-pairing it to slowing down the "aging process" of hair. Of course, many hair-care products contain a large amount of panthenol, and there is indeed a great deal of evidence that panthenol is a good conditioning agent for hair. It can cling to the hair cuticle as well as absorb somewhat into the hair cortex, temporarily smoothing out split ends and holding moisture in the hair. While panthenol does that well, lots of conditioning ingredients can do the same thing. Plus, it is all temporary; nothing has been permanently changed or altered in the least. There are some very good products in this line, but don't let its claims go to your head—it will waste your money and won't help your hair. For more information on Lange, call (800) 227-1406.

☺ **Baby Shampoo and Bath** *($8.10 for 10 ounces)* is a very good shampoo that contains mostly water, detergent cleansing agent, lather agent, water, thickeners, conditioning agent, preservatives, and fragrance. There isn't much chelating agent in here and the conditioning agent used leaves a deposit on the hair shaft. Still, this is a good shampoo for normal to dry hair of any thickness.

☹ **Elastin Shampoo and Body Cleanser** *($12.99 for 8 ounces)* uses sodium C14-16 olefin sulfonate and TEA-lauryl sulfate as the main detergent cleansing agents, which makes it too drying for all hair types.

☺ **Panthenol C3 Shampoo for Clarifying and Chelating** *($7.49 for 8 ounces)* is a very good shampoo that contains mostly water, detergent cleansing agent, lather agent, water, thickeners, conditioning agent, preservatives, and fragrance. There isn't much chelating agent here and the conditioning agent in here doesn't make this clarifying. Still, this is a good shampoo for normal to dry hair of any thickness.

☹ **Panthenol Formula II Shampoo for Dry Hair and Sensitive Scalps** *($10.99 for 8 ounces)* uses sodium C14-16 olefin sulfonate and TEA-lauryl sulfate as the main detergent cleansing agents, which makes it too drying for all hair types but especially for dry hair or sensitive scalps.

☹ **Panthenol Protein Shampoo for Dehydrated Damaged Hair** *($8.49 for 8 ounces)* uses TEA-lauryl sulfate and sodium C14-16 olefin sulfonate as the main detergent cleansing agents, which makes it too drying for all hair types but especially for dry hair.

☹ **Panthenol Shampoo Hair Thickener for Normal to Oily Hair** *($6.99 for 8 ounces)* uses sodium C14-16 olefin sulfonate and TEA-lauryl sulfate as its main detergent cleansing agents, which makes it too drying for all hair types.

☺ **Elastin Conditioning Rinse** *($13.49 for 8 ounces)* contains mostly water, thickeners, conditioning agents, detangling agent, silicone, detangling agent/film former, plant oil, and preservatives. This is a good conditioner for normal to slightly dry hair of any thickness. It does have a minimal sticky feel, but that can help hair feel thicker. The elastin is useless, but I am concerned that this product contains a tiny amount of sulfur, which can strip hair color, though I suspect there isn't enough to have any effect on the hair.

☺ **Panthenol Conditioning Rinse for Normal and Oily Hair** *($7.50 for 8 ounces)* is similar to the Elastin Conditioning version above and the same comments apply. This conditioner is not appropriate for oily hair or oily scalp.

☺ **Panthenol Protein Conditioning Rinse for Dehydrated, Damaged Hair** *($8.49 for 8 ounces)* is similar to the Elastin Conditioning version above and the same comments apply.

☺ **Panthenol Protein Hair Moisturizer for Dehydrated Hair** *($8.50 for 4 ounces)* contains mostly water, conditioning agents, thickeners, detangling agent, preservatives, and fragrance. This is a good conditioner for dry hair of any thickness.

☺ **CVS: Conditioner Volumizer Styler Leave-in Conditioner** *($14.50 for 8 ounces)* is a good leave-in conditioner that is more like a styling spray than a conditioner. It works well for normal to slightly dry hair that is fine or thin, and can have a slight sticky, stiff feel. It contains mostly water, detangling agent/film former, conditioning agents, preservatives, and fragrance.

☺ **Elastin Panthenol Protein Pak** *($32 for 8 ounces)* contains mostly water, conditioning agents, thickeners, detangling agent, preservatives, and fragrance. This is a good conditioner for dry hair of any thickness.

☺ **Panthenol 5% Treatment Hair and Skin Fixative** *($11.49 for 8 ounces)*. If you want to consider panthenol as the answer for your hair, this is the product to try. It does contain 5% panthenol and that's it except for preservatives and a thickening agent. That means it's 94.9% thickener, 5% panthenol, and 0.1% preservatives. It's just a good conditioner for normal to dry hair, but you could find out if panthenol is the be-all and end-all for your hair.

☺ **Spray Shine for Hair** *($11.99 for 4 ounces)* is a standard silicone spray that can leave a silky-smooth feel on hair.

☺ **Designing Gelee Form Styler** *($6.99 for 8 ounces)* is a fairly liquidy gel with a light to medium hold and minimal stiff or sticky feel. It contains mostly water, alcohol, detangling agents/film formers, slip agent, conditioning agents, and fragrance.

☺ **Super Shaper Gel Extra Firm Hold** *($7.49 for 3 ounces)* contains mostly water, alcohol, film former, conditioning agent, thickener, preservatives, slip agent, silicone, and fragrance. This standard gel has a medium hold and a slight stiff, sticky feel.

☺ **Styling Creme with Marine Collagen** *($9.49 for 8 ounces)* has marine collagen, but that doesn't have any effect on this standard, medium-hold styling cream with a slight sticky, stiff feel. It is a good for styling stubborn frizzies and curls. It contains mostly plant water, film former, thickeners, conditioning agents, detangling agent, silicone, plant oil, preservatives, and fragrance.

☺ **Elastin Configuration 1, Fine, Limp Hair Thickener** *($14.50 for 8 ounces)* is a good styling spray for normal to dry fine or thin hair that has minimal- to light-hold and no stiff or sticky feel. It contains mostly water, alcohol, detangling agent/film former, conditioning agents, preservatives, and fragrance.

☺ **Panthenol Thermal Styling Spray** *($6.49 for 8 ounces)* is a standard soft- to light-hold styling spray with minimal to no stiff or sticky feel. It contains mostly water, alcohol, film former, conditioning agents, fragrance, and slip agents.

☺ **Texturizing Spray with Marine Collagen** *($8.49 for 8 ounces)* is a standard medium-hold styling spray with minimal stiff and sticky feel. It contains mostly plant water, film formers, conditioning agents, fragrance, and preservatives.

☺ **Ultra-Hold Finishing Spray** *($8.99 for 8 ounces)* is a standard hairspray with medium to firm hold and a slight sticky, stiff feel that can be brushed through easily. It contains mostly alcohol, water, film formers, conditioning agent, silicone, and fragrance.

L'anza

L'anza's approach to hair care is like that of many salon lines—filled with claims to make its products seem superior to all others when, in the long run, there really aren't many or any differences—or at least no differences that the hair or scalp will notice. L'anza's Straight & Smooth, for example, "is a cysteine enhanced non-chemical temporary curl relaxer that has a heat activated style memory built into the formula." While that sounds good, cysteine is an amino acid that doesn't cling well to hair. The product ends up containing the same film-forming ingredients that every other styling product does; these can help hair bounce back, but they're not unique to this product.

"Volume Formula hair care is a genuine breakthrough in hair chemistry! The secret: anti-oxidants, natural vitamins and nutrients that help slow down the aging process." There are no secrets! The ingredients are fully disclosed on the label. And there is no research or data anywhere proving that antioxidants of any kind can "protect the hair and scalp from free radicals, the toxins produced by smoke, fumes, alcohol, fatty foods and even sunlight." Green tea and vitamins, even if they could provide benefit for hair, don't have the ability to cling to the hair shaft during rinsing or styling. There are more claims, too—but the individual product reviews and the ingredient labels speak for themselves.

For more information on L'anza, call (800) 423-0307, or visit its Web site at www.lanzahair.com.

Colors & Curls by L'anza

☹ **Moisturizing Shampoo, Shampoo for Color-Treated Hair** *($4.95 for 8.5 ounces)* uses TEA-lauryl sulfate as its main detergent cleansing agent, which makes it too drying for the hair and too irritating and drying for the scalp.

☺ **Protein Plus Shampoo, Shampoo for Bleached and Permed Hair** *($7.50 for 10.1 ounces)* contains mostly water, detergent cleansing agent, lather agent, conditioning agents, plant oil, thickeners, plant extracts, preservatives, and fragrance. This is a good shampoo for normal to dry hair of any thickness.

☺ **Detangler Weightless Rinse Out Conditioner** *($5.95 for 8.5 ounces)* contains mostly water, thickeners, detangling agent, conditioning agent, plant extracts, silicone, preservatives, and fragrance. This is a good conditioner for normal to dry hair of any thickness.

☺ **Moisture Treatment Super Hydrating Treatment** *($28 for 16.1 ounces)* contains mostly water, detangling agent, conditioning agent, plant extracts, thickeners, water-binding agents, preservatives, and fragrance. This is a good conditioner for normal to dry hair that is normal to fine or thin.

☺ **Reconstructor Intensive Hair Repair Treatment** *($12.90 for 4.2 ounces)* contains mostly water, conditioning agent, detangling agents, thickeners, plant extracts, plant oils, water-binding agents, preservatives, and fragrance. This is a good conditioner for dry hair of any thickness. This product can't repair or reconstruct hair. It does contain glycolic acid, which could eat away at the hair shaft, but there isn't enough of it and the pH isn't low enough for it to have that effect. At this amount it's just a water-binding agent.

☺ **Leave-in Protector, Daily Color and Perm Protector** *($6.50 for 4.2 ounces)* contains mostly water, detangling agent, conditioning agent, plant extracts, silicone, water-binding agents, preservatives, and fragrance. This is a standard, but good, leave-in conditioner for normal to dry hair of any thickness. It won't protect a perm.

☺ **Hair Polish** *($9.99 for 3.3 ounces)* contains mostly water, thickeners, plant oil, slip agent, conditioning agent, preservatives, and fragrance. This is a good conditioner for dry hair. It isn't much of a polish, though it can help smooth hair and that can add shine and control.

☺ **Liquid Gel** *($8.90 for 6.7 ounces)* contains mostly water, film former, thickeners, silicone, plant extracts, conditioning agent, preservatives, fragrance, and coloring agents. This is basically a good standard gel that has a light to medium hold and a slight stiff, sticky feel. It also has silvery glitter, which can flake all over the place every time you brush your hair.

☺ **Spray Gel** *($8.95 for 10.1 ounces)* contains mostly water, alcohol, thickeners, film former, silicone, conditioning agent, water-binding agent, plant extracts, silicone, fragrance, and coloring agents. This is a good standard spray gel that has a light hold and minimal to no stiff or sticky feel.

☺ **Bodifying Foam, Moisturizing Setting Foam** *($8.95 for 7.1 ounces)* is a standard mousse with a medium hold and a somewhat sticky feel. It contains mostly water, propellant, film formers, alcohol, silicone, detangling agent, conditioning agent, water-binding agent, plant extracts, silicone, fragrance, and preservatives.

☺ **Bodifying Foam, Super Hold and Shine** *($9.40 for 7 ounces)* is almost identical to the Moisturizing Setting Foam above and the same comments apply.

☺ **Finishing Freeze** *($9.80 for 10.1 ounces)* is a standard hairspray with medium hold and a slight stiff feel that easily brushes through. It contains mostly alcohol, film formers, water, conditioning agent, plant extracts, and fragrance.

☺ **Dramatic F/X Super Hold Hairspray** *($9.90 for 10.6 ounces)* is a medium-to firm-hold aerosol hairspray with a slightly stiff feel that can easily be brushed through. It contains mostly alcohol, propellant, film former, conditioning agent, silicones, plant extracts, and fragrance.

Long Hair Formula by L'anza

☹ **Cleanse** *($10.95 for 13.5 ounces)* uses TEA-lauryl sulfate as the main detergent cleansing agent, which makes it too drying for the hair and too irritating and drying for the scalp.

☺ **Condition** *($12.95 for 13.5 ounces)* contains mostly water, detangling agent, thickeners, conditioning agent, plant extracts, silicone, preservatives, and fragrance. This is a good basic conditioner for normal to slightly dry hair of any thickness.

☺ **Strengthen** *($12.95 for 5.07 ounces)* contains mostly water, conditioning agent, plant oils, detangling agent, more conditioning agent, thickeners, plant extracts, water-binding agents, preservatives, and fragrance. There's nothing in here that will strengthen hair any more than any other conditioner can. This one is suitable for dry hair of any thickness.

☺ **$$$ ProtecShine** *($14.95 for 1.7 ounces)* is a standard silicone serum that works well to make hair look shiny and feel silky. This one is just absurdly overpriced given the versions with identical ingredients being sold at the drugstore.

Rebalance by L'anza

☺ **Deep Cleansing Shampoo, Shampoo for Fine Hair and Oily Scalp** *($7 for 10.1 ounces)* includes a conditioning agent that makes this shampoo better for normal to dry hair. It contains mostly water, detergent cleansing agents, lather agent, conditioning agent, plant extracts, thickeners, preservatives, and fragrance.

☺ **Remedy Shampoo, Shampoo for Problem Scalps and Dry Hair** *($8.60 for 8.5 ounces)* is similar to the Deep Cleansing one above, only with slightly more gentle detergent cleansing agents, and the same basic comments apply. This product does contain salicylic acid, but the pH isn't low enough for it to work as an exfoliant.

☹ **Shampoo Plus, Daily Conditioning Shampoo** *($4.95 for 8.5 ounces)* contains mostly water, detergent cleansing agents, lather agent, plant extract, conditioning agents, silicone, thickeners, preservatives, detangling agent, and fragrance. It also contains clove and peppermint extract, which can be irritating for the scalp.

☺ **Strait-Line Curl Relaxing Shampoo** *($8.96 for 8.5 ounces)* won't straighten hair, but it is a good shampoo for normal to dry fine or thin hair to give it some thickness. It contains mostly water, detergent cleansing agents, lather agent, thickeners, silicone, plant oil, conditioning agents, film former, preservatives, and fragrance.

☹ **Clarifying Treatment Build-Up and Deposit Remover** *($7.95 for 4.2 ounces)* is a basic conditioner containing sodium thiosulfate, an ingredient used in perms to straighten or curl hair. It also swells the hair shaft. It is more gentle than many perm ingredients but it's still a reducing agent and using it to remove buildup and mineral deposits seems drastic given that it can strip color and break down hair.

☺ **Power Treatment, Active Conditioning Formula** *($12.40 for 4.2 ounces)* contains mostly water, conditioning agents, detangling agent, thickeners, plant oils, plant extracts, water-binding agent, preservatives, and fragrance. This is a good conditioner for dry to very dry hair of any thickness.

☹ **Revitalizer, Stimulating Hair and Scalp Moisturizer** *($9.85 for 8.5 ounces)* contains peppermint, menthol, and eucalyptus oil, which are all stimulating, as well as irritating and drying for the scalp.

☺ **Strait-Line Curl Relaxing Conditioner** *($9.96 for 6.7 ounces)* contains mostly water, thickeners, castor oil, detangling agent, plant oils, silicones, conditioning agents, more thickeners, emollient, preservatives, and fragrance. This is a very emollient, heavy conditioner for dry to very dry thick or coarse hair. It absolutely will help to smooth and weight down curls, and it can also have a slight stiff, sticky feel.

☺ **Leave-in Conditioner, Light Daily Conditioning Treatment** *($6.50 for 4.2 ounces)* contains clove and peppermint, which can be irritating for the scalp. If you avoid the scalp this is a good basic detangling leave-in conditioner for normal hair of any thickness.

☺ **Gel Mist, Light Control Gel** *($9.70 for 10.1 ounces)* contains mostly water, thickeners, conditioning agent, film former, silicone, plant extracts, fragrance, slip agent, and preservatives. This is a good light-hold spray gel with minimal stiff, sticky feel.

☺ **Mega Gel, Flexible Style Control Gel** *($9.90 for 8.5 ounces)* contains mostly water, film former, silicone, plant extracts, fragrance, thickeners, conditioning agent, more silicone, more plant extracts, more fragrance, and preservatives. This is a good light-hold gel with minimal to no stiff feel.

☺ **Shine Gel Controls and Softens Frizzy Hair** *($13.49 for 3.3 ounces)* is just silicone with a thickening agent. It is the same as any other silicone serum, and it can add a silky feel and soft shine to hair.

☹ **Styling Foam, Medium Hold Styling Foam** *($8 for 7.1 ounces)* is a standard mousse with a light hold and minimal to no stiff or sticky feel. It contains mostly water, film formers, propellant, slip agents, thickeners, detangling agent, conditioning agent, plant extracts, fragrance, and preservatives. This product does contain clove extract and peppermint, which can be a problem for the skin, so keep it far away from the scalp.

☺ **Strait-Line Temporary Curl Relaxer and Smoother** *($11 for 6.7 ounces)* contains mostly water, silicones, slip agents, thickeners, conditioning agents, detangling agent, plant oil, preservatives, and fragrance. This is a good styling serum to help straighten hair. It has minimal hold but works well with styling tools and has no stiff or sticky feel.

☺ **Special F/X, Light Styling Spray** *($9.80 for 10.6 ounces)* is a standard aerosol hairspray with a medium hold and a slight stiff feel that can easily be brushed through. It contains mostly alcohol, water, propellant, film former, conditioning agent, slip agents, plant extracts, and fragrance.

☺ **Styling Spritz, for Curling Iron Styling** *($8.95 for 10.1 ounces)* is a light-to medium-hold hairspray with a slight stiff feel that can be used when styling or as a hairspray. It is similar to the Special FX above, only in nonaerosol form.

☹ **Hairspray, All-Day Hold Hairspray** *($9.40 for 10.1 ounces)* is a standard hairspray with medium hold that has a slight stiff feel that easily brushes through. And yes, you guessed it, it is incredibly similar to most all of the hairsprays in the L'anza arsenal. It contains mostly alcohol, film formers, water, conditioning agent, silicone, preservatives, and fragrance.

Volume Formula by L'anza

☺ **Bodifying Shampoo** *($7.96 for 12.6 ounces)* contains mostly water, plant extracts, detergent cleansing agents, lather agent, conditioning agent, vitamins, preservatives, and fragrance. There is nothing about this that will add body, but it is a good basic shampoo for normal to slightly dry hair of any thickness.

☺ **Weightless Rinse** *($8.96 for 12.6 ounces)* contains mostly water, detangling agent, thickeners, castor oil, conditioning agents, plant extracts, silicone, preservatives, vitamins, and fragrance. The amount of vitamins in here is negligible and hardly worth mentioning. This is not a weightless conditioner, but it is a good one for normal to dry hair that is fine or thin. It can easily build up on hair.

☺ **Zero Weight Gel** *($9.89 for 8.5 ounces)* is a relatively standard gel with medium hold and minimal stiff or sticky feel. The twist is that this one contains gold glitter. The glitter part is a your personal preference, but I would think twice about shining during the day, and every time you brush your hair you tend to sprinkle sparkles all over yourself. The gel contains mostly water, film formers, slip agents, silicone, conditioning agents, plant extracts, thickeners, preservatives, fragrance, and coloring agents.

☺ **Body Styling Cream** *($8.96 for 8.5 ounces)* is more of a gel lotion than a cream, but it has a silky finish and can help in smoothing curls and frizzies without hold or stiffness. It can get greasy and heavy, so use it sparingly. It contains mostly water, detangling agent, thickeners, slip agents, plant oils, vitamins, silicones, preservatives, and fragrance. It has minimal to no stiff or sticky feel.

☺ **Root Effects** *($9.72 for 7.1 ounces)* contains mostly water, propellant, alcohol, film formers, slip agents, conditioning agents, thickeners, plant extracts, and fragrance. This is a strange mix between a mousse and an aerosol styling spray. Either way it has light to medium hold with minimal stiff or sticky feel and it can help with any aspect of styling hair, not just dealing with the roots.

☺ **Finishing Protector Dryspray** *($9.96 for 8.5 ounces)* contains mostly alcohol, water, film former, silicones, conditioning agent, slip agent, plant extracts, and fragrance. This is a standard hairspray with medium hold and minimal stiff feel that easily brushes through.

☺ **Anti-Oxidant Replenisher** *($14.96 for 8.5 ounces)* is a lightweight styling gel with no hold, though it can help smooth frizzies and curls when styling. It contains mostly water, thickeners, silicones, slip agents, conditioning agents, vitamins, preservatives, and fragrance. The antioxidants in here can't protect hair.

L'Oreal

L'Oreal has a number of lines represented at the drugstore, including FortaVive, ColorVive, VitaVive, HydraVive, BodyVive, and its Studio Line. Strangely enough, there is very little difference between the Vive lines, and the differences that do exist don't help produce the results promised by the names. ColorVive isn't the answer if you have color-treated hair that is dried out or damaged, HydraVive isn't great if your hair needs extra moisture, VitaVive won't feed hair, BodyVive doesn't add all that much body (at least not any more than the other Vives do), and FortaVive doesn't fortify hair. There are still some good products to consider, but the marketing direction isn't reflected in formulation differences. For example, BodyVive contains ceramide, a good water-binding agent that can help as a conditioning agent. However, there is nothing about ceramide that is better than any other conditioning agents for helping hair feel fuller or softer. Studio Line is a group of styling products that have some great options to consider.

For more information on L'Oreal, call (212) 818-1500, (800) 322-2036, or visit its Web site at www.lorealcosmetics.com.

BodyVive by L'Oreal

☺ **BodyVive Daily Body for Fine Hair, Volumizing Shampoo plus Ceramide-R & Protein, Regular** *($3.79 for 13 ounces)* contains mostly water, detergent cleansing agent, lather agent, silicone, thickeners, fragrance, detangling agent/film former, and preservatives. This is a good shampoo for dry hair of any thickness, though it can build up on hair. The amount of "ceramide R" in here is so minimal that it is practically nonexistent.

☺ **BodyVive Daily Body for Fine Hair, Thickening Shampoo plus Ceramide-R & Protein, Thin/Extra Fine** *($3.79 for 13 ounces)* contains mostly detergent cleansing agents, fragrance, lather agent, detangling agent, preservatives, and thickeners. This is a good basic shampoo for all hair types, but there is nothing in here that will provide body or much of any conditioning.

☺ **BodyVive Daily Body for Fine Hair, No Weight Conditioner plus Ceramide-R & Protein, All Fine Hair** *($3.79 for 13 ounces)* contains mostly water, thickeners, conditioning agents, silicones, detangling agent, lanolin, silicone, film former, and preservatives. This is a good conditioner for dry hair that is normal to fine or thin.

☺ **BodyVive Daily Body for Fine Hair, Add-in Body plus Ceramide-R** *($3.79 for 8.5 ounces)* contains mostly water, alcohol, slip agent, film formers, fragrance, silicone, castor oil, and conditioning agent. This is an OK standard styling spray that has a light to medium hold with a slight stiff, sticky feel.

ColorVive by L'Oreal

☺ **ColorVive Daily Care for Color-Treated Hair Gentle Shampoo plus UV Filter, Regular Colored or Highlighted** *($2.99 for 13 ounces)* is just shampoo, and that's great for all hair types. It contains mostly water, detergent cleansing agents, lather agents, fragrance, thickener, and preservatives. There is nothing in here to protect hair color, and the UV filter claim is meaningless without an SPF number.

☺ **ColorVive Daily Care for Color-Treated Hair Gentle Shampoo plus UV Filter, for Dry Hair Colored or Highlighted** *($3.79 for 13 ounces)* is almost identical to the one above and the same comments apply.

☺ **ColorVive Weekly Protective Conditioning, Dry Defense Plus UV Filter 5-Minute Treatment** *($1.59 for 1 ounce)* contains mostly water, thickeners, detangling agents, silicone, fragrance, conditioning agent, and preservatives. There is really nothing special in here; this is just a basic conditioner for dry hair of any thickness. If you keep any conditioner in the hair for five minutes, it will be better for the hair.

☺ **ColorVive Daily Care for Color-Treated Hair, Creme Conditioner plus UV Filter, Regular Colored or Highlighted** *($2.99 for 13 ounces)* is almost identical to the 5-Minute Treatment above and the same comments apply.

☺ **ColorVive Daily Care for Color-Treated Hair, Creme Conditioner plus UV Filter, for Dry Hair Colored or Highlighted** *($3.79 for 13 ounces)* is almost identical to the 5-Minute Treatment above and the same comments apply.

FortaVive by L'Oreal

☺ **FortaVive Daily Care for Damaged Hair, Repairing Shampoo plus Ceramide-R** *($3.79 for 13 ounces)* contains mostly water, detergent cleansing agents, silicone, lather agents, thickeners, fragrance, preservatives, and detangling agent. This is a good silicone-based shampoo that would work great for dry hair of any thickness.

☺ **FortaVive Weekly Ceramide Replacement, Pure Strength with Ceramide-R 5-Minute Treatment** *($1.59 for 1 ounce)* contains mostly water, thickeners, conditioning agent, detangling agent, lanolin, silicones, more thickeners, fragrance, and preservatives. There is nothing special in here; it is just a basic conditioner for very dry hair that is thick or coarse. If you keep any conditioner in the hair for five minutes it will be better for the hair.

☺ **FortaVive Daily Care for Damaged Hair, Repairing Conditioner plus Ceramide-R** *($3.79 for 13 ounces)* contains mostly water, thickeners, conditioning agent, film former/detangling agents, slip agent, fragrance, and preservatives. This is a basic conditioner for normal to slightly dry hair that is normal to fine or thin in thickness.

HydraVive by L'Oreal

☺ **HydraVive Daily Care for Dry Hair, Shampoo + Conditioner plus Hydra-Protein Two-in-One** *($3.79 for 13 ounces)* is almost identical to the FortaVive Daily Care shampoo above and the same comments apply.

☺ **HydraVive Daily Care for Dry Hair, Moisture Shampoo plus Hydra-Protein, Dry/Damaged** *($3.79 for 13 ounces)* contains mostly water, detergent cleansing agent, lather agent, thickeners, slip agent, fragrance, conditioning agent, detangling agent/film former, and preservatives. This is a good shampoo for normal to slightly dry hair that is fine or thin to normal in thickness.

☺ **HydraVive Weekly Protein Conditioning Moisture Solution with Hydra-Protein 5-Minute Treatment** *($1.59 for 1 ounce)* contains mostly water, thickeners, slip agent, detangling agent, silicone, fragrance, preservatives, and conditioning agent. This is a very standard conditioner for normal to dry hair of any thickness. Leaving it on for five minutes will help, but that's true for any conditioner.

☺ **HydraVive Daily Care for Dry Hair, Moisture Conditioner plus Hydra-Protein, Dry/Damaged** *($3.79 for 13 ounces)* contains mostly water, thickeners, detangling agent, fragrance, slip agent, film former, preservatives, and conditioning agent. This is a very standard conditioner for normal to slightly dry hair that is fine or thin to normal.

VitaVive by L'Oreal

☺ **VitaVive Daily Care for Normal Hair, Multi-Vitamin Clear Shampoo** *($3.79 for 13 ounces)* is just a shampoo that would be great for hair types. It contains mostly water, detergent cleansing agent, lather agent, thickeners, fragrance, preservatives, vitamins, conditioning agent, and more preservatives. The amounts of vitamins and conditioning agent in here are insignificant.

☺ **VitaVive Daily Care for Normal Hair 2-in-1, Multi-Vitamin Shampoo + Conditioner** *($4.29 for 13 ounces)* is similar to the one above, only with silicone. That can help dry hair, though it can also cause buildup.

☺ **VitaVive Daily Care for Normal Hair, Multi-Vitamin Conditioner** *($3.79 for 13 ounces)* contains mostly water, thickeners, conditioning agent, silicone, detangling agent, fragrance, more thickeners, preservatives, lanolin, more silicone, and vitamins. This is a good conditioner for normal to slightly dry hair of any thickness. The lanolin and silicone are barely present in this formulation.

Studio Line by L'Oreal

☺ **Studio Line Anti-Frizz Alcohol-Free** *($2.99 for 6 ounces)* contains mostly water, slip agent, thickener, conditioning agents, silicone, fragrance, preservatives, and castor oil. This is a good lightweight styling gel for smoothing curls and frizzies. It has no hold and therefore no stiff or sticky feel.

☺ **Studio Line Anti-Sticky Invisi-Gel Alcohol-Free Extra Body** *($2.99 for 6.8 ounces)* is a standard gel with medium hold that definitely has a somewhat sticky feel. It contains mostly water, film formers, conditioning agents, thickeners, fragrance, preservatives, and silicone.

☺ **Studio Line Anti-Sticky Invisi-Gel Alcohol-Free Mega Body** *($2.99 for 6.8 ounces)* is almost identical to the Extra Body version above and the same comments apply.

☺ **Studio Line Total Control Clean Gel Alcohol Free Multi-Vitamin Formula Extra Hold** *($2.99 for 6.8 ounces)* is similar to the Extra Body version above and the same basic comments apply.

☺ **Studio Line Mega Gel Multi-Vitamin Formula Mega Hold** *($2.99 for 6.8 ounces)* is similar to the Extra Body version above and the same basic comments apply.

☺ **Studio Line Lasting Curls Gel** *($2.99 for 6 ounces)* is similar to the Extra Body version above and the same comments apply.

☺ **Studio Line Pumping Curls** *($2.99 for 8 ounces)* is more of a leave-in conditioner than anything else. It has almost no hold, but a slippery, soft feel. That can help when styling, but it offers no hold or support for hair. It contains mostly water, alcohol, conditioning agents, fragrance, film formers, silicones, and detangling agent. This is very good for smoothing curls and frizzies without weight or stiffness.

☺ **Studio Line Mega Mousse Mega Body** *($2.99 for 6.9 ounces)* is a standard mousse with a light hold and minimal to no stiff or sticky feel. It contains mostly water, alcohol, propellant, film formers, conditioning agents, silicone, detangling agent, and fragrance.

☺ **Studio Line Springing Curls Mousse** *($2.99 for 6 ounces)* is almost identical to the Mega Mousse above and the same comments apply.

☺ **Studio Line Mega Spritz Multi-Vitamin Formula Mega Hold** *($2.99 for 8.5 ounces)* is a standard hairspray with a medium hold and a somewhat stiff feel that can easily be brushed through. It contains mostly alcohol, water, film former, conditioning agents, fragrance, and silicone. It has a slight stiff, sticky feel.

☺ **Studio Line Mighty Mist Hair Spray Extra Hold** *($2.99 for 8 ounces)* is almost identical to the Mega Spritz above and the same comments apply.

☺ **Studio Line Mighty Mist Hair Spray Mega Hold** *($2.99 for 8 ounces)* is almost identical to the Mega Spritz above and the same comments apply.

☺ **Studio Senses The Feel for Better Hair Texture** *($3.99 for 8 ounces)* contains mostly water, silicone, thickeners, fragrance, film former, and preservatives. This is a good lightweight silicone gel with minimal to almost no hold that can help with styling hair smooth and adding shine and softness.

☺ **Studio Senses The Shiny Look Liquid Shine & Hold** *($6.31 for 6 ounces)* is a very standard but good silicone spray that can add shine and a silky feel to hair. This one does have a small amount of film former, but it is so minimal it gives no noticeable hold.

☺ **Studio Senses The Touch Define & Shine Pomade** *($4.49 for 2 ounces)* is a standard pomade with no stiff or sticky feel, though it can feel greasy and heavy, so use it sparingly. It contains mostly Vaseline, mineral oil, wax, silicone, thickeners, and preservatives. It has no film formers, so there is less hold—but that's what prevents it from having a stiff feel on hair.

☹ **Studio Senses The Warm Scent for Hair Freshness** *($6.31 for 3.5 ounces)* is just cologne for the hair; it has no other purpose.

☹ **Studio Senses The Cool Scent for Hair Freshness** *($6.31 for 3.5 ounces)* is just cologne for the hair; it has no other purpose.

L'Oreal Kids

☺ **Extra Gentle 2-in-1 Shampoo, Extra Conditioning, Burst of Cherry-Almond** *($3.49 for 9 ounces)* is a standard shampoo with nothing to make it particularly better for children. It is a good shampoo with lots of detergent cleansing agents, thickeners, fragrance, film former, preservatives, and coloring agents, which makes it good for normal hair that is fine ofr thin.. Don't rely on this product to help comb out snarls in children's hair or be extra conditioning in any way.

☺ **Extra Gentle 2-in-1 Shampoo, Extra Manageability, Burst of Tropical Punch** *($3.49 for 9 ounces)* is almost identical to the Cherry Almond version above and the same comments apply.

☺ **Extra Gentle 2-in-1 Shampoo, Fine Hair, Burst of Banana-Melon** *($3.49 for 9 ounces)* is almost identical to the Cherry Almond version above and the same comments apply.

☺ **Extra Gentle 2-in-1 Shampoo, Normal Hair, Burst of Fruity Apricot** *($3.49 for 9 ounces)* is almost identical to the Cherry Almond version above and the same comments apply.

☺ **Extra Gentle 2-in-1 Shampoo, Thick or Curly or Wavy Hair, Burst of Watermelon** *($3.49 for 9 ounces)* is almost identical to the Cherry Almond version above and the same comments apply.

☺ **Extra Gentle Conditioner Plus Detangler, Hard to Manage Hair, Burst of Juicy Grape** *($3.49 for 9 ounces)*. You kind of wonder, if the 2-in-1 shampoos above really worked, why would you need this conditioner? This is a good basic conditioner for normal to slightly dry hair of any thickness; it contains mostly water, thickeners, slip agents, detangling agents, silicone, fragrance, plant oil, and preservatives.

☺ **Extra Gentle Styling Gel Plus Manager, All Hair Types, Burst of Cherry-Almond, No Alcohol** *($3.49 for 9 ounces)* is a standard gel that contains mostly water, silicone, slip agents, film former, preservatives, thickeners, and fragrance. It has a light hold and works great for dry hair of any thickness.

M.A.C.

For more information on M.A.C., call (905) 470-7877, (800) 387-6707, or visit its Web site at www.elcompanies.com.

☺ **Clarifying Shampoo** *($7 for 8 ounces)* is about as good a standard shampoo as you will find. It contains mostly water, detergent cleansing agents, glycerin, preservatives, fragrance, and preservatives. This works great for most hair types.

☺ **Maintain Shampoo** *($7 for 8 ounces)* is similar to the one above, with the addition of minimal conditioning agents that would mostly be washed away. It does contain fragrance and coloring agents. It would be fine for most all hair types as a basic shampoo.

☺ **Retain Shampoo** *($7 for 8 ounces)* contains mostly water, foaming agent, detergent cleansing agent, glycerin, conditioning agents, preservatives, detangling agent, fragrance, and some water-binding agents. The water-binding agents would be rinsed away before they could have a moisturizing effect. This is a good shampoo for most hair types, with minimal chance of buildup.

☺ **Intensive Conditioner** *($8 for 5 ounces)* isn't all that intensive, but it is a good conditioner for normal to dry hair. It contains mostly water, plant oils, thickeners, glycerin, detangling agents, panthenol, protein, fragrance, and preservatives. There is a tiny bit of alcohol in here, but not enough to be a problem for hair.

☺ **Moisture Rinse** *($10 for 8 ounces)* is a lightweight detangling conditioner for normal to slightly dry or damaged hair. It contains mostly water, thickeners, detangling agents, fragrance, and preservatives. The amount of silicone, panthenol, and water-binding agents in here is minimal, so they won't help much.

☺ **Protective Spray** *($8 for 8 ounces)* isn't all that protective, but it is a good lightweight, leave-in conditioner that would work well for most hair types. The claim is that this is supposed to be a low pH sealant for use after chemical processing of the hair. The pH is 4 (not 3 as the label states). But even if it were lower, part of the dye or perm process itself is to neutralize the pH of the hair to return it to a healthy level and stop the processing step, so this product is completely unnecessary. It contains mostly water, detangling agents, silicone, thickeners, fragrance, and preservatives.

☹ **Texturizing Lotion** *($8 for 8.4 ounces)* contains mostly water, film former, alcohol, plant extract, silicone, detangling agents, protein, panthenol, preservatives, and fragrance. The amount of alcohol in here makes it a problem for hair and scalp, plus the squeeze bottle makes it hard to apply to hair. A spray bottle would have been far better.

☺ **Styling Gel** *($7.60 for 5 ounces)* is a standard gel with light hold and minimal stiff or sticky feel. It contains water, film former, silicone, thickeners, fragrance, detangling agents, more fragrance, and preservatives.

☺ **Curl Enhancer** (*$8 for 8.4 ounces*) contains mostly water, glycerin, silicones, thickeners, detangling agents, protein, panthenol, preservatives, and fragrance. This is more of a styling cream to straighten hair or smooth frizzies than something to enhance curls. It has a slight sticky feel and minimal hold. Use it minimally or it can feel heavy and greasy.

☺ **Hair Gloss** (*$8 for 2.5 ounces*) contains mostly water, slip agent, thickeners, castor oil, silicones, fragrance, and preservatives. This is a good styling gel with a minimal hold and an emollient, almost greasy feel. It can help smooth frizzies and stubborn curls, but use it minimally or it can get heavy and greasy looking.

☺ **Holding Spray** (*$7 for 8 ounces*) contains mostly alcohol, water, film former, conditioning agents, panthenol, detangling agents, silicone, and fragrance. This is a good, light-hold hairspray with minimal to no stiff or sticky feel.

Mastey

Henri Mastey happens to be a chemist. While that is an impressive status for the owner of a cosmetics or hair-care company, and while there are indeed some good products in the Mastey group, the line also provides some appalling misinformation. What a shame—because it clouds an otherwise interesting line, and Mastey disseminates some of the most misleading notions about hair-care ingredients and the evil lurking in other manufacturers' bottles. Of course the source for the information is rarely given, or if a source is cited it is just a snippet that sounds impressive but doesn't portray the complete story. For example, Mastey states, "Propylene glycol is often called 'industrial strength anti-freeze'." First, it's ethylene glycol that's antifreeze, not propylene glycol. Moreover, while propylene glycol does have problems in pure or 100 percent concentrations, the cosmetics industry uses only minute fractions of that. Many cosmetics ingredients, like some of those in Mastey's own products, would be deadly in pure concentrations.

Another Mastey warning about ingredients concerns nitrosamines. I've written about this issue in "DEA in Cosmetics," in Chapter 3, *Hair-Care Basics*. While the ingredients Mastey points to in this regard include DEA (diethanolamine), his own products use MEA (monoethanolamine). The issue here is about amines in general and their effect in a product. While research was done on DEA, researchers have estimated that the same would be true for MEA.

Mastey also wants you to be afraid of glycerin because it draws "moisture from the deeper skin layers to rehydrate the surface. Obviously, this is like drying the hair & skin from the inside out!" That's not true. Glycerin is a direct component of skin and hair. In the amounts used in cosmetics, it cannot remove moisture but it can reinforce the structure of the skin and hair. The problem stated by Mastey does occur, but only when glycerin is used in concentrations of 50 percent or greater.

You also are told you need to worry about the cleansing agents other companies use, ranging from "sodium lauryl sulfate, ammonium lauryl sulfate, and sodium laureth sulfate," because they strip away the skin's lipids, and sodium lauryl sulfate can even "cause hair loss." Mastey then provides a chart of irritation showing how this is true. The source of the ratings is not mentioned and of course Mastey's ingredients are not included. While sodium lauryl sulfate is indeed a potentially irritating ingredient, this other information is completely without validation. There isn't proof for this anywhere. Further, if the fear is that these ingredients remove lipids (oils), are we to assume that because Mastey products are free of them they leave oil on your hair?

I could go on, but you get the idea. This is such a shame, because this misleading hysteria detracts from some otherwise well formulated products. For more information on Mastey, call (805) 257-4814, (800) 6 MASTEY, or visit its Web site at www.mastey.com.

☺ **Clarte Normalizing Creme Shampoo** *($9 for 10.2 ounces)* contains mostly water, detergent cleansing agents, thickeners, lather agent, slip agent, conditioning agent, water-binding agent, preservatives, and fragrance. This is a good basic shampoo for all hair types. The amount of conditioning agent in here is so tiny it wouldn't be a problem for buildup.

☺ **Enove Volumizing Creme Shampoo** *($9 for 10.2 ounces)* is almost identical to the Clarte above and the same comments apply.

☺ **Traite Moisturizing Creme Shampoo Nutrient Rich Cleansing Complex** *($9 for 10.2 ounces)* is almost identical to the Clarte above and the same comments apply.

☺ **Le Remouver Deep Cleansing Clarifier** *($9 for 10.2 ounces)* is almost identical to the Clarte above, only with slightly more detergent cleansing agents, but the same comments apply.

☺ **Color Refreshing Shampoo Ash Blonde** *($8 for 8 ounces)* is almost identical to the Clarte above and the same comments apply.

☺ **Color Refreshing Shampoo Blue-Brown** *($8 for 8 ounces)* is almost identical to the Clarte above and the same comments apply.

☺ **Color Refreshing Shampoo Cinnamon** *($8 for 8 ounces)* is almost identical to the Clarte above and the same comments apply.

☺ **Color Refreshing Shampoo Golden Blonde** *($8 for 8 ounces)* is almost identical to the Clarte above and the same comments apply.

☺ **Color Refreshing Shampoo Golden Brown** *($8 for 8 ounces)* is almost identical to the Clarte above and the same comments apply.

☺ **Color Refreshing Shampoo Golden Henna** *($8 for 8 ounces)* is almost identical to the Clarte above and the same comments apply.

☺ **Color Refreshing Shampoo Red Copper** *($8 for 8 ounces)* is almost identical to the Clarte above and the same comments apply.

☺ **Color Refreshing Shampoo Red Flame** *($8 for 8 ounces)* is almost identical to the Clarte above and the same comments apply.

☺ **Color Refreshing Shampoo Red Wine** *($8 for 8 ounces)* is almost identical to the Clarte above and the same comments apply.

☺ **Color Refreshing Shampoo Silver-Violet** *($8 for 8 ounces)* is almost identical to the Clarte above and the same comments apply.

☺ **Basic Superpac Protein Complex Reconstructor** *($16.20 for 10.2 ounces)* contains mostly water, thickeners, detangling agent, conditioning agents, water-binding agents, vitamins, preservatives, and fragrance. This is a good basic conditioner for normal to dry hair that is fine to thin or normal in thickness. It can't reconstruct a hair on your head.

☺ **Frehair Finishing Creme Rinse** *($9 for 10.2 ounces)* contains mostly water, thickeners, detangling agent, conditioning agents, vitamins, preservatives, and fragrance. This is a good lightweight conditioner for normal hair of any thickness.

☺ **HC Formula +B5 Hair & Scalp Mender** *($9 for 10.2 ounces)* contains mostly water, conditioning agents, thickeners, water-binding agent, slip agents, vitamins, preservatives, and fragrance. This is a good conditioner for dry hair of any thickness. There is nothing in here that can mend hair or scalp.

☺ **Liquid Pac Revitalizing Reconstructor** *($5.90 for 5.1 ounces)* is almost identical to the HC Formula above and the same comments apply. This one does have a tiny amount of film former, which makes it slightly better for dry hair that is normal to fine or thin.

☺ **Moisturee Revitalizing Hydrating Complex** *($13.80 for 10.2 ounces)* contains mostly water, thickeners, detangling agent, conditioning agents, water-binding agents, vitamins, preservatives, and fragrance. This is a good basic conditioner for normal to dry hair that is fine to thin or normal.

☺ **Enplace Hair Sculpting Liquid Gel Alcohol-Free** *($9 for 10.2 ounces)* is a standard styling spray that contains mostly water, film formers, conditioning agents, water-binding agent, thickeners, preservatives, and fragrance. It has a light hold with minimal stiff or sticky feel.

☺ **Enplace Sculpting Lotion with Sunscreen** *($5.90 for 5.1 ounces)* is a standard styling spray with a light hold and minimal to no stiff or sticky feel. It contains mostly water, film formers, conditioning agents, water-binding agent, thickeners, preservatives, and fragrance.

☺ **Le Gel Firm Hold Styling Gel Alcohol Free** *($5.90 for 5.1 ounces)* is a standard gel that contains mostly water, film formers, thickeners, conditioning agents, water-binding agent, vitamins, preservatives, and fragrance. It has a medium hold with a somewhat sticky feel, though it can easily be brushed through. The sunscreen in here can't protect from sun damage. Without an SPF number you can't tell if this is even an SPF 2 or if it will stay on the hair after brushing or styling.

☺ **Le Gel Soft Hold Hair Styling Gel with Sunscreen** *($5.90 for 5 ounces)* is almost identical to the Le Gel Firm Hold above, only with a light to medium hold.

☺ **Shine Naturel Wet & Shine with Sunscreen** *($5.90 for 5.1 ounces)* contains mostly water, film formers, slip agents, conditioning agents, thickeners, vitamins, and fragrance. This liquid gel has a light hold with minimal stiff or sticky feel.

☺ **Direction Shaper Spray** *($5.90 for 5.1 ounces)* is a very light-hold standard hairspray with no stiff or sticky feel. It would work great to style hair. It contains mostly alcohol, water, film formers, conditioning agents, slip agents, silicone, and fragrance.

☺ **Designer Firm Hold Volumizing Liquid Mousse with Sunscreen** *($5.90 for 5.1 ounces)* is a standard styling spray that has nothing to with the styling properties of most mousses. It has light to medium hold with minimal stiff or sticky feel that contains water, film former, conditioning agents, slip agents, preservatives, and fragrance. Without an SPF number you can't tell if this is even an SPF 2 or if it will stay on the hair after brushing or styling.

☺ **Designer Soft Hold Volumizing Liquid Mousse with Sunscreen** *($5.50 for 5.1 ounces)* is almost identical to the Firm Hold version above and the same comments apply.

☺ **Fixe Firm Hold Finishing Hair Spray with Sunscreen** *($5.90 for 5.1 ounces)* is a standard hairspray with light to medium hold that contains mostly alcohol, water, film formers, conditioning agents, slip agents, silicone, and fragrance. It has a slight sticky, stiff feel, though it can be easily brushed through. The sunscreen claim is bogus; though this product does contain a sunscreen ingredient, it can't protect the hair from sun damage or it would be rated with an SPF.

☺ **Fixe Soft Hold Finishing Hair Spray with Sunscreen** *($5.90 for 5.1 ounces)* is similar to the Fixe Firm Hold above and the same comments apply.

☺ **Rigide Spritz for Maximum Hold with Sunscreen** *($5.50 for 5.1 ounces)* is similar to the Fixe Firm Hold above and the same comments apply.

☺ **Activateur Curl Enhancer with Sunscreen** *($5.50 for 5.1 ounces)* contains mostly water, conditioning agents, slip agents, detangling agent/film former, water-binding agents, and fragrance. This is a very lightweight, leave-in conditioner with minimal to no stiff feel that would work great for normal to dry hair that is normal to fine or thin in thickness. It doesn't revitalize curls any more than most leave-in conditioners can.

☺ **Lumineux Hair Shine Mist** *($10 for 5.1 ounces)* is a standard silicone serum that can add a silky shine and softness to hair.

Matrix

Matrix is now owned by Bristol-Myers Squibb. Over the years, Matrix has had its share of owners. Having been bought and sold a few times, it has now grown to be a huge group of products with varying lines for different niche markets. Its Amplify Volumizing System is supposed to use technology that "is so new it could only come from the leader in professional hair care. In fact, it is so breakthrough, we took it to the patent office." Whether or not these products are patented is unclear, but with no patent number provided there's no way to confirm that. What is clear from the ingredient listing is that these products use the same film formers that show up in most products that make claims about making hair thicker.

Biolage is supposed to be "a rejuvenating collection of hair care products based on a unique botanical ingredient system. These natural extracts bring back the silky, healthy shine nature gave your hair." Vital Nutrients is supposed to be "daily nutrition for healthy hair." Actually, almost no plant extracts or vitamins appear in either of these product lines, and the ones that do show up have no real effect on hair. The major ingredients in these products are the same that show up in almost every hair-care product being sold.

For the enormous number of women who color their hair, Logics is Matrix's answer to the dilemma of color fading. The line is "fortified" with something called "Photogard 4" to prevent that from happening. However, that claim just doesn't hold up in the wash. The ingredients in these products are as standard as they get, and the sunscreen is ineffective. As long as product isn't rated with an SPF, the claims about sun protection for the hair are as bogus as they would be for an unrated product for the skin.

For more information on Matrix, call (440) 248-3700, (800) 6 MATRIX, (800) 282-2822, or visit its Web site at www.matrixbeautiful.com.

Amplify Volumizing System by Matrix

☹ **Shampoo** *($12.75 for 13.5 ounces)* uses sodium lauryl sulfate as one of the main detergent cleansing agents, which makes it too drying for the hair and scalp.

☺ **Conditioner** *($13.75 for 13.5 ounces)* is a good, basic conditioner for normal to slightly dry hair of any thickness. It contains mostly water, thickeners, detangling agents, conditioning agents, fragrance, slip agent, preservatives, and coloring agents.

☺ **Liquid Gel** *($12.75 for 5.1 ounces)* is a good, basic styling gel with a light hold and minimal sticky feel. It contains mostly water, film formers, thickeners, silicone, conditioning agents, fragrance, preservatives, and coloring agents.

☺ **Root Lifter** *($13.75 for 8.5 ounces)* is a good styling spray in an awkward container with a nozzle that looks like it can direct the spray right where you need it, meaning the roots. But it tends to concentrate too much in one area and that isn't as helpful as you would think. It takes a knack to get used to this kind of application, which is more gimmick than an improvement. You can count on a light to medium hold with a slight sticky feel, though it can easily be brushed through. It contains mostly water, film formers, conditioning agents, castor oil, fragrance, preservatives, and coloring agents.

☺ **Volumizing System Hair Spray** *($13.75 for 10 ounces)* is a standard hairspray with medium to firm hold and a slight stiff feel, though it does let you brush through hair. It contains mostly alcohol, propellant, film formers, conditioning agents, silicone, and fragrance.

Icon for Men by Matrix

☺ **Body Building Shampoo** *($3.99 for 8 ounces)* is a good basic shampoo with minimal conditioning agents and no film formers, so it would work for all hair types. It does contain about 1 to 2 percent salicylic acid (BHA), which can be a problem for the hair, but the pH of this shampoo is around 6, and that it isn't low enough for the BHA to denature hair or exfoliate the scalp. It is still of concern and is out of place in a hair-care product.

☺ **Conditioning Shampoo** *($3.99 for 8 ounces)* is similar to the Body Building version above, only with slightly more conditioning agents. It is still a good basic shampoo for all hair types and the comment about the BHA applies here as well.

☹ **Dandruff Shampoo** *($7.49 for 8 ounces)* uses sodium C14-16 olefin sulfonate as the main detergent cleansing agent, which is too drying and irritating for the scalp. It also contains 2 percent BHA, and while that may be able to exfoliate the scalp it can also denature the hair by eroding the cuticle, though the pH of this shampoo isn't low enough for the BHA to have that effect.

☺ **Lite Conditioner** *($5.99 for 8 ounces)* is a good basic conditioner for normal to dry hair of any thickness; it contains mostly water, thickener, conditioning agents, detangling agents, slip agents, silicone, preservatives, and fragrance. It does contain about 2 percent salicylic acid, and that is of concern, though the pH does appear to be too high to make it an effective exfoliant, which would denature the hair shaft's cuticle layer.

☺ **Controlling Gel** *($5.99 for 4 ounces)* is a good basic gel with a light to medium hold and minimal stiff or sticky feel. It contains about 1 to 2 percent BHA, which raises the same concerns as mentioned for the shampoos and conditioners above.

☺ **Grooming Cream** *($7.99 for 4 ounces)* also has salicylic acid, though it's probably not enough to be a problem for hair and the pH is definitely not high enough either. It would be a good styling cream with no stiffness or sticky feel, but it also has minimal hold.

☺ **Controlling Spray (Aerosol)** *($8.99 for 10 ounces)* is a standard medium- to firm-hold aerosol hairspray that has a slight stiff feel, though it can be brushed through. It contains mostly alcohol, propellant, film formers, fragrance, slip agents, silicone, and conditioning agents.

☺ **Natural Holding Spray** *($8.99 for 8 ounces)* is similar to the Controlling Spray above, only in nonaerosol form, and the same basic comments apply.

Logics by Matrix

☹ **Balancing Shampoo** *($11.95 for 13.5 ounces)* uses sodium lauryl sulfate as one of its main detergent cleansing agents, which makes it too drying for the hair and scalp.

☹ **Clarifying Shampoo** *($11.95 for 13.5 ounces)* uses sodium lauryl sulfate as one of its main detergent cleansing agents, which makes it too drying for the hair and scalp.

☹ **Remoisturizing Shampoo** *($11.95 for 13.5 ounces)* uses sodium lauryl sulfate as one of its main detergent cleansing agents, which makes it too drying for the hair and scalp.

☺ **Color Refresher Revitalizing Conditioner Charcoal, Dark Cool Brown** *($11.75 for 6 ounces)* contains mostly water, detangling agent, thickeners, silicone, conditioning agent, preservatives, fragrance, and dye agents. This is a good color-enhancing conditioner for normal to dry hair of any thickness.

☺ **Color Refresher Revitalizing Conditioner Crimson, Red/Violet** *($11.75 for 6 ounces)* is almost identical to the version above and the same comments apply.

☺ **Color Refresher Revitalizing Conditioner Earth, Ash Brown** *($11.75 for 6 ounces)* is almost identical to the version above and the same comments apply.

☺ **Color Refresher Revitalizing Conditioner Fire, Red/Orange** *($11.75 for 6 ounces)* is almost identical to the version above and the same comments apply.

☺ **Color Refresher Revitalizing Conditioner Quartz, Violet** *($11.75 for 6 ounces)* is almost identical to the version above and the same comments apply.

☺ **Color Refresher Revitalizing Conditioner Redwood, True Red** *($11.75 for 6 ounces)* is almost identical to the version above and the same comments apply.

☺ **Color Refresher Revitalizing Conditioner Sand, Neutral Blond** *($11.75 for 6 ounces)* is almost identical to the version above and the same comments apply.

☺ **Color Refresher Revitalizing Conditioner Sun, Gold** *($11.75 for 6 ounces)* is almost identical to the version above and the same comments apply.

☺ **Colorsure Conditioner** *($14.95 for 13.5 ounces)* contains mostly water, thickeners, glycerin, detangling agent, film former, silicones, conditioning agent, preservatives, fragrance, and coloring agents. This is a good basic conditioner for dry hair that is normal to fine or thin in thickness.

☺ **Leave-in Protector** *($13.95 for 13.5 ounces)* is a good leave-in conditioner for dry hair of any thickness but coarse. It contains mostly water, silicone, conditioning agents, slip agents, detangling agents, film former, fragrance, and preservatives.

☺ **$$$ Shine FX** *($17.50 for 3.1 ounces)* contains mostly alcohol, propellant, silicone, film former, conditioning agent, slip agent, and fragrance. This is a light-hold styling spray that has minimal to no stiff or sticky feel.

☺ **$$$ Smooth FX** *($12.50 for 1.7 ounces)* is just an overpriced silicone serum that can add shine and make hair feel silky soft.

☺ **Bodifying Spray Gel** *($12 for 13.5 ounces)* is a good, light-hold spray gel with a slight sticky feel, though it can easily be brushed through. It contains mostly water, film formers, slip agents, conditioning agents, castor oil, preservatives, and fragrance.

☺ **Designing Glissage Gel** *($9.95 for 4.5 ounces)* contains mostly water, film formers, castor oil, conditioning agents, thickeners, preservatives, and fragrance. This is a good, light- to medium-hold gel with a somewhat sticky feel that does easily brush through.

☺ **Forming Foam** *($12.95 for 10 ounces)* is a good but basic mousse with a light hold and minimal stiff or sticky feel. It contains mostly water, propellant, film formers, conditioning agents, slip agents, silicone, fragrance, and preservatives.

☺ **Performance Spray** *($10.94 for 10 ounces)* is a standard medium- to firm-hold aerosol hairspray that has a slight stiff, sticky feel, though it is easily brushed through. It contains mostly alcohol, propellant, film formers, conditioning agents, silicone, and fragrance.

☺ **Thermal Fixative** *($11.99 for 13.5 ounces)* is a standard medium-hold hairspray that has a minimal stiff, sticky feel and is easily brushed through. It contains mostly water, film formers, conditioning agents, silicone, castor oil, preservatives, and fragrance. There's nothing about it that is "activated by heat" anymore than any other hairspray.

☺ **Total Hold Spritz** *($12.95 for 13.5 ounces)* is a standard, light-hold hairspray that has minimal to no stiff, sticky feel. It contains mostly alcohol, water, film formers, conditioning agents, and fragrance.

☹ **Perfecting Clay Complex** *($12.95 for 4.3 ounces)* does contain clay, which is drying for hair; it can also chip away at the cuticle.

Essentials by Matrix

☹ **Actrol Dandruff Clarifying Shampoo** *($13.75 for 12 ounces)* is a standard zinc pyrithione–based dandruff shampoo that is quite similar to Head & Shoulders, only this one is more expensive. This also contains menthol, which adds unnecessary irritation for the scalp.

☹ **Alternate Action Clarifying Shampoo** *($12.95 for 16 ounces)* uses TEA-lauryl sulfate and sodium lauryl sulfate among its main detergent cleansing agents, which makes it too drying for the hair and scalp.

☺ **Essential Color Therapy Shampoo** *($12.95 for 16 ounces)* contains mostly water, detergent cleansing agents, lather agent, conditioning agents, preservatives, fragrance, and coloring agents. The amount of conditioning agents is negligible, so they have little impact on the hair. That makes this a good basic shampoo for all hair types and that won't cause buildup.

☺ **Nourishing Shampoo** *($12.95 for 16 ounces)* contains mostly water, detergent cleansing agents, lather agent, fragrance, conditioning agents, detangling agent, thickeners, preservatives, film former, and coloring agents. This is a good shampoo for dry hair that is normal to fine or thin in thickness. The list of specialized conditioning agents comes well after the preservatives, which makes them barely present and unlikely to have any effect on hair.

☺ **Perm Fresh Shampoo** *($12.95 for 16 ounces)* contains mostly water, detergent cleansing agents, lather agents, lots of detangling agent, silicone, water-binding agents, silicones, conditioning agents, thickeners, film former, slip agents, preservatives, fragrance, and coloring agents. This would be a good shampoo for hard-to-comb, dry hair.

☺ **Simply Clean Shampoo** *($11.75 for 16 ounces)* contains mostly water, detergent cleansing agents, lather agents, conditioning agents, detangling agents, water-binding agents, thickeners, and preservatives. This would be a good shampoo for normal to dry hair of any thickness.

☺ **SoSilver Shampoo** *($12.95 for 16 ounces)* is similar to the Simply Clean above, although this one contains violet dye agents; still, that can only minimally help to make silver hair look less yellow.

☺ **Essential Body & Strength Reconstructor** *($14 for 8 ounces)* won't repair one hair on your head, but it is a good conditioner for normal to slightly dry hair of any thickness. It contains mostly water, thickening agents, detangling agent, conditioning agents, fragrance, and preservatives.

☺ **Essential Color Therapy Revitalizing Conditioner** *($10.25 for 4 ounces)* contains mostly water, thickeners, detangling agent, conditioning agents, silicones, plant oils, film former, water-binding agents, preservatives, fragrance, and coloring agents. This is a very good conditioner for dry to extremely dry hair of any thickness.

☺ **Nutrient Rich Conditioner** *($10.95 for 4 ounces)* contains mostly water, slip agent, thickeners, detangling agents, conditioning agents, plant oil, water-binding agents, preservatives, and fragrance. This is a good basic conditioner for normal to dry hair of any thickness.

☺ **Perm Fresh Moisture Supply** *($10.95 for 4 ounces)* contains mostly water, thickeners, detangling agents, conditioning agents, thickeners, plant oils, fragrant oil, water-binding agents, silicones, slip agents, preservatives, fragrance, and coloring agents. This is a very good conditioner for dry hair of any thickness.

☺ **Simply Silk Detangling Rinse** *($8.99 for 13.5 ounces)* contains mostly water, thickeners, conditioning agents, detangling agents, slip agents, silicones, water-binding agent, preservatives, and fragrance. This is a good leave-in conditioner for normal to dry hair of any thickness.

☺ **Essential Color Therapy Leave-in Conditioner** *($14.95 for 12 ounces)* contains mostly water, pH adjuster, sunscreen agents, conditioning agents, water-binding agents, detangling agents, silicone, thickeners, preservatives, plant oil, fragrance, and coloring agents. This is a good leave-in conditioner for normal to slightly dry hair of any thickness. Without an SPF number there is no way to know how much sun protection this product has, and sunscreen agents do not hold up under brushing or styling treatments.

☺ **Instacure Leave-in Treatment** *($18.95 for 12 ounces)* contains mostly water, thickeners, water-binding agents, silicone, detangling agent, film former, slip agents, preservatives, and fragrance. This is a good leave-in conditioner for someone with normal to slightly dry hair that is normal to fine or thin in thickness.

☺ **Perm Fresh Leave-in Treatment** *($11.75 for 12 ounces)* contains mostly water, detangling agents/film formers, conditioning agents, water-binding agents, silicone, preservatives, and fragrance. This is a good leave-in conditioner for normal to dry hair that is normal to fine or thin in thickness.

☺ **5 + Protopak Restructurizing Treatment** *($4.75 for 1 ounce)* won't reconstruct hair, but it is a good conditioner for normal to dry hair that is fine or thin. Using it as instructed, under a dryer for five to eight minutes, would help any conditioner make hair feel better. It contains mostly water, thickener, film former, water-binding agents, conditioning agents, detangling agents, thickeners, slip agents, preservatives, and fragrance.

☺ **Glossifier Hair Polish** *($9.95 for 4 ounces)* turns out to be more of a styling lotion with a lot of silicone, some extra water-binding agents, thickeners, fragrance, and preservatives. It has no film formers so there is no stiff or sticky hold, but it can help smooth frizzies and curls and add shine and a silky feel to hair.

☺ **Sculpting Glaze** *($10.95 for 13.5 ounces)* contains mostly water, slip agents, film formers, detangling agents, alcohol, thickeners, silicones, water-binding agents, preservatives, and fragrance. This is a good styling spray with a medium hold and minimal stiff or sticky feel that can easily be brushed through.

☺ **Styling Gel** *($9.95 for 4 ounces)* contains mostly water, film formers, slip agents, water-binding agents, silicones, thickeners, preservatives, and fragrance. This is a good, standard, light- to medium-hold gel with minimal to no stiff or sticky feel.

☺ **Moussette Styling Foam** *($12.95 for 9 ounces)* is a standard, medium- to firm-hold mousse with a slight stiff, sticky feel, though it can be brushed through easily. It contains mostly water, alcohol, propellant, film formers, detangling agents, silicone, thickeners, and fragrance.

☺ **Finishing Spray** *($7.50 for 14 ounces)* is a standard, light- to medium-hold aerosol hairspray with minimal to no stiff, sticky feel that contains mostly alcohol, propellant, film formers, silicones, and fragrance.

☺ **Proforma Hair Spray Aerosol** *($12.95 for 12 ounces)* is similar to the Finishing Spray above, only this one has more of a medium hold and a slightly more sticky feel.

☺ **Vital Control Hair Spray** *($12.95 for 14.8 ounces)* is similar to the Freeze Spray above, only with medium to firm hold, but the same basic comments apply.

☺ **Freeze Spray** *($12.95 for 12 ounces)* is similar to the Finishing Spray above, only in nonaerosol form.

Biolage by Matrix

☹ **Anti-Dandruff Shampoo** *($12.50 for 12 ounces)* contains sodium C14-16 olefin sulfonate, which can be drying and irritating for the hair and scalp. It also contains tea tree oil, which may have some antimicrobial properties against dandruff, but the amount may not be enough for it to have an effect.

☺ **Color Care Shampoo** *($12.99 for 16 ounces)* contains mostly water, detergent cleansing agents, lather agents, conditioning agents, detangling agent/film former, preservatives, thickeners, fragrance, and coloring agents. This is a good shampoo for normal to slightly dry hair that is normal to fine or thin in thickness.

☹ **Energizing Shampoo** *($12.99 for 16 ounces)* uses sodium lauryl sulfate as one of the main cleansing agents, which makes it too drying for the hair and scalp.

☹ **Hydrating Shampoo** *($12.99 for 16 ounces)* uses sodium lauryl sulfate as one of the main cleansing agents, which makes it too drying for the hair and scalp.

☹ **Normalizing Shampoo** *($11.95 for 16 ounces)* uses sodium lauryl sulfate as one of the main cleansing agents, which makes it too drying for the hair and scalp.

☺ **Conditioning Balm** *($10.95 for 4 ounces)* contains mostly water, slip agent, thickeners, detangling agent, plant extract, film former, preservatives, and fragrance. This is a good, lightweight conditioner for normal to slightly dry hair that is normal to fine or thin in thickness.

☺ **Detangling Solution** *($12.75 for 13.5 ounces)* contains mostly water, thickeners, detangling agent, plant extracts, silicones, thickeners, fragrance, and coloring agents. This is a very good detangling agent for dry hair of any thickness.

☹ **Pre-Shampoo Conditioner** *($10.85 for 4 ounces)* is supposed to be applied to hair before you shampoo, but that would be like applying dirt to the skin before you wash it. If the shampoo you are using is any good, this would all be washed away, so all this ends up being is a conditioner with film formers.

☺ **Daily Leave-in Tonic** *($12.75 for 13.5 ounces)* is a leave-in conditioner that works well for normal to slightly dry hair that is normal to fine or thin in thickness. It contains mostly water, plant extracts, film formers, conditioning agents, detangling agents, silicone, slip agents, and preservatives.

☺ **Shine Renewal** *($12 for 3.9 ounces)* is a standard silicone serum that contains mostly silicone, plant extracts, and fragrance. It works great for adding shine and a silky feel to hair. However, there are far less expensive, identical versions at the drugstore.

☺ **Defining Elixir Texturizing Jelly** *($11 for 4 ounces)* contains mostly water, film formers, thickeners, plant extracts, silicone, detangling agent, slip agents, preservatives, and coloring agents. This is a good light- to medium-hold gel with a slight stiff, sticky feel.

☺ **Gelee** *($12.75 for 13.5 ounces)* contains mostly water, film formers, slip agents, thickeners, plant extracts, silicone, castor oil, fragrance, and preservatives. It's a good, light- to medium-hold gel with a minimal amount of stiff sticky feel, and it can be brushed through.

☺ **Hydro-Foaming Styler** *($13.99 for 9 ounces)* is a standard mousse that contains mostly water, propellant, film formers, thickeners, plant extracts, silicone, conditioning agents, castor oil, fragrance, and preservatives. This has a light to medium hold with a slight stiff, sticky feel that does let you brush through hair.

☺ **Hydro-Glaze Soft Styling Spray** *($14.95 for 8.5 ounces)* contains mostly plant water, propellant, film formers, conditioning agents, slip agents, more film former, silicone, detangling agent, preservatives, and fragrance. This aerosol styling spray has a light to medium hold with minimal stiff feel, and it can easily be brushed through.

☺ **Glaze** *($12.75 for 13.5 ounces)* contains mostly water, film formers, plant extracts, thickeners, fragrance, and preservatives. This is a good styling spray with a light hold and minimal stiff or sticky feel that is easily brushed through. It is quite similar to the Hydro-Glaze above only in nonaerosol form.

☺ **Thermal-Active Setting Spray** *($14.50 for 8 ounces)* contains mostly water, film former, castor oil, conditioning agents, plant extracts, silicone, slip agents, fragrance, and preservatives. This is a good, light- to medium-hold styling spray that can have a slight stiff feel and that is easily brushed through. It will definitely hold a set, but not any better than any other styling spray.

☺ **Complete Control Hair Spray Firm Hold** *($13.50 for 10 ounces)* is a standard aerosol hairspray that has a medium hold with a somewhat stiff feel that can easily be brushed through. It contains mostly alcohol, propellant, film formers, plant extracts, silicone, slip agents, and fragrance.

☺ **Firm-Active Hair Spray Extra Firm** *($14.25 for 8.5 ounces)* is almost identical to the Complete Control above, only in nonaerosol form.

☺ **Natural Finish Hair Spray** *($8.50 for 10 ounces)* isn't all that natural. Rather, it is almost identical to the Complete Control above, only in nonaerosol form.

☺ **Finishing Spritz** *($14.50 for 13.5 ounces)* is almost identical to the Complete Control above, only in nonaerosol form.

☹ **Hydroactive Hair Masque** *($35 for 16 ounces)* has magnesium aluminum silicate as one of the main ingredients, which has drying properties, and is not best for hair.

Vavoom by Matrix

☹ **Shampooing** *($11.75 for 16 ounces)* uses TEA-lauryl sulfate and sodium C14-16 olefin sulfonate as its main cleansing agents, which makes it too drying for the hair and scalp.

☺ **Styling Shampoo** *($11.75 for 16 ounces)* contains mostly water, detergent cleansing agents, lather agents, conditioning agent, detangling agent, fragrance, and preservatives. This is mostly just shampoo with a tiny amount of conditioning agent that shouldn't cause buildup. This shampoo does contain some amount of sodium polystyrene sulfonate, which can be drying and possibly strip dyed hair color with repeated use.

☺ **Conditioning** *($11.95 for 16 ounces)* contains mostly water, thickeners, detangling agent, plant oil, more detangling agent, conditioning agent, silicones, preservatives, and fragrance. This is a very good conditioner for dry hair of any thickness.

☺ **Styling Conditioner** *($11.95 for 16 ounces)* is similar to the Conditioning above and the same comments apply.

☺ **$$$ Liquid Shine** *($17.95 for 1.25 ounces)* is a standard silicone serum with an absurd price tag. The silicone ingredients—cyclomethicone and dimethicone—that it contains are identical to those in the $6 versions at the drugstore. It adds a silky-soft shine to hair.

☺ **Spray Shine** *($14.75 for 4 ounces)* is similar to the Liquid Shine above, only in spray form.

☺ **Forming Gel** *($10.95 for 12 ounces)* contains mostly water, film formers, slip agent, silicone, detangling agents, thickeners, preservatives, and fragrance. This is a good standard gel that has a light hold with minimal to no stiff or sticky feel.

The Reviews M

☺ **Smoothing Gel** *($14 for 9.75 ounces)* is similar to the one above, only with a light hold and minimal to no stiff or sticky feel.

☺ **Glazing** *($10.95 for 4 ounces)* contains mostly water, film formers, detangling agents, silicones, thickeners, preservatives, and fragrance. This is a liquidy gel that has a light to medium hold with minimal stiff or sticky feel.

☹ **Pomousse** *($20 for 3.75 ounces)* is a mousse that contains mostly water, castor oil, thickeners, slip agents, propellant, preservatives, fragrance, and coloring agents. It has a medium hold with a somewhat sticky, heavy feel. Be careful how much you apply—this can weigh hair down and feel thick and greasy.

☺ **Volumizing Foam** *($13.50 for 9 ounces)* is a standard mousse with a medium hold and a somewhat sticky feel. It contains mostly water, propellant, film formers, silicones, thickeners, slip agent, preservatives, and fragrance.

☺ **Sculpting Spray Gel** *($12.75 for 12 ounces)* is a standard styling spray with a light to medium hold and a slight stiff, sticky feel. It contains mostly alcohol, water, film formers, slip agents, silicone, preservatives, and fragrance.

☺ **Freezing Spray** *($12.25 for 14.8 ounces)* is a standard aerosol hairspray that contains mostly alcohol, propellant, film formers, silicone, and fragrance. It has a medium to firm hold with a slight stiff, sticky feel, but can be brushed through.

☺ **Professional Styling Spray** *($17.50 for 15 ounces)* is similar to the Freezing Spray above, only with a slightly firmer hold and a slightly stiffer feel.

☺ **Shaping Spray (Aerosol)** *($12.75 for 10 ounces)* is similar to the Freezing Spray above and the same comments apply.

☺ **Spritzing Spray Extra** *($12.75 for 12 ounces)* is similar to the Freezing Spray above, only in nonaerosol form and with a firmer hold and a slightly stiffer feel.

☹ **Quality Control Conditioning Styler** *($12.45 for 13.5 ounces)* uses sodium polystyrene sulfonate as the main film former, which can be drying and can potentially strip hair color.

Vital Nutrients by Matrix

☹ **BodyFusion Extra Volume Shampoo** *($11.75 for 13.5 ounces)* uses sodium lauryl sulfate as one of its main cleansing agents, which makes it too drying for the hair and scalp.

☹ **MoistureRich Fusion Shampoo** *($11.75 for 13.5 ounces)* uses sodium lauryl sulfate as one of its main cleansing agents, which makes it too drying for the hair and scalp.

☹ **ShineFusion Shampoo** *($11.75 for 13.5 ounces)* uses sodium lauryl sulfate as one of its main cleansing agents, which makes it too drying for the hair and scalp.

☺ **BodyFusion Extra Volume Conditioner** *($12.75 for 13.5 ounces)* contains mostly water, thickeners, detangling agents, more thickeners, conditioning agents, silicone, fragrance, preservatives, and coloring agents. This is a very good conditioner for dry hair of any thickness.

☺ **MoistureRich Fusion Conditioner** *($12.75 for 13.5 ounces)* is similar to the Body Fusion above and the same basic comments apply.

☺ **BodyFusion Designing Gel** *($9.99 for 8 ounces)* contains mostly water, film formers, conditioning agents, thickeners, silicone, fragrance, preservatives, and coloring agents. This is a good standard gel with a light to medium hold and minimal stiff, sticky feel.

☺ **BodyFusion Spray Gel** *($9.96 for 8.5 ounces)* contains mostly water, film formers, conditioning agents, plant oil, castor oil, thickeners, fragrance, and preservatives. This standard spray gel has a light hold and minimal to no stiff, sticky feel.

☹ **BodyFusion Volumizer** *($9.86 for 8.5 ounces)* has sodium polystyrene sulfonate as the second ingredient, which can be drying for hair and possibly strip hair color.

☺ **MoistureRich Fusion Defining Cream** *($9.99 for 4 ounces)* is a good styling cream to smooth frizzy or curly hair. It has no hold and therefore no stiff or sticky feel, though be careful how much you use—it can easily build up and look and feel greasy and heavy. It contains mostly water, thickeners, silicone, conditioning agents, plant oil, fragrance, and preservatives.

☺ **BodyFusion Styling Spray** *($9.86 for 10 ounces)* contains mostly alcohol, water, propellant, film formers, conditioning agents, plant oil, slip agents, and silicone. This is a standard but good light-hold hairspray with minimal stiff feel, and it can easily be brushed through.

Motions at Home

This is a line of hair-care products intended for use by African Americans. It does have some of the standard mineral oil–based products that can have a greasy feel on hair, but it also has products with silicone, and they can create more of a silky-soft feel. For more information on Motions at Home, call (708) 450-3000, (800) 333-6666, or visit its Web site at www.alberto-culver.com.

☹ **Lavish Conditioning Shampoo with Polymeric Conditioning and Silk Protein/Keratin Protein** *($3.63 for 6 ounces)* uses sodium lauryl sulfate as one of the main cleansing agents, which makes it too drying for the hair and scalp.

☺ **After Shampoo Moisture Plus Conditioner** *($2.99 for 6 ounces)* contains mostly water, mineral oil, detangling agents/film formers, silicones, thickeners, conditioning agent, preservatives, and fragrance. This would work for extremely dry hair that is normal to fine or thin in thickness, but it can easily build up and leave a greasy feel on hair.

☺ **Critical Protection and Repair Treatment** *($6.99 for 15 ounces)* contains mostly water, mineral oil, thickeners, conditioning agent, plant extracts, silicone, preservatives, and fragrance. It is similar to the Moisture Plus version above, only without the film formers, so it would work for any hair thickness.

☺ **Hair and Scalp Daily Moisturizing Hair Dressing** *($4.62 for 6 ounces)* contains mostly water, mineral oil, slip agent, silicones, thickeners, Vaseline, film former, preservatives, and fragrance. It can have a greasy feel on hair but it is a good conditioner for extremely dry hair.

☺ **Salon Sheen** *($7.69 for 4 ounces)* is a very good standard silicone serum that can add a silky-soft shine to hair.

☺ **Light Hold Working Spritz for Curling and for Hold** *($3.16 for 10 ounces)* contains mostly alcohol, water, film formers, slip agent, and fragrance. This is a good, very standard, medium-hold hairspray with a slight stiff feel that can easily be brushed through.

☺ **Oil Sheen and Conditioning Spray for Superb Sheen and Softness** *($3.86 for 11.25 ounces)* contains mostly wax, propellant, plant oil, plant extracts, alcohol, and fragrance. This performs just as the name implies: it places a coating of oil over the hair and that can make it look shiny, but it can also make it look greasy, so use it sparingly.

M Professional Hair

M Professional has many designer makeup lines worried because the inexpensive eyeshadows, blushes, lipsticks, and pencils it makes are some of the best around! Capitalizing on its success, M Professional has launched a line of hair-care products. How do they stack up? I think you'll find that the products, despite the varied names, are really only most suitable for normal hair that is thin or fine—which is great, but first you have to get around the names to find what is best for your hair. For more information on M Professional, call (310) 453-2566, (800) 662-6776, or visit its Web site at www.mprofessional.com.

☺ **Abuse Shampoo Tormented, Permed or Color Treated Hair** *($4.60 for 13 ounces)* is simply shampoo with a good amount of film former (the main ingredient in hairspray). Film former leaves hair feeling stiffer and, with only a few shampooings, can easily build up. This shampoo is definitely not appropriate for someone with any amount of hair damage, or someone whose hair is at all coarse. But it could work well for someone with fine, thin, normal hair if they wanted a feel of more thickness. It would need to be alternated with a shampoo that contained no styling agents.

☺ **Big Shampoo** *($4.60 for 13 ounces)* is similar to the one above and can be an option for someone with fine, thin hair; the same warnings apply.

☺ **Just Shampoo Regular, Dry or Just Dirty Hair** *($4.60 for 13 ounces)* this isn't just shampoo, it is a shampoo that contains film former, which is a problem for dry hair, but it can an option for someone with thin, fine, normal hair, but that's about it.

☺ **Just Conditioner Regular, Dry or Just Needy Hair** *($4.60 for 13 ounces)* is a fairly standard but rather heavy conditioner with wax and film formers, though it does have plenty of antistatic agents. That makes it best for those who want their hair to lie flat and who are also looking for thickness. It isn't suitable for dry or damaged hair in the least.

☺ **Abuse Conditioner, Extra-Dry, Permed, or Chemically Treated Hair** *($4.60 for 13 ounces)* contains mostly water, detangling agent, thickeners, film former, conditioning agents, preservatives, fragrance, and coloring agents. This is a good conditioner for normal to dry hair but it is not emollient enough for someone with extra dry hair.

☺ **Serious Memory Gel** *($4.60 for 9.5 ounces)* is merely film former and silicone, and that makes it a great lightweight styling gel for normal to fine, thin hair, or minimally thick, curly hair.

☺ **Shaping Memory Gel Any Kind of Hair Don't Lose Control** *($4.60 for 9.5 ounces)* is almost identical to the one above, and the same comments apply.

☺ **Leave On Conditioner for the Truly Demented Hair** *($4.60 for 13 ounces)* is mostly silicone and lightweight emollient conditioning agents, with a small amount of film former. That makes it good for normal to thin hair, but it would be too heavy for fine or limp hair, and could make dry or damaged hair feel brittle.

☺ **Shine On Laminate Brilliant Shine Finish** *($4.60 for 2 ounces)* is a very standard but very excellent silicone serum! Just the tiniest drop can make coarse, damaged hair feel like silk.

☺ **Defrizzer Elixer, Makes Hair Behave** *($4.60 for 2 ounces)* is almost identical to the Shine On above and the same comments apply.

Nano
(see Proxiphen & Nano)

Neutrogena

For more information on Neutrogena, call (310) 642-1150, (800) 217-1136, or visit its Web site at www.neutrogena.com.

☺ **Anti-Residue Shampoo** *($5.29 for 6 ounces)* is just a shampoo with no ingredients that could build up on hair. It contains mostly water, detergent cleansing agent, lather agent, slip agent, preservatives, and fragrance. This would work well on all hair types.

☺ **Clean Balancing Shampoo for Normal Hair** *($4.99 for 10.1 ounces)* is a standard two-in-one shampoo that contains mostly water, detergent cleansing agents, lather agent, conditioning agent, silicone, detangling agent/film former, preservatives, coloring agents, and fragrance. This would work well for dry hair that is normal to fine or thin in thickness. It can create buildup with repeated use.

☺ **Clean Replenishing Shampoo for Dry, Damaged Hair** *($4.99 for 10.1 ounces)* is almost identical to the Normal Hair version above and the same comments apply.

☺ **Clean Volumizing Shampoo for Fine, Thin Hair** *($4.99 for 10.1 ounces)* is almost identical the Normal Hair version above and the same comments apply.

☹ **Healthy Scalp Anti-Dandruff Shampoo** *($7.39 for 6 ounces)* uses sodium C14-16 olefin sulfonate, which can irritate and dry the scalp. It also contains 1.8 percent salicylic acid, which can exfoliate a flaky scalp; however, it can also denature the hair, though the pH of this product is probably too high for it to be effective either way.

☹ **Maximum Strength Therapeutic T/Sal Therapeutic Shampoo** *($5.41 for 4.5 ounces)* is almost identical to the Healthy Scalp shampoo above, only this version contains 3.0 percent salicylic acid, and the same comments apply.

☺ **Moisturizing Shampoo for Permed or Color Treated Hair** *($5.29 for 6 ounces)* isn't moisturizing in the least, it is just shampoo that contains mostly water, detergent cleansing agents, lather agents, preservatives, coloring agents, and fragrance. That makes it a good basic shampoo for all hair types.

☺ **Clean Balancing Conditioner for Normal Hair** *($4.99 for 10.1 ounces)* contains mostly water, thickeners, conditioning agents, detangling agents, silicone, preservatives, fragrance, and coloring agents. This is a good conditioner for normal to dry hair of any thickness.

☺ **Clean Replenishing Conditioner for Dry, Damaged Hair** *($4.99 for 10.1 ounces)* is similar to the one above, with slightly more conditioning agents. It would be slightly better for dry hair of any thickness, but only slightly.

☺ **Clean Volumizing Conditioner for Fine Hair** *($4.99 for 10.1 ounces)* is similar to the Dry, Damaged version above and the same comments apply. There is nothing in here that would add volume to thin or fine hair.

☺ **Conditioner Detangling Formula** *($5.29 for 6 ounces)* contains mostly water, thickeners, detangling agents, silicones, preservatives, and fragrance. This is a very good conditioner for dry hair of any thickness.

☺ **Conditioner Revitalizing Formula for Permed or Color Treated Hair** *($5.29 for 6 ounces)* contains mostly water, thickeners, detangling agents, silicone, preservatives, fragrance, and coloring agents. This is a very basic conditioner that would work for normal to slightly dry hair of any thickness. There is nothing in here helpful for hair damaged by chemical treatments.

☺ **Hairspray for Permed or Color-Treated Hair, Natural Hold** *($5.29 for 7 ounces)* has nothing in it that would make this standard hairspray better for color-treated hair. It contains mostly alcohol, water, film formers, conditioning agent, silicone, fragrance, and coloring agents. It has a light to medium hold with a slight stiff feel, and is easily brushed through.

☺ **Hairspray for Permed or Color-Treated Hair, Super Hold** *($5.29 for 7 ounces)* is almost identical to the Natural Hold above and the same comments apply.

☹ **HeatSafe Instant Heat-Activated Hair Treatment for Dry or Damaged Hair, Fine, Thin Hair Formula** *($8.49 for 6 ounces)* implies by its name that if you use it, the heat from styling tools won't hurt your hair, yet there is absolutely nothing in this lightweight, leave-in conditioner that makes styling hair any less damaging. If your styling tools heat up to over 200 degrees Fahrenheit, which most do, you put the hair at risk. There are no products that can prevent that from happening. This leave-in conditioner does contain sodium polystyrene sulfonate, which can be drying to hair with repeated use.

☺ **HeatSafe Instant Heat-Activated Hair Treatment for Dry or Damaged Hair, Regular Formula** *($8.49 for 6 ounces)* merits the same comments as given above for the Thin Hair version of this product. This lightweight leave-in conditioner is suitable for normal hair of any thickness; it isn't conditioning or emollient enough for dry, damaged hair. It contains mostly water, slip agent, conditioning agents, preservatives, and fragrance.

☺ **Therapeutic T/Gel Shampoo Extra Strength Formula** *($8.49 for 6 ounces)* is a very good 2 percent coal-tar shampoo for fighting seborrhea or psoriasis. It contains a tiny amount of detangling agent, but other than that it is just detergent cleansing agents and lather agents with preservatives and coloring agents.

☹ **Therapeutic T/Gel Shampoo Fine/Oily Hair** *($ 5.24 for 4.4 ounces)* uses sodium lauryl sulfate as one of its main cleansing agents, which makes it too drying for the hair and scalp.

☺ **Therapeutic T/Gel Shampoo Original Formula** *($4.50 for 4.4 ounces)* is a very good 0.5% coal-tar shampoo for fighting seborrhea or psoriasis. It contains no other ingredients but detergent cleansing agents, lather agents, preservatives, and coloring agents.

☹ **Therapeutic T/Gel Shampoo Stubborn Itch Control** *($4.49 for 4.4 ounces)* is similar to the one above, only with menthol, which can be irritating and drying for the scalp.

☹ **T/Scalp Shampoo, Anti-Itch Liquid** *($8.49 for 2 ounces)* contains 1 percent hydrocortisone, which can be helpful for an itchy scalp; unfortunately this product also contains 45 percent alcohol, plus camphor and menthol, which are all extremely drying and irritating, and that's bad for an itchy scalp.

The Reviews N

☺ **Therapeutic T/Gel Conditioner** *($4.50 for 4.4 ounces)* is a standard coal-tar conditioner for seborrhea or psoriasis. As a conditioner it can more easily be left on the scalp, but the thickeners, conditioning agents, and film former can be a problem for some hair types. This wouldn't work well for oily scalp or thick, coarse hair.

☺ **T/Scalp Antipruritic Anti-Itch Liquid** *($6.36 for 2 ounces)* is a standard 1 percent hydrocortisone liquid and would work well to calm an itchy scalp.

Nexxus

Nexxus is owned by the Jheri Redding company (the original Jheri Redding products are owned by Conair Corporation). For more information on Nexxus, call (805) 968-6900, (800) 444-6399, or visit its Web site at www.nexxusproducts.com.

☹ **Aloe Rid Clarifying Shampoo** *($11.49 for 16.9 ounces)* contains sodium thiosulfate, a reducing agent used in perms, which can be drying and damaging to hair.

☹ **Assure Polymeric Shampoo** *($17 for 16.9 ounces)* contains a small amount of sodium styrene, which can be drying and possibly strip hair color with repeated use.

☺ **Botanoil Treatment Shampoo** *($5.50 for 8.4 ounces)* contains mostly water, detergent cleansing agent, lather agent, plant oils, conditioning agents, water-binding agents, film former, vitamins preservatives, fragrance, and coloring agents. This can be a good shampoo for dry hair, though it does contain a tiny amount of sodium styrene, which can be drying and possibly strip hair color with repeated use.

☺ **Dandarrest Dandruff Shampoo** *($11.50 for 16.9 ounces)* is a standard zinc pyrithione–based dandruff shampoo that is quite similar to Head & Shoulders, only this one is more expensive.

☺ **Diametress Hair Thickening Shampoo** *($9.50 for 8.4 ounces)* contains mostly water, detergent cleansing agent, conditioning agents, lather agent, plant extract, preservatives, fragrance, and coloring agents. This is a good shampoo for normal to dry hair of any thickness. It doesn't contains ingredients that add much thickness to hair, but it does contain witch hazel, though in a very minute amount so it wouldn't have much of a drying effect on hair or scalp.

☺ **Exoil Deep Cleansing Shampoo** *($4.50 for 8.4 ounces)* is similar to the one above and the same comments apply. The conditioning agents in here are not appropriate for oily hair or scalp.

☹ **Pep'r'Mint Herbal Shampoo** *($5 for 8.4 ounces)* contains peppermint, just as the name says it does, as well as lemon, and both can be irritating and drying for the scalp.

☺ **Rejuv-a-Perm Vitalizing Shampoo** *($11.50 for 16.9 ounces)* contains mostly water, detergent cleansing agent, lather agent, film former, thickeners, water-binding agents, preservatives, and fragrance. This would be a good shampoo for dry hair that is normal to fine or thin in thickness but it can't "rejuvenate" a perm.

☺ **Simply Silver Toning Shampoo** *($6.50 for 8.4 ounces)* contains mostly water, detergent cleansing agent, lather agent, conditioning agent, water-binding agent, plant oil, preservatives, fragrance, and coloring agents. This would be a good shampoo for dry hair of any thickness. The violet coloring agents in here can help minimally reduce the yellow overtones of gray hair.

☺ **Therappe Moisturizing Shampoo** *($9 for 16.9 ounces)* contains mostly water, detergent cleansing agent, lather agent, plant oils, conditioning agents, water-binding agents, film former, vitamins, preservatives, fragrance, and coloring agents. This can be a good shampoo for dry hair, though it does contain a tiny amount of sodium styrene, which can be drying and possibly strip hair color with repeated use.

☺ **Vita Tress Biotin Shampoo** *($13 for 16.9 ounces)* contains mostly water, detergent cleansing agents, lather agent, plant oil, water-binding agents, preservatives, fragrance, and coloring agents. This can be a good shampoo for dry hair of any thickness. It does contain an insignificant amount of RNA and DNA, which are window dressing to create the illusion that this shampoo can change hair; however, these ingredients can't do that.

☺ **Aloe Rid Clarifying Treatment** *($5.50 for 5 ounces)* does contain a chelating agent high up on the ingredient listing, which would help to prevent minerals from binding to hair. It has no conditioning agents or detangling agents, so you would still need to apply a conditioner after using this.

☹ **Emergencee Polymeric Reconstructor** *($14 for 3.3 ounces)* contains a form of sulfonic acid, which can be drying to hair and possibly strip hair color with repeated use.

☹ **E Acidifying Conditioner** *($14 for 16.9 ounces)* contains mostly plant water, conditioning agent, detangling agent, fragrance, preservatives, and coloring agents. This conditioner does contain grapefruit juice, which can be drying to hair and scalp.

☹ **Epitome Botanical Reconstructor** *($15 for 10.1 ounces)* contains mostly water, plant extracts, conditioning agents, vitamins, mineral salts, enzymes, preservatives, and fragrance. The minerals can bind to hair and chip away at the hair shaft, and the papain (enzyme) can also denature hair.

☺ **Humectress Moisturizing Conditioner** *($16 for 16.9 ounces)* contains mostly water, slip agent, thickeners, conditioning agents, detangling agent, mineral oil, castor oil, preservatives, Vaseline, fragrance, and coloring agents. This is a good conditioner for very dry, coarse hair, but it can cause buildup with repeated use.

☺ **Keraphix Creme Reconstructor** *($22 for 16.9 ounces)* contains mostly water, conditioning agents, slip agent, detangling agents, thickeners, mineral oil, plant oil, film former, preservatives, Vaseline, and fragrance. This is a good conditioner for coarse hair that is dry to very dry.

☹ **Vita Tress Cystine Conditioner** *($10 for 5 ounces)* contains a form of sulfonic acid, which can be drying to hair and possibly strip hair color.

☺ **Rejuv-a-Perm Curl Rejuvenator** *($10 for 5 ounces)* contains mostly water, plant extracts, plant oils, lanolin, thickeners, conditioning agent, vitamins, minerals, preservatives, and fragrance. This is a good leave-in conditioner for dry hair of any thickness, but it doesn't tighten curls, it just adds emollient and a slight sticky feel to the hair. This is also a very watery product, and the dispenser can make a mess, so be careful when you open it (this would have been far better in a spray bottle). I also have some concern about the papain and minerals in here. I suspect there's not enough of them to be a problem, but the papain (an enzyme) can denature the cuticle and the minerals can chip away at it.

☺ **Rejuv-a Perm Curl Enhancer** *($9 for 10.1 ounces)* is a lightweight styling spray with a soft hold and no stiff or sticky feel. It contains mostly water, alcohol, plant extract, film former, silicone, preservatives, and fragrance. It can help hold curl or can be used to smooth hair—it's the styling technique that affects how this product works on your hair.

☺ **Vita Tress Biotin Creme** *($11.50 for 2.1 ounces)* contains mostly water, thickeners, detangling agents, conditioning agents, water-binding agents, vitamins, preservatives, and fragrance. This is a good conditioner for normal to dry hair of any thickness. The vitamins and RNA and DNA in here provide no extra help for hair. The claim about hair growth is bogus and completely unsubstantiated; there is nothing in this product that can stimulate or alter hair growth in any way.

☺ **VitaTress Hair Volumizer** *($10 for 10.1 ounces)* contains mostly water, detangling agents, film formers, silicones, conditioning agents, thickeners, preservatives, and fragrance. This can add a feel of thickness to dry, fine hair that is thin to normal.

☺ **Headress Leave-in Conditioner** *($22 for 16.9 ounces)* contains mostly water, conditioning agents, thickeners, detangling agents, preservatives, and fragrance. This basic conditioner can be very good for normal to dry hair of any thickness.

☺ **$$$ Headress Design Shine** *($14 for 1 ounce)* is a standard (though extremely overpriced) silicone serum that can leave hair feeling soft and silky.

☺ **$$$ Headress Hair Glow** *($14 for 3.3 ounces)* is almost identical to the Design Shine above and the same comments apply.

☺ **Botanic Oil Natural Oil** *($8.50 for 8.4 ounces)* is mostly safflower oil, sesame oil, sunflower seed oil, and corn oil. You would be fine just using the safflower oil from your kitchen as an extra conditioning step, without the expense. The extra oils offer no extra help for hair. The product's directions say to apply this to dry ends, wait three minutes, and then shampoo. That would wash away any benefit. For very dry hair the better option would be to apply a drop and smooth it over extremely dry ends before styling, or to leave it on dry ends overnight and then shampoo the next morning.

☺ **Versastyler Designing Lotion** *($10 for 16.9 ounces)* is a standard styling-liquid gel that contains mostly water, film formers, slip agents, silicone, preservatives, and fragrance. It has a medium hold and minimal stiff or sticky feel, and can be brushed through.

☺ **Retexxtur Transforming Pomade** *($14 for 4 ounces)* contains mostly water, thickeners, conditioning agent, film former, silicone, preservatives, fragrance, and coloring agents. This standard styling lotion can help to smooth out coarse, frizzy, and stubborn curls with a light hold and minimal to no stiff or sticky feel. It can easily become too heavy and make hair look greasy or limp, so use it sparingly.

☺ **Spray Gel Maxxistyler** *($10 for 10.1 ounces)* contains mostly water, film formers, conditioning agents, thickeners, silicone, preservatives, and fragrance. This is a good, standard styling spray with a light to medium hold and minimal stiff or sticky feel that can be brushed through.

☹ **Exxtra Gel Super Hold** *($8 for 8.4 ounces)* contains a form of sulfonic acid, which can be drying to hair and possibly strip hair color with repeated use.

☹ **Styling Gel Regular Hold** *($5.99 for 8.4 ounces)* contains a form of sulfonic acid, which can be drying to hair and possibly strip hair color with repeated use.

☺ **Fluid Styling Potion Liquid Gel** *($8 for 8.4 ounces)* contains mostly water, film formers, conditioning agents, thickeners, silicone, preservatives, and fragrance. This is a good, standard styling gel with a medium hold and minimal stiff or sticky feel.

☺ **Mousse Plus Alcohol Free** *($11.50 for 10.6 ounces)* contains mostly water, film formers, propellant, detangling agent, silicone, plant oil, mink oil, preservatives, and fragrance. This is a good light- to medium-hold mousse with minimal stiff or sticky feel. The mink oil in here is a good conditioning agent but it is no better for the hair than any other conditioning agent.

☺ **Comb Thru Hair Spray** *($7.50 for 10.6 ounces)* is a standard aerosol hairspray with a medium to firm hold and a somewhat stiff, sticky feel, though it can be brushed through. It contains mostly alcohol, propellant, film formers, plant oil, and fragrance.

☺ **Firmist Hair Spray** *($7.50 for 10.6 ounces)* is almost identical to the Comb Thru above and the same comments apply.

☺ **Headress Shaping Spray** *($7.50 for 10.6 ounces)* is almost identical to the Comb Thru Hair Spray above, only with a more medium than firm hold; the same basic comments apply.

☺ **Hairspray Styling Versatility** *($7.50 for 10.1 ounces)* is almost identical to the Headress Shaping Spray above and the same comments apply.

☺ **Maxximum Super Holding Hair Spray** *($7.50 for 10.1 ounces)* is almost identical to the Comb Thru Hair Spray above and the same comments apply.

☺ **Sculpting and Finishing Spray Maxximum** *($7.50 for 10.1 ounces)* is almost identical to the Headress Shaping Spray above, only in nonaerosol form, and the same comments apply.

☺ **Hair Spray Body Building Firm Hold** *($7.50 for 10.1 ounces)* is almost identical to the Headress Shaping Spray above only in nonaerosol form, and the same comments apply.

☺ **Styling and Finishing Hair Spray Natural Hold** *($7.50 for 10.1 ounces)* is a standard styling spray that contains mostly alcohol, water, film formers, slip agents, silicone, preservatives, and fragrance. It has a light hold and minimal to no stiff or sticky feel.

Nick Chavez Perfect Plus

In the world of advertising, every hair-care product is wonderful and works perfectly to create your dream head of hair. This is even more poignantly demonstrated with the praise and glory attributed to the products presented in infomercials or on any TV shopping channel. I am well aware that all the miracles and enthusiasm for otherwise standard or ordinary products are nothing more than slick snake-oil sales pitches, but clearly there are customers ready and willing to believe every half truth and bit of hyperbole, and the all rest of the misleading information presented. I often wonder if the viewers ever notice that if they only wait a week or two, a different line on a different channel, or even the same channel, will have similar miraculous promises.

Having said all that, Nick Chavez is a hair-care line sold on QVC. There are definitely some good products to consider, but they are exceptionally overpriced for what you get and can easily be replaced with less expensive but just as well formulated drugstore versions. The explanations given to defend the natural origin of the ingredients are misleading. Does anyone really believe that dicetyldimonium chloride has a vegetable origin that makes it less "chemical" for the hair? Whether or not sodium cocoyl isethionate, cocamidopropyl betaine, or cocamide DEA come from coconut doesn't mean you could eat this stuff without drastic repercussions. In fact DEA is a fairly controversial ingredient right now, but Chavez doesn't seem to want to talk about that. (I've discussed this issue in the section on "DEA in Cosmetics" in Chapter Three, *Hair-Care Basics*).

For more information on Nick Chavez, call (800) 345-1515 or visit its Web site at www.iqvc.com.

☺ **Shampoo 1, Clarifier, for Normal to Oily Hair** *($8 for 8 ounces)* contains mostly water, cleansing agents, lather agent, thickeners, conditioning agents, detangling agent, preservatives, and fragrance. This very standard shampoo is the same as most in the industry. It would work well for normal to dry hair, though the conditioning agents make it inappropriate for an oily scalp.

☺ **Shampoo 2, Moisture Booster, Colored and Chemically Treated Hair** *($8 for 8 ounces)* contains mostly water, cleansing agents, lather agent, thickeners, conditioning agents, plant oils, detangling agent, vitamins, preservatives, and fragrance. This very standard shampoo would work well for dry hair of any thickness.

☺ **Conditioner, Adds Body and Shine while It Detangles** *($10 for 8 ounces)* contains mostly plant water, thickeners, detangling agent, conditioning agents, plant oils, vitamins, silicone, preservatives, and fragrance. This standard conditioner would work well for dry hair of any thickness.

☺ **Daily Detangler** *($12 for 8 ounces)* is a good leave-in conditioner for dry hair that is normal to fine or thin. It contains mostly water, detangling agents/film former, conditioning agents, plant oils, vitamins, plant extracts, silicones, preservatives, and fragrance. The film former can help make hair feel thicker.

☺ **Spray Gel, for Lift and Volume, Locks in Curl, Smoothes Frizzies** *($12 for 8 ounces)* contains mostly water, alcohol, film formers, thickeners, slip agents, and fragrance. This standard styling spray has a light hold and minimal to no stiff or sticky feel.

☺ **Aloe Mousse** *($12 for 6 ounces)* is a standard mousse that contains mostly plant water, propellants, film formers, alcohol, vitamins, conditioning agent, silicone, slip agents, fragrance, and preservatives. It has light to medium hold with minimal stiff or sticky feel and easily be brushed through.

☺ **Straightening Pomade** *($14 for 8 ounces)* contains mostly plant water, slip agent, mineral oil, thickeners, conditioning agents, vitamins, preservatives, and fragrance. This is a good, basic lotion-style pomade to smooth frizzies and curls with no stiff or sticky hold. It has no film formers so it gives less hold, but that is also why there is no stiff feel on hair. Be sure to use this sparingly; it can easily look greasy and heavy on hair.

☺ **Volumizing Mist for Fine, Thin and Thinning Hair** *($14 for 8 ounces)* contains mostly plant water, film former, conditioning agents, vitamins, conditioning agents, slip agents, detangling agents, more film former, silicone, preservatives, coloring agents, and fragrance. This is a good styling spray that can add thickness to fine or thin hair, but it can also be used as a lightweight styling spray for a soft hold and minimal to no stiff or sticky feel. It would work for hair of any type—it just depends on the styling you want to do.

☹ **Omega 6 Re-Activator, Extends the Life of Your Style** *($13.75 for 4 ounces)* is a huge waste of money. It contains 99 percent water, with a little alcohol, rose water, and preservatives. That makes this mostly fragrant water for the hair. The rest of the ingredients following the preservative are there in such minuscule amounts almost shocking. Moreover, what is Omega 6 anyway? Perhaps the company was thinking of Omega-3 from fish oil? Either way, it has no effect on the health of hair.

☺ **$$$ Shine** *($16 for 2 ounces)* is a standard and exceptionally overpriced silicone serum. Many similar serums in the drugstore work just as well for a fraction of the price.

☺ **Hairspray, Quick Drying, Super Hold** *($10 for 8 ounces)* is a good standard hairspray with a medium to firm hold and a slight stiff, sticky feel, though it does let you brush through it. It contains mostly alcohol, water, film formers, slip agents, silicone, and fragrance.

☹ **Cello-Gloss** *($20 for 10 ounces)* contains mostly water, slip agent, thickeners, conditioning agent, plant extracts, preservatives, coloring agents, and film former. This is a conditioner with dye agents meant to temporarily enhance hair color. The application is what makes it different from most other color-enhancing products. You're supposed to apply it all over your head, then cover your hair with a plastic cap, sit under a hairdryer for ten minutes, and then rinse and shampoo. That's a lot of trouble when most color-enhancing shampoos or conditioners can provide the same amount of color saturation (which isn't much) without all the bother. You also have to be careful of getting this one on your skin, clothing, and towels or it will cause some staining.

Nioxin

There's no doubt about it: Nioxin sells lots of hair-care products. Its claim to fame is centered around the belief that there are "natural" hair-care remedies, albeit expensive ones, for growing hair. "Nioxin Research Labs are committed to the continual investigation of environmental and physiological causes of baldness and thinning hair." Who wouldn't want to believe that this company has the answer if you're suffering from hair loss?

It turns out that Nioxin's natural treatment utilizes several standard plant extracts and some vitamins. The claims about hair growth are, to say the least, pretty spectacular. While the company references clinical results, none were ever made available to me, nor are there any in print. It takes incredible marketing skill to convince consumers that extracts of balm mint, nettle, chamomile, yarrow, sage, rosemary, and hops, to mention some of the plant extracts in Nioxin, can grow hair. There is also a tiny amount of saw palmetto in some of these products; for that, see my comments about this ingredient in the review for Hair Genesis products.

According to Nioxin, "The leading cause of hair loss is a toxin known as DHT (dihydrotestosterone). DHT causes a deterioration of the hair follicle, rendering it unable to produce hair. If this toxin is not removed, the damage can be irreparable. Nioxin has proven to be effective in reversing the damage caused by DHT." There are several problems with this description. First, DHT is hardly a toxin. Second, it doesn't explain why in addition to making scalp hair fall out, DHT makes your mustache, beard, chest hair, back hair, and pubic hair grow. It's a mystery why DHT makes some hairs grow and other hairs miniaturize.

Nioxin wants to cover all the bases of hair loss and has come up with another problem, "demodex folliculorum in the hair follicle," for which it has the answer. *Demodex folliculorum* is a fancy name for a type of mite that can be present in the hair shaft and oil gland. According to the *Ohio State University Fact Sheet*, 1991, "These microscopic mites [demodex folliculorum] live in the hair follicles or sebaceous glands of most humans. Very few persons are allergic to them. Those who are may lose their eyelashes or develop acne." Moreover, the possible presence of this mite is true for people of all ages, so why isn't it making children bald? While it can cause problems, diagnosis is often difficult because mite specimens must be collected and identified by trained specialists before treatment can be made. When it comes to baldness, it doesn't make sense to select a treatment for organisms that may not exist or even be causing your problem.

There are many other claims about feeding the hair and preventing baldness lurking in the Nioxin brochures. None of the products will hurt you, but nothing can substantiate its claim to help stop hair loss either.

For more information about Nioxin call (800) 628-9890 or visit its Web site at www.nioxin.com.

☹ **1 Bionutrient Cleanser for Normal Hair** *($10.50 for 8 ounces)* uses TEA-lauryl sulfate as the main cleansing agent, which can be irritating and drying for the scalp.

☹ **1C Bionutrient Cleanser for Chemically Treated or Dry Hair** *($10.50 for 8 ounces)* uses TEA-lauryl sulfate as the main cleansing agent, which can be irritating and drying for the scalp.

☺ **Fit Cleanser Normal to Dry** *($5 for 5 ounces)* contains plant water, conditioning agents, detergent cleansing agent, lather agent, plant oils, and preservatives. This cleanser is good for dry hair of any thickness. It does contain papain and bromelain, enzymes that can exfoliate skin and also exfoliate the hair shaft, but the amount is probably not enough to have this effect.

☺ **Nioxin Fit Cleanser Normal to Oily** *($4.95 for 5 ounces)* is almost identical to the Normal to Dry version above and the same comments apply. The plant oil in this product is a problem for oily scalp or hair.

☹ **Semodex Sebolytic Cleanser for Men** *($9.95 for 6 ounces)* uses TEA-lauryl sulfate as its main cleansing agent, which can be irritating and drying for the scalp. This shampoo is supposed to be effective for ridding the scalp of hair mites, yet there are no ingredients in it that can have an effect against this type of infestation.

☹ **Semodex Sebolytic Cleanser for Women** *($9.95 for 6 ounces)* contains an amazing number of plants, all supposed to be beneficial for women and hair loss. There's everything from wild yam (which is supposed to be a source of progesterone) to saw palmetto and a host of other plants. Wild yam is a poor source of progesterone and saw palmetto is controversial for growing hair. Other than that, the main cleansing agent is TEA-lauryl sulfate, which can be drying and irritating on the scalp.

☺ **2 Bionutrient Treatment for Fuller Thicker Healthier Hair, Regular Formula** *($28.74 for 4 ounces)* contains mostly water, aloe, conditioning agents, water-binding agents, vitamins, thickeners, plant extracts, antioxidant, and preservatives. This is a good conditioner for normal to dry hair of any thickness, but that's about it. The antioxidant and plant extracts are in such minuscule amounts they couldn't do much for even one hair. This product does contain peppermint oil, which can be irritating to the scalp; the tingle it produces, though, probably makes a person feel like they are growing hair.

☺ **$$$ 2C Bionutrient Treatment for Chemically Treated Hair, for Fuller, Thicker, Healthier Hair** *($53 for 8 ounces)* is similar to the one above, only with silicone and a detangling agent. That can be better for very dry hair, but the other comments above also apply.

☺ **Bliss Triple Action Instant Reconditioner** *($8 for 8 ounces)* contains mostly water, film former, silicones, conditioning agents, detangling agent, preservatives, and fragrance. This standard conditioner is very good for dry hair that is normal to fine or thin in thickness. An interesting twist for this product is that it contains propolis extract, which is resin from a beehive. It can coat the hair shaft like any film former to add a feel of thickness.

☺ **Cytogen Advanced Scalp Treatment for Thinning Hair for Chemically Treated Hair** *($26.95 for 4 ounces)* contains mostly water, silicones, conditioning agents, detangling agent, water-binding agents, vitamins, thickeners, plant extracts, preservatives, and fragrance. This standard conditioner is very good for dry hair of any thickness. It does contain peppermint oil, which can be a scalp irritant, but perhaps that could be mistaken as indicating this product is working to grow hair, when it isn't!

☺ **NX3 Nutrient Booster for Thinning Hair** *($19.90 for 1 ounce)* contains mostly water, conditioning agent, plant extracts, slip agent, thickeners, silicone, film former, and preservatives. The belief that these plant extracts can grow hair is up to you. Other than that, this is a good leave-in conditioner for dry hair of any thickness.

☺ **Scalp Therapy Scalp Massage and Botanical Hair Conditioner** *($16.80 for 12 ounces)* contains mostly water, plant extracts, conditioning agents, thickeners, detangling agents, film former, silicone, preservatives, and coloring agents. Again the belief in plant stuff for hair growth is up to you; there is nothing in here that can do anything for hair growth. Other than that, this is a good conditioner for dry hair that is normal to fine or thin.

☺ **Semodex Scalp Serum for Men** *($29.95 for 2 ounces),* like the version below for women, does contain a tiny amount of tea tree oil. Tea tree oil is a disinfectant, though, with no reported benefit against mites.

☹ **Semodex Scalp Serum for Women** *($29.95 for 2 ounces)* is similar to the version for men above, only this one contains wild yam and saw palmetto extract.

☺ **Structure & Strength Triple Bonding Reconstructor for Damaged Hair, Fine to Fragile** *($12.54 for 6 ounces)* contains mostly plant water, conditioning agents, silicones, thickener, detangling agents, water-binding agents, film former, preservatives, and fragrance. This can't reconstruct hair but it is a good conditioner for dry hair of any thickness.

☺ **Structure & Strength Triple Bonding Reconstructor for Damaged Hair, Medium to Coarse** *($12.54 for 6 ounces)* contains mostly plant water, conditioning agents, silicones, thickeners, detangling agents, preservatives, and fragrance. This won't reconstruct one hair on your head but it is a good conditioner for dry hair of any thickness.

☺ **Lift Volumizing Mist for Root Support** *($10 for 8 ounces)* contains mostly water, film formers, conditioning agents, vitamins, slip agents, preservatives, and fragrance. It is a standard, lightweight styling spray that can add a feel of thickness to the hair and help lightly control styling. It has a light hold with minimal to no stiff or sticky feel.

☹ **$$$ NIOgel Weightless Styling Enhance** *($87.96 for 6 ounces)* contains mostly plant water, film formers, conditioning agents, thickeners, silicones, vitamins, and preservatives. It's an exceptionally standard styling gel that has medium hold and a sticky feel. This is hardly weightless.

☹ **Fit Styling Energizer** *($9.96 for 5 ounces)* is hard to place in any clear category. It is basically just a lightweight styling lotion with light to medium hold and a slight stiff, sticky feel. If it was just that. it would be fine, but the catch for this product is that it contains the supplement DHEA (a male sex hormone produced by the adrenal glands) as well as pregnenolone (a precursor of DHEA). There are huge claims attached to these substances by the vitamin/supplement industry for all kinds of benefits from weight loss to enhancing memory. Regardless of all the claims, objective observers such as the Mayo Clinic's Mayo Foundation for Medical Education and Research Web site, and Dr. Andrew Weil, the guru of health supplements who teaches at the University of Arizona in Tucson, both express concern about DHEA. According to Dr. Weil, "evidence for DHEA's benefits is inconclusive. There was one small, six-month study at the University of California-San Diego that reported improved energy and feelings of well-being." He continues, "I'm cautious about using any hormones on a regular basis without good reason and without medical supervision. We don't know what the downside of taking supplemental DHEA may be over time." Having said all that, and while it's unlikely that any of this product can be absorbed through the scalp, you should know the health concerns; the rest is up to you.

☺ **NIOspray Climate Control (Aerosol)** *($9.50 for 10 ounces)* is a standard aerosol hairspray with a firm hold and a somewhat stiff feel that does not easily allow hair to be brushed through.

☺ **NIOspray Climate Control Extra (Aerosol)** *($9.50 for 10 ounces)* is almost identical to the version above and the same comments apply.

☺ **NIOspray Power Hold (Aerosol)** *($10 for 10 ounces)* is similar to the Climate Control version above, only with medium hold and a less stiff feel; it can be brushed through.

☹ **Recharging Complex Dietary Supplement for Women** *($29.96 for 90 caplets)*. If you want to believe that this supplement can grow hair, there's no stopping you from taking this. But taking a product with progesterone (which is what this pill contains) is problematic and at best controversial without the consent of a physician.

☹ **Recharging Complex Dietary Supplement for Men** *($29.96 for 90 caplets)* is similar to the one above for women and the same comments apply.

Origins

Estee Lauder created Origins as its way of getting part of the natural cosmetics business. To meet this contrived need, Origins has thrown plants of all kinds into itsproducts among the standard ingredients. For potential allergic or sensitizing reactions, a lot of these plants are extremely problematic. For the scalp, lots of the plants can be an itchy, irritating problem. But other than that, these are just the same basic hair-care formulations that show up in lots of other hair-care products. For more information on Origins, call (800) ORIGINS or visit its Web site at www.origins.com.

☹ **Clear Head Shampoo for Everyday** *($10 for 8.5 ounces)* contains peppermint, spearmint, and mint, which can be irritating for the scalp.

☺ **Last Straw Conditioning Shampoo** *($17.50 for 7 ounces)* is, aside from the complicated list of plant extracts, just a shampoo with minimal to almost nonexistent conditioning agents. It contains mostly plant water, detergent cleansing agents, thickeners, plant extracts, fragrant oils, and preservatives. The price is absurd for what you get.

☹ **No Deposit If Your Hair Acts Bored** *($10 for 8.5 ounces)*. The claim that this shampoo wouldn't leave a deposit is nonsense: it contains film former, resin, and castor oil. It also contains peppermint and menthol, which can be an irritating problem for the scalp.

☹ **Snow Removal Dandruff Shampoo** *($10 for 8.5 ounces)* uses sodium C14-16 olefin sulfonate as the main detergent cleansing agent, which can be drying and possibly strip color from the hair. It also contains salicylic acid, and that has the potential to exfoliate the scalp and can also denature the hair shaft.

☹ **Happy Ending Conditioner** *($11 for 8.5 ounces)* has sodium lauryl sulfate as one of the main ingredients (used in conditioners as emulsifying agents, not cleansing agents), which makes it too drying for the hair and scalp. This product also contains grapefruit, orange, and lemon, which can be drying and irritating to the scalp.

☺ **Knot Free Finishing Rinse** *($11 for 8.5 ounces)* contains peppermint and lemon, so keep it away from the scalp. Other than that, it is just a standard leave-in conditioner that would work well for normal to slightly dry hair of any thickness. It contains mostly plant water, thickeners, detangling agents, conditioning agents, plant extracts, slip agents, silicones, and preservatives.

☺ **Take Control Styling Gel to Put Hair in Its Place** *($11 for 5 ounces)* contains mostly plant water, film former, slip agents, plant extracts, conditioning agents, castor oil, silicone, and preservatives. It has a light hold with a slight stiff, sticky feel that does let you brush through the hair. It also contains peppermint, spearmint, and orange, which can be irritating for skin, so keep it away from the scalp.

☹ **Don't Get Stiffed Alcohol Free Hair Spray Non-Aerosol** *($11 for 6.7 ounces)* is a fairly wet hairspray, so it can collapse a style before it sets in place. It also has a fairly sticky feel with a medium to firm hold. It contains mostly plant water, film formers, castor oil, plant extracts, conditioning agents, silicone, and preservatives.

☺ **Supermane Grooming Mist** *($12.50 for 6.7 ounces)* contains mostly plant water, castor oil, slip agent, plant extracts, fragrant oils, conditioning agent, film formers, and preservatives. This has a slight sticky feel but it can help smooth out hair when styling; it has a light hold that does let you brush through hair.

Ouidad

Ouidad products are specifically aimed at those with curly and frizzy hair. Do these products make a difference for that hair condition? Not any more than lots of other hair-care products do. Strangely, Ouidad's brochure warns against the dangers of silicone, yet its Shine Hair Glaze is almost all silicone. Didn't they read their own ingredient lists? It also states that silicone attracts dust and builds up more than other conditioning agents. It simply isn't true. Many of the ingredients in the Ouidad products, however—plant oils, mineral oil, thickeners, and film formers—do attract dust, and then hold on to it. Regardless, all conditioning agents and all hairstyling agents can build up on hair, making it appear dull and heavy.

The brochure also claims the ingredients in these products are "small enough to penetrate the hair shaft and rebuild hair's weakened infrastructure." This is a completely impossible, unsubstantiated claim. The ingredients in these products are no different from those found in hundreds of other hair-care products. And even if the ingredients could get into the hair shaft, keeping them in there is an entirely different story (after all, hair is like a two-way door; what goes in easily comes out easily).

Aside from the hype, which is standard in the world of beauty, there are some good products here—it's just that some of the prices are way out of line. For more information on Ouidad, call (800) 677-HAIR or visit its Web site at www.ouidad.com.

☺ **Clear Shampoo** *($7.50 for 8 ounces)* is a standard, detergent-based shampoo that contains some conditioning agents and plant oils as well as some sulfur, which can be extremely drying for the scalp and is indicated only for dandruff. The conditioning agents in this shampoo can build up on hair with repeated use.

☺ **$$$ Deep Treatment** *($30 for 4 ounces)* won't go all that deep, but it is deeply overpriced. It contains mostly water, thickeners, detangling agents, conditioning agents, plant oils, water-binding agents, and preservatives. This is a good but extremely standard moisturizer for dry hair of any thickness. The price is just absurd for a commonplace conditioner.

☺ **Balancing Rinse** *($9 for 8 ounces)* contains mostly water, thickeners, detangling agent, conditioning agents, preservatives, and fragrance. This is a lightweight leave-in conditioner for normal hair to help with combing.

☺ **Botanical Boost** *($10 for 8 ounces)* is a standard leave-in conditioner that contains a handful of plant extracts. The plants can't boost hair, but the lightweight detangling agents and conditioning agents can help make normal to slightly dry hair of any thickness easier to comb.

☺ **Styling Mist** *($9 for 8 ounces)* is just a standard hairstyling spray that can have a soft to medium hold.

☺ **Tress F/X** *($8 for 8 ounces)* is a styling gel that has a light hold with minimal to no sticky feel. It contains mostly water, detangling agents/film formers, slip agents, conditioning agents, thickeners, fragrance, and preservatives.

☺ **$$$ Clear Control** *($15 for 2 ounces)* contains mostly water, mineral oil, thickeners, glycerin, more thickeners, and preservatives. This is a gel-like pomade that adds minimal control and can help smooth frizzies and stubborn curls, but that's hardly worth this price tag. This can make hair look greasy and heavy, so use it sparingly.

☺ **$$$ Shine Hair Glaze** *($20 for 1 ounce)* is just an overpriced silicone serum. There are identical and far cheaper versions at the drugstore.

Pantene

Pantene is one of the most popular hair-care product lines being sold. Pantene would like you to believe this is the case because "every product in the Pantene

Pro-V hair care range contains a special pro-vitamin complex. This vitamin complex contains Pro-Vitamin B5, which penetrates the hair shaft and the root to nourish from within, whilst the products also aim to strengthen the outer hair cuticle for increased protection. A test on shampoo and conditioner proved that nothing penetrates the inner world of your hair deeper than Pro-Vitamin B5." Well, that last statement is actually true in a bizarre sort of way. Panthenol, the hair-care ingredient name for vitamin B5, does penetrate as well as any other conditioning agent, which isn't very much. But even if panthenol were some kind of miracle for hair, it turns out most hair-care products use it, so it isn't exclusive to this line. It seems Pantene's popularity is due to the millions and millions of dollars it spends on advertising. Those ads are enough to convince anyone to give these products a try.

For more information on Pantene, call (800) 723-9569 or in Canada (800) 668-0151. You can also visit the Procter & Gamble Web site at www.pg.com.

☹ **Progressive Treatment Shampoo for Dry Hair** *($3.47 for 7 ounces)* contains ammonium xylenesulfonate, a solvent that can be drying for the scalp and hair. This is also a high pH shampoo that can be a problem for the hair and scalp for dryness and irritation. I suspect the purpose is to create a feel of thicker hair, which this kind of formulation can do; on the downside are the problems it can cause for the hair shaft and the scalp in the long run.

☹ **Progressive Treatment Shampoo for Permed or Color Treated Hair, Revitalizing Formula** *($3.47 for 7 ounces)* is similar to the one above for Dry Hair and the same comments apply.

☹ **Progressive Treatment Shampoo, Vitamin Therapy for Overworked or Damaged Hair** *($3.69 for 7 ounces)* is similar to the one above for Dry Hair and the same comments apply.

☹ **Pro-Vitamin Daily Clarifying Shampoo** *($4.49 for 13 ounces)* is similar to the one above for Dry Hair and the same comments apply.

☹ **Pro-Vitamin Shampoo Extra Body for Fine Hair** *($3.39 for 13 ounces)* is similar to the one above for Dry Hair and the same comments apply.

☹ **Pro-Vitamin Shampoo for Normal Hair** *($3.39 for 13 ounces)* is similar to the one above for Dry Hair and the same comments apply.

☹ **Pro-Vitamin Shampoo Plus Conditioner in One Extra Body for Fine Hair** *($3.39 for 13 ounces)* is similar to the one above for Dry Hair and the same comments apply.

☹ **Pro-Vitamin Shampoo Plus Conditioner in One Moisturizing for Dry or Damaged Hair** *($4.49 for 13 ounces)* is similar to the one above for Dry Hair and the same comments apply.

☹ **Pro-Vitamin Shampoo Plus Conditioner in One for Normal Hair** *($4.49 for 13 ounces)* is similar to the one above for Dry Hair and the same comments apply.

☺ **Pro-Vitamin Shampoo Plus Conditioner, Revitalizing for Permed, Color Treated Hair** *($4.49 for 13 ounces)* is similar to the one above for Dry Hair and the same comments apply.

☺ **Pro-Vitamin Shampoo Revitalizing for Permed/Color Treated Hair** *($3.39 for 13 ounces)* is similar to the one above for Dry Hair and the same comments apply.

☺ **Pro-Vitamin Pyrithione Zinc Anti-Dandruff Shampoo** *($3.39 for 13 ounces)*. Given that Procter & Gamble created the technology for the zinc pyrithione used in its Head & Shoulders line, this one is as good as any in that category and quite similar to the original. This one may be a little bit easier on the hair.

☺ **Progressive Treatment Creme Conditioner, for Dry Hair, Moisture Replenishing Formula** *($3.47 for 7 ounces)* contains mostly water, silicones, thickeners, detangling agent/film former, conditioning agents, fragrance, thickeners, preservatives, and coloring agents. This is a good basic conditioner for dry hair that is normal to fine or thin in thickness.

☺ **Progressive Treatment Creme Conditioner, Extra Body for Fine or Normal Hair** *($3.47 for 7 ounces)* is almost identical to the Moisture Replenishing version above and the same comments apply.

☺ **Progressive Treatment Creme Conditioner for Permed or Color Treated Hair, Revitalizing Formula** *($3.47 for 7 ounces)* is almost identical to the Moisture Replenishing version above and the same comments apply.

☺ **Progressive Treatment Creme Conditioner, Vitamin Therapy** *($3.47 for 7 ounces)* is almost identical to the Moisture Replenishing version above and the same comments apply.

☺ **Pro-Vitamin Daily Heat Activated Conditioner** *($3.39 for 10.2 ounces)* is supposed to work with heat to improve the condition of heat-styled hair. It would be great if this were true, but it isn't. This is a good, basic styling spray that can also be used as a leave-in conditioner for normal to dry hair of any thickness. However, this product will not stop typical blow-dryer or curling iron heat of 200 degrees Fahrenheit or greater from doing damage.

☺ **Pro-Vitamin Daily Treatment Conditioner, Extra Body for Fine Hair** *($3.39 for 13 ounces)* contains mostly water, silicones, thickeners, detangling agent/film former, conditioning agents, fragrance, and preservatives. This is a good basic conditioner for dry hair that is normal to fine or thin in thickness.

☺ **Pro-Vitamin Daily Treatment Conditioner, Moisturizing for Dry or Damaged Hair** *($3.39 for 13 ounces)* is almost identical to the Extra Body version above and the same comments apply.

☺ **Pro-Vitamin Daily Treatment Regular Conditioning for Normal Hair** *($3.39 for 13 ounces)* is almost identical to the Moisture Replenishing version above and the same comments apply.

☺ **Pro-Vitamin Daily Treatment Conditioner, Revitalizing for Permed or Color Treated Hair** *($3.39 for 13 ounces)* is almost identical to the Moisture Replenishing version above and the same comments apply.

☺ **Pro-Vitamin Daily Light Spray Conditioner** *($3.39 for 10.2 ounces)* contains mostly water, detangling agent, film formers, slip agents, conditioning agents, silicone, preservatives, and fragrance. This is a good leave-in conditioner for normal to slightly dry hair that is normal to fine or thin in thickness.

☺ **Pro-Vitamin Deep Fortifying Hair Treatment** *($3.39 for 13 ounces)* contains mostly water, thickeners, silicones, conditioning agents, fragrance, and preservatives. This isn't a special treatment in the least but it is a good conditioner for dry hair of any thickness.

☺ **Pro-Vitamin Sculpting Gel, Extra Hold, Alcohol Free** *($2.79 for 7.1 ounces)* is a standard, light-hold gel with no stiff or sticky feel. It contains mostly water, detangling agent/film former, conditioning agents, thickeners, preservatives, and fragrance.

☺ **Pro-Vitamin Styling Spray Gel, Extra Hold** *($2.79 for 8.5 ounces)* is similar to the Sculpting Gel above, only this one is in spray form.

☺ **Pro-Vitamin Styling Mousse, Extra Hold for Control** *($2.79 for 8 ounces)* is a standard mousse that gives a light, combable hold and that contains mostly water, propellant, detangling agent/film former, conditioning agents, slip agents, preservatives, and fragrance.

☺ **Pro-Vitamin Hairspray Flexible Hold with Elastesse (Aerosol)** *($2.79 for 8.25 ounces)* is just an aerosol hairspray that contains mostly alcohol, water, propellant, film former, conditioning agent, and fragrance. It has a light to medium hold with minimal stiff or sticky feel.

☺ **Pro-Vitamin Hairspray Flexible Hold with Elastesse for Fine Hair (Aerosol)** *($2.79 for 8.25 ounces)* is similar to the one above and the same basic comments apply.

☺ **Pro-Vitamin Hairspray Flexible Hold with Elastesse Unscented (Non-Aerosol)** *($2.79 for 10 ounces)* is similar to the two above, only in nonaerosol form.

☺ **Pro-Vitamin Wet or Dry Styling and Holding Spray, Extra Firm Hold (Non-Aerosol)** *($2.79 for 8.5 ounces)* is similar to the Flexible Hold Non-Aerosol version above, and the same basic comments apply.

☺ **Pro-Vitamin Hairspray Ultra Firm Hold (Aerosol)** *($2.79 for 8.25 ounces)* is a standard aerosol hairspray that contains mostly alcohol, water, propellant, film former, conditioning agent, and fragrance. It has a firm hold with a somewhat stiff, sticky feel, though it does allow you to brush through the hair.

☺ **Pro-Vitamin Hairspray Ultra Firm Hold (Non-Aerosol) (Scented and Unscented)** *($2.79 for 10.2 ounces)* is similar to the Ultra Firm aerosol version above, only this one is nonaerosol; the same basic comments apply. The unscented version still contains a masking fragrance.

☺ **Pro-Vitamin Fixation Spritz, Maximum Hold** *($2.79 for 8.5 ounces)* is almost identical to the Ultra Firm Hold Non-Aerosol above and the same comments apply.

☺ **Pro-Vitamin Hair Strengthening Complex** *($9.64 for 3.4 ounces)* is just a conditioner for normal to dry hair that is normal to fine or thin in thickness. It contains mostly water, slip agent, conditioning agents, film former, castor oil, preservatives, and fragrance. It is a leave-in conditioner that can be helpful with combing for normal hair. It has no ability to strengthen hair.

Pro-V Color

This is Pantene's attempt to convince you it has developed products that can keep hair color from fading. It isn't possible; none of these products can affect either your natural hair color or your dyed hair color. There isn't one ingredient in any of these products that isn't present in similar combinations in the other Pantene products.

☺ **Pro-V Color Color Protector Pre-Wash Spray for Color Treated and Highlighted Hair** *($5.49 for 5.1 ounces)* a pre-wash (meaning before you shampoo) is like applying dirt to your skin before you wash your face. These are conditioning agents and film formers that work for conditioning the hair, which is useless if you are then going to wash your hair.

☺ **Pro-V Color Gentle Cleansing Shampoo for Color Treated and Highlighted Hair** *($5.49 for 13 ounces)* is a standard shampoo that contains mostly water, detergent cleansing agents, slip agents, thickeners, silicone, vitamins, conditioning agent, preservatives, and fragrance. It would work well for someone with normal to slightly dry hair that is fine or thin.

☺ **Pro-V Color Vitalizing Care Conditioner for Color Treated and Highlighted Hair** *($5.49 for 12 ounces)* is a good conditioner for normal to dry hair of any thickness. It contains mostly water, silicone, conditioning agents, vitamins, thickeners, detangling agent/film former, silicone, fragrance, and preservatives.

☺ **Pro-V Color Intensive Care Masque for Color Treated and Highlighted Hair** *($7.59 for 5.1 ounces)* is just a good conditioner for normal to dry hair of any thickness, but it isn't as good as the Vitalizing Care Conditioner above. This one contains mostly water, thickeners, silicones, conditioning agents, vitamins, fragrance, and preservatives.

☺ **Pro-V Color Leave-in Finishing Spray with UV Filters for Color Treated and Highlighted Hair** *($5.49 for 3.4 ounces)* is a standard styling spray with light hold and minimal stiff or sticky feel. It contains mostly water, slip agent, conditioning agents, film former, castor oil, preservatives, and fragrance. Without an SPF number the sun protection is bogus and misleading.

Paul Mitchell

Paul Mitchell, one of the oldest and best-known of salon lines, is famous for its diverse products and professional decorum. One hallmark of the Paul Mitchell line is awapuhi, the Hawaiian ginger plant. Of course, the claim here is that this is a very special species of Hawaiian ginger with unique properties. It may have unique properties, but none have been substantiated when it comes to hair. However, it does lend a nice fragrance to many of the products. In the long run, this is a good line of hair-care products to consider and the prices aren't as outlandish as some salon brands'. For more information on Paul Mitchell, call (514) 335-7135 or (800) 793-8790.

☺ **Awapuhi Shampoo** *($8.50 for 16 ounces)* contains mostly water, detergent cleansing agents, lather agent, plant extracts, plant oil, detangling agent/film former, thickeners, and preservatives. This is a good shampoo for normal to slightly dry hair that is normal to thin or fine. The film former in here can build up on hair.

☺ **Baby Don't Cry Shampoo** *($7.50 for 16 ounces)* is just detergent cleansing agent, lather agent, thickeners, and fragrance. This is actually a very good basic shampoo for any hair type; if it didn't have fragrance, it would even be great for a baby's sensitive skin.

☺ **Shampoo One** *($7.50 for 16 ounces)* contains mostly plant water, detergent cleansing agent, lather agent, thickeners, plant extracts, plant oils, conditioning agents, film former/detangling agent, preservatives, and fragrance. This is a good shampoo for normal to dry hair that is normal to fine or thin in thickness. The film former and conditioning agents can build up on hair, just as the henna in this shampoo can.

☺ **Shampoo Two** *($7.50 for 16 ounces)* is almost identical to version One above, only minus the film former. That makes this better for normal to dry hair of any thickness and reduces the chances for buildup.

☺ **Shampoo Three** *($11.50 for 16 ounces)* is just shampoo, and that's great for all hair types. It contains mostly water, detergent cleansing agent, lather agent, thickeners, preservatives, and fragrance. It also contains a chelating agent that can help prevent minerals from attaching to hair.

☹ **Tea Tree Special Shampoo** *($16 for 16 ounces)* does contain tea tree oil, which could have an effect on dandruff, but this product also contains a good amount of peppermint oil, which can just make scalp problems worse.

☺ **The Wash Moisture Balancing Shampoo** *($13 for 16 ounces)* contains mostly water, detergent cleansing agents, lather agent, conditioning agents, slip agents, plant extracts, water-binding agents, detangling agents, silicone, preservatives, and fragrance. This is a good shampoo for normal to dry hair of any thickness.

☺ **Beige Blonde** *($10.50 for 8.5 ounces)* is a good color-enhancing shampoo that contains mostly water, detergent cleansing agents, lather agent, thickeners, plant extract, conditioning agents, detangling agents, silicone, preservatives, dye agents, and fragrance. It would work well for any hair type.

☺ **Cool Blue** *($10.50 for 8.5 ounces)* is almost identical to the Beige Blonde above and the same basic comments apply.

☺ **Cool Brown** *($10.50 for 8.5 ounces)* is almost identical to the Beige Blonde above and the same basic comments apply.

☺ **Golden Blonde** *($10.50 for 8.5 ounces)* is almost identical to the Beige Blonde above and the same basic comments apply.

☺ **Golden Brown** *($10.50 for 8.5 ounces)* is almost identical to the Beige Blonde above and the same basic comments apply.

☺ **Platinum Blonde** *($10.50 for 8.5 ounces)* is almost identical to the Beige Blonde above and the same basic comments apply.

☺ **Red** *($10.50 for 8.5 ounces)* is almost identical to the Beige Blonde above and the same basic comments apply.

☺ **Red Brown** *($10.50 for 8.5 ounces)* is almost identical to the Beige Blonde above and the same basic comments apply.

☺ **Red Orange** *($10.50 for 8.5 ounces)* is almost identical to the Beige Blonde above and the same basic comments apply.

☺ **Awapuhi Moisture Mist** *($7 for 8 ounces)* contains mostly water, water-binding agent, plant extracts, detangling agent/film former, castor oil, fragrance, and preservatives. This is a good leave-in conditioner for dry hair that is normal to fine or thin in thickness. It can leave a slight sticky feel on hair but it will smooth out frizzies.

☹ **The Conditioner** *($7 for 6 ounces)* contains mostly plant water, thickeners, detangling agents, conditioning agents, plant extracts, plant oil, slip agents, fragrance, preservatives, and coloring agents. This is a good basic conditioner for normal to slightly dry hair of any thickness. It does contain spearmint oil, a skin irritant, so keep it away from the scalp.

☺ **The Detangler Instant Condition and Shine** *($7.95 for 8 ounces)* contains mostly water, slip agents, conditioning agents, thickeners, plant oil, preservatives, and fragrance. This is a very lightweight conditioner for normal to slightly dry hair that needs only a little help in combing.

☺ **Hair Repair Treatment** *($9 for 6 ounces)* contains mostly plant water, lots of thickening agents, detangling agents, film former, silicones, water-binding agent, plant oil, preservatives, and fragrance. This won't repair anything, but it is a very good conditioner for normal to dry hair that is normal to fine or thin in thickness. It does contain a tiny amount of sulfur, though probably not enough to be a problem for the hair.

☺ **Lite Detangler** *($9 for 8 ounces)* is, just as the name implies, a light, leave-in conditioner for normal to slightly dry hair. It contains mostly water, plant extracts, slip agents, conditioning agents, silicone, detangling agent, and preservative.

☺ **The Rinse Balancing Conditioner** *($12.95 for 16 ounces)* is a light, leave-in conditioner for normal to slightly dry hair that is normal to fine or thin in thickness. It contains mostly water, detangling agent, film former, slip agents, plant extracts, conditioning agents, thickeners, silicone, preservatives, fragrance, and coloring agents.

☹ **Seal and Shine** *($5.50 for 8 ounces)* contains sodium polystyrene sulfonate, which can be drying for hair and has the potential to strip color from hair.

☺ **Super Charged Conditioner** *($8.50 for 4 ounces)* contains mostly plant water, thickeners, conditioning agents, detangling agents, preservatives, slip agents, plant oil, and fragrance. This is hardly supercharged, but it is a good conditioner for normal to dry hair of any thickness.

☹ **Tea Tree Special Conditioner** *($10 for 8 ounces)* does contain tea tree oil, which can be helpful against dandruff, but it also contains peppermint oil, and that can make matters worse.

☺ **$$$ Gloss** *($20 for 5.1 ounces)* is a standard, though overpriced, silicone serum in a gel form. It adds shine and a silky feel to hair.

☺ **$$$ The Shine** *($13.50 for 4.2 ounces)* is similar to the Gloss above, only in spray form, and the same basic comments apply.

☺ **The Cream Condition with Style** *($10.95 for 5.1 ounces)* contains mostly water, film former, slip agents, silicone, thickeners, conditioning agents, detangling agents, plant oils, preservatives, and fragrance. This is a good, leave-in conditioner in a gel-lotion form that can also be a styling aid to help smooth out curls or frizzies. It has minimal to no stiff or sticky feel but it can easily build up and make hair feel greasy and heavy, so use it sparingly.

☺ **Extra-Body Sculpting Gel** *($6.95 for 6 ounces)* contains mostly water, film formers, thickeners, preservatives, and fragrance. This extremely basic styling gel has a light hold and minimal sticky feel.

☺ **Soft Sculpting Spray Gel** *($7 for 8 ounces)* contains mostly aloe water, alcohol, film formers, thickeners, castor oil, and fragrance. This extremely basic spray gel has a light hold with minimal to no stiff or sticky feel.

☺ **Fast Drying Sculpting Spray** *($8 for 8 ounces)* is a standard medium-hold hairspray with a slight stiff, sticky feel that can easily be brushed through. It is best when used to hold a hairstyle rather than for styling. It contains mostly alcohol, water, film former, conditioning agent, silicone, and fragrance.

☺ **Super Clean Sculpting Gel** *($6.50 for 6 ounces)* contains mostly plant water, detangling agent/film former, thickeners, plant extracts, plant oil, conditioning agents, preservatives, and fragrance. This basic styling gel has a light hold with minimal stiff or sticky feel.

☺ **Extra Body Sculpting Foam** *($9 for 6 ounces)* is a standard mousse with a light to medium hold and minimal stiff or sticky feel. It contains mostly water, film formers, propellant, plant extract, thickeners, silicones, preservatives, and fragrance.

☺ **Sculpting Foam** *($8.50 for 6 ounces)* is almost identical to the Extra Body version above and the same basic comments apply.

☺ **Foaming Pomade** *($10 for 5.1 ounces)* doesn't foam; rather, it is just a creamy lotion that contains mostly water, mineral oil, Vaseline, thickeners, propellant, film former, fragrance, and preservatives. This can keep frizzy, coarse hair smooth with minimal to no hold and no stiff or sticky feel, but it can have a greasy texture and appearance, so use it sparingly.

☺ **The Heat Humidity Resistant Styling Spray** *($11 for 8.5 ounces)* contains mostly water, film formers, detangling agents, silicones, conditioning agent, plant extracts, slip agents, preservatives, and fragrance. This is just a lightweight styling spray that can help hold a soft to light style with almost no stiff or sticky feel. It can't protect against humidity or heat any more than any other styling hair product can.

☺ **Volumizing Spray** *($11 for 8 ounces)* is a light- to medium-hold styling spray with a slight stiff, sticky feel. It can help when styling hair but the volume comes from your styling technique, not this product. It contains mostly plant water, film former, slip agents, plant extracts, conditioning agents, thickeners, fragrance, and preservatives.

☺ **Hair Sculpting Lotion** *($5.50 for 8 ounces)* is a light-hold liquid gel with minimal to no stiff or sticky feel. It can smooth out frizzies and curls when styling. It contains mostly plant water, detangling agent/film former, plant extracts, plant oil, conditioning agents, slip agents, preservatives, and fragrance.

☺ **Super Sculpt Styling Glaze** *($6.50 for 8 ounces)* is similar to the Sculpting Lotion above, only with slightly more hold and slightly more sticky feel, but just slightly.

☺ **Slick Works Definition with Shine** *($12 for 5.1 ounces)* contains mostly water, mineral oil, thickeners, slip agents, film former, plant extracts, silicones, fragrance, and preservatives. This is a standard, light-hold gel with a slight greasy finish, but it can be great for smoothing out coarse, thick, dry hair. Use it sparingly or it can make hair look heavy.

☺ **Wax Works Control with Shine** *($11.95 for 5 ounces)* contains mostly water, mineral oil, slip agents, film former, thickeners, plant extracts, fragrance, and preservatives. This is a standard gel for smoothing stubborn, hard-to-hold hair; it has a medium to firm hold and a somewhat stiff, sticky finish. It can easily leave a greasy, heavy look on hair, so use it sparingly.

☺ **Super Clean Spray with Awapuhi** *($9.50 for 10 ounces)* is a standard aerosol hairspray with a medium to firm hold and a somewhat stiff feel, though it can be brushed through. It contains mostly alcohol, propellant, water, film formers, slip agents, plant extracts, silicones, and fragrance.

☺ **Super Clean Extra Firm Holding Spray** *($10 for 10 ounces)* is almost identical to the Super Clean Spray above and the same basic comments apply.

☺ **Freeze and Shine Super Spray** *($9 for 8 ounces)* is almost identical to the Super Clean Spray above only in nonaerosol form, and the same basic comments apply.

☺ **Soft Spray** *($7 for 8 ounces)* is almost identical to the Super Clean Spray above only in nonaerosol form, and the same basic comments apply.

☺ **The Masque Intensive Therapy Treatment** *($15.50 for 4.2 ounces)* contains mostly water, slip agents, film formers, plant extracts, more slip agents, silicones, conditioning agents, plant oils, thickeners, fragrance, and preservatives. On the one hand, this is an exceptionally standard conditioner for normal to dry hair that is thin or fine. On the other, the long ingredient list includes sulfur, which can strip hair color. It also contains a trace amount of colloidal gold, though it's anyone's guess what that can do for hair.

☺ **Rogaine Complete Treatment Kit** *($36.75 for this and the Botanical Prep Shampoo and Body Building Treatment below).* If you are looking for the active ingredient minoxidil at 5 percent, this is as good as any, though it's definitely not any different from similar ones at the drugstore that contain the exact same ingredient. This kit also comes with the two following products, though they serve no purpose for helping the hair to grow.

☹ **Botanical Prep Shampoo** uses sodium C14-16 olefin sulfonate as the main cleansing agent, which is too drying for both hair and scalp, and can be irritating for the scalp.

☺ **Botanical Body-Building Treatment** is just a standard, lightweight, leave-in conditioner using slip agents and detangling agent. This one also contains a tiny amount of saw palmetto and wild yam extracts. I discuss saw palmetto in the review on Hair Genesis products and wild yam in the review of Nioxin products.

Pert

When it comes to two-in-ones—shampoo combined with conditioner—Pert is state of the art. Procter & Gamble invented the process of using silicone (dimethicone) with standard detergent cleansing agents. Why was this so amazing and revolutionary? Because of dimethicone's unique ability to cling to hair even during the process of shampooing and rinsing. Since 1985, when Pert first took the drugstore shelves by storm, Procter & Gamble has spent quite a bit of money and time perfecting the amount of silicone oil needed for different hair types. I still feel strongly that two-in-ones have limitations because of buildup (if the silicone doesn't wash out, it can indeed build up on the hair shaft), and also because if you are someone with an oily scalp you don't need the silicone (which has a silky though slightly greasy feel) on the scalp. But if you have normal to slightly dry hair, if you prefer a flatter rather than a fuller look, or especially if your hair is short, and you are considering a two-in-one, Pert isn't a bad place to start.

For more information on Pert, call (800) 723-9569 or in Canada (800) 668-0151. You can also visit the Procter & Gamble Web site at www.pg.com.

☺ **Pert Plus Shampoo Plus Conditioner in One, Dry or Damaged Hair** *($3.71 for 15 ounces)* contains mostly water, detergent cleansing agents, thickeners, silicone, lather agent, film former, fragrance, preservatives, and coloring agents. This is a good shampoo/conditioner for normal to slightly dry hair that is normal to fine or thin in thickness.

☺ **Pert Plus Shampoo and Conditioner in One, Extra Body for Fine Hair** *($3.71 for 15 ounces)* is almost identical to the version above for Dry or Damaged hair and the same comments apply.

☺ **Pert Plus Shampoo Plus Conditioner in One, Normal Hair** *($3.71 for 15 ounces)* is almost identical to the version above for Dry or Damaged hair and the same comments apply.

☺ **Pert Plus Shampoo and Conditioner in One, Oily Hair** *($3.71 for 15 ounces)* is almost identical to the version above for Dry or Damaged hair and the same comments apply.

☺ **Tear-Free Pert Plus for Kids, Light Conditioning** *($3.49 for 15 ounces)* is almost identical to the version above for Dry or Damaged hair and the same comments apply.

☺ **Tear-Free Pert Plus for Kids, Normal Conditioning** *($3.71 for 15 ounces)* is almost identical to the version above for Dry or Damaged hair and the same comments apply.

☹ **Pert Plus Dandruff Control Shampoo and Conditioner in One, Extra Body for Fine or Oily Hair** *($3.49 for 15 ounces)* is the same type of shampoo as Head & Shoulders, also owned by Proctor & Gamble. It contains zinc pyrithione as the active ingredient to fight dandruff along with detergent cleansing agents, lather agent, fragrance, silicone, preservatives, and coloring agents. The silicone can be a problem for someone with oily hair or scalp.

☹ **Pert Plus Dandruff Control Shampoo and Conditioner in One for Normal to Dry Hair** *($3.71 for 15 ounces)* is almost identical to the version above for Extra Body only this one doesn't contain silicone, which makes it better for all hair types for controlling dandruff.

philosophy

Philosophy has come up with an intriguing twist on the same old cosmetics theme, and in some ways it's the most amazing marketing campaign I've ever seen. It has a quality of upscale, department-store élan, with a touch of Zen, family values, and a heavy dose of twenty-something attitude thrown into the mix. It's hard to tell if you are shopping a cosmetics and hair-care line or looking for a new religious experience. In many ways, this is the least cosmetics-oriented line I've ever seen. That's not to say philosophy isn't in the business of selling cosmetics, because that is exactly what it does, and with expensive price tags to boot. (Who says a philosophical point of view has to be inexpensive? Although that happens to be my philosophy.)

Most of the basic information in the philosophy brochure is actually quite good, such as advice about weight loss, sun care, exercise, relaxation, and basic facts about skin aging. But there's also a fair share of nonsense about vitamins and botanicals being the beneficial ingredients in its products. Although there are definitely some very good products in this line, many are overpriced for what you get. Skin care is really the most significant part of philosophy's product lineup. The hair-care products almost seem an afterthought. There are few options to consider here, but for the most part these are just the same old same old.

For more information on philosophy call (888) 2-NEW-AGE (doesn't that phone number just figure?), (800) 736-5155, (800) LOVE 151, or visit its Web site at www.philosophy.com.

☺ **clearing the hair deep cleansing shampoo** *($12 for 8 ounces)* contains mostly water, detergent cleansing agents, lather agent, plant extracts, detangling agent/film former, fragrant oils, and preservatives. This is a good shampoo for most all hair types, though the film former may cause buildup.

☹ **it's all in your head everyday shampoo** *($12 for 8 ounces)* uses sodium C14-16 olefin sulfonate as the main cleansing agent, which can be irritating for the scalp and hair and drying for the hair, and may possibly strip hair color.

☺ **the big blow off liquid protein hair conditioner** *($12 for 6 ounces)* is a good simple conditioner for dry hair of any thickness. It contains mostly, water, detangling agents, silicone, conditioning agents, and preservatives. The price is a "big blow" for this standard formulation.

☺ **the breaking point overnight intensive hair conditioner** *($12 for 2 ounces)* contains mostly plant oils, thickeners, vitamins, and fragrant oils. This is mostly sunflower oil, and that's great for dry hair of any thickness, but you can get the same results from the sunflower oil in your kitchen cupboard. The vitamins in here have no ability to benefit hair or scalp.

☺ **entangled daily conditioner** *($12 for 8 ounces)* contains mostly water, silicones, conditioning agent, thickeners, plant oil, fragrant oils, slip agent, preservatives, and coloring agents. This is a very good, silicone-based conditioner that would work well for dry to very dry hair of any thickness.

☹ **headtrip weekly deep conditioning hair treatment** *($13 for 4 ounces)* contains lemon oil, orange oil, and eucalyptus oil, which can be irritating and drying for the scalp.

☺ **shear splendor daily conditioner for chemically treated hair** *($13 for 8 ounces)* contains mostly plant water, silicones, thickeners, detangling agents, castor oil, plant oil, conditioning agents, plant extracts, and preservatives. This is a good conditioner for dry hair that is coarse or thick.

☺ **memory styling gel** *($12 for 4 ounces)* is a standard styling gel with a light hold and minimal to no stiff or sticky feel that contains mostly water, film former, thickeners, conditioning agent, plant extracts, slip agent, preservatives, and fragrance.

☺ **let's get something straight straightening balm for humid climates** *($12 for 4 ounces)* is a liquidy styling gel that has a light hold and minimal to no stiff or sticky feel. It can help in straightening and smoothing hair. It contains mostly water, detangling agent, slip agents, thickener, conditioning agents, fragrant oils, silicone, and preservatives.

☺ **hold that thought anti-frizz hair spray** *($14 for 8 ounces)* is a standard medium-hold hairspray with a slight stiff feel that can easily be brushed through. It contains mostly alcohol, film former, water, slip agent, fragrance, and silicone.

☺ **$$$ curly head silicone hair serum for frizzy hair** *($11 for 2 ounces)* is a standard silicone serum, the same as any at the drugstore for half the price. This can leave a silky feel and a soft shine on hair.

Phytotherathrie

For all the promise of plants and natural ingredients in its name, this line turns out to be a very straightforward, standard group of hair-care products. The plant extracts are the usual amalgam, and accompany all the standard formulations. The claims for what the plants can do are bogus—there is nothing unique or special in here—but you have to do a lot of explaining to convince a woman to spend $16.50 on 3.3 ounces of dandruff shampoo that isn't all that different from Head & Shoulders, which is $3.39 for 15.2 ounces. Actually, there is something quite ironic about a line that sells a Moisturizing Sun Gel claiming (rather indirectly) that it can protect the hair from the sun, as well as an After Sun Repair cream. Wouldn't you assume that if the Sun Gel worked you wouldn't need the Sun Repair? For more information about Phytotherathrie, call (800) 648-0349 or in Canada (800) 363-1660.

☺ **Phytargent Whitening Shampoo for Grey and White Hair with Azulene from Camomile** *($15 for 6.8 ounces)* contains mostly water, detergent cleansing agents, lather agent, thickeners, detangling agent/film former, fragrance, preservatives, and dye agents. The deep-red dye agents in here can slightly reduce the yellow overtones of gray hair but not much. This is just a basic shampoo that can work well for normal hair that is normal to fine or thin.

☺ **Phytocadamia Restoring Shampoo for Very Dry Hair with Macadamia Oil and Illipe Butter** *($15 for 6.8 ounces)* contains mostly plant water, detergent cleansing agents, lather agent, emollients, thickeners, vitamins, conditioning agents, detangling agent/film former, slip agents, and preservatives. This is indeed a good shampoo for very dry, coarse hair.

☺ **Phytocidre Restoring Shampoo with Cider Vinegar for Colored or Permed Hair** *($15 for 6.8 ounces)* is an interesting option for shampooing. It contains mostly water, detergent cleansing agents, vinegar, thickener, and preservatives. This simple shampoo contains very gentle cleansing agents so it wouldn't be very effective for washing out hairstyling or conditioning buildup, though it would be great for gentle cleansing. The vinegar lowers the pH of the product, which can help shut down layers on the cuticle. However, for the money, you can shampoo with any shampoo that doesn't contain conditioning agents or film formers and then rinse your hair with plain old vinegar to see if you liked the effect.

☺ **$$$ Phytocoltar Dandruff Cream Shampoo for Dandruff** *($16.50 for 3.3 ounces)* is a standard zinc pyrithione–based dandruff shampoo that also contains coal tar as well as tea tree oil. This definitely covers a few bases for fighting dandruff, but I would start with Head & Shoulders (which also uses zinc pyrithione) before jumping into this expense.

☺ **Phytojoba Gentle, Regulating Milk Shampoo for Dry Hair with Jojoba Oil (1%)** *($15 for 6.8 ounces)* contains mostly detergent cleansing agents, plant water, lather agents, plant oil, thickeners, conditioning agents, detangling agent/film former, fragrance, and preservatives. This is a good shampoo for normal to slightly dry hair that is normal to fine or thin in thickness.

☺ **$$$ Phytolactum Scalp-Cleansing Shampoo for Normal Hair/Sensitive Scalp with Phytolactine and Almond Milk Extract** *($15 for 3.3 ounces)* contains mostly plant extract, detergent cleansing agents, lather agent, thickeners, water-binding agents, film former, preservatives, and fragrance. It would be a good shampoo for normal hair that is fine or thin. Nothing in here makes this one better for sensitive skin. There is no actual ingredient called phytolactine, it's just a made-up name used to represent some plant extracts and a conditioning agent. The film former in this shampoo is what can build up on hair and make it feel thicker.

☺ **$$$ Phytomiel "Le Petit Phyto" Hypoallergenic Plant Based Shampoo for Baby's Hair with Honey Absolute and Apricot** *($15 for 2.5 ounces)* is a standard "baby" shampoo that contains plant extracts, detergent cleansing agents, conditioning agent, plant oil, thickeners, fragrance, and preservatives. There is nothing about this that makes it better than Johnson & Johnson's baby shampoo at a fraction of this price.

☹ **Phytoneutre Concentrated Cream Shampoo for Normal Hair with Plant Extracts** *($14.50 for 3.3 ounces)* contains eucalyptus oil, which can be a scalp irritant.

☺ **Phytopanama Mild Shampoo for Frequent Washing for All Hair Types, Contains 65% Quillaja Decoction** *($15 for 6.8 ounces)* contains mostly plant water—65 percent tea water of quillaja bark, also called soap bark tree. According to the *Encyclopedia of Common Natural Ingredients*, Second Edition, by Foster and Leung, 1996, quillaja has some antimicrobial properties and is used to treat dandruff. There are no published studies demonstrating its effectiveness, but there would be no reason to use it for normal scalp conditions. It contains mostly detergent cleansing agents, lather agent, thickener, detangling agent, plant oil, and preservatives.

☺ **Phytorhum Fortifying Shampoo for Lifeless Hair with Egg Yolk and Rum** *($15 for 6.8 ounces)* does include egg yolk and rum, and while they may be good for eggnog they have no impact on hair. This standard shampoo contains mostly plant water, detergent cleansing agents, lather agents, egg yolk, plant oil, conditioning agent, detangling agent/film former, preservatives, fragrance, and coloring agents. It would work well for normal to dry hair that is also normal to fine or thin in thickness. The film former is what adds thickness to hair, not the other stuff in here.

☹ **Phytosatine Nourishing Shampoo for Dry Hair/Sensitive Scalp with Camelina Sativa Oil (1%) and Phytolactine 1%** *($16.50 for 6.8 ounces)* contains nothing that makes it better for a sensitive scalp. Fragrance and preservatives are the number-1 and -2 causes of irritation, so this product loses on both counts, along with 99 percent of all hair-care products. Other than that, it contains mostly plant water, detergent cleansing agents, lather agent, plant oil, water-binding agents, plant extracts, detangling agent/film former, fragrance, preservatives, and coloring agents. It is a pretty standard shampoo for dry hair that is normal to fine or thin. It also contains something called "gold of pleasure oil," but that turns out to be just a plant oil. Its name is better than its benefit for hair, which is the same as any other plant oil.

☺ **Phytosteine Sebum Cleansing Shampoo for Oily Hair/Sensitive Scalp with Plant Extracts Enriched with a Derivative of Cysteine 2.3% and Phytolactine 1%** *($16.50 for 6.8 ounces)*. The cysteine derivatives in here are about as far removed from cysteine as the paper in this book is from a tree. Nonetheless, even if it were pure cysteine, which is an important amino acid in hair, in a hair-care product it is just a conditioning agent and can't replenish the cysteine loss in your own hair. Other than that, this is just shampoo containing mostly plant water, detergent cleansing agent, plant extracts, thickeners, conditioning agents, preservatives, and fragrance. The conditioning agents in here make it a problem for oily hair and scalp, though it would be fine for normal hair of any thickness.

☹ **Phytosylic Dermatological Shampoo for Dandruff with Salicylic Compound and Essential Oils** *($16.50 for 6.8 ounces)* contains tea tree oil and salicylic acid as the components to fight dandruff. Tea tree oil can have an effect, but probably not at this concentration. Salicylic acid is a poor option because though it can exfoliate the scalp, it can also denature the hair shaft.

☺ **Phytovolume Volumizer Shampoo for Fine Limp Hair with Yarrow Extract** *($15 for 6.8 ounces)* contains mostly plant water, detergent cleansing agents, lather agent, thickeners, conditioning agent, detangling agents/ film formers, preservatives, and fragrance. This is a good standard shampoo for normal to slightly dry hair that is fine or thin.

☺ **$$$ Phytherose Revitalizing Treatment for Dry Hair with Abyssinian Rose Tea (20%)** *($18 for 5 ounces)* contains mostly plant water, emollients, plant oil, castor oil, detangling agent, silicone, film former, conditioning agent, fragrance, and preservatives. This is a very good emollient conditioner for dry hair that is coarse or thick.

☺ **$$$ Phyto 7 Plant Based Treatment Cream for Dry Hair with Extracts of Plants** *($15 for 1.7 ounces)* definitely does contain plant extracts, but not much "cream"; this is just an overpriced but good conditioner for normal hair to help with combing.

☺ **$$$ Phyto 9 Vegetal Hydrating Cream for Very Dry Hair with Macadamia Oil** *($18 for 1.7 ounces)* is similar to the one above, only with plant oil; it is slightly better for slightly dry hair.

☺ **Phytobaume Untangling Balm for All Hair Types with Mallow** *($15 for 6.8 ounces)* contains mostly plant water, thickeners, silicone, detangling agent, conditioning agent, film former, preservatives, and fragrance. This can work for frizzy or curly normal to slightly dry hair that is fine or thin, to help smooth it out.

☺ **Phytodefrisant Plant Based Relaxing Balm for All Hair Types** *($15 for 3.3 ounces)* is similar to the Mallow version above and the same comments apply.

☺ **Phyto Style Heat-Protective Spray with Wheat Amino-Acids (Non-Aerosol)** *($15 for 5 ounces)* contains nothing that can protect hair from heat. It is more of a leave-in conditioner than a styling spray, with minimal to no hold and no stiff or sticky feel. It can be used either way—it just depends on how you want to style your hair.

☺ **$$$ Phytovolume Actif Volumizer Spray for Fine and Limp Hair, Enriched with Hair Protein** *($16 for 3.3 ounces)* contains mostly alcohol, water, film formers, plant extracts, conditioning agents, and fragrance. This is a good styling spray with a medium hold and a slight stiff feel, though it can be brushed through easily.

☺ **$$$ PhytoFix Setting Gel for All Hair Types** *($15 for 3.3 ounces)* is a standard (and extremely overpriced) gel that contains mostly water, thickeners, alcohol, plant extract, film former, slip agent, and preservatives. It has a good light hold with minimal stiff or sticky feel.

☺ **$$$ Phyto Style Finishing Gel** *($13.50 for 3.3 ounces)* is similar to the PhytoFix above, only this one has a medium hold with a somewhat stiff, sticky feel.

☺ **Phyto Style Volumizing Mousse** *($15 for 5 ounces)* is a standard mousse that contains mostly water, propellant, alcohol, plant extracts, detangling agent/film former, conditioning agents, fragrance, and preservatives. This has a light hold with no stiff or sticky feel.

☺ **$$$ Phytolaque Hair Spray for All Hair Types with Vegetal Lacquer Proteins (Non-Aerosol)** *($15 for 3.3 ounces)* contains mostly alcohol, film formers, fragrance, and silicone. The primary film-former is the one used in thousands of styling products. As to the vegetable lacquer, this product does contain shellac, but that is a minute portion of the contents. This hairspray does give a good light to medium hold with minimal stiff or sticky feel.

☺ **$$$ Phytolaque Hair Spray for Sensitive Hair with Silk Proteins (Non-Aerosol)** *($15 for 3.3 ounces)* is similar to the All Hair Types above, only with a lighter hold and minimal to no stiff or sticky feel. This version does contain silk amino acids, but in this minute amount, as a standard conditioning agent, they don't help something called "sensitive" hair.

☺ **$$$ Phyto Style Holding Spray (Non-Aerosol)** *($15 for 5 ounces)* is similar to the Hair Spray for All Hair Types and the same comments apply.

☹ **Huile D'Ales Revitalizing Botanical Oil for Dry Hair, with Essential Plant Oils** *($18 for 5 packets of 0.33-ounce treatments)* contains mostly castor oil, plant oils, fragrant oil, conditioning agents, vinegar, slip agent, and preservatives. This can have a slight sticky feel on hair, but, in the long run, you would be far better off applying plain sunflower oil as a treatment to the hair, then washing, and then following up with a vinegar rinse and conditioner; it would do the same thing for pennies.

☹ **$$$ Phytophanere Dietary Supplement for Hair and Nails** *($45 for 120 caplets).* It's unbelievable—there isn't one thing in this that can have any effect on hair, nails, or health for that matter. It is just assorted plant oils and some yeast.

☹ **$$$ Phytocyane Revitalizing Lotion with Procyanidins and Gingko Biloba for Thinning Hair Women** *($45 for 12 0.25-ounce ampoules)* includes nothing to help hair growth. For that, women need to consider effective, proven options, not this group of unproven plant extracts.

☺ **$$$ Phytolait Beauty Milk for Hair** *($15 for 1.3 ounces)* doesn't happen to include any milk, but it does have water, mineral oil, plant oils, thickeners, conditioning agents, preservatives, fragrance, and coloring agents. This is the most expensive mineral oil–based hair conditioner around, and its not even remotely worth the price. However, it is good for dry, coarse hair.

☺ **$$$ Phytomoelle Restorative and Rehydrating Mask for Very Dry Hair with Vegetal Marrow** *($29 for 3.3 ounces)* is just water, plant extracts, corn oil, conditioning agent, thickeners, fragrance, and preservatives. A thin layer of corn oil from your kitchen cupboard would work just as well if not better for extremely dry hair. There is nothing in here that can repair hair; it is just an emollient cream that can be a good conditioner for hair.

☹ **Phytopolleine Botanical Scalp Stimulant for Lifeless Hair with Fortifying Essential Oils** *($28 for 0.8 ounce)* contains lemon oil, cypress oil, and eucalyptus oil, all of which can be irritating and drying for the scalp.

☺ **$$$ Phytopolleine Hair Root Stimulant for All Types of Hair Botanical Stimulant of the Scalp** *($28 for 0.8 ounce)* is just fragrance and wheat germ oil. It also contains a trace amount of animal placental lipids, but there is nothing in the placenta that can help hair.

☹ **Phytopolleine Plus Capillary Oil Solution for Thinning Hair with Essential Vert and Essential Oils** *($40 for five 0.13-ounce ampoules)* contains lemon oil, cypress oil, and eucalyptus oil, all of which can be irritating and drying for the scalp.

☹ **Phytosquame Intensive Scalp Treatment Oil Based Soothing and Purifying Solution for Dandruff, Itching and Flaking** *($42 for box of five 0.17-ounce tubes)* contains lemon oil rather high up on the ingredient list, and that can be irritating and drying for the scalp.

☹ **Phytosquare Oily Based Soothing and Purifying Solution Intensive Scalp Treatment for Dandruff, Itching, and Flaking** *($42 for five 0.17-ounce tubes)* is almost identical to the Intensive Scalp version above and the same comments apply.

☺ **$$$ Phyyto Men Hair and Body Shampoo with Burdock** *($17 for 5 ounces)* contains mostly plant water, detergent cleansing agent, detangling agent/film former, fragrance, conditioning agent, preservatives, and coloring agents. There is nothing in here special for men's hair, it's just an overpriced standard shampoo for normal to slightly dry hair that is normal to fine or thin.

☺ **Phyyto Men Revitalizing Hair Lotion with Alcoholic Extract of Burdock** *($17 for 6.76 ounces)* is just water, conditioning agents, thickeners, and fragrance. It works well for normal to dry hair that is normal to fine or thin in thickness.

PhytoPlage by Phytotherathrie

☺ **Sun Shampoo for Hair and Body with Bancoulier Oil** *($15 for 3.3 ounces)* contains mostly water, detergent cleansing agents, conditioning agents, lather agent, plant oil, fragrance, and preservatives. This standard shampoo would work well for normal to slightly dry hair of any thickness.

☺ **After-Sun Repair Dual Usage Cream or Mask with Bancoulier Oil and Marsh Mallow** *($17 for 2.5 ounces)* is just thickeners, with plant water and plant oils. That's great for dry hair, but hardly worth the price.

☺ **High-Protection Sun Oil for Weakened Hair** *($19.50 for 3.3 ounces)* includes nothing that will protect one hair on your head from sun damage. Without an SPF, all claims about sun protection are completely bogus and deceptive.

☺ **$$$ Moisturizing Sun Gel for All Types of Hair** *($13 for 2.5 ounces)* includes nothing that will protect one hair on your head from sun damage. Without an SPF, all claims about sun protection are completely bogus and deceptive.

☺ **$$$ Sun Protection Oil for All Hair Types, "The Original" Since 1975** *($17 for 3.3 ounces)* includes nothing that will protect one hair on your head from sun damage. Without an SPF, all claims about sun protection are completely bogus and deceptive.

☺ **$$$ After Sun Repair Cream or Mask** *($18 for 2.5 ounces)* is just a cream conditioner for dry hair; it can't repair one hair strand on your head. And with all these "sun protecting" products, it's a bit shocking you would still need anything to repair hair!

PhytoSpecific by Phytotherathrie

☺ **Hydra-Repairing Shampoo with Shea Butter** *($18 for 5.07 ounces)* contains mostly water, detergent cleansing agents, thickeners, emollient, slip agents, conditioning agent, detangling agent/film former, fragrance, and preservatives. This is a good basic shampoo for dry, coarse hair that is fine or thin. The film former makes it a problem for thick hair that doesn't need any additional thickness.

☺ **Multi-Regenerating Creme Bath with Jojoba Oil, Deep-Down Treatment for Very Dry, Brittle and Damaged Hair** *($19 for 6.75 ounces)*. If you believe this conditioner can regenerate hair, I have a bridge I'd love to sell you! This standard conditioner is great for dry hair that is coarse or thick but it is hardly the only one. It contains mostly water, thickeners, detangling agents, emollients, silicone, plant oils, castor oil, film former, conditioning agents, preservatives, fragrance, and coloring agents. It can leave a slight sticky feel on hair.

☺ **$$$ Revitalizing Treatment with Vegetal Oils for Dry Hair and Scalp** *($19 for 3.35 ounces)* contains mostly plant oils, castor oil, mineral oil, thickeners, fragrance, preservatives, and coloring agents. This is a lot of money for peanut oil, castor oil, and mineral oil! It is a good conditioner for dry, coarse hair, but it could easily be replaced by similar ones from other lines, or by oil in your kitchen cupboard.

☺ **Beauty Styling Creme for Normal to Dry Hair with Shea Butter** *($13 for 3.38 ounces)* contains mostly Vaseline, thickeners, emollients, plant oil, conditioning agents, fragrance, preservatives, and coloring agents. It is a very good and somewhat greasy pomade for straightening or smoothing coarse thick hair, frizzies, or stubborn curls. It has no film formers, which means no hold and no stiff or sticky feel, but be careful—this can easily make hair look greasy and heavy; use it sparingly.

☺ **Restructuring Milk with Canola Oil for Normal to Dry Hair** *($17 for 5.07 ounces)* contains mostly water, thickeners, detangling agents, plant oil, mineral oil, silicone, thickeners, conditioning agents, fragrance, preservatives, and coloring agents. This is a very good styling lotion for smoothing or straightening coarse, thick hair without leaving a stiff or sticky feel.

Prell

For more information about Prell, call (800) 723-9569 or in Canada (800) 668-0151. You can also visit the Procter & Gamble Web site at www.pg.com.

☹ **Extra Body Shampoo for Fine or Oily Hair** *($2.60 for 15.2 ounces)* contains ammonium xylenesulfonate, a solvent that can be drying for the scalp and hair. This is also a high pH shampoo. That can temporarily swell the hair shaft to make it feel thicker, but in the long run will dry out the hair and cause damage, as well as dry out and irritate the scalp.

☹ **Moisturizing Shampoo Formula for Dry/Damaged Hair** *($2.60 for 15.2 ounces)* is almost identical to the Extra Body version above and the same warning applies.

☹ **Original Shampoo for Normal to Oily Hair** *($2.60 for 15.2 ounces)* is almost identical to the Extra Body version above, only it contains even more ammonium xylenesulfonate, and the same warning applies.

☺ **Conditioner Moisturizing Formula for Dry/Damaged Hair** *($2.60 for 15.2 ounces)* contains mostly water, silicone, thickeners, detangling agent/film former, thickeners, fragrance, and preservatives. This would be a very good basic conditioner for dry hair that is fine or thin.

Principal Secret

There is nothing secret about these products. They are all exceptionally standard and have nothing to do with the flowing mane of this line's namesake. Victoria Principal had great hair way before these products ever came along! One word of warning: the fragrance in all these products consists of orange, tangerine, and lime oils, which are all particularly irritating for the scalp and skin. For more information on Principal Secret, call (800) 367-9444 or visit its Web site at www.iqvc.com. (Note: the first price is retail, the second is for club members.)

☺ **Gentle Daily Shampoo** *($11, $7.75 for 10 ounces)* contains mostly water, detergent cleansing agents, lather agent, thickeners, conditioning agents, plant extracts, slip agents, detangling agent, preservatives, and fragrance. This is a good shampoo for normal to dry hair of any thickness if you don't have a problem with the fragrance.

☺ **Deep Cleansing Shampoo** *($11, $7.75 for 6 ounces)* is similar to the one above only with more film former. The same basic comments apply.

☺ **Tangle-Free Moisturizing Conditioner** *($13, $9 for 10 ounces)* contains mostly water, thickener, detangling agents, slip agent, plant extracts, conditioning agents, preservatives, fragrance, and coloring agents. This is a good lightweight conditioner for normal to slightly dry hair of any thickness.

☺ **No-Rinse Condition With Sun Protection** *($13, $9 for 6 ounces)* mentions sun protection, but without an SPF the claim is bogus. Other than that, this is a good, but standard, leave-in conditioner for normal to slightly dry hair that is fine or thin. It contains mostly water, glycerin, detangling agents/film formers, thickeners, conditioning agents, silicones, plant extracts, preservatives, and fragrance.

☺ **Perfect Styling Gel** *($11, $7.75 for 6 ounces)* is a standard styling gel that contains mostly water, film former, slip agent, water-binding agent, silicones, plant extracts, thickeners, preservatives, fragrance, and coloring agent. It works well for a light to medium hold with minimal to slight stiff or sticky feel.

☺ **Super Control Hair Spray** *($13, $9 for 10 ounces)* is a firm-hold hairspray that contains mostly water, film formers, slip agents, conditioning agents, silicone, plant extracts, and preservatives.

☹ **High Protein Hair Mask** *($24, $17 for 6 ounces)* contains peppermint oil, orange oil, tangerine oil, and lime oil, which can all be irritating and drying for the scalp.

Professional

This line is the knock-off king—all these products clearly indicate on the label that they are meant to be identical to the designer versions. There are several problems with this type of advertising and marketing. First, it assumes the designer line is better because of the name on the label, and that is never automatically the case. Second, these products don't compare to the lines they say they do. And third, it is unethical to capitalize on someone else's marketing efforts. Either establish a name on your own merits or don't go into business. For more information on Professional, call (813) 910-7675 or (800) 382-3609.

☹ **Daily Botanical Shampoo** *($3.62 for 16 ounces)* uses sodium C14-16 olefin sulfonate as the main cleansing agent, which can be too drying and irritating for the scalp and too drying for the hair. It can also potentially strip hair color.

☺ **Hawaiian Ginger Shampoo** *($3.62 for 16 ounces)* is a good basic shampoo for all hair types except oily hair and scalp. It contains mostly water, detergent cleansing agent, lather agent, plant extracts, slip agent, conditioning agents, thickeners, and preservatives.

☺ **Luxury Shampoo** *($3.62 for 16 ounces)* contains mostly water, detergent cleansing agent, lather agent, conditioning agents, plant extracts, film former, preservatives, and fragrance. This is a good shampoo for normal to dry hair that is fine or thin. It can build up on hair.

☹ **Shampoo for Processed Hair** *($3.62 for 16 ounces)* uses sodium lauryl sulfate as one of the main cleansing agents, which makes it too drying for the hair and scalp.

☹ **Shampoo for Treated Hair** *($3.62 for 16 ounces)* uses TEA-lauryl sulfate as one of the main cleansing agents, which makes it too drying for the hair and scalp.

☺ **Shine Extraordinaire** *($3.62 for 16 ounces)* contains mostly water, detergent cleansing agent, lather agent, conditioning agents, slip agents, plant extracts, thickeners, preservatives, and fragrance. This is a good shampoo for normal to slightly dry hair of any thickness.

☺ **Uniquely for Normal to Fine Hair** *($3.62 for 16 ounces)* contains mostly water, detergent cleansing agents, lather agent, fragrance, plant extracts, plant oil, conditioning agent, detangling agent/film former, and preservatives. This is a good shampoo for normal to slightly dry hair that is normal to fine or thin. It can build up on hair.

☺ **Balm Revitalisant** *($4.60 for 16 ounces)* contains mostly plant water, slip agent, detangling agent, thickeners, film former, conditioning agent, preservatives, and fragrance. This is a good styling balm for smoothing out curls and frizzies with a light hold and minimal stiff or sticky feel.

☺ **Detangling Conditioner** *($4.60 for 16 ounces)* contains mostly water, thickeners, detangling agent, castor oil, slip agents, silicone, plant extracts, and fragrance. This is a good leave-in conditioner for dry hair that is coarse and needs extra control. It can have a slight sticky feel.

☺ **Moisture Potion** *($4.60 for 16 ounces)* contains mostly water, slip agent, thickeners, mineral oil, detangling agent, conditioning agents, castor oil, vitamins, preservatives, Vaseline, fragrance, silicone, more preservatives, and coloring agents. This is a very good conditioner for dry hair that is coarse or thick.

☺ **Polymeric Reconstructor** *($4.60 for 16 ounces)* won't reconstruct anything, but it is a good conditioner for normal to dry hair that is normal to fine or thin. It contains mostly water, thickeners, detangling agent, conditioning agents, slip agent, plant oil, film former, preservatives, and fragrance. There is a tiny amount of DNA in here for window dressing, but it provides no benefit for the hair.

☺ **Special Treatment** *($4.60 for 16 ounces)* contains mostly water, thickeners, slip agents, detangling agent, castor oil, plant extracts, conditioning agents, plant oil, silicones, preservatives, fragrance, and coloring agents. This is a very good conditioner to help with control for dry hair that is coarse or thick.

☺ **Ultimate Reconstructor** *($4.60 for 4 ounces)* contains mostly water, conditioning agents, thickeners, mineral oil, fragrance, plant oils, and preservatives. This can't reconstruct hair but it is a good conditioner for dry hair that is thick or coarse.

☺ **Wearable Treatment** *($4.60 for 16 ounces)* is a lightweight styling gel that has minimal hold and no stiff or sticky feel, but it can help smooth hair when styling. It contains mostly water, thickeners, detangling agents, preservatives, plant oils, fragrance, film former, and coloring agents.

☺ **Forming Gel Coiffure** *($3.29 for 12 ounces)* contains mostly water, lots of film formers, silicone, detangling agents, thickeners, preservatives, and fragrance. It is a good, light- to medium-hold gel with minimal to no stiff or sticky feel.

☺ **Gel with Awapuhi** *($3.29 for 12 ounces)* is a light- to medium-hold gel with minimal stiff, sticky feel. It contains mostly plant water, detangling agent/film former, conditioning agent, thickeners, preservatives, and fragrance.

☺ **Brilliant Shine/Firm Hold Hairspray (Non-Aerosol)** *($3.62 for 12 ounces)* is a standard, medium-hold hairspray with a minimal stiff feel that does allow you to brush through hair. It contains mostly alcohol, plant water, film former, silicone, conditioning agents, and fragrance. It doesn't provide any more shine than a thousand other hairsprays.

☺ **Extra Hold Finishing Spray (Non-Aerosol)** *($3.62 for 12 ounces)* is almost identical to the Brilliant Shine version above and the same comments apply.

☺ **Sculpting Shaping Spray (Non-Aerosol)** *($3.62 for 12 ounces)* is almost identical to the Brilliant Shine one above, only with firmer hold and a slightly stiffer feel.

☺ **Ultra-Shaping Hair Spray (Aerosol)** *($4.34 for 10 ounces)* is a medium-hold aerosol hairspray with a minimal stiff feel that can easily be brushed through. It contains mostly alcohol, propellant, film formers, silicones, slip agents, conditioning agents, and fragrance.

☺ **Ultra-Shaping Hair Spray Plus (Aerosol)** *($4.34 for 10 ounces)* is virtually identical to the version above and the same comments apply.

Progaine

The Progaine hair-care products are meant to be used with Rogaine, the original hair treatment for male-pattern baldness that launched the use of minoxidil as the first over-the-counter, FDA-approved treatment for growing hair. There is nothing special or different about Progaine shampoo and conditioner that makes it helpful if you are using Rogaine. Although Progaine shampoo and conditioner have no effect on hair growth, they both happen to be quite good and quite inexpensive, and definitely worth considering. For more information on Progaine, call (800) 253-8600.

☺ **Progaine 2 in 1 Shampoo** *($3.76 for 10 ounces)* contains mostly water, detergent cleansing agents, silicone, thickeners, lather agent, conditioning agents, detangling agent, plant extracts, fragrance, and preservatives. This is a standard, silicone-based shampoo with conditioner that would work well for dry hair of any thickness, though it can easily build up on hair. There is nothing about this product that makes it helpful if you are using Rogaine (minoxidil).

☹ **Progaine Shampoo, Extra Body and Volumizing Formula** *($3.79 for 10 ounces)* uses sodium lauryl sulfate as one of the main cleansing agents, which makes it too drying for the hair and scalp.

☺ **Progaine Shampoo for Permed or Color Treated Hair** *($3.79 for 10 ounces)* contains mostly water, detergent cleansing agents, lather agents, thickeners, detangling agent/film former, conditioning agents, plant extracts, detangling agent, fragrance, and preservatives. This is a good shampoo for normal to slightly dry hair that is fine or thin. There is nothing about this product that makes it helpful if you are using Rogaine (minoxidil).

☺ **Progaine Conditioner** *($3.79 for 10 ounces)* contains mostly, water, thickeners, conditioning agents, detangling agent, plant extracts, fragrance, and preservatives. This is a good conditioner for normal to slightly dry hair of any thickness. There is nothing about this product that makes it helpful if you are using Rogaine (minoxidil).

Pro-Vitamin

Pro-Vitamin products are, according to the company, "the next generation in hair treatments and are formulated with the most advanced ingredients available. Our treatments wrap themselves around each hair strand from root to tip repairing and restoring your hair to its healthiest. All Pro-Vitamin products contain an exclusive blend of 14 essential vitamins linked with high performance silk amino proteins." There are definitely vitamins in these products, but are they helpful for hair or skin? While vitamins are essential for health, they don't work on their own. The various vitamins are not chemically related, and most differ in their physiological actions. Generally, vitamins are catalysts, and combine with proteins to create metabolically active enzymes that in turn produce hundreds of important chemical reactions throughout the body. Without vitamins, many of these reactions would slow down or cease. The intricate ways in which vitamins act on the body, however, are still far from clear. It takes a network of complex chemical interactions to get vitamins to do their thing, which no hair-care or skin-care product could possibly mimic. However, vitamins can be good moisturizing agents and conditioning agents in their pure form, though most don't hold up under water so they don't cling well to hair or scalp when added to shampoo and conditioner, and definitely not when styling. There are good products in this line, but it's not because of their vitamin content.

For more information on Pro-Vitamin, call (813) 855-8035 or visit its Web site at www.pro-vitamin.com.

☹ **Anti-Frizz Hydrating Shampoo** *($3.99 for 10 ounces)* uses TEA-lauryl sulfate as the main detergent cleansing agent, which can be too drying and irritating for the scalp and too drying for the hair.

☹ **Hair Loss Treatment Shampoo for Fine, Limp, Thinning Hair** *($4.99 for 10 ounces)* uses TEA-lauryl sulfate as the main cleansing agent, which can be too drying and irritating for the scalp and too drying for the hair. It also contains menthol and spearmint, which are also irritating and drying for the scalp.

☹ **Instant Repair Corrective Shampoo** *($3.29 for 16 ounces)* uses TEA-lauryl sulfate as its main cleansing agent, which can be too drying and irritating for the scalp and too drying for the hair.

☹ **Maximum Body Shampoo** *($3.99 for 10 ounces)* uses TEA-lauryl sulfate as its main cleansing agent, which can be too drying and irritating for the scalp and too drying for the hair.

☹ **MegaShine Shampoo** *($3.99 for 10 ounces)* uses TEA-lauryl sulfate as its main cleansing agent, which can be too drying and irritating for the scalp and too drying for the hair.

☹ **Perm and Color, Corrective Shampoo** *($4.19 for 12.5 ounces)* uses TEA-lauryl sulfate as its main cleansing agent, which can be too drying and irritating for the scalp and too drying for the hair.

☺ **Special Effects Fat Hair Thickening Shampoo** *($4.19 for 12.5 ounces)* works the same as any "thickening" shampoo does—with film former. This standard shampoo contains mostly water, detergent cleansing agents, slip agent, lather agent, film former, thickeners, vitamins, plant extracts, silicone, castor oil, fragrance, and preservatives.

☹ **Special Effects Straighten Out Straightening Shampoo** *($4.19 for 12.5 ounces)* uses TEA-lauryl sulfate as the main cleansing agent, which can be too drying and irritating for the scalp and too drying for the hair.

☹ **Split-Ends Mender Shampoo** *($3.99 for 10 ounces)* uses TEA-lauryl sulfate as the main cleansing agent, which can be too drying and irritating for the scalp and too drying for the hair. This can't make split ends grow back together.

☺ **Anti-Frizz Hydrating Conditioner** *($3.99 for 10 ounces)* contains mostly water, slip agent, thickeners, detangling agents, silicone, vitamins, plant extracts, film former, fragrance, and preservatives. This is a very good conditioner for normal to dry hair of any thickness. The tiny amount of film former in here is not going to add much thickness.

☹ **Hair Loss Treatment Conditioner for Fine, Limp, Thinning Hair** *($4.99 for 10 ounces)* includes nothing that can affect hair loss. It does contain spearmint oil and menthol, which are irritating for the scalp. That tingling sensation could lead a consumer to believe this product was doing something to stimulate hair growth when all it was doing was causing irritation.

☺ **Instant Repair Corrective Conditioner** *($3.29 for 16 ounces)* contains mostly water, thickeners, castor oil, vitamins, detangling agent, mineral oil, silicone, conditioning agents, preservatives, and fragrance. This is a good conditioner for dry, coarse, or thick hair to gain control. It can have a slight sticky feel.

☺ **Maximum Body Conditioner** *($3.99 for 10 ounces)* is almost identical to the Instant Repair above and the same comments apply.

☺ **MegaShine Conditioner** *($3.99 for 10 ounces)* is almost identical to the Instant Repair above and the same comments apply.

☺ **Perm and Color Corrective Conditioner** *($4.19 for 12.5 ounces)* is almost identical to the Instant Repair above and the same comments apply.

☺ **Special Effects Fat Hair Thickening Conditioner** *($4.19 for 12.5 ounces)* is almost identical to the Instant Repair above and the same comments apply.

☺ **Special Effects Straighten Out Straightening Conditioner** *($4.19 for 12.5 ounces)* is almost identical to the Instant Repair above and the same comments apply.

☹ **Split-Ends Mender Leave-in Conditioner** *($3.99 for 10 ounces)* uses TEA-lauryl sulfate as a main ingredient, probably as an emulsifier, but it can still cause problems for the hair and scalp in terms of irritation and dryness. This can't make split ends grow back together.

☺ **Hot Oil Instant Repair** *($3.62 for two capsules and two vials)* definitely contains lots of plant oil, which is mostly canola oil. There is nothing in this that canola oil in your kitchen cupboard can't replace. The vitamins in the capsules are a nice touch, but they don't benefit the hair.

☺ **Hot Oil Plus Vitamins, Perm/Color Repair** *($3.62 for two capsules and two vials)* is similar to the Instant Repair above, only this one contains macadamia nut oil as the main oil, but the same comments above still apply. There is nothing about macadamia nut oil that is better for dry hair than canola oil.

☺ **5-Minute Blow-Dry Miracle** *($5.45 for 5 ounces)* is just a good styling spray with a light hold that can have minimal to no stiff or sticky feel. Definitely do not expect any miracles of any kind—this doesn't make blow-drying go any faster. It contains mostly water, film former, detangling agent, castor oil, conditioning agent, preservatives, and fragrance.

☺ **Hair Loss Treatment Hair-Thickening Leave-in Volumizer** *($4.99 for 10 ounces)* contains nothing that can grow or replace lost hair; it is just a good, standard, leave-in styling spray with a light to medium hold and a slight stiff feel. It contains mostly alcohol, water, film formers, silicone, detangling agents, vitamins, conditioning agents, slip agent, castor oil, and preservatives. It does contain spearmint oil, which can be a skin irritant, so keep it away from the scalp.

☹ **Hair Loss Treatment Stimulator** *($8.99 for 2 ounces)* is completely bogus; this is just alcohol with traces of vitamins, and it won't grow hair.

☺ **Hair Treatment Capsules, Instant Repair** *($3.99 for 12 0.41-ounce treatments)* is just vitamins with some conditioning agents and silicone. Your hair will not be repaired instantly, as the package claims. If that was the case, why would they need to sell 12 in a package—wouldn't just one have done the trick?

☺ **Hair Treatment Capsules, Maximum Body** *($3.99 for 12 0.41-ounce treatments)* is almost identical to the Instant Repair version above and the same comments apply.

☺ **Hair Treatment Capsules, Mega Shine** *($3.99 for 12 0.41-ounce treatments)* is almost identical to the Instant Repair version above and the same comments apply.

☺ **Hair Treatment Capsules, Perm/Color Repair** *($3.99 for 12 0.41-ounce treatments)* is almost identical to the Instant Repair version above and the same comments apply.

☺ **Hair Treatment Capsules, Split-Ends Mender** *($3.99 for 12 0.41-ounce treatments)* is almost identical to the Instant Repair version above and the same comments apply.

☺ **Pro-Vitamin C Anti-Frizz Hair Serum** *($5.99 for 2.75 ounces)* is a standard silicone serum that would work well for making hair feel silky and smooth as well as adding shine. The amount of vitamin C is so insignificant as to hardly warrant a comment.

☺ **Pro-Vitamin E Instant Repair Hair Serum** *($5.99 for 2.75 ounces)* is almost identical to the Pro-Vitamin C Anti-Frizz above and the same comments apply. I suspect Pro-Vitamin didn't think anyone would notice that these two products were equal except for the product's different colors.

☺ **Special Effects ColorShield, Color Extender/UV Protector** *($5.99 for 5 ounces)* is a standard silicone serum and works well to add a silky, soft feel to hair as well as adding shine. It won't protect hair color in the least, and contains nothing that will protect from sun damage in any way, shape, or form.

☺ **Special Effects Extreme Shine, Weightless Shine and Anti-Frizz Treatment** *($5.99 for 5 ounces)* is almost identical to the ColorShield above and the same comments apply.

☺ **Special Effects Fat Hair Thickening and Strengthening Serum** *($5.99 for 5 ounces)* is a good silicone gel that can help smooth out coarse, curly, or frizzy hair with minimal hold and minimal to no sticky or stiff feel. It contains mostly water, silicone, thickeners, conditioning agents, plant oils, castor oil, slip agents, preservatives, and fragrance. It has less hold because there are no film formers, but that is also why there is no stiff feel on hair. It does contain a tiny amount of sulfur, but I suspect it isn't enough to be a problem for hair. There is nothing in here that can make hair feel thick or fat.

☺ **Special Effects Hair Control Hair Glossing and Styling Stick** *($5.45 for 2.5 ounces)* is a good straightening-wax balm with a light hold and minimal to no stiff or sticky feel. It contains mostly water, thickeners, film former, silicone, plant extracts, preservatives, fragrance, and coloring agents. This isn't an easy product to use because the stick is inconvenient. Regardless, be careful how much you do use—it can easily look heavy and greasy on hair.

☺ **Special Effects Straighten Out Hair Straightener and Anti-Frizz Serum** *($5.99 for 5 ounces)* is a standard silicone serum with a slight amount of hold. It works great for adding shine and a silky-smooth feel to hair when styling.

Proxiphen & Nano

Nano Shampoo and Conditioner, Proxiphen, and Proxiphen-N are topical products for hair growth created and sold by a Dr. Peter Proctor. Proctor is a physician with a Ph.D. in pharmacology. He is also the resident guru of an Internet hair-loss chat group. While the doctor's credentials are impressive, there are some serious questions regarding his hair-growth systems. As is often the case with non-FDA-approved hair-regrowth products such as these (and because there are no studies supporting any of the claims), the authority of the endorsements is also questionable.

Nano Shampoo and Conditioner contains nicotinic acid N-Oxide (that's where the name Nano comes from) and superoxide dismutase (an antioxidant) for hair regrowth. As with any product touted to grow hair, Nano also has a following of users. Yet the claims made for this product are surprising, because it is only supposed to be "as effective as minoxidil." You would wonder, if Nano is only as good as minoxidil, why not just use minoxidil, which has extensive substantiated claims and is approved by the FDA for hair regrowth? The cost for Nano Shampoo and Conditioner is $39.95 for a three-month supply, although they rarely last three months.

Proxiphen, also developed by Proctor, is a topical prescription medication for hair regrowth, but it only takes a phone call to Proctor's office to obtain yours. Proxiphen contains a variety of ingredients, including minoxidil, retinoic acid (Retin-A), phenytoin (trade name Dilantin, an anticonvulsant and antiseizure medication), spironolactone (a potent, topically effective antiandrogen), copper peptides (similar to those in Tricomin, reviewed later in this chapter), Nano (superoxide dismutase, an antioxidant, plus pyrmidine n-oxides, an amino acid), arginine (another amino acid), butylated hydroxytoluene (a preservative), and ascorbyl palmitate (a form of vitamin C). I discuss some of these in Chapter Two, *To the Root of the Matter*, in the section on "Hair Growth—Scams or Solutions?"

It is interesting to note that some people have reported loss of hair they gained with minoxidil when they began using Proxiphen, which has a lower concentration of commercial minoxidil. Others have reported that Proxiphen irritates the scalp, not surprising given the Retin-A and toluene it contains. Proctor says that Proxiphen stops hair loss, thickens hair, enlarges miniaturized hairs, and produces regrowth at the front of the hairline. And while the product has been prescribed by Proctor in various formulations for ten years, no independent, published clinical studies on its effectiveness are available. It costs $59.95 for two months.

There is also a nonprescription version of Proxiphen, called Proxiphen-N. The ingredients include superoxide dismutase, copper-binding peptides, and pyrmidine n-oxide, but none of the other more serious prescription-only ingredients in the Proxiphen mentioned above. Again, this product is promoted with no substantiating research or clinical data.

It is important to note that Proctor does hold several patents for some of the ingredients used in his products for hair regrowth. However, keep in mind that a patent doesn't have anything to do with efficacy. It simply establishes that Proctor is the one who can use these ingredients in hair-regrowth products. In other words, you could take a patent out establishing that you use tomatoes in your hair-regrowth products. The patent would then establish that you are the only one who can use tomatoes for that purpose—but it wouldn't in any way prove that tomatoes grow hair.

I would love to discuss the impact of these ingredients on the scalp in great detail, but the focus of this book isn't on balding, and it would take pages. Again, please refer to "Hair Growth—Scams or Solutions?" in Chapter Two of this book.

Proctor's Web site at www.drproctor.com is worth a visit. His information is all based on some very interesting hypotheses that are worth looking at with an objective eye. The notion that his products are the answer for balding is questionable at best, but in the world of hair hope, that never stops the consumer from spending money.

Quantum

For more information on Quantum, call (800) 621-3379.

☹ **Clarifying Shampoo for Deep Cleansing to Remove Build-Up** *($4.49 for 15 ounces)* uses sodium lauryl sulfate as one of the main cleansing agents, which makes it too drying for the hair and scalp.

☹ **Daily Cleansing Shampoo for All Hair Types** *($4.99 for 15 ounces)* uses sodium lauryl sulfate as one of the main cleansing agents, which makes it too drying for the hair and scalp.

☺ **Moisturizing Shampoo for Permed, Color-Treated and Dry Hair** *($4.49 for 15 ounces)* contains mostly water, detergent cleansing agent, lather agent, slip agent, thickeners, detangling agent/film former, fragrance, and preservatives. This is a good standard shampoo for normal to slightly dry hair that is normal to fine or thin. This would not be emollient for very dry hair. There is a tiny amount of sodium lauryl sulfate in this shampoo, but not enough to be a problem for the hair or scalp.

☺ **Volumizing Shampoo for Fine, Limp, and Lazy Hair** *($8.99 for 33.8 ounces)* contains mostly water, detergent cleansing agent, lather agent, thickeners, fragrance, preservatives, detangling agent, conditioning agents, film former, water-binding agents, and coloring agents. This is a good standard shampoo for normal to slightly dry hair that is normal to fine or thin. The tiny amount of conditioning agents, water-binding agents, and film former are here in such minute amounts that they won't have much impact on hair, which can be good for preventing buildup.

☺ **Moisturizing Conditioner for Permed, Color-Treated and Dry Hair** *($4.99 for 15 ounces)* contains mostly water, thickeners, detangling agent, fragrance, film former, and preservatives. This is a boring, mostly detangling formula for normal hair. This is not at all appropriate for dry hair of any kind.

☺ **Daily Moisturizer Leave-in Detangler and Conditioner** *($4.29 for 12 ounces)* contains mostly water, conditioning agent, detangling agents, slip agent, fragrance, film former, and preservatives. This is a good, basic, leave-in conditioner for normal to slightly dry hair that is normal to fine or thin.

☺ **Lustre Finish for Instant Shine** *($5.99 for 6.25 ounces)* is an aerosol silicone spray that can add shine to hair and make it feel soft. It contains mostly alcohol, propellant, silicone, slip agents, and fragrance.

☺ **Smoothing Gel Thermal Activated** *($5.99 for 7 ounces)* contains mostly water, detangling agent, thickeners, conditioning agents, silicone, slip agents, preservatives, and fragrance. This is a good minimal- to no-hold styling gel with no stiff or sticky feel, but it can help in smoothing most hair types when styling.

☺ **Styling Gel Natural Hold for Sculpt, Style or Set** *($4.99 for 7 ounces)* is a standard, light- to medium-hold gel with minimal stiff or sticky feel. It contains mostly water, film former, slip agents, thickeners, preservatives, fragrance, and coloring agents.

☺ **Volumizing Foam for Instant Volume and Body** *($5.49 for 9 ounces)* is a standard mousse with a light to medium hold and minimal stiff or sticky feel. It contains mostly water, propellant, detangling agents/film formers, preservatives, and fragrance.

☺ **Finishing Spray for Firm, Flexible Hold** *($4.99 for 11 ounces)* has a medium to firm hold with a slight stiff feel that does let you brush through hair. It contains mostly alcohol, propellant, water, film formers, conditioning agents, fragrance, and silicone.

☺ **Spritz for Firm Hold** *($4.99 for 8 ounces)* is similar to the Finishing Spray above, only in nonaerosol form.

☺ **Perm Revitalizer to Revive and Moisturize Curls** *($3.99 for 8 ounces)* is just a basic leave-in styling spray that has a light hold and minimal to no stiff or sticky feel. It would work on any hair type, it just depends what style you were going after. It contains mostly water, alcohol, film formers, slip agent, fragrance, conditioning agent, detangling agent, water-binding agent, and silicone.

Queen Helene

Queen Helene has been on the scene since 1930, selling hair-care products for African-American hair care. That's a long time. It has grown since then, and now has more than a hundred products for the face, body, feet, hair, and scalp. While the time-honored name may sound like a harbinger of superior quality, this ends up being just another hair-care line, and a somewhat dated line at that—for example, see the huge vats of styling gels. The sizes are generous and the prices more than reasonable, but the oversize jars make for awkward application, as you have to dig into the container to get the product out—not the best idea when there are a lot of better packaging alternatives available. What is truly unique is that these products are far less greasy than many hair-care lines marketed for African-American hair problems. Several of its products do contain cholesterol, which is just a fat that can be emollient for hair. It doesn't mend, repair, or provide any special benefit other than the usual conditioning. For more information on Queen Helene, call (800) 645-3752 or visit its Web site at www.queenhelene.com.

☺ **Cholesterol Conditioning Shampoo** *($3 for 16 ounces)* contains mostly water, detergent cleansing agents, lather agent, detangling agent/film former, thickeners, conditioning agents, more film formers, more thickeners, preservatives, and fragrance. This shampoo can leave a stiff feel on hair but it can help add a feeling of thickness to fine hair.

☺ **Cocoa Butter Shampoo** *($3.59 for 21 ounces)* is similar to the Cholesterol version above, only with slightly fewer film formers, which makes it better for dry to very dry hair that is fine or thin.

☺ **Dandruff Shampoo** *($3.19 for 16 ounces)* has a disinfectant in it, but it's not the type used in dandruff treatments known to fight dandruff. This is just a good basic shampoo with no conditioning agents (so it won't build up on hair), so the claim about fighting dandruff is dubious.

☺ **Garlic Shampoo Unscented** *($3 for 21 ounces)*. I am glad to hear a garlic shampoo is unscented because I'm not sure anyone wants their head smelling like an Italian restaurant. Nevertheless, there is nothing about garlic that is helpful for scalp or hair. This is just a gentle shampoo with no conditioning agents or film formers that can weigh hair down, but there is absolutely nothing in this shampoo that will prevent excessive breakage or loss of hair!

☺ **Mint Julep Shampoo with Protein, Concentrated** *($2.99 for 16 ounces)* is almost identical to the Garlic one above, only without the garlic; it actually doesn't contain mint either, which is good, because that would be a problem for the scalp.

☺ **Placenta Acid-Balanced Conditioning Shampoo Concentrate with Panthenol, Pearlescent Formula** *($3.99 for 16 ounces)* is just a standard shampoo with some conditioning agents and minimal problems for buildup, and that makes it good for most all hair types. There is nothing in a placenta from any animal that can help hair.

☺ **Rum Scented Shampoo Concentrate Plus Egg, Triple Lathering Formula Conditioning Shampoo for Dry and Brittle Hair** *($3.19 for 16 ounces)* does have a rum scent, and that may be nice for some, but the egg powder is just a conditioning agent and not better than many others. This is just standard shampoo with some conditioning agents and minimal problems for buildup, and that makes it good for most all hair types.

☺ **RX-18 Shampoo, Removes Build-Up and Residue** *($3.19 for 16 ounces)* is just standard, gentle shampoo with some conditioning agents and minimal problems for buildup, and that makes it good for most all hair types. It probably doesn't have a strong enough detergent base to remove most of the greasy conditioners and styling products in this line.

☺ **Cholesterol Creamy Hair Conditioner** *($2.99 for 16 ounces)* contains mostly water, slip agents, detangling agents, film former, preservatives, fragrance, and coloring agents. This isn't a deep conditioner, it is actually just a good, rather ordinary conditioner for normal to slightly dry hair of any thickness.

☺ **Cholesterol Hair Conditioning Cream** *($2.59 for 15 ounces)* is a far more emollient version than the one above. It contains mostly water, thickeners, mineral oil, cholesterol, lanolin, slip agents, fragrance, and coloring agents. This would be good for very dry hair that is thick or coarse.

☺ **Cholesterol with Ginseng Conditioning/Strengthening Cream** *($2.92 for 15 ounces)* is similar to the Cholesterol Hair version above, only with ginseng (which doesn't help hair in the least) and detangling agent, and the same basic comments apply.

☺ **Placenta Cream Hair Conditioner with Panthenol** *($3.49 for 15 ounces)* is similar to the Cholesterol Hair version above and the same comments apply. The placenta enzymes in here provide no benefit for hair.

☺ **Cocoa Butter Hair Conditioner** *($3.59 for 21 ounces)* is a basic conditioner that would be good for normal to slightly dry hair that is fine to thin or normal. It contains mostly water, slip agents, thickeners, detangling agent/film former, conditioning agent, preservatives, and fragrance.

☺ **Super Cholesterol Hair Conditioning Cream for Extremely Damaged Hair** *($6.29 for 2 pounds)* is similar to the Cholesterol Hair version above and the same comments apply.

☺ **Cholesterol Instant Leave-in Hair Conditioner** *($3 for 16 ounces)* contains mostly water, slip agent, film former, conditioning agents, detangling agent, lanolin oil, preservatives, and fragrance. This is a very good leave-in conditioner for dry hair that is fine or thin.

☺ **Cholesterol Hot Oil Treatment** *($5.49 for 8 ounces)* contains mostly water, slip agents, lanolin oil, conditioning agent, detangling agent/film former, preservatives, and fragrance. This is a good basic conditioner for dry hair, whether you heat it up or not.

☺ **Jojoba Hot Oil Treatment** *($5.49 for 8 ounces)* is almost identical to the Cholesterol Hot Oil version above, only this one has a tiny amount of jojoba extract, which has no benefit for hair (if it was jojoba oil, it would be as good as any nonfragrant plant oil, but this product just has the extract).

☺ **Placenta Hot Oil Treatment** *($5.49 for 8 ounces)* is almost identical to the Cholesterol Hot Oil version above, only this one has a tiny amount of placental enzymes, which have no benefit for hair.

☺ **Designing Lotion, Maximum Hold** *($3.29 for 16 ounces)* doesn't have maximum hold; rather, it is a soft-hold styling spray with minimal to no stiff or sticky feel.

☺ **Cholesterol Conditioning Styling Gel** *($3.29 for 16 ounces)* is a basic styling gel that contains mostly water, film former, thickeners, conditioning agents, slip agents, preservatives, fragrance, and coloring agents. It has light to no hold with minimal to no stiff or sticky feel. It can help when styling hair smooth but it offers no control or hold.

☺ **Crystalene Clear Moisturizing Styling Gel for All Types of Hair Design** *($3 for 16 ounces)* is a fairly basic styling gel that contains mostly water, thickeners, film former, conditioning agent, slip agents, preservatives, and fragrance. It has a light to medium hold with a slight sticky feel.

☺ **Designing Gel for Maximum Hold and Extra Volume** *($2.99 for 16 ounces)* is almost identical to the Crystalene Clear above and the same basic comments apply.

☺ **Styling Gel Normal** *($3 for 16 ounces)* is almost identical to the Crystalene Clear above and the same basic comments apply.

☺ **Styling Gel Superhold** *($3.19 for 16 ounces)* is almost identical to the Crystalene Clear above and the same basic comments apply.

☺ **Styling Gel Hard to Hold** *($3.19 for 16 ounces)* is similar to the Crystalene Clear above and the same basic comments apply.

☺ **Sculpturing Gel & Glaze** *($3 for 12 ounces)* is similar to the Crystalene Clear above, only with slightly more hold and a slightly more sticky feel.

☺ **Super Protein 4 in 1 Hair Conditioner and Styling Gel** *($3.20 for 16 ounces)* is similar to the Crystalene Clear above only with slightly more hold and a slightly more sticky feel.

☺ **Liquid Styling Gel for Extra Control, Contouring and Shaping** *($2.89 for 12 ounces)* is similar to the Crystalene Clear above and the same basic comments apply.

☺ **Pro-Rich Protein Conditioning and Styling Gel** *($3 for 16 ounces)* is similar to the Crystalene Clear above and the same basic comments apply.

Rave

Rave's styling products are more impressive than one might assume for its more-than-reasonable prices. Don't overlook this line because it's cheap—there are some good products to consider that perform with the best of them. For more information on Rave, call (800) 626 RAVE or (800) 423-5369.

☺ **Frizz Taming Spray Ultra Smoothness** *($1.89 for 9 ounces)* contains mostly water, slip agent, detangling agents, fragrance, and preservatives. It can only minimally help to smooth frizzies, but works as a leave-in conditioner to make combing easier for normal, healthy hair.

☺ **Bodifying Gel Ultra Hold** *($1.99 for 10 ounces)* is a standard styling gel that contains mostly water, film former, thickeners, fragrance, preservatives, and silicone. It has a good, light-to-medium hold with a slight sticky feel.

☺ **Sculpting Gel Mega Hold Alcohol Free** *($1.49 for 4 ounces)* is almost identical to the Bodifying Gel above, only with a slightly softer hold and minimal to no stiff or sticky feel.

☺ **Bodifying Gel Spray Ultra Hold Alcohol Free** *($1.79 for 7.1 ounces)* is almost identical to the Sculpting Gel above, only this one is in spray form. The same basic comments apply.

☺ **Bodifying Mousse Ultra Hold for Control** *($1.99 for 13 ounces)* is a standard mousse with a light to medium hold and minimal stiff or sticky feel that contains mostly water, propellant, detangling agent/film former, silicones, preservatives, and fragrance.

☺ **Volumizing Mousse + Gel Volume & Lasting Control** *($1.89 for 6 ounces)* comes out like a gel and then turns into a foam, the same as any mousse. It has a light to medium hold with minimal to no stiff or sticky feel. It contains mostly water, propellant, film formers, silicones, thickeners, preservatives, and fragrance.

☺ **Sculpting Spritz Mega Hold** *($1.99 for 14 ounces)* is a good, light- to medium-hold hairspray with a minimal stiff feel that can easily be brushed through. It contains mostly alcohol, water, film formers, conditioning agent, and fragrance.

☺ **Hairspray 2 Super Hold Non-Aerosol** *($1.49 for 7 ounces)* is a good medium-hold hairspray with a slight stiff feel, though it can be brushed through. It contains mostly alcohol, water, film formers, conditioning agent, and fragrance.

☺ **Hairspray 2 Super Hold Aerosol Scented or Unscented** *($1.49 for 7 ounces)* is almost identical to the 2 Super Hold Non-Aerosol above, only in aerosol form. It does have a slightly softer hold, though the general basic comments apply.

☺ **Hairspray 3 Ultra Hold Aerosol Scented or Unscented** *($1.99 for 14 ounces)* is almost identical to the 2 Super Hold Aerosol above and the same comments apply.

☺ **Hairspray 3 Ultra Hold Unscented Non-Aerosol** *($0.89 for 7 ounces)* is almost identical to the 2 Super Hold Non-Aerosol above and the same comments apply.

☺ **Hairspray Plus Conditioning Nutrients 3+ Ultra Hold** *($1.49 for 7 ounces)* doesn't include much conditioning; it's just a hairspray with a light to medium hold and a slight stiff feel.

☺ **Microspray 3 Ultra Hold Micro Droplet Technology Aerosol** *($1.59 for 3.5 ounces)* has a light to medium hold with a minimal stiff feel that can easily be brushed through. It contains mostly alcohol, propellant, water, film former, conditioning agents, silicones, and fragrance.

☺ **Microspray 4 Mega Hold Micro Droplet Technology Aerosol** *($1.59 for 3.5 ounces)* is almost identical to the Microspray 3 above and the same basic comments apply.

☺ **Hairspray 4 Mega Hold Fresh Fragrance Non-Aerosol** *($0.89 for 7 ounces)* has a medium to firm hold and can't easily be brushed through. It contains mostly alcohol, water, film formers, slip agent, preservatives, and fragrance.

☺ **Hairspray 4 Mega Hold Aerosol Scented and Unscented** *($1.50 for 14 ounces)* is almost identical to the 2 Super Hold Aerosol above and the same comments apply.

Ready to Wear
(see John Frieda)

Redken

Redken has been around as an independent hair-care company for a long time. It was purchased back in 1995 by the L'Oreal company. As one L'Oreal insider confided to me, "We need to get Redken up to speed." That could just be ego talking, but the notion that Redken has secrets no one else knows about just can't hold water anymore. Assuredly both Redken and L'Oreal know what the other party is doing. Regardless, Redken has a vast range of products and while some just have overblown claims, others are absolutely worth considering.

What isn't overblown here is Redken's new Active Express Shampoo and Conditioner, which is not only supposed to help hair dry faster but does! (Personally, for my thick, curly hair, that's one hour faster than usual.) It appears that these products work due to their increased alcohol content. What that ends up doing is leaving the hair more dry and flyaway. Unfortunately, unless you use the entire Redken Active Express system, you won't get the benefit. Using other styling products, especially smoothing lotions and silicone serums, slows the drying process back down to normal time. There's no denying that this group helps cut drying time, but the question is, will you like the results as much as the time you save?

Redken Color Extend can't extend the length of time hair dye will stay in your hair. These are just shampoos and conditioners that are as standard as they come. I discuss this more in the section on "Sunscreen in Hair-Care Products" in Chapter Three, *Hair-Care Basics.*

The CAT products line, says the company, "incorporates patented Taurine Technology to strengthen all hair types by as much as 65%." Taurine and cysteine are two important amino acids in the human body and these do show up in the hair. And in much the same way that skin-care products would like you to believe that you can take a single component present in the human body, like collagen, stick it in a cream, and have it resupply what your skin has lost from damage, this product adds taurine. But adding taurine back to hair can't be done. It can help as a moisturizing agent, but it can't replace what the hair has lost. Taurine is a good ingredient for conditioning hair, but not any better than lots of other conditioning agents. Some lines want you to believe their vitamins do the trick, others that panthenol or silk amino acids are the answer. None of these are the miracle you're hoping for, just good standard conditioning agents. Beside, if taurine was such a great ingredient, why would Redken have to come out with so many new products?

CAT stands for Cationic Protein Polypeptide, an ingredient in some of the Redken products, and refers to a positively charged protein (the protein is just a standard conditioning agent with a positive charge). That process makes the conditioner repel water so it can better cling to the hair. But this is nothing unique, it's a basic concept used in most hair products to keep conditioning agents clinging to the right places on the hair shaft instead of being washed away.

Redken's small group of One 2 One products "is formulated with Redken's unique complex of anti-oxidant vitamins, essential minerals and natural protein to preserve and protect hair." That sounds great, but minerals and antioxidants have no proven ability to do that.

Another group of Redken products (recently being called 5TH Avenue NYC) uses a unique rating system. The container for each styling product has a numbered ruler that ranks the amount of hold you can expect: 1–4 is soft hold, 5–15 is regular hold, and 16–26 is for a firm hold. I wish the numbering system were more reliable, but it ends up being as confusing as in the rest of the hair-care world, where there is little to no difference between Flexible, Firm, Mega, or Ultra hold.

For more information on Redken, call (212) 818-1500, (800) 423-5369, or visit its Web site at www.redkenhair.com.

☹ **Hair Cleansing Creme Alternate Clarifying Shampoo** *($9.95 for 10.1 ounces)* uses sodium lauryl sulfate as one of the main cleansing agents, which makes it too drying for the hair and scalp.

☺ **Solve, Anti-Dandruff Shampoo** *($9.90 for 8.5 ounces)* is a good, standard, zinc pyrithione–based shampoo, similar to Head & Shoulders, only this one is more expensive.

☺ **Vivagen Thinning Hair Enrichment Shampoo** *($8.50 for 8.5 ounces)* is a standard shampoo with conditioning agents, plus a long-drawn-out list of "hair hopeful" ingredients ranging from yeast and vitamins to hops and minerals. These can't help hair grow, but they do sound impressive. It contains mostly water, detergent cleansing agent, lather agent, thickeners, conditioning agents, slip agents, vitamins, minerals, preservatives, fragrance, and coloring agents. It would work well for normal to dry hair of any thickness, with minimal risk of buildup.

☹ **Vivagen Hair Enrichment Treatment for Thinning Hair** *($19.95 for 5 ounces)* contains menthol, which is a scalp irritant; it may make you feel like you're growing hair, but it isn't doing a thing except causing irritation.

☺ **$$$ Glass Smoothing Complex 1** *($12 for 2 ounces)* is a standard (though overpriced) silicone serum that can add a silky-soft feel and shine to hair.

☺ **Details Conditioning Styling Complex 2** *($10 for 5 ounces)* is a minimal-hold lotion with no stiff or sticky feel for smoothing frizzies and curls. It contains mostly water, slip agent, thickeners, conditioning agents, detangling agent/film former, fragrance, and preservatives.

☺ **Shine Design Weightless Finishing Gel 2L** *($9 for 2.85 ounces)* contains mostly water, thickeners, slip agent, mineral oil, preservatives, fragrance, and coloring agents. This thick, waxy-feeling gel has no hold and therefore no stiff or sticky feel. It can help when styling to smooth frizzies and curls, but it can also easily look greasy and heavy, so use it sparingly.

☺ **Undone Weightless Finishing Creme 2** *($14.95 for 3.4 ounces)* is a minimal- to no-hold creamy lotion that has minimal to no sticky feel. It works well for smoothing frizzies and curls. It contains mostly water, thickeners, slip agent, silicone, conditioning agents, preservatives, and fragrance.

☺ **Water Wax Water Based Pomade 3** *($12.95 for 1.7 ounces)* is a standard waxlike pomade that contains mostly water, castor oil, thickeners, slip agents, conditioning agents, preservatives, and coloring agents. This is good for controlling stubborn frizzies with minimal hold, but it can have a slight sticky, heavy feel, so use it sparingly. Because it has no film formers there's less hold, but also no stiff feel on hair.

☺ **Guts Volume Boosting Spray Foam 10** *($9.95 for 10.58 ounces)* is a very standard mousse with a medium to firm hold and a somewhat sticky feel that contains mostly water, propellant, film former, conditioning agents, silicone, slip agent, preservatives, and fragrance.

☺ **Touch Control Texture Whip Styling 5** *($9.95 for 6.7 ounces)* is a standard mousse with a medium hold and a somewhat sticky feel. It contains mostly water, propellant, film former, detangling agent, conditioning agent, thickeners, silicone, preservatives, and fragrance.

☺ **Contour Shaping Lotion 8** *($6.95 for 8.5 ounces))* is a medium- to firm-hold liquid gel with a somewhat stiff or sticky feel. It contains mostly water, film formers, alcohol, conditioning agents, thickeners, preservatives, and fragrance.

☺ **Creatif Contour Shaping Lotion 8L** *($13 for 16.9 ounces)* is identical to the Contour Shaping Lotion above, only with a packaging and identity change.

☺ **Centigrade Thermactive Gel 4** *($11 for 8.5 ounces)* is a medium-hold gel that contains mostly water, film formers, thickeners, conditioning agents, castor oil, slip agent, fragrance, and preservatives. It has a minimal sticky, stiff feel.

☺ **Hardwear Super Strong Gel 16** *($10 for 8.5 ounces)* contains mostly water, alcohol, film formers, thickeners, silicone oil, fragrant oil, conditioning agent, and preservatives. This is a good, firm-hold gel with a somewhat stiff, sticky feel.

☺ **Outline Fixing Gel 12** *($6.95 for 8.5 ounces)* is almost identical to the Hardwear Super Strong Gel above, only with slightly less hold and a slightly less sticky feel.

☺ **Amino Pon Hairspray Firm Hold 16** *($8 for 11 ounces)* is a standard aerosol hairspray with medium to firm hold and a stiff, sticky feel that can be brushed through. It contains mostly alcohol, water, propellant, conditioning agent, and fragrance.

☺ **Body & Bounce Sculpting Spray Gel 6** *($7.50 for 8.5 ounces)* contains mostly water, film formers, silicone, thickener, conditioning agents, fragrance, and preservatives. This is a good standard hairspray with a light to medium hold and minimal stiff or sticky feel.

☺ **Airset Heat Styling Protectant Soft Control 3** *($6.95 for 8.5 ounces)* is a very standard styling spray with a light hold and minimal stiff or sticky feel. It contains mostly water, alcohol, film formers, conditioning agents, slip agent, preservatives, and fragrance.

☺ **Hot Sets Thermal Setting Mist 22** *($6.95 for 5 ounces)* is a standard, light-hold styling spray with minimal stiff or sticky feel. It would work as well as any to hold the shape from curling irons or hot rollers. It contains mostly alcohol, water, film formers, silicone, conditioning agents, more silicone, and fragrance.

☺ **Lift & Shine Finishing Spritz 15** *($7.50 for 8.5 ounces)* is a standard, light-to medium-hold hairspray with a minimal stiff feel, and it can be brushed through. It contains mostly alcohol, water, film formers, conditioning agents, silicone, and fragrance.

☺ **Quick Dry Shaping Mist 18** *($9.90 for 11 ounces)* is a standard aerosol hairspray with a medium to firm hold and a slight stiff feel that does let you brush through hair. This doesn't dry any faster than any other aerosol hairspray. It contains mostly alcohol, water, film formers, conditioning agents, silicone, and fragrance.

☺ **Framework Designing Spray 20** *($10 for 11 ounces)* is similar to the Quick Dry above and the same comments apply.

☺ **Suspend Forming and Mending Spray Firm Control 16** *($7 for 5 ounces)* is a standard, firm-hold hairspray with a somewhat stiff, sticky feel that can be brushed through. It contains mostly water, alcohol, film formers, and fragrance.

☺ **Direct Airosol Mist Ultra Hold 26S** *($6.95 for 8.5 ounces)* is a standard firm-hold hairspray with a stiff, sticky feel that can be brushed through with some effort. It contains mostly water, alcohol, film formers, and fragrance.

Active Express by Redken

☺ **Active Express Flash Wash Fast-Drying Shampoo** *($7.50 for 10.1 ounces).* I tried to find out from Redken why its Active Express works—because it does—but after several calls I couldn't get anyone to help me out. According to its press release, these products work because they contains "blends [of] witch-hazel extract and fruit acids.... The acids cause the hair's cuticle to lock down flat, thus minimizing water absorption and accelerating runoff. (Picture feathers that allow water to run off a duck's back.)" But duck feathers allow water to run off because they hold oil, not because their cuticle is locked down! Redken's "picture" is weirdly misleading, but who said hair-care marketing wasn't misleading?

Further fruit acids in a low pH formulation can lock down the cuticle, but not as well as other ingredients with low pHs that don't have the hair-exfoliating properties of a low pH fruit acid. Exfoliating the hair shaft is not a good thing! But not to worry, because these products do not have a low enough pH to allow the fruit acids to hurt the hair shaft. They're also no lower in pH than those in lots of other hair-care products. What really causes the improved drying time is the amount of alcohol in the shampoo and conditioner (witch hazel contains a good percentage of alcohol). In the testing done at my office, it improved air-drying time by at least 40 minutes to an hour (I did not test drying time for blow-dryers). As great as this sounds, there is one word of warning: it can make hair dry and more flyaway, which makes sense when you think about it, and that can make problems for some hair types. It contains mostly water, detergent cleansing agents, witch hazel, lather agent, silicone, thickeners, fragrance, detangling agent/film former, preservatives, slip agent, conditioning agents, lots more thickeners, more preservatives, and coloring agents. I suspect it's worth a try for those in a hurry, but unless you use the entire Redken Active Express system you won't get the benefit. Using other styling products, especially smoothing lotions and silicone serums, slows the drying process back down to normal time. There's no denying that this group helps cut drying time, so the question is whether you will like the results as much as the time you save.

☺ **Active Express Split Second Rinse-Out Conditioner** *($7.95 for 8.5 ounces).* The same comments as for the shampoo above about helping hair dry faster apply to this conditioner as well, and again, pure alcohol is rather high up on the ingredient listing. Still, this is a good conditioner for most hair types, though it can make hair more flyaway if your hair is dry or coarse.

☺ **Active Express Quick Treat Treatment & Styler** *($12.95 for 8.5 ounces)* contains mostly water, film former, detangling agents, preservatives, fragrance, conditioning agents, plant extracts, and coloring agents. It's more of a leave-in conditioner than a styling spray. It has a soft to almost nonexistent hold and minimal no stiff or sticky feel.

All Soft by Redken

☺ **All Soft Shampoo** *($7.50 for 10.1 ounces)* contains mostly water, detergent cleansing agent, lather agent, silicone, thickeners, plant oil, conditioning agents, preservatives, slip agent, coloring agents, and fragrance. This is a good shampoo for dry hair, but what's providing that benefit is mostly just silicone technology.

☺ **All Soft Concentrate** *($13.95 for 5 ounces)* contains mostly water, detangling agents, slip agents, thickeners, plant oil, conditioning agents, preservatives, and fragrance. This is a good but very standard conditioner for normal to slightly dry hair of any thickness. The directions describe towel-drying hair and then applying the conditioner, waiting five minutes, and then rinsing. Like any conditioner, the longer you leave it on, the better it makes hair feel—that isn't special to this product.

☺ **All Soft Conditioner** *($8 for 8.5 ounces)* contains mostly water, thickeners, silicone, detangling agents, slip agents, plant oil, conditioning agents, preservatives, detangling agents, coloring agents, and fragrance. This is a good standard conditioner for dry hair of any thickness.

☺ **All Soft Hair Masque** *($9.95 for 5 ounces)* is almost identical to the All Soft Conditioner above and the same basic comments apply.

CAT by Redken

☺ **CAT Revitalizing Shampoo** *($5.50 for 10.1 ounces)* contains mostly water, detergent cleansing agents, lather agent, thickeners, conditioning agents, preservatives, detangling agent, and silicone. This is a fairly standard shampoo that would work well for most hair types with minimal risk of buildup.

☺ **Fat CAT Body Booster Shampoo for Fine Hair** *($6.50 for 10.1 ounces)* is similar to the Revitalizing version above, only this one contains more silicone. That won't do much for fine hair, but it's better for drier hair.

☺ **CAT Protein Reconstructing Treatment** *($11.95 for 5 ounces)* won't reconstruct one hair on your head, but it is a good conditioner for normal to slightly dry hair that is normal to fine or thin. It contains mostly water, thickeners, conditioning agents, detangling agent/film former, and preservatives.

☺ **CAT Replenishing Conditioner** *($6.25 for 6 ounces)* contains mostly water, thickeners, conditioning agents, detangling agents, silicone, preservatives, and fragrance. This is a good standard conditioner for normal to slightly dry hair of any thickness.

☺ **Fat CAT Body Booster Detangler** *($7.25 for 6 ounces)* is similar to the Replenishing Conditioner above and the same comments apply.

☺ **CAT Polishing Shine** *($7.95 for 2 ounces)* is a standard silicone serum that works great for adding shine and a silky feel to hair.

☺ **CAT Styling Gel** *($7.50 for 6 ounces)* is a good standard gel with a light to medium hold and minimal stiff or sticky feel. It contains mostly water, alcohol, film formers, thickeners, silicone, preservatives, fragrance, and conditioning agents.

☺ **Fat CAT Body Booster Fine Hair Thickening Lotion** *($8.95 for 6 ounces)* is a good styling lotion for straightening frizzies or curly hair; it gives a light to medium hold and has minimal to no sticky feel. This can feel heavy, so use it sparingly. It contains mostly water, witch hazel, film formers, thickeners, silicone, conditioning agents, preservatives, and fragrance.

☺ **CAT Finishing Spritz** *($7.75 for 10.1 ounces)* is a standard hairspray with a light to medium hold and minimal stiff feel; it can easily be brushed through. It contains mostly alcohol, water, film formers, fragrance, silicone, and conditioning agents.

☺ **Fat CAT Body Booster Plump Spray for Fine Hair** *($10 for 11 ounces)* is similar to the Finishing Spritz above, only in aerosol form.

☹ **Fat CAT Body Booster Volumist for Fine Hair** *($8.95 for 6 ounces)* contains mostly water, alcohol, film formers, conditioning agents, slip agents, detangling agent, preservatives, and fragrance. This is just a styling spray with a medium hold and a somewhat sticky, stiff feel.

☺ **CAT Sculpting Mousse** *($9.50 for 7 ounces)* is a good standard mousse with a medium to firm hold and a slight stiff, sticky feel. It contains mostly water, propellant, film formers, thickeners, silicone, fragrance, preservatives, and conditioning agents.

☺ **Fat CAT Body Booster Treatment for Fine Hair** *($8.95 for 5 ounces)* contains mostly water, conditioning agents, thickeners, slip agents, detangling agents, preservatives, and fragrance. This is just a lightweight styling spray with a light hold and good hair-conditioning agents. It would work for most hair types to create a soft styling hold.

Climatress by Redken

☺ **Climatress Shampoo Normal to Dry Hair** *($7.50 for 10.1 ounces)* contains mostly water, detergent cleansing agents, lather agent, thickeners, plant oil, conditioning agents, preservatives, and fragrance. This is a good shampoo for someone with dry hair of any thickness.

☺ **Climatress Conditioner for Normal to Dry Hair** *($8 for 8.5 ounces)* contains mostly water, thickeners, mineral oil, detangling agents, plant oil, conditioning agents, preservatives, and fragrance. This is a very good standard conditioner for dry hair that is coarse or thick.

☺ **Climatress Treatment** *($9.95 for 5 ounces)* is similar to the Conditioner above and the same comments apply.

☺ **Climatress High Humidity Hairspray** *($7.95 for 11 ounces)* is just a standard aerosol hairspray with a medium to firm hold and a slight stiff sticky feel; it contains mostly alcohol, water, propellant, film formers, conditioning agents, silicone, and preservatives.

Color Extend Redken

☺ **Color Extend Shampoo** *($7.50 for 10.1 ounces)* won't extend hair color and cannot protect from sun damage in the least. Without an SPF number, there is no way to know how much, if any, real protection is in here. Besides, these products don't contain one unique ingredient when compared to any of the other Redken products not making this claim! This contains mostly water, detergent cleansing agent, lather agent, thickeners, conditioning agents, preservatives, detangling agent/film former, and fragrance. This is a good shampoo for dry hair of any thickness, but that's it.

☺ **Color Extend Conditioner** *($8 for 8.5 ounces)* contains mostly water, thickeners, detangling agents/film former, thickeners, silicone, conditioning agents, preservatives, and fragrance. This is a good conditioner for normal to dry hair that is normal to fine or thin.

☺ **Color Extend Leave-in Sealer** *($13 for 6.7 ounces)* is just a silicone-based leave-in conditioner for normal to slightly dry hair. It dispenses from an aerated container so you spread the conditioner over the hair in mousse form. This product won't hold in color and the sunscreen in here can't protect from sun damage; because there's no SPF, any claim about sun protection is meaningless. This does contain mostly water, thickener, silicone, more thickeners, detangling agents, conditioning agents, preservatives, and fragrance—the same standard ingredients that show up in thousands of products—and none of them can protect from the sun either.

Extreme Redken

☹ **Extreme Shampoo for Damaged Hair** *($7.50 for 10.1 ounces)* uses TEA-lauryl sulfate as its main cleansing agent, which is too drying for the hair and potentially irritating for the scalp.

☺ **Extreme Conditioner for Damaged Hair** *($7.50 for 8.5 ounces)* isn't extreme in the least; it's actually quite similar to many of the Redken conditioners. This one contains mostly water, thickeners, detangling agents, conditioning agents, preservatives, film former, more preservatives, and fragrance. It would be good for someone with normal to dry hair of any thickness.

☺ **Extreme Treatment** *($12.95 for 5 ounces)* contains mostly water, slip agent, thickeners, detangling agent/film former, silicone, conditioning agents, preservatives, and fragrance. This is a good lightweight conditioner for normal to slightly dry hair that is normal to fine or thin.

Glypro by Redken

☺ **Glypro+ Shampoo for Fine Delicate Hair** *($6.99 for 10.1 ounces)* contains mostly water, detergent cleansing agents, lather agent, conditioning agent, thickeners, more conditioning agents, preservatives, fragrance, and coloring agents. This is a good shampoo for normal to dry hair of any thickness, but there is nothing about this that would be helpful for delicate hair.

☺ **Glypro+ Conditioner for Fine/Delicate Hair** *($7.95 for 8.5 ounces)* contains mostly water, thickeners, silicone, conditioning agent, slip agent, more thickeners, more conditioning agents, preservatives, fragrance, and coloring agents. This is a good standard conditioner for normal to dry hair of any thickness, but it isn't better in any way for delicate hair.

One 2 One by Redken

☺ **One 2 One Moisturizing Shampoo** *($8.75 for 10.1 ounces)* contains mostly water, detergent cleansing agents, lather agent, vitamins, minerals, conditioning agent, thickener, preservatives, fragrance, film former, and plant oil. This is a good shampoo for normal to dry hair of any thickness, but the vitamins and minerals in here won't help hair anymore than they do in hundreds of other products.

☺ **One 2 One Volumizing Shampoo** *($8.75 for 10.1 ounces)* is almost identical to the Moisturizing version above and the same comments apply.

☺ **One 2 One Daily Recovery Conditioner** *($8.75 for 10.1 ounces)* contains mostly water, thickeners, detangling agents, vitamins, minerals, conditioning agents, silicone, fragrance, preservatives, coloring agents, and plant oil. This is a good standard conditioner for normal to slightly dry hair of any thickness.

☺ **One 2 One Groom Brushing Gloss** *($12.50 for 3.4 ounces)* is a good, no-hold straightening gel serum that contains mostly alcohol, thickeners, conditioning agents, plant oil, and fragrance. It can help when styling frizzy hair smooth.

☺ **One 2 One Stay Firm Hold Treatment Spray** *($9.50 for 5 ounces)* is a standard, medium- to firm-hold hairspray with a slight stiff feel that can easily be brushed through. It contains mostly alcohol, water, film former, vitamins, conditioning agents, plant oil, and fragrance. The vitamins provide no extra treatment.

☺ **One 2 One Smooth Anti-Frizz Creme** *($12.50 for 3.4 ounces)* is a good styling cream that is more of a lotion for smoothing frizzies and curls. It has minimal hold and a slight greasy finish but it works well, especially for coarse dry hair. It contains mostly water, thickeners, vitamins, minerals, conditioning agents, water-binding agent, plant oil, detangling agent, preservatives, and fragrance.

☺ **One 2 One Straight Hair Straightening Balm** *($12.50 for 5 ounces)* is a minimal-hold gel lotion with no stiff or sticky feel. It contains mostly water, witch hazel, thickener, detangling agent, vitamins, conditioning agents, more thickeners, plant oil, preservatives, and fragrance.

Shades EQ by Redken

☺ **Shades EQ, Color Care Shampoo, Clear** *($6.35 for 10.1 ounces)* contains mostly water, detergent cleansing agent, lather agent, detangling agents/film formers, silicone, conditioning agents, fragrance, and preservatives. This is a good basic shampoo for normal to slightly dry hair that is fine or thin. The film formers in here can cause buildup.

☺ **Shades EQ, Color Enhancing Shampoo, Bonfire Red** *($5.90 for 5 ounces)* contains mostly water, detergent cleansing agents, lather agent, thickeners, preservatives, fragrance, and dye agents. This is a good, basic, color-enhancing shampoo with no ingredients that can cause buildup or make hair limp.

☺ **Shades EQ, Color Enhancing Shampoo, Espresso** *($5.90 for 5 ounces)* is identical to the version above and the same comments apply.

☺ **Shades EQ, Color Enhancing Shampoo, Platinum Ice Violet** *($5.90 for 5 ounces)* is almost identical to the version above and the same comments apply.

☺ **Shades EQ, Color Enhancing Shampoo, Rocket Fire Red** *($5.9 for 5 ounces)* is almost identical to the version above and the same comments apply.

The Reviews R

☺ **Shades EQ, Color Enhancing Shampoo, St. Tropez Gold** *($5.90 for 5 ounces)* is almost identical to the version above and the same comments apply.

☺ **Shades EQ, Color Enhancing Shampoo, Vanilla Cream** *($5.90 for 5 ounces)* is almost identical to the version above and the same comments apply.

☺ **Shades EQ, Color Care Protector, Leave-in** *(6.407 for 5 ounces)* contains mostly water, detangling agent, conditioning agents, silicones, fragrance, and preservatives. This is a great leave-in conditioner for dry hair of any thickness.

Revlon

Revlon is a huge cosmetics company with a wide range of products. Its strength is in its makeup lines, where it has some of the best technologies for makeup, particularly for foundations (its stay-put technology for ultra-matte foundations, and its use of sunscreen in foundations is unsurpassed in the industry). Its hair-care products have some good selections, they just aren't exciting. But that's OK, because there really isn't much excitement in the world of hair-care formulations. For more information on Revlon, call (212) 572-5000, (800) 4 REVLON, or visit its Web site at www.revlon.com.

ColorStay by Revlon

☹ **Stay Blonde Shampoo for Blonde Color Treated Hair Locks Color in the First Critical Week After You Color** *($3.29 for 10 ounces)* uses sodium lauryl sulfate as one of the main cleansing agents, which makes it too drying for the hair and scalp.

☹ **Stay Brunette Shampoo for Brunette Color Treated Hair Locks Color in the First Critical Week After You Color** *($3.29 for 10 ounces)* uses sodium lauryl sulfate as one of the main cleansing agents, which makes it too drying for the hair and scalp.

☹ **Stay Red Shampoo for Red Color Treated Hair Locks Color in the First Critical Week After You Color** *($3.29 for 10 ounces)* uses sodium lauryl sulfate as one of the main cleansing agents, which makes it too drying for the hair and scalp.

☺ **Stay Blonde Conditioner for Blonde Color Treated Hair Locks Color in the First Critical Week After You Color** *($3.29 for 10 ounces)*, like the other ColorStay conditioners that follow, is a far better option for a color-enhancing boost, but none of these has any ability to lock in color. As one Revlon chemist told me, if someone could figure out how to prevent hair dye from fading, that company would be the only one selling products. These would work well for normal to dry hair of any thickness. They contain mostly water, detangling agents, thickeners, silicones, water-binding agents, conditioning agents, slip agents, vitamins, fragrance, preservatives, and dye agents.

B.Dalton Bookseller
Meadowbrook Parkway
Garden City, NY 11530
(516)747-2727
02-03-02 S00169 R008

Don't Go Shopping For Ha   19.95
187796826X

SUB TOTAL   19.95
SALES TAX   1.70
TOTAL   21.65
AMOUNT TENDERED
CASH   22.00

TOTAL PAYMENT   22.00
CHANGE   .35
        Thank you for shopping at
         B. Dalton Booksellers
Shop online 24 hours a day www.bn.com
#146466 02-03-02 12:52P mahima

 Thank you for shopping at B. Dalton

Full refund issued for new and unread books and unopened music within 30 days with a receipt from any Barnes & Noble store.
Store Credit issued for new and unread books and unopened music after 30 days or without a sales receipt. Credit issued at <u>lowest sale price</u>.
We gladly accept returns of new and unread books and unopened music from bn.com with a bn.com receipt for store credit at the bn.com price.

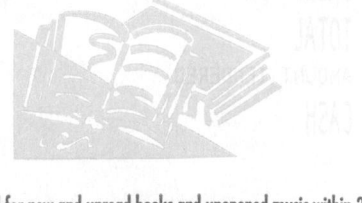

Full refund issued for new and unread books and unopened music within 30 days with a receipt from any Barnes & Noble store.
Store Credit issued for new and unread books and unopened music after 30 days or without a sales receipt. Credit issued at <u>lowest sale price</u>.
We gladly accept returns of new and unread books and unopened music from bn.com with a bn.com receipt for store credit at the bn.com price.

☺ **Stay Brunette Conditioner for Brunette Color Treated Hair Locks Color in the First Critical Week After You Color** *($3.29 for 10 ounces)* is almost identical to the version above and the same comments apply.

☺ **Stay Red Conditioner for Red Color Treated Hair Locks Color in the First Critical Week After You Color** *($3.29 for 10 ounces)* is identical to the version above and the same comments apply.

Flex by Revlon

☹ **Triple Action Extra Body Shampoo Balsam & Protein Protects, Nourishes, Fortifies** *($2.39 for 15 ounces)* uses sodium C14-17 alkyl sec sulfonate as one of the detergent cleansing agents, which can be drying for hair and scalp and potentially strip hair color. It also contains balsam, which can build up on hair and make it feel stiff and brittle.

☹ **Triple Action Frequent Use Shampoo for All Hair Types** *($2.39 for 15 ounces)* is almost identical to the Extra Body one above and the same comments apply.

☹ **Triple Action Moisturizing Shampoo Balsam & Protein Fortifies, Nourishes Protects** *($1.84 for 15 ounces)* is almost identical to the Extra Body one above and the same comments apply.

☹ **Triple Action Normal to Dry Shampoo Balsam & Protein Fortifies, Nourishes, Protects** *($2.39 for 15 ounces)* is almost identical to the one above and the same comments apply.

☹ **Triple Action Ultra Clean Shampoo Balsam & Protein; Fortifies, Nourishes, Protects** *($2.06 for 15 ounces)* is almost identical to the one above and the same comments apply.

☹ **Two in One Original Balsam Scent for All Hair Types Shampoo & Conditioner in One** *($2.39 for 11 ounces)* uses sodium lauryl sulfate and sodium C14-17 alkyl sec sulfonate as the main cleansing agents, which makes it too drying for the hair and scalp.

☺ **Fresh Scent Extra Body Flex Light and Free Conditioner Maximizes** *($2.09 for 15 ounces)* contains mostly water, thickeners, slip agents, conditioning agents, water-binding agent, detangling agent, silicone, fragrance, preservatives, and coloring agents. This is a very good conditioner for normal to dry hair of any thickness.

☺ **Fresh Scent Moisturizing Flex Light and Free Conditioner** *($2.09 for 15 ounces)* is almost identical to the one above and the same comments apply.

☺ **Fresh Scent Normal Flex Light and Free Conditioner** *($2.09 for 15 ounces)* is almost identical to the ones above and the same comments apply.

☺ **Triple Action Extra Body Conditioner Balsam & Protein Fortifies, Nourishes, Protects** *($2.39 for 15 ounces)* is similar to the versions above, only this one contains balsam, and that can build up on the hair and make it feel brittle and stiff.

The Reviews R

☺ **Triple Action Frequent Use Conditioner Balsam & Protein Fortifies, Nourishes, Protects** *($2.39 for 15 ounces)* is almost identical to the one above and the same comments apply.

☹ **Triple Action Moisturizing Conditioner Balsam & Protein Fortifies, Nourishes, Protects** *($1.84 for 15 ounces)* is almost identical to the ones above and the same comments apply.

Outrageous by Revlon

☺ **Daily Beautifying Shampoo for Normal Hair** *($2.34 for 15 ounces)* contains mostly water, detergent cleansing agents, lather agent, thickeners, conditioning agents, water-binding agent, fragrance, and preservatives. This is a good shampoo for normal to dry hair of any thickness.

☹ **Moisture-Rich Shampoo for Dry, Permed Hair or Color-Treated Hair** *($3.70 for 15 ounces)* uses sodium lauryl sulfate and sodium C14-17 alkyl sec sulfonate as the main cleansing agents, which makes it too drying for the hair and scalp.

☺ **Two-in-One Shampoo Plus Conditioner Extra Body** *($2.99 for 15 ounces)* is a standard, silicone-based shampoo that contains mostly water, detergent cleansing agents, silicones, lather agent, detangling agent, thickeners, film former, fragrance, preservatives, and coloring agents. This is a good shampoo for dry hair that is fine or thin. It can easily cause buildup.

☺ **Two-in-One Shampoo Plus Conditioner Moisturizing** *($2.34 for 15 ounces)* is similar to the Extra Body version above and the same comments apply.

☹ **Volumizing Shampoo for Fine Hair** *($2.34 for 15 ounces)* uses sodium lauryl sulfate and sodium C14-17 alkyl sec sulfonate as the main cleansing agents, which makes it too drying for the hair and scalp.

☺ **Outrageous Daily Beautifying Conditioner for Normal Hair** *($2.34 for 15 ounces)* contains mostly water, thickeners, detangling agent, conditioning agents, slip agents, silicone, fragrance, and preservatives. This is a good conditioner for normal to dry hair of any thickness.

☺ **Moisture-Rich Conditioner for Dry, Permed or Color-Treated Hair** *($2.34 for 15 ounces)* is similar to the Normal Hair version above, only this one contains more silicone, which does make it better for dry hair of any thickness.

☺ **Volumizing Conditioner for Fine Hair** *($3.19 for 15 ounces)* is similar to the Beautifying Conditioner above and the same comments apply.

Robert Craig

Robert Craig is a hairstylist with an interesting group of hair-care products. "His shampoos are based on the varying degrees of hardness of the water with which they are used rather than hair type, and the rest of the line is water soluble. This allows the hair to receive the right amount of gentle cleansing with no buildup of product even on chemically treated hair fiber." That's a unique claim, but nothing in these formulations is supporting it. These are very standard shampoos and conditioners with no chelating agents (ingredients that prevent minerals from binding to hair). There are some good products in this line but they won't help you with whatever problems your water supply delivers.

For more information on Robert Craig, call (212) 627-1404, (800) 91 SALON, or visit its Web site at www.robertcraig.com.

☹ **Shampoo for Extremely Hard Water** *($9 for 8 ounces)* uses sodium lauryl sulfate as one of the main detergent cleansing agents, which can be drying for the hair and drying and irritating for the scalp. It also contains peppermint, which is a skin irritant.

☹ **Shampoo for Hard Water** *($9 for 8 ounces)* is almost identical to the Extremely Hard Water version above and the same concerns apply.

☹ **Shampoo for Soft Water** *($9 for 8 ounces)* is almost identical to the Extremely Hard Water version above and the same concerns apply.

☺ **Conditioner** *($12 for 8 ounces)* contains mostly water, conditioning agents, thickeners, slip agent, detangling agent/film former, plant extracts, preservatives, coloring agent, and fragrance. This is a good conditioner for dry hair that is normal to fine or thin. This does contain peppermint, so keep it off the scalp.

☺ **Conditioning Spray 3-in-1 Formulation** *($12 for 8 ounces)* contains mostly plant water, detangling agents, slip agents, conditioning agents, vitamins, preservatives, coloring agent, and fragrance. This is a good, leave-in conditioner for dry hair that is normal to fine or thin.

☺ **Spray Shine 3-in-1 Formulation** *($18 for 8 ounces)* contains mostly plant water, silicones, slip agents, vitamins, and fragrance. This is a very good, silicone-based spray that can be used for styling or as a leave-in conditioner for normal to dry hair of any thickness.

☺ **Spray Gel 3-in-1 Formulation** *($10 for 8 ounces)* is a standard spray gel that contains mostly water, alcohol, film formers, detangling agents, thickeners, and fragrance. The claim about sun protection is bogus, but this does have a good light hold with minimal to no stiff or sticky feel.

☺ **Mousse 3-in-1 Formulation** *($12 for 7 ounces)* dispenses like a gel and then becomes a mousse. It contains mostly plant water, film formers, propellant, conditioning agents, silicone, thickeners, and fragrance. The claim about sun protection is bogus, but this does have a good light hold with a minimal to slight sticky feel.

☺ **Pomade** *($8 for 2 ounces)* is a standard pomade with no film formers, so it can smooth hair without stiffness or a sticky feel, though it also provides little hold.

It contains mostly water, mineral oil, thickeners, preservatives, and fragrance. It can easily look greasy and heavy if you use too much, so use it sparingly.

☺ **Spray Finishing 3-in-1 Formulation** *($10 for 8 ounces)* can't protect from sun damage in the least, but it is a good standard hairspray with a light to medium hold and a slight stiff feel that can easily be brushed through. It contains mostly alcohol, plant water, film formers, conditioning agents, plant oil, silicone, and fragrance.

Rusk

For more information on Rusk, call (800) 829 RUSK or visit its Web site at www.rusk1.com.

☺ **Look Gentle Cleanse for Normal Hair** *($5 for 8 ounces)* contains mostly water, detergent cleansing agents, lather agent, thickeners, conditioning agents, detangling agents, film former, fragrance, and preservatives. This is a standard shampoo that would work well for normal to slightly dry hair that is normal to fine or thin in thickness.

☺ **Moist Wash Luxurious Moisturizing Cleanse** *($5 for 8 ounces)* contains mostly water, detergent cleansing agents, lather agent, thickeners, detangling agents/ film formers, conditioning agents, fragrance, preservatives, and coloring agents. This standard shampoo would work well for normal to slightly dry hair that is fine or thin in thickness. It can easily build up on the hair.

☹ **Sensories Brilliance Grapefruit & Honey Color Protect Shampoo** *($8.80 for 13.5 ounces)* uses sodium lauryl sulfate and sodium C14-17 alkyl sec sulfonate as the main cleansing agents, which makes it too drying for the hair and scalp.

☹ **Sensories Calm Guarana & Ginger Nourishing Shampoo** *($8.80 for 13 ounces)* uses TEA-lauryl sulfate and sodium C14-17 alkyl sec sulfonate as the main cleansing agents, which makes it too drying for the hair and scalp.

☺ **Sensories Full Green Tea & Alfalfa Shampoo** *($8.80 for 13 ounces)* contains mostly water, detergent cleansing agents, lather agent, conditioning agents, detangling agent/film former, fragrance, slip agent, preservatives, and coloring agents. The plant extracts have no effect on hair. This is a standard shampoo that would work well for normal to dry hair that is normal to fine or thin in thickness.

☺ **Sensories Moist Sunflower & Apricot Shampoo** *($8.50 for 13 ounces)* contains mostly water, detergent cleansing agents, lather agents, conditioning agents, plant extracts, detangling agents, film former, fragrance, slip agent, preservatives, and coloring agents. This is a standard shampoo that would work well for normal to dry hair that is normal to fine or thin in thickness.

☺ **Sensories Smoother Passionflower & Aloe Shampoo** *($8.80 for 13 ounces)* is almost identical to the Sunflower & Apricot version above and the same comments apply.

☺ **ResQ Intensive Hair Treatment** *($10.96 for 6 ounces)* contains mostly water, thickeners, detangling agent, conditioning agents, detangling agent, silicone, slip agent, fragrance, and preservatives. This isn't intensive in the least; it is just a good conditioner for normal to dry hair of any thickness.

☺ **ResQ Restorative Conditioner Normal to Dry Hair** *($9 for 12 ounces)* is almost identical to the Intensive Hair Treatment above and the same comments apply.

☺ **Sensories Calm Guarana & Ginger 60 Second Hair Revive** *($8.95 for 13 ounces)* is almost identical to the Intensive Hair Treatment above and the same comments apply.

☺ **Sensories Invisible Hibiscus & Kukui Foaming Detangler** *($9.90 for 13 ounces)* contains mostly water, detangling agents, conditioning agents, plant oil, plant extract, silicones, thickeners, fragrance, preservatives, and coloring agents. This is a good leave-in conditioner that would work well for normal to dry hair of any thickness.

☺ **Treatment Ultra Rich Conditioner** *($11 for 5 ounces)* contains mostly water, detangling agent/film former, thickeners, conditioning agents, silicone, preservatives, and fragrance. This isn't all that rich, but it is a good conditioner for normal to dry hair of any thickness.

☺ **Sensories Brilliance Grapefruit & Honey Leave-in Color Protector** *($9.90 for 8 ounces)* contains mostly water, silicones, conditioning agents, plant extracts, detangling agents, film former, slip agent, fragrance, preservatives, and coloring agents. This is a good, lightweight, leave-in conditioner that would work well for normal hair of any thickness, mostly to help with combing.

☺ **Sheer Brilliance Polisher for Smooth, Refining & Shining** *($13 for 4 ounces)* is a standard silicone serum that is overpriced, but it would work well to add shine and a silky feel to hair.

☺ **Shining Sheen & Movement Mist** *($12.10 for 4 ounces)* is similar to the Sheer Brilliance version above, only this one is in spray form.

☺ **Radical Sheen Texturizing Polishing Gel** *($15.35 for 3 ounces)* contains mostly slip agents, silicone, water, film former, thickeners, and preservatives. This is mostly a silicone serum in gel form. It has minimal to no hold and no stiff or sticky feel. It works well to smooth coarse, curly, or frizzy hair.

☺ **Jel Fx** *($5.84 for 5 ounces)* contains mostly water, film former, thickeners, conditioning agents, silicones, slip agents, fragrance, and preservatives. This is a good standard styling gel with a light to medium hold and minimal stiff or sticky feel.

☺ **Jele Gloss Bodifying Lotion** *($8.80 for 12 ounces)* contains mostly water, film former, castor oil, thickeners, fragrance, slip agents, silicone, conditioning agents, more fragrance, and preservatives. This is a good standard styling lotion with a medium hold that can have a somewhat stiff, sticky feel.

☺ **Blofoam Spray-on Texturizing Foam** *($11 for 10 ounces)* is a standard mousse that contains mostly plant water, propellants, alcohol, film formers, silicone, slip agents, thickeners, and fragrance. It has a light to medium hold with minimal to no stiff, sticky feel.

☺ **Mousse Volumizing Foam** *($12.10 for 8 ounces)* is similar to the Blofoam one above, only with slightly more hold and a slightly more sticky feel.

☺ **Wired Internal Restructure Multiple Personality Styling Cream** *($10.10 for 6 ounces)*. What a great name for a standard styling cream! This contains mostly water, thickener, detangling agents, film formers, castor oil, alcohol, conditioning agents, silicone, plant extracts, slip agents, fragrance, and preservatives. It has minimal hold and minimal to no stiff or sticky feel. It can control stubborn curls and frizzies, but use it sparingly—it can look heavy and greasy if overdone.

☺ **Str8 Anti-Frizz/Anti-Curl Lotion** *($9.50 for 6 ounces)* contains mostly water, film former, castor oil, silicones, conditioning agents, detangling agents, fragrance, thickeners, and preservatives. This is a styling lotion that has a light hold and minimal to no stiff or sticky feel. It would work well to straighten coarse, thick hair and smooth frizzies.

☹ **Radical Hair Creme Thickening Styling Creme** *($14 for 5 ounces)* is a heavy, waxy, gel-like cream that can leave a white, spackle-like coating on the hair that feels like . . . well, wax. That may be radical for some, but I don't think they're reading this book.

☺ **Thick Body and Texture Amplifier** *($10.90 for 6 ounces)* contains mostly water, alcohol, detangling agents/film formers, conditioning agents, silicone, slip agents, fragrance, and preservatives. It's a lightweight styling spray with a light hold and minimal stiff or sticky feel.

☺ **Radical Hold** *($9.95 for 8 ounces)* is a standard hairspray with a medium to firm hold and a stiff feel, though it can be brushed through. It contains mostly alcohol, water, film formers, silicone, and fragrance.

☺ **Worx Atomizer Fixing/Finishing Spray** *($12.50 for 10 ounces)* is almost identical to the Radical Hold above, only in aerosol form, and the same comments apply.

☺ **Worx Working/Finishing Spray** *($12.50 for 10 ounces)* is almost identical to the Radical Hold above, only in aerosol form, and the same basic comments apply.

☺ **W8less Plus Extra Hold Shaping and Control Myst** *($11 for 10 ounces)* is almost identical to the Radical Hold above, only this one is in aerosol form; the same basic comments apply.

☺ **W8less Shaping and Control Myst** *($10 for 2 ounces)* is almost identical to the Radical Hold above, only this one is in aerosol form, and the same basic comments apply.

☺ **Spray Bombe Working/Finishing Spray** *($8 for 8 ounces)* is almost identical to the Radical Hold above and the same comments apply.

☹ **Sensories Masque Balm Mint & Babassu Treatment** *($11 for 6 ounces)* contains clay as the second ingredient, which is drying for hair and scalp. Plus, when the clay dries it can chip away at the cuticle layer of hair.

Salon Selectives

Assuming that salons set the standard for product formulations (they don't, but assuming they do), a number of the products here would not be the ones they would choose, at least not if they knew better. Some of these are among the most consistently poorly formulated hair-care products I've reviewed. Either the formulations contain problematic ingredients, or else they are just so ordinary and standard that they make you wonder, "Why bother?" If you only need hairsprays or gels, there are some good inexpensive options here, but if you need more serious help this is not the line to consider. For more information on Salon Selectives, call (800) 621-3379.

☺ **Botanical Blends Shampoo Nourishing with Aloe Mango** *($1.96 for 15 ounces)* contains mostly water, detergent cleansing agents, lather agent, silicone, plant extract, slip agent, thickeners, detangling agent, preservatives, fragrance, vitamins, and alcohol. This shampoo also has a small amount of TEA-dodecylbenzenesulfonate, which can be drying to hair and scalp. It may not be enough to be a problem, but why have this in here at all?

☹ **Botanical Blends Shampoo Strengthening with Melon Rose** *($1.96 for 15 ounces)* contains ammonium xylenesulfonate, which can be drying for the hair and drying and irritating for the scalp.

☹ **Botanical Blends Shampoo Volumizing with Citrus Peach** *($1.96 for 15 ounces)* contains ingredients with some of the same problems as the Aloe Mango version above, as well as lemon oil and orange oil, all of which can be problems for the scalp.

☹ **Shampoo Level 1 Frequent Use Formula** *($1.96 for 15 ounces)* contains ammonium xylenesulfonate, which can be drying for the hair and drying and irritating for the scalp. It also contains peppermint, which can be irritating for the scalp and skin as well.

☹ **Shampoo Level 3 Revitalizing** *($1.96 for 15 ounces)* contains ammonium xylenesulfonate, which can be drying for the hair and drying and irritating for the scalp.

The Reviews S

☺ **Shampoo Level 4 Extra Moisturizing** *($1.96 for 15 ounces)* is just a basic, silicone-based shampoo, which makes this an extremely standard two-in-one shampoo. It also contains a tiny amount of TEA-dodecylbenzenesulfonate, which can be drying for hair and scalp.

☺ **Shampoo Level 5 Balanced** *($1.96 for 15 ounces)* contains ammonium xylenesulfonate, which can be drying for the hair and drying and irritating for the scalp.

☺ **Shampoo Level 6 Bodifying** *($1.96 for 15 ounces)* is similar to the Level 4 above, only with film former. It also contains a tiny amount of TEA-dodecyl-benzenesulfonate, which can be drying for hair and scalp.

☺ **Shampoo Level 7 Daily Clarifying** *($1.96 for 15 ounces)* contains ammonium xylenesulfonate, which can be drying for the hair and drying and irritating for the scalp.

☺ **Botanical Blends Conditioner Nourishing with Aloe Mango** *($1.96 for 15 ounces)* contains mostly water, thickeners, silicones, conditioning agent, plant extract, more thickeners, preservatives, fragrance, castor oil, and slip agents. This product isn't nourishing, but it is an OK basic conditioner for normal to slightly dry hair of any thickness. It does contain a tiny amount of sulfur, which adds a small risk of stripping hair color.

☺ **Botanical Blends Conditioner Strengthening with Melon Rose** *($1.96 for 15 ounces)* contains mostly water, thickeners, silicones, detangling agent, slip agent, plant extracts, more thickeners, preservatives, and fragrance. This is a good basic conditioner for normal to slightly dry hair of any thickness, but it won't strengthen a hair on your head.

☺ **Botanical Blends Conditioner Volumizing with Citrus Peach** *($1.96 for 15 ounces)* contains lemon oil and orange oil, so do not use this near the scalp. Other than that, it is similar to the Strengthening version above and the same comments apply.

Conditioner Type B Body Building *($1.96 for 15 ounces)* is similar to the Strengthening version above and the same comments apply.

☺ **Conditioner Type E Shine Enhancing** *($1.96 for 15 ounces)* is similar to the Strengthening version above and the same comments apply.

☺ **Conditioner Type F Deep Fortifying** *($1.96 for 15 ounces)* contains a tiny amount of sulfur, which still adds a small risk of stripping hair color.

☺ **Conditioner Type M Moisturizing** *($1.96 for 15 ounces)* contains mostly water, thickeners, silicones, conditioning agents, fragrance, more thickeners, preservatives, water-binding agents, slip agents, and vitamins. This is a good basic moisturizer for normal to slightly dry hair of any thickness. The minuscule amounts of vitamins and water-binding agents in here are almost not worth mentioning.

☺ **Conditioner Type P Protective** *($1.96 for 15 ounces)* won't protect a hair on your head—it is just an extremely standard conditioner that would work OK for normal to slightly dry hair of any thickness. It contains mostly water, thickeners, detangling agent, silicone, conditioning agents, fragrance, more thickeners, and preservatives.

☺ **Conditioner Type L Light Conditioning Spray** *($1.67 for 7 ounces)* contains mostly water, silicones, conditioning agent, detangling agents, slip agent, thickeners, fragrance, and preservatives. This is a good leave-in conditioner for normal to dry hair of any thickness.

☺ **Smoothing Gel Flexible Control Gel Level 10** *($1.67 for 7 ounces)* contains mostly water, film former, thickeners, more film formers, silicone, slip agent, preservatives, and fragrance. It is a good, light- to medium-hold gel with minimal stiff or sticky feel.

☺ **Texturizing Gel Max Control Level 15 Alcohol-Free** *($1.67 for 7 ounces)* is almost identical to the Smoothing Gel above and the same comments apply.

☺ **Sculpting Gel Ultra Control Level 20 Alcohol Free** *($1.67 for 7 ounces)* is almost identical to the Smoothing Gel above and the same comments apply.

☺ **Botanical Blends Texturizing Gel Extra Control Kiwi Jasmine Blend Alcohol-Free** *($1.67 for 7 ounces)* is almost identical to the Smoothing Gel Flexible above and the same comments apply.

☺ **Spray Gel Max Control Level 15** *($1.67 for 7 ounces)* is a good basic spray gel with a light hold and minimal stiff or sticky feel. It contains mostly water, alcohol, film formers, detangling agent, slip agents, fragrance, and preservatives.

☺ **Styling Foam Flexible Control Level 10 Air Infused Alcohol-Free** *($1.67 for 7 ounces)* is a standard nonpropellant mousse (the foam comes from a packaging technique that aerates the ingredients). It contains mostly water, film formers, detangling agent, fragrance, and preservatives. It has a medium hold and a slight stiff, sticky feel.

☺ **Botanical Blends Bodifying Mousse Extra Control Kiwi Jasmine Alcohol-Free** *($1.67 for 7 ounces)* is a standard mousse with a light hold and a slight sticky feel that contains mostly water, propellant, plant extracts, slip agents, fragrance, detangling agents/film formers, preservatives, and castor oil.

☺ **Shaping Mousse Maximum Control Level 15 Alcohol-Free** *($1.67 for 7 ounces)* is a standard mousse with a medium hold and a somewhat sticky feel that contains mostly water, propellant, detangling agents/film formers, slip agents, fragrance, silicone, and preservatives.

☺ **Volumizing Mousse Flexible Control Level 10 Alcohol-Free** *($1.67 for 7 ounces)* is a standard mousse with a light hold and minimal stiff feel that contains mostly water, propellant, detangling agents/film formers, slip agents, fragrance, silicone, and preservatives.

☺ **Perfect Curls Flexible Control Level 10** *($1.67 for 7 ounces)* is a standard hairspray with a light hold and minimal stiff feel. It contains mostly alcohol, water, film formers, fragrance, slip agents, and silicone.

☺ **Finishing Spray Flexible Hold Level 10 Non-Aerosol** *($1.67 for 7 ounces)* is a standard hairspray with a medium hold and a somewhat stiff feel. It contains mostly alcohol, water, film formers, fragrance, slip agents, and silicone.

☺ **Finishing Spray Flexible Hold Level 10 Aerosol** *($1.67 for 7 ounces)* is almost identical to the Flexible Hold Level 10 above, only in aerosol form, and the same basic comments apply.

☺ **Finishing Spray Maximum Hold Level 15 Non-Aerosol Scented and Unscented** *($1.67 for 7 ounces)* is almost identical to the Flexible Hold Level 10 version above and the same comments apply.

☺ **Finishing Spray Maximum Hold Level 15 Aerosol** *($1.67 for 7 ounces)* is almost identical to the Flexible Hold Level 10 above, only this one is in aerosol form. The same basic comments apply.

☺ **Spritz Fixx Ultra Hold Level 20 Non-Aerosol** *($1.67 for 7 ounces)* is almost identical to the Flexible Hold Level 10 version above and the same comments apply.

☺ **Style Freeze Ultra Hold Level 20 Aerosol** *($1.67 for 7 ounces)* is almost identical to the Flexible Hold Level 10 version above and the same comments apply.

☺ **Botanical Blends Finishing Spray Extra Hold Kiwi Jasmine Blend Aerosol Dual Usage** *($1.67 for 7 ounces)* is almost identical to the Flexible Hold Level 10 version above only this one is in aerosol form; the same comments apply.

☺ **Botanical Blends Finishing Spray Extra Hold Kiwi Jasmine Blend Non-Aerosol** *($1.67 for 7 ounces)* is similar to the version above except in nonaerosol form, and the same basic comments apply.

Salon Style by Lamaur

For more information about Salon Style by Lamaur, call (612) 571-1234 or (800) 444-0699.

☺ **Conditioning Shampoo, Hydration with Detangling Silks** *($2.22 for 15 ounces)* contains mostly water, detergent cleansing agent, lather agent, film former, silicone, detangling agent, conditioning agents, plant extracts, thickeners, preservatives, and fragrance. This is a good shampoo for normal to dry hair that is fine or thin. It can cause buildup.

☺ **Moisture Potion Shampoo** *($2.22 for 15 ounces)* is similar to the one above and the same basic comments apply.

☺ **Nutrishine Shampoo** *($2.22 for 15 ounces)* contains mostly water, detergent cleansing agent, lather agent, thickeners, conditioning agent, plant extracts, detangling agents, film former, slip agent, and preservatives. This can't nourish anything, but it is a good basic shampoo for normal to slightly dry hair that is normal to fine or thin.

☺ **Strengthening Shampoo** *($2.22 for 15 ounces)* can't strengthen hair, but it is good for normal to slightly dry hair that is normal to fine or thin. It contains mostly water, detergent cleansing agent, lather agent, thickeners, conditioning agents, plant oil, vitamins, detangling agent/film former, slip agents, and preservatives.

☺ **Therapy Shampoo** *($2.22 for 15 ounces)* is similar to the Strengthening Shampoo above and the same comments apply.

☺ **Botanical Reconstructor Conditioner** *($2.22 for 20 ounces)* contains mostly water, detangling agents, thickeners, silicones, slip agents, film former, plant oil, conditioning agents, plant extracts, preservatives, and fragrance. This is a good standard conditioner for normal to slightly dry hair that has normal to fine or thin thickness.

☹ **Detangling Conditioner with Balsam and Biotin** *($2.22 for 15 ounces)* is almost identical to the Botanical Reconstructor above and the same basic comments apply. This version does contain balsam, which can build up on hair and feel stiff.

☺ **Moisture Potion Conditioner** *($2.22 for 20 ounces)* is almost identical to the Botanical Reconstructor above and the same basic comments apply.

☺ **Deep Conditioner, Hydrobalance Hair Masque** *($2.22 for 15 ounces)* is a standard conditioner for normal to slight dry hair that is normal to fine or thin in thickness. It contains mostly water, thickeners, detangling agents, film former, slip agent, conditioning agents, preservatives, and fragrance. This conditioner does contain a tiny amount of balsam, which can build up with repeated use and make hair feel stiff.

☺ **Design Elements Spray-on Styling Gel, Extra Hold** *($2.27 for 10 ounces)* is a standard spray gel with a light hold and minimal to no stiff or sticky feel. It contains mostly water, film former, slip agents, plant extracts, conditioning agent, thickeners, silicone, preservatives, and fragrance.

☺ **Shaping Elixxer Alcohol-Free Spray Gel, Natural Hold** *($2.29 for 8 ounces)* is a standard spray gel with a light hold and minimal to no stiff or sticky feel. It contains mostly water, film former, slip agents, plant extracts, conditioning agent, thickeners, silicone, preservatives, and fragrance.

☺ **Body Boost Alcohol-Free Mousse with Botanicals, Extra Hold** *($2.22 for 7 ounces)* is a standard mousse with a light to medium hold and minimal stiff or sticky feel. It contains mostly water, propellant, film formers, slip agents, conditioning agents, thickeners, detangling agent, silicone, preservatives, and fragrance.

☺ **Design Elements Non-Aerosol Hair Spray Flexible Hold** *($2.27 for 10 ounces)* is a standard hairspray with a light to medium hold and minimal stiff feel. It contains mostly alcohol, water, film former, silicone, conditioning agents, coloring agents, and fragrance.

☺ **ProMist Quick Drying Hairspray, Mega Hold** *($2.22 for 9.5 ounces)* is a standard aerosol hairspray with a medium hold and a slight stiff feel that can be brushed through. It contains mostly alcohol, propellant, film former, conditioning agent, silicone, and fragrance.

☺ **Protect 'N Shine Fixxer Hair Spray, Mega Hold with UVA Protectant** *($2.22 for 10.5 ounces)* is a standard nonaerosol hairspray with a light hold and minimal to no stiff feel that can easily be brushed through. It contains mostly alcohol, propellant, film former, conditioning agent, silicone, and fragrance. This spray cannot protect from UVA or any kind of sun exposure.

Schwarzkopf

This line goes way back to when Hans Schwarzkopf invented his first shampoo in 1903. Today Schwarzkopf is recognized in the salon trade as one of the major trendsetting and education sources in the industry. It has a large range of products and there's some incredible repetition between lines. Some good options are available here, but think twice about believing the claims—they just don't live up to the formulations.

For more information on Schwarzkopf, call (310) 604-0777, (800) 326-2855, or visit its Web site at www.schwarzkopf.com.

Bonacure by Schwarzkopf

☺ **Basic Beauty Shampoo for Frequent Use, Basic Formula** *($7.60 for 8.5 ounces)* contains mostly detergent cleansing agent, water, lather agent, thickeners, fragrance, detangling agent/film former, slip agents, castor oil, and preservatives. This is a good basic shampoo for normal hair that is fine or thin. It can easily build up on hair and feel stiff or sticky.

☺ **Extra Rich Repair Shampoo, Repair Formula** *($8.40 for 8.5 ounces)* is almost identical to the Basic Beauty version above, minus the castor oil; it is far less likely to cause buildup, but it won't repair anything. This is a good basic daily shampoo to prevent buildup for all hair types.

☺ **Volume Shampoo for Fine Hair, Volume Formula** *($7.90 for 8.5 ounces)* is almost identical to the Basic Beauty version above and the same comments apply.

☹ **Basic Beauty Spray Conditioner** *($8 for 6.8 ounces)* is a fairly ordinary leave-in conditioner that contains mostly water, alcohol, film former, silicone, detangling agent, and fragrance. The alcohol can be a problem for dry hair and you wouldn't want to get this on the scalp.

☺ **Extra Rich Repair Conditioner, Repair Formula** *($9.50 for 8.5 ounces)* isn't rich in the least; it is just a standard conditioner that would be OK for normal to slightly dry hair that is fine or thin. It contains mostly water, thickeners, detangling agent/film former, fragrance, and conditioning agent.

☺ **Intensive Moisturizing Treatment, Repair Formula** *($14.90 for 5.1 ounces)* isn't intensive by anyone's definition. It is just an extremely ordinary conditioner that would be OK for normal to dry hair of any thickness. It contains mostly water, thickeners, mineral oil, more thickeners, preservatives, and a tiny amount of plant oil.

☺ **Volume Spray Conditioner for Fine Hair, Volume Formula** *($8 for 6.8 ounces)* is just water, alcohol, film former, detangling agent, and fragrance. This is a very lightweight, leave-in conditioner that can help with combing and add a bit of thickness, but not much. It would work well for normal hair. The amount of alcohol in here can be problematic in a conditioner and won't work well for dry hair.

☺ **Gloss Tonic, Specific Formula** *($8 for 5.1 ounces)* is a standard silicone spray that works well to add a silky feel and shine to hair.

☹ **Hair Body Volume, Support and Care for All Hair Types** *($9.90 for 6.8 ounces)* is almost identical to the Volume Spray above and the same warning applies.

Igora Color Care by Schwarzkopf

☺ **Shampoo** *($8.10 for 10.1 ounces)* contains mostly water, thickeners, detergent cleansing agent, detangling agent, more thickeners, mineral oil, fragrance, plant oil, and preservatives. There is nothing in this shampoo that can protect hair color, though it would be good for extremely dry hair that is coarse or thick.

☺ **Conditioner** *($9.90 for 10.1 ounces)* contains mostly water, thickeners, detangling agent, mineral oil, fragrance, plant oil, conditioning agent, preservatives, and coloring agents. This is a good standard conditioner for dry hair of any thickness.

☺ **Intensive Treatment** *($14.90 for 5.1 ounces)* isn't that intense; it's almost identical to the Conditioner above, and the same comments apply.

☺ **Rinse for Color-Treated Hair** *($9.50 for 8.45 ounces)* is almost identical to the Conditioner above and the same basic comments apply.

Natural Styling by Schwarzkopf

☺ **Conditioning Shampoo** *($5.90 for 6.8 ounces)* contains mostly water, detergent cleansing agent, lather agent, thickeners, conditioning agent, preservative, fragrance, and detangling agent. This is a good basic shampoo for everyday use with minimal risk of buildup; it also provides minimal to no conditioning as a result.

☺ **Conditioning Rinse** *($6.40 for 6.8 ounces)* contains mostly water, detangling agent/film former, thickener, silicones, fragrance, and preservatives. This is a very basic but good conditioner for dry hair that is fine or thin.

☺ **Shaping Gel** *($7.90 for 8.11 ounces)* is a good basic gel that contains mostly water, film former, thickeners, and fragrance. It has a medium hold and a somewhat sticky feel that can still be brushed through.

☺ **Setting Lotion** *($8.20 for 8.45 ounces)* contains mostly water, alcohol, film former, fragrance, thickeners, and castor oil. This standard styling spray has a light hold and minimal to no stiff or sticky feel.

☺ **Curl Revitalizer** *($7.50 for 8.45 ounces)* contains mostly water, alcohol, detangling agent/film former, and fragrance. This is a lightweight styling spray that has a soft hold and minimal to no stiff feel.

Silhouette Styling System by Schwarzkopf

☺ **Style Care Shampoo #1** *($6 for 6.8 ounces)* contains mostly water, detergent cleansing agents, lather agent, slip agent, thickeners, fragrance, detangling agent/film former, castor oil, preservatives, and coloring agent. This is a good shampoo for normal hair that is fine or thin. It can easily build up on hair.

☺ **Style Care Conditioner #2** *($7.90 for 6.8 ounces)* is a simple conditioner that contains mostly water, thickeners, detangling agent, fragrance, and conditioning agents. It can work well for normal hair of any thickness to help with combing, but that's it.

☺ **Intensive Treatment #3** *($9.30 for 4.1 ounces)* is a simple conditioner in aerosol form that contains mostly water, propellant, thickeners, detangling agent, plant oil, and film former. It can work well for normal hair of any thickness to help with combing, but it is hardly intensive.

☺ **Gloss Creme Control & Shine** *($11.90 for 1.8 ounces)* is a standard silicone serum that can add a silky-soft feel and shine to hair.

☺ **Moulding Creme Ultra Control** *($13 for 5.3 ounces)* isn't a cream but a good standard gel with a minimal to light hold and minimal to no stiff or sticky feel. It contains mostly water, film former, thickeners, slip agents, silicone, preservatives, fragrance, and coloring agents.

☺ **Styling Gel Super Hold** *($7.90 for 8.75 ounces)* is a good standard styling gel with a medium hold and minimal stiff or sticky feel. It contains mostly water, film formers, alcohol, thickeners, silicone, fragrance, preservatives, and coloring agents.

☺ **Non-Aerosol Styling Mousse Natural Hold** *($13.90 for 6.8 ounces)*. The ingredients for this mousse are aerated in a pump delivery that creates a wet-feeling foam. It contains mostly water, film formers, alcohol, detangling agent, and fragrance. This ordinary group of ingredients gives a soft, light hold with minimal to stiff or sticky feel.

☺ **Non-Aerosol Styling Mousse Super Hold** *($13.90 for 6.8 ounces)* is almost identical to the Natural Hold above, with slightly more hold and a slightly more sticky feel, but only slightly.

☺ **Styling Mousse Natural Hold** *($8.50 for 6.5 ounces)* is similar to the Non-Aerosol Natural Hold above, only this one is a real mousse delivered with propellant. It has a light to medium hold and minimal to no stiff or sticky feel.

☺ **Styling Mousse Super Hold** *($8.50 for 6.5 ounces)* is almost identical to the one above and the same comments apply.

☺ **Hairspray Super Hold (Aerosol)** *($15 for 13.6 ounces)* is a standard aerosol hairspray with a medium to firm hold and a stiff feel that does allow you to brush through hair. It contains mostly alcohol, propellant, film former, silicone, and fragrance.

☺ **Non-Aerosol Hairspray Natural Hold** *($9.50 for 8.45 ounces)* is a standard hairspray with a medium hold and a slight stiff feel that can be brushed through. It contains mostly alcohol, propellant, film former, silicone, and fragrance.

☺ **Non-Aerosol Hairspray Super Hold** *($8.80 for 8.45 ounces)* is almost identical to the Natural Hold version above and the same comments apply.

Scruples

For more information on Scruples, call (800) 457-0016 or visit its Web site at www.scrupleshaircare.com.

☹ **Hair Clearifier Shampoo** *($3.50 for 4 ounces)* uses sodium C14-16 olefin sulfate as the main cleansing agent, which can be drying for the hair and irritating and drying for the scalp. It also contains menthol, and that can also cause scalp problems.

☹ **Moisture Bath Moisture Replenishing Shampoo** *($3.50 for 4 ounces)* uses sodium C14-16 olefin sulfate as the main cleansing agent, which can be drying for the hair and irritating and drying for the scalp.

☺ **Renewal Shampoo for Color Treated Hair** *($3.50 for 4 ounces)* contains mostly water, detergent cleansing agent, lather agent, thickeners, water-binding agents, silicones, detangling agents/film formers, slip agents, preservatives, and fragrance. This is a good basic shampoo for someone with normal to slightly dry hair that is normal to fine or thin. There is nothing in here to help color-treated hair.

☺ **Smooth Out Shampoo** *($5.95 for 8.5 ounces)* contains balm mint, which can be a problem for the scalp. Other than that, it is almost identical to the Renewal Shampoo above and the same comments apply.

☹ **Structure Bath Extra Body Strengthening Shampoo** (*$3.50 for 4 ounces*) uses sodium C14-16 olefin sulfate as the main cleansing agent, which can be drying for the hair and irritating and drying for the scalp.

☺ **Cohesion Intercellular Hair Binder** (*$5.95 for 4 ounces*) contains mostly water, thickeners, detangling agent, water-binding agents, silicone, conditioning agents, castor oil, slip agents, preservatives, and fragrance. This can be helpful for coarse or very dry hair.

☺ **ER Emergency Repair for Damaged Hair** (*$9.95 for 6 ounces*) contains mostly water, thickeners, detangling agents, water-binding agents, silicone, conditioning agents, film former, slip agents, preservatives, and fragrance. It can't repair one hair on your head, but it is a good conditioner for normal to slightly dry hair of any thickness.

☺ **Moisturex Intensive Moisturizing Hair Treatment** (*$5.95 for 4 ounces*) contains mostly water, thickeners, detangling agents, water-binding agents, silicone, conditioning agents, castor oils, slip agents, preservatives, and fragrance. This can be helpful for coarse or very dry hair.

☺ **Quickseal Fortifying Creme Conditioner** (*$5.95 for 4 ounces*) contains mostly water, thickeners, castor oil, detangling agent, conditioning agents, water-binding agents, fragrance, and preservatives. This conditioner can be effective for dry hair that is coarse, but it can easily build up.

☺ **Renewal Hair Conditioner for Color Treated Hair** (*$5.95 for 4 ounces*) contains mostly water, thickeners, detangling agent, conditioning agents, water-binding agents, silicones, slip agents, preservatives, and fragrance. This is a good conditioner for normal to dry hair of any thickness.

☹ **Smooth Out Conditioner** (*$9.95 for 8.5 ounces*) won't smooth out anything. It is almost identical to the Renewal Hair Conditioner above, and the same basic comments apply. This product does contain balm mint, a potential skin irritant, so keep it off the scalp.

☺ **Reconstruct Leave-in Protein Spray** (*$9.95 for 8.5 ounces*) is a good leave-in conditioner for normal to dry hair that is fine or thin. It contains mostly, water, conditioning agents, water-binding agents, silicones, thickeners, detangling agents, film formers, preservatives, and fragrance.

☺ **$$$ Renewal Hair Therapy Polish** (*$19.95 for 4 ounces*) is a standard but very overpriced silicone serum that would indeed leave the hair feeling silky and soft as well as adding shine.

☺ **Spray Lites Hair Glosser** (*$8.95 for 4.2 ounces*) has too much alcohol, so the positives of the silicone in here are diminished. The gimmick with this spray is that it adds a small amount of glitter to the hair. That may be worth considering, but a silkier feel would have been preferable.

☺ **Tea Tree Sculpting Glaze Concentrate** *($7.95 for 8.5 ounces)* is a good styling gel that contains mostly water, film formers, thickeners, plant extract, conditioning agents, water-binding agent, silicones, castor oil, slip agents, preservatives, and fragrance. It has a light to medium hold with a slight stiff, sticky feel that can be brushed through. It does contain some amount of tea tree oil, but that serves no purpose for hair; it only has benefit for the scalp to fight dandruff or other scalp dermatitis.

☺ **Enforce Sculpting Glaze Concentrate** *($5.95 for 4 ounces)* is almost identical to the Tea Tree Sculpting Glaze above, just minus the tea tree oil.

☺ **Total Accents Precision Creme** *($9.95 for 5 ounces)* is more of a gel lotion than a cream but it does help smooth stubborn curls and frizzies with minimal to no hold and no stiff or sticky feel. It contains mostly water, thickeners, silicones, castor oil, more thickeners, film former, conditioning agents, water-binding agent, slip agents, fragrance, and preservatives.

☺ **Smooth Out Non-Chemical Straightening Gel** *($11.95 for 8.5 ounces)* is a next-to-no-hold gel, and that can help when styling hair smooth. It also has no stiff or sticky feel. It contains mostly water, thickeners, detangling agent, conditioning agents, silicone, preservatives, and fragrance.

☺ **Renewal Forming Gel for Color Treated Hair** *($6.50 for 6 ounces)* contains nothing specific for color-treated hair, though it is a good, basic, medium-hold styling gel with a somewhat sticky feel that can be brushed through. It contains mostly water, thickeners, film former, conditioning agents, water-binding agents, silicones, preservatives, and fragrance.

☺ **Creme Parfait Ultra Thick Styling Mousse** *($9.95 for 10.6 ounces)* is a good standard mousse that has a light to medium hold and minimal stiff or sticky feel. It contains mostly water, propellant, film formers, thickeners, conditioning agents, water-binding agent, silicones, and fragrance.

☺ **Emphasis Texturizing Styling Mousse** *($5.95 for 6 ounces)* is almost identical to the Creme Parfait above and the same comments apply.

☺ **More Emphasis Extra Body Styling Mousse** *($5.95 for 6 ounces)* is almost identical to the Creme Parfait above and the same basic comments apply.

☺ **Ultra Form Molding Spray** *($6.95 for 8.5 ounces)* is a standard hairspray that contains mostly alcohol, water, propellant, film former, water-binding agent, conditioning agent, slip agent, silicones, and fragrance. This has a medium to firm hold with a slight stiff or sticky feel.

☺ **High Definition Extra Dry Hair Spray** *($4.95 for 1.5 ounces)* is almost identical to the Ultra Form Molding Spray above only this one is in aerosol form, but the same comments apply.

☺ **Effects Fast Drying Styling Spray** *($5.95 for 10.6 ounces)* is almost identical to the Ultra Form Molding Spray above only this one is in aerosol form, but the same comments apply.

☺ **Effects Super Hold Finishing Spray** *($5.95 for 10.6 ounces)* is almost identical to the Ultra Form Molding Spray above only this one is in aerosol form, but the same comments apply.

☺ **Renewal Styling Spray for Colored Treated Hair** *($6.50 for 8.5 ounces)* is almost identical to the Ultra Form Molding Spray and the same comments apply.

☺ **Enforce Fast Drying Styling Spray** *($7.50 for 8.5 ounces)* is almost identical to the Ultra Form Molding Spray and the same comments apply.

☺ **Enforce Plus Extra Firm Holding Spray** *($7.50 for 8.5 ounces)* is almost identical to the Ultra Form Molding Spray, only this one does have a firmer hold and a stiffer feel, though it does allow you to brush through hair.

☺ **V2 Double Volume for Hair** *($9.95 for 8.5 ounces)* is a standard hairspray that has a light to medium hold and minimal stiff or sticky feel. It contains mostly alcohol, water, film formers, water-binding agent, conditioning agent, silicone, detangling agent, and fragrance.

Sebastian

Sebastian has an incredible array of products—it's a virtual playground of hair-care choices. Of course, a lot of the line is redundant and unnecessarily complicated; after all, how many shampoos with standard detergent cleansing agents are needed in any one line? The same goes for the huge selection of hairsprays, gels, and conditioners. There are good products to be found in the Sebastian line, but sifting through the arsenal isn't easy, either for you or the hairstylist!

For more information on Sebastian, call (800) 829-7322 or visit its Web site at www.sebastian-intl.com.

Collectives by Sebastian

☹ **Blue Mint Shampoo for Oily Hair** *($6.30 for 10.2 ounces)* contains mint, and that can cause a problem with skin irritation, although mint has no effect on oil whatsoever. This shampoo also contains conditioning agents, which can be a problem for oily hair or an oily scalp.

☺ **Cello Shampoo Extraordinary Shine for Normal to Slightly Oily Hair** *($6.30 for 10.2 ounces)* is inappropriate for oily hair because it contains far too many conditioning agents. However, it would work fine for someone with normal to dry hair that is normal to fine or thin. It contains mostly water, detergent cleansing agents, lather agent, thickeners, conditioning agents, detangling agent/film former, plant extracts, vitamins, fragrance, preservatives, and coloring agents.

☺ **Cello Shampoo for Normal to Dry Hair** *($6.30 for 10 ounces)* is almost identical to the Slightly Oily Hair version above and the same comments apply.

☺ **Green Apple Shampoo for Normal Hair** *($5.80 for 10.2 ounces)* contains mostly water, detergent cleansing agents, lather agent, slip agent, conditioning agents, detangling agent, thickeners, fragrance, preservatives, and coloring agents. This is a good basic shampoo for normal to slightly dry hair of any thickness.

☺ **Misty Rose Shampoo for Dry Hair** *($6.30 for 10.2 ounces)* contains mostly water, detergent cleansing agents, lather agent, thickener, conditioning agents, detangling agent/film former, plant oil, fragrance, preservatives, and coloring agents. This is a good basic shampoo for normal to slightly dry hair that is normal to fine or thin.

☺ **Moisture Shampoo for Normal to Dry Hair** *($7.30 for 10.2 ounces)* contains mostly water, detergent cleansing agents, lather agent, detangling agents, thickener, conditioning agents, preservatives, fragrance, and coloring agents. This is a good basic shampoo for normal to slightly dry hair of any thickness.

☺ **Potion 5 Shampoo Revitalizing Treatment Shampoo for Hair and Scalp** *($4.25 for 8.5 ounces)* contains mostly water, detergent cleansing agents, lather agent, plant oil, plant extracts, water-binding agent, conditioning agents, thickeners, detangling agent/film former, castor oil, preservatives, fragrance, and coloring agents. This is a good basic shampoo for normal to slightly dry hair that is normal to fine or thin. It is supposed to wash out Potion 7, but with the number of film formers in this shampoo that is unlikely. With repeated use you would get buildup.

☺ **Cello-Primer Detangler Build-Up Remover** *($5.50 for 5.1 ounces)* contains mostly water, conditioning agent, thickeners, detangling agent/film former, preservatives, and fragrance. This is just a good leave-in conditioner for normal hair but the film former in here can lead to buildup; this doesn't remove anything from hair except tangles.

☺ **Formulating Creme Deep Conditioner 5-Minute Conditioning Treatment** *($17.50 for 10.2 ounces)* is just a standard conditioner and, like most every other conditioner, if you leave it on your hair for five minutes or longer, it will penetrate better and help hair to feel softer. It contains mostly water, thickeners, detangling agents, conditioning agents, film formers, more thickeners, silicone, vitamins, preservatives, fragrance, and coloring agents. This is a good conditioner for dry hair that has normal to fine or thin thickness.

☺ **Moisture Base Moisturizing Conditioner** *($7.75 for 5.1 ounces)* contains mostly water, detangling agents, thickeners, conditioning agents, film former, Vaseline, preservatives, fragrance, and coloring agents. This is a good conditioner for dry hair that is normal to fine or thin.

The Reviews S

☺ **Sheen Instant Conditioner** *($11.30 for 10.2 ounces)* contains mostly water, slip agent, detangling agent, alcohol, plant oil, thickeners, film former, conditioning agents, preservatives, fragrance, and coloring agents. This is a good conditioner for dry hair that is normal to fine or thin.

☺ **Cello-Fix Leave On Conditioner Spray for Damaged Hair** *($12 for 10.2 ounces)* contains mostly water, slip agents, detangling agents, film former, conditioning agents, silicone, preservatives, and fragrance. This is a good, standard, leave-in conditioner for normal to dry hair that is normal to fine or thin. It has no special properties for damaged hair.

☺ **Thick-Ends: An Ends Conditioner** *($11.30 for 5.1 ounces)* contains mostly water, slip agent, conditioning agents, thickeners, water-binding agents, preservatives, fragrance, and coloring agents. This is a good, liquidy gel that is meant to be a leave-in conditioner, but it is actually more of a very lightweight styling liquid. It has a minimal sticky feel and can work well to add a feel of thickness and help with styling.

☺ **Potion 7 Restructure and Reconditioning Treatment** *($17.50 for 5.1 ounces)* is more of a styling gel than reconditioning treatment, and the standard formula doesn't warrant the price. It contains mostly water, slip agents, conditioning agent, detangling agents, thickeners, film former, emollient, plant extracts, preservatives, fragrance, and coloring agent. This is a good lightweight styling gel with an extremely light hold and minimal to no stiff or sticky feel. It can help smooth out frizzies or form curls.

☺ **Potion 9 Wearable Treatment to Restore and Restyle, Super Concentrated** *($13.50 for 5.1 ounces)* contains mostly water, slip agents, conditioning agent, detangling agents, thickeners, film former, plant oils, fragrant oils, plant extracts, preservatives, fragrance, and coloring agent. This is a good lightweight styling gel with an extremely light hold and minimal stiff or sticky feel. It can help smooth out frizzies or form curls. It is actually quite similar to the Thick-Ends Conditioner above and similar to Potion 7 as well.

☹ **$$$ 2 + 1 Interim Reconstructor Home Maintenance Reconstructor Treatment** *($28.99 for 12 1-ounce foil packs)* is just an extremely overpriced, extremely standard conditioner. It contains mostly water, thickeners, detangling agent/film former, slip agent, conditioning agents, more film former, plant oil, vitamins, fragrance, and preservatives. Like any conditioner that you leave on for more than a minute, it can penetrate better and make the hair feel softer, but nothing is repaired. If it was, why would you need 12 packets? Wouldn't your hair be fixed with the first or the second "treatment"?

☹ **Hi-Contrast Gel Reinforcing Gel** *($9.80 for 5.1 ounces)* contains mostly water, film former, conditioning agents, thickeners, silicone, detangling agent/film former, preservatives, fragrance, and coloring agents. For some reason this gel contains hydrogen peroxide, which can bleach hair with repeated use. If that doesn't bother you, this is a good gel with a medium hold and a somewhat sticky feel that does let you brush through hair.

☺ **Wet Liquid Sculpting Gel** *($7.80 for 10.2 ounces)* contains mostly water, detangling agent/film former, conditioning agents, thickeners, more detangling agent, preservatives, and fragrance. This is a standard but good liquidy gel with a light hold and little to no stiff or sticky feel.

☺ **Fizz Styling Foam** *($12.80 for 8 ounces)* is a standard mousse with a light to medium hold and a somewhat sticky feel that does allow you to brush through hair. It contains mostly water, alcohol, film former, propellant, conditioning agents, thickeners, silicone, detangling agents, fragrance, and coloring agents.

☺ **Fizz Extra Extra Firm Styling Foam** *($13.40 for 8 ounces)* is almost identical to the Fizz Styling Foam above and the same comments apply.

☺ **$$$ Grease Flexible Fixative** *($8.10 for 1.5 ounces)* contains mostly Vaseline, mineral oil, thickeners, silicone, fragrance, and preservatives. This is indeed "flexible" grease in wax form, with no hold—just slick control to smooth stubborn frizzies and curls. It can look greasy and heavy, so use it sparingly.

☺ **Molding Mud Sculpting Bonder** *($14.30 for 4 ounces)* contains mostly water, thickeners, slip agent, preservatives, film former, silicone, fragrance, and coloring agents. This has a light hold but a heavy, sticky, wax base that can help smooth stubborn curls and frizzies. It can look heavy and greasy, so use it sparingly.

☺ **Shpritz Light Finishing Spray** *($8 for 10.2 ounces)* contains mostly water, film former, conditioning agents, slip agents, preservatives, coloring agent, and fragrance. This has a soft, light hold and minimal to no stiff or sticky feel.

☺ **Shpritz Forte Extra Strength Finishing Spray** *($8.50 for 10.2 ounces)* doesn't add extra strength; it's just a standard hairspray with a medium hold and minimal stiff feel that can easily be brushed through. It contains mostly alcohol, water, film former, conditioning agents, slip agent, and fragrance.

☺ **Hold & Mold Spray Gel Styling and Finishing Spray** *($10.30 for 10.2 ounces)* is similar to the Shpritz Forte Extra above and the same basic comments apply.

Laminates by Sebastian

☺ **Shampoo Polishing Shampoo** *($8.50 for 8.5 ounces)* is a standard, silicone-based shampoo similar to any two-in-one shampoo. This one contains mostly water, detergent cleansing agent, lather agent, conditioning agents, slip agent, silicone, thickeners, detangling agent/film former, plant extracts, preservatives, fragrance, and coloring agents. This is a good shampoo for someone with normal to dry hair of any thickness. It can cause buildup.

☺ **Conditioner** *($12 for 8.5 ounces)* contains mostly water, thickeners, silicone, detangling agent, slip agent, more silicones, mineral oil, plant oil, conditioning agents, detangling agent/film former, preservatives, and fragrance. This is a good conditioner for dry to extremely dry hair of any thickness.

☺ **$$$ Hi Gloss Spray** *($9.50 for 1.7 ounces)* is a standard silicone spray that contains mostly silicone, fragrance, and coloring agents. It can add a soft, silky feel and shine to hair.

☺ **$$$ Drops** *($9.50 for 1.7 ounces)* is a standard silicone serum that contains mostly silicone and fragrance. It can add shine and a soft, silky feel to hair.

☺ **$$$ Gel** *($17.80 for 5.1 ounces)* is mostly a silicone serum in gel form. It contains silicones, detangling agent, detangling agent/film former, alcohol, conditioning agent, preservatives, fragrance, and coloring agents. It has no hold but it can help to add a soft feel and shine to hair, and can smooth out stubborn frizzies.

☺ **$$$ Get a Grip Liquid Texture** *($16 for 5.1 ounces)* contains mostly water, detangling agent/film former, conditioning agents, silicone, more detangling agent, more film former, plant extract, thickeners, preservatives, fragrance, and coloring agents. There is menthol in here, a skin irritant, so keep this away from the roots of the hair. Other than that, this is a medium- to firm-hold gel-like lotion with a somewhat sticky feel that allows you to brush through hair.

☺ **$$$ Get It Straitt** *($17 for 8.5 ounces)* contains mostly water, slip agents, conditioning agents, silicones, plant extract, film former, thickeners, detangling agent, preservatives, and fragrance. This is just an overpriced, light-hold, liquidy gel with no stiff or sticky feel. It can help to smooth hair or to create any style that doesn't need much control. There are far less expensive versions than this to consider.

☺ **Hair Spray (Aerosol)** *($10.50 for 8.5 ounces)* is a standard aerosol hairspray with a light hold and minimal stiff feel. It contains mostly alcohol, water, film former, plant extracts, silicone, slip agents, conditioning agent, and fragrance.

Performance Active by Sebastian

☺ **Cleanser: A Hair and Body Wash** *($8.30 for 8.5 ounces)* contains mostly water, detergent cleansing agents, lather agent, detangling agent/film former, plant extracts, vitamin, more detangling agents, conditioning agents, preservatives, fragrance, and coloring agents. Though I am definitely someone who believes in streamlining skin- and hair-care routines, this product won't do it. There is no reason to use detangling agents other than on your hair, they serve no purpose for skin. Other than that, this is a good basic shampoo for normal to dry hair that is normal to thin or fine.

☹ **Shampoo and Treatment** *($7 for 8.5 ounces)* contains menthol, a skin irritant, which can be a problem for the scalp.

☺ **Conditioner: A One Minute Conditioning Masque for Hair** *($20 for 8.5 ounces)* contains mostly water, silicones, thickeners, conditioning agents, detangling agents, film formers, plant extracts, plant oil, preservatives, fragrance, and coloring agents. This is a good standard conditioner for dry hair that is normal to fine or thin. The film formers in here can cause buildup.

☺ **Gelee** *($17.50 for 5.1 ounces)* contains mostly water, detangling agent/film former, slip agents, conditioning agents, plant extract, preservatives, fragrance, and coloring agents. This is a good conditioner for normal to slightly dry hair that is normal to fine or thin.

☺ **Gelee and Conditioner** *($22 for 8.5 ounces)* contains mostly plant water, thickeners, slip agents, conditioning agents, preservatives, fragrance, and coloring agents. This is a good, leave-in conditioner for normal to slightly dry hair of any thickness. It has no stiff or sticky feel but also doesn't add much hold or thickness.

☺ **Texturizer & Body Builder** *($16.50 for 8.5 ounces)* contains mostly water, thickeners, slip agents, conditioning agents, film former, plant extracts, preservatives, detangling agent, fragrance, and coloring agents. This is a standard gel that has a light to medium hold with a somewhat stiff or sticky feel that does let you brush through the hair.

☺ **Volumizer & Finishing Spray** *($13 for 8.5 ounces)* is a good standard hairspray with a light to medium hold and minimal to no stiff, sticky feel. It contains mostly alcohol, water, film formers, slip agents, plant extracts, conditioning agents, fragrance, and coloring agents.

Shaper Slipline by Sebastian

☺ **Shampoo, Conditioning Shampoo for all Hair Types** *($5.80 for 10.2 ounces)* contains mostly water, detergent cleansing agents, lather agent, slip agent, plant oil, silicone, thickeners, conditioning agents, detangling agents/film formers, plant extracts, preservatives, and fragrance. This is a good basic shampoo for normal to slightly dry hair of any thickness. The silicone, plant oil, and conditioning agents make this a problem for oily hair and scalp. The film formers make it a problem for coarse, thick hair.

☺ **Conditioner, Body Building Conditioner for All Hair Types** *($8.50 for 10.2 ounces)* contains mostly water, thickeners, detangling agents, conditioning agents, plant oil, silicone, detangling agent/film former, preservatives, fragrance, and coloring agents. This is a good conditioner for normal to dry hair of any thickness. The plant oil, silicone, and conditioning agents make this a problem for oily scalp and hair.

☺ **Clean Gel** *($10.50 for 10.2 ounces)* contains mostly water, film formers, slip agents, conditioning agents, plant oil, silicone, thickeners, preservatives, fragrance, and coloring agents. This standard gel has a light to medium hold with a slight stiff, sticky feel.

☺ **Liquid Shaper Styling Gel and Fast Drying Hair Spray** *($10.80 for 8.5 ounces)* is a standard aerosol hairspray with a medium to firm hold and a slight stiff feel that can easily be brushed though. It contains mostly alcohol, water, film formers, slip agents, conditioning agents, and fragrance.

☺ **Liquid Shaper Plus, Extra Hold Hair Spray and Spray Gel** *($9.95 for 8.5 ounces)* is similar to the Shaper Styling Gel above and the same comments apply.

☺ **Shaper Hair Spray Styling Mist for Hold and Control** *($9.95 for 10 ounces)* is similar to the Liquid Shaper Styling Gel above, only with a more light-to-medium hold, but the same basic comments apply.

☺ **Shaper Plus Hair Spray Styling Mist for Super Hold and Extra Control** *($18.30 for 18 ounces)* is similar to the Liquid Shaper Styling Gel above and the same comments apply.

☺ **Shaper Zero g Weightless Hair Spray** *($14.95 for 14.1 ounces)* is similar to the Liquid Shaper Styling Gel above and the same comments apply.

XTAH by Sebastian

This contemporary styling line will probably be gone from the shelves by the time this book goes to press. Most likely the idea was to compete with some of the "extreme" styling lines like Fudge or Rusk's Radical. The results here were difficult-to-use packaging (the shape of the bottles were unusually wide and the tops hard to get off), hard-to-understand directions, absurd prices, and some OK to poor formulations.

☺ **$$$ XTAH Twisted Taffy Free-Former** *($17.50 for 4.4 ounces)* is a sticky, thick, liquid gel—well, sort of. The texture is hard to describe, but it gives a light hold and a sticky feel. It can help form hair, but the weight and feel on the hair leaves much to be desired.

☺ **$$$ XTAH Crude Clay Modeler** *($17.50 for 4.4 ounces)* is mostly Vaseline, thickeners, and slip agent. For some reason there is also clay in here, but that probably won't be much of a problem. This greasy wax pomade works well to smooth frizzies and curls, but it can easily look greasy and heavy, so use it sparingly.

☺ **$$$ XTAH Primer Pre-Fixxer** *($15.96 for 8.5 ounces)*. Once you figure out how to get the cap off, this is just a standard styling spray with a light hold and minimal to no stiff or sticky feel.

☺ **$$$ XTAH Vinyl Fabricator** *($18.86 for 4.4 ounces)* has a name that's more intimidating than what you actually get. This is just a medium-hold gel with a slight stiff, sticky feel that can be brushed though. The container is hard to use but the contents are just standard stuff.

Selsun Blue

For more information on Selsun Blue, call (800) 227-5767 or in Canada (800) 361-7852.

☺ **2-in-1 Treatment Dandruff Shampoo and Conditioner in One** (*$6.64 for 11 ounces*) is only a very basic two-in-one shampoo for normal to slightly dry hair of any thickness. There's nothing in this version to fight dandruff! It's just shampoo (meaning detergent cleansing agents and lather agent) with silicone.

☹ **Balanced Treatment Dandruff Control for All Hair Types** (*$6.64 for 11 ounces*) is a basic shampoo of just detergent cleansing agents and lather agent that uses selenium sulfide as the ingredient to fight dandruff. The sulfur in the selenium sulfide can strip hair color, so using this one is best for those who have not had success with other dandruff treatments or who have short hair.

☹ **Medicated Treatment Dandruff Shampoo** (*$6.64 for 11 ounces*) is almost identical to the Balanced version above and the same comments apply.

☹ **Moisturizing Treatment Dandruff Shampoo** (*$6.64 for 11 ounces*) is almost identical to the Balanced version above and the same comments apply.

Senscience

For more information on Senscience, call (800) 242-9283 or in Canada (800) 626-3684.

☹ **Complete Clarifier Pre-Shampoo Treatment** (*$6.99 for 8 ounces*). Using a pre-shampoo is sort of like putting dirt on your body before taking a shower. This just gets washed away before you shampoo. My concern about this product is that it contains sodium thiosulfate, an ingredient often used in perms. That can denature hair or strip hair color and that's a problem.

☺ **Energy Shampoo for Dry Hair** (*$8.63 for 16.9 ounces*) contains mostly water, detergent cleansing agents, lather agent, thickeners, fragrance, detangling agent/film former, silicone, conditioning agents, and preservatives. This is a good shampoo for normal to slightly dry hair of any thickness. There is nothing about this shampoo that energizes hair.

☺ **Energy Shampoo for Normal Hair** (*$8.63 for 16.9 ounces*) is almost identical to the Dry Hair version above and the same basic comments apply.

☺ **Inner Conditioner for Coarse Hair** (*$12.39 for 16.9 ounces*) contains mostly water, silicone, thickeners, detangling agent, conditioning agent, more thickeners, slip agent, preservatives, and fragrance. This is a good, basic, silicone-based conditioner that would work well for dry, coarse, or thick hair.

☺ **Inner Conditioner for Fine Hair** (*$12.39 for 16.9 ounces*) is almost identical to the one above for Coarse Hair only with slightly less silicone. That doesn't make it all that much better for fine hair, but it does make it better for normal to dry hair of any thickness.

☺ **Inner Conditioner for Medium Hair** *($12.39 for 16.9 ounces)* is almost identical to the one above for Fine Hair and the same comments apply.

☺ **Inner Repair Leave-in Conditioner** *($7.20 for 8 ounces)* contains mostly water, alcohol, silicone, film formers, conditioning agents, detangling agent, fragrance, and preservatives. Because of its alcohol content, this is far better used as a light-weight styling spray with a minimal hold and no stiff or sticky feel. It can add a slight thickness to hair but just minimally.

☹ **Shiatsu Scalp Spray Invigorating Scalp Spray** *($19.99 for 6.7 ounces)* has nothing invigorating in it. This is just water, alcohol, slip agent, conditioning agents, slip agents, fragrance, and preservatives. It isn't even a good leave-in conditioner—the alcohol will only dry and be irritating to the scalp.

☹ **Shiatsu Scalp Toner Soothing Scalp Toner** *($15.99 for 7.6 ounces)* is similar to the Spray version above and the same warnings apply.

☺ **Simply Shine Lustre** *($14.99 for 3.4 ounces)* is a standard silicone spray that adds shine and a silky feel to hair. Basically, this is just a pricey version of the same silicone serums available at the drugstore for less than half this price.

☺ **VitalEsse Repair and Shine** *($11.99 for 1.8 ounces)* is a standard silicone serum that adds shine and a silky-soft feel to hair, and there are definitely far less expensive, identical versions available at the drugstore.

☺ **VitalRich Moisturizing Hairdress** *($7.99 for 3.55 ounces)* is just a silicone-based lotion that can help with styling and that has minimal to no hold and only a slight sticky feel. It contains mostly water, slip agent, silicones, alcohol, thickeners, fragrance, conditioning agents, preservatives, and castor oil. It can help smooth out stubborn frizzies and curls.

☺ **Straighten Out Smoothing Gel** *($9.99 for 6.8 ounces)* is a no-hold gel with minimal to no sticky feel that simply contains water, detangling agents, slip agents, conditioning agents, preservatives, fragrance, and silicone. It can help when styling hair straight but it doesn't offer control or molding.

☺ **Energel Shaping Gel** *($7.20 for 7.6 ounces)* contains mostly water, alcohol, film former, thickeners, silicone, conditioning agents, fragrance, and preservatives. This is a good standard spray gel with a medium to firm hold and a definite sticky feel that can be brushed through.

☺ **Styling Froth Conditioning Gel** *($10.80 for 6 ounces)* contains mostly water, slip agents, film former, propellant, thickeners, fragrance, and preservatives. This is a fairly frothy mousse that has a medium hold and a somewhat sticky feel.

☺ **Effervesse Soft Styling Foam** *($9.99 for 7.7 ounces)* is a standard mousse that contains mostly water, alcohol, propellant, film former, slip agent, silicones, fragrance, detangling agent, and preservatives. It has a light hold with minimal to no stiff or sticky feel.

☺ **Volumesse Body Building Foam** *($9.95 for 7 ounces)* is an aerated foam (rather than one with propellant) that contains mostly water, film former, slip agent, detangling agent/film former, conditioning agents, fragrance, more detangling agent, and preservatives. It has a light to medium hold with a somewhat stiff, sticky feel that can be brushed through.

☺ **Fine Design Volumizing Treatment** *($7.99 for 8 ounces)* is a simple, liquidy gel with a light to medium hold that has a slight stiff sticky feel. It contains mostly water, slip agent, alcohol, film former, thickener, conditioning agents, fragrance, and preservatives.

☺ **Maximum Memory Firm Holding Spray** *($8.99 for 6.5 ounces)* is a standard aerosol styling spray with a medium to firm hold and a slight stiff feel that does allow you to brush through hair. It contains mostly alcohol, propellant, film former, silicone, and fragrance.

☺ **Energy Spritz** *($8.05 for 8 ounces)* is similar to the Maximum Memory above only in nonaerosol form, and the same comments apply.

☺ **Memory Mist Brushable Holding Spray** *($7.99 for 6.5 ounces)* is almost identical to the Maximum version above and the same comments apply.

☺ **Swing Thermal Setting Spray** *($8.10 for 7.6 ounces)* can be used as a styling spray, but it is more of a medium hold-hairspray with a somewhat stiff, sticky feel that can be brushed though. It contains mostly water, alcohol, film former, silicone, fragrance, and conditioning agent.

Sheenique

This line of products created for the African-American hair-care market uses silk amino acids as the cornerstone of many of its products. The tiny amount of this standard conditioning agent used cannot make the hair feel like silk, nor does it perform any better than many other conditioning ingredients. What is true for many African-American hair-care lines is also the case here: you need to watch out for the greasy stuff. Ingredients like this won't get you the smooth, soft look you want; rather, they just tend to look greasy and heavy. For more information on Sheenique, call (800) 782-8729.

☹ **Silk Braid Shampoo** *($0.99 for 8 ounces)* uses sodium C14-16 olefin sulfate as the main cleansing agent, which can be drying for the hair and drying and irritating for the scalp. If the goal is to only affect synthetic braids, this basic detergent cleansing formulation would work well.

☹ **Silk Moisturizing Shampoo** *($4.79 for 16 ounces)* uses sodium C14-16 olefin sulfate, sodium lauryl sulfate, and TEA-lauryl sulfate as most of the detergent cleansing agents, and that makes this too potentially irritating for the scalp and drying for the hair.

☺ **Silk Neutralizing Shampoo** *($4.49 for 16 ounces)* contains silk amino acids, which act as a conditioning agent, but that won't make your hair feel like silk. This shampoo contains mostly water, detergent cleansing agent, lather agent, thickeners, detangling agent/film former, conditioning agents, preservatives, fragrance, and coloring agents. It would work well for dry hair of any thickness.

☺ **Just Beautiful Creme Hairdressing and Conditioner, Children's Formula for All Hair Textures** *($3.99 for 4 ounces)* contains mostly water, Vaseline, mineral oil, thickeners, conditioning agents, fragrance, and preservatives. This thick, greasy conditioner would be OK for very dry, damaged hair, but the film it leaves on hair and scalp can easily build up.

☺ **Nubian Results Moisturizing Conditioner** *($5.99 for 16 ounces)* contains mostly water, thickeners, conditioning agents, detangling agents, and preservatives. This is a good conditioner for normal to dry hair of any thickness. This is one of the few products from Sheenique that doesn't have greasy ingredients.

☹ **Nubian Silk Herbal Gro Hairdress** *($4.79 for 8 ounces)* contains mostly Vaseline, thickeners, plant oil, castor oil, fragrance, lanolin oil, conditioning agents, plant extracts, and preservatives. This conditioner does contain sulfur, which can strip hair color, so this is not a good option for dyed hair. Other than that, it works for very dry, damaged hair but it can leave a greasy film on the hair and scalp that can easily build up.

☺ **Silk Reforming Complex, Stops Breakage** *($7.99 for 16 ounces)* won't stop breakage of any kind—it is simply an emollient cream that can be good for dry hair to help smooth out frizzies and curl with no hold and no sticky, stiff feel. It contains mostly thickeners, fragrance, conditioning agents, preservatives, Vaseline, slip agent, more preservatives, and detangling agent.

☹ **Silk Sensitive Scalp Protection Creme** *($4.99 for 14 ounces)* is greasy stuff and can easily build up on hair and make it look greasy. It contains mostly mineral oil, thickener, Vaseline, lanolin, conditioning agent, and coloring agent. This product also contains camphor and menthol, two highly irritating ingredients that would be completely inappropriate for any scalp problem, but doubly so for someone with sensitive skin.

☺ **Botanical Potion Wearable Treatment Highly Concentrated Botanical Leave-in Conditioner and Style Finisher** *($5.99 for 5.1 ounces)* contains mostly water, slip agent, detangling agents, thickeners, silicone, film former, more slip agents, coloring agent, conditioning agents, plant oils, fragrant oils, fragrance, and preservatives. The minimal amount of plant oils in this product aren't what makes it good;

rather, it is just a good, silicone-based styling spray that has a light hold and works well for styling dry hair that is fine or thin.

☺ **Stayz-N Leave-on Treatment** *($2.99 for 8 ounces)* is similar to the Botanical Potion above and the same basic comments apply.

☺ **Nubian Silk Oil Treatment** *($2.99 for 2 ounces)* is mostly mineral oil, with some slip agents, lanolin oil, fragrance, preservatives, and coloring agents. This is greasy stuff, but if this really was the direction you wanted for your hair, you would be far better off with just plain mineral oil.

☺ **Silk Braid Oil** *($2.99 for 8 ounces)* is similar to the Nubian Silk Oil version above and the same basic comments apply.

☺ **Silk Braid Sheen Spray** *($3.69 for 8 ounces)* contains mostly water, slip agents, film former, preservatives, fragrance, and plant oils. The Silk Sheen Spray On Hair Polish below is a far better way to add shine and softness; this is more of a lightweight styling spray than a product to add shine.

☺ **Silk Sheen Spray On Hair Polish** *($4.99 for 4 ounces)* is just a standard silicone spray and it would work great to add shine and soft, silky feel to hair.

☺ **Silk Oil Sheen Spray (Aerosol)** *($3.19 for 10 ounces)* is just an aerosol version of putting mineral oil on the hair. Mineral oil can help extremely dry hair, but the performance of silicone on the hair is far better. Consider the Silk Sheen Spray On Hair Polish above instead of this one.

☺ **Silk Freez Style Gel** *($3.99 for 16 ounces)* is a good basic gel with a light to medium hold and a somewhat sticky feel. It contains mostly water, film formers, silicone, thickeners, preservatives, fragrance, and coloring agents.

☺ **Silk Styling Gel Ultimate Hold** *($3.99 for 16 ounces)* is a good basic gel with a light hold and minimal sticky feel. It contains mostly water, film formers, silicone, thickeners, preservatives, fragrance, and coloring agents.

☺ **Soft 'N Clear Styling Gel** *($3.99 for 16 ounces)* has no hold, but that eliminates any stiff or sticky feel, and this gel can help when styling hair smooth. It contains mostly water, conditioning agents, thickeners, preservatives, fragrance, and coloring agents.

☹ **Bodifi Setting Lotion Concentrated, Extra Hold** *($4.49 for 16 ounces)* is a light-hold styling lotion with a slight sticky feel. It would have been far better if this liquid had been in a spray bottle, as is it is difficult to apply without making a mess. The recommendation is to dilute the product, but that would mean little to no hold, and for a setting lotion that isn't the best idea. It contains mostly water, detangling agent/film former, slip agents, preservatives, fragrance, and coloring agent. The teeny amount of silk amino acids in here barely provides any conditioning benefit.

☺ **Silk Freez Spritz (Non-Aerosol)** *($2.99 for 8 ounces)* is a good basic hairspray with a medium hold that has a somewhat stiff feel that does allow you to brush through hair. It contains mostly alcohol, film former, water, slip agent, fragrance, and conditioning agent. The teeny amount of silk amino acids in here barely provides any conditioning benefit.

☺ **Super Hold Hair Spray (Aerosol)** *($2.89 for 10 ounces)* is a standard aerosol hairspray with a light to medium hold and minimal stiff feel that contains mostly alcohol, propellant, film formers, slip agents, silicone, fragrance, and conditioning agent.

Soft & Beautiful

For more information on Soft & Beautiful, call (214) 631-4247 or (800) 527-5879.

☺ **Color Code Neutralizing Decalcifying Shampoo** *($3.50 for 16 ounces)* is just a basic shampoo that would work well for normal to slightly dry hair that is normal to fine or thin. It doesn't contain any chelating ingredients that would help remove buildup from hair. It contains mostly water, detergent cleansing agents, lather agent, detangling agent/film former, fragrance, thickeners, and preservatives.

☺ **Moisturizing Shampoo, Pro-Vitamin Formula** *($3.95 for 16 ounces)* is a basic shampoo that would work well for normal to dry hair that is normal to fine or thin. It contains mostly water, detergent cleansing agents, lather agent, thickener, conditioning agents, fragrance, detangling agents, film former, more fragrance, preservatives, and coloring agents. The teeny amounts of vitamins in here have no effect on hair.

☺ **Creme Moisturizer, Extra Light** *(3.59 for 4 ounces)* contains mostly water, mineral oil, Vaseline, thickeners, slip agent, lanolin, lanolin oil, silicone, fragrance, preservatives, and coloring agents. This is not extra-light; it can be greasy and heavy on the hair and can easily build up. It can be an option for extremely dry hair that is coarse or thick.

☺ **Hair Moisturizing Complex** *($3.95 for 16 ounces)* is just water, mineral oil, some conditioning agents, and thickeners. This is a good conditioner for extremely dry hair that is thick or coarse, but it can leave a greasy film.

☺ **Oil Moisturizing Lotion** *($3.72 for 8 ounces)* has a name that fits: this is oily stuff. It contains mostly water, mineral oil, lanolin, thickeners, Vaseline, lanolin oil, fragrance, preservatives, and coloring agent. It is an option for extremely dry hair, but be careful or you can end up with an oily look instead of a soft, smooth appearance.

☺ **Perm Repair Leave-in Conditioner** *($2.95 for 2 ounces)* won't repair one strand of hair; it is just a good, but standard, lightweight styling spray with minimal stiff or sticky feel, and can work well for normal to dry hair that is normal to fine or thin. It contains mostly water, slip agents, detangling agents/film former, silicones, fragrance, conditioning agents, and preservatives. The minuscule amounts of vitamins and silk amino acids in here aren't enough for even one hair, much less a whole head of hair.

☺ **Vitamin Enriched Oil Sheen with Sunscreen** *($4.19 for 17.2 ounces)* doesn't have an SPF, and without that, the allusion to sun protection is deceptive. Aside from that, this is just a good silicone spray that can help add shine and softness to hair. It contains mostly slip agents, propellant, silicone, and fragrance.

☺ **Herbal Aloe Therapy Creme** *($4.95 for 4 ounces)* contains mostly Vaseline, lanolin, mineral oil, plant oils, silicone, plant extracts, fragrance, and preservatives. This is greasy stuff and can easily build up on hair and scalp. It can work for extremely dry hair that is coarse or thick, but be careful.

☹ **3-in-1 Dry Scalp Treatment** *($5.95 for 4 ounces).* The menthol in here can be irritating for the scalp and should not be used anywhere on skin.

☺ **Botanical Oil** *($4.95 for 4 ounces)* is just plant oils, mineral oil, lanolin oil, fragrance, and silicone. It would work well for extremely dry hair or scalp but, for the money, and given that this is about 80 percent safflower oil, you would do just as well using some safflower oil from your kitchen cupboard.

☺ **Sculpting Gel** *($4.95 for 8 ounces)* is a good basic gel that offers little hold but can help smooth hair with minimal to no stiff or sticky feel. It contains mostly water, slip agents, thickeners, plant extracts, preservatives, and fragrance.

☺ **Oil Sheen with Sunscreen (Aerosol)** *($3.19 for 10 ounces)* is primarily a silicone spray in aerosol form. This is a good way to add shine and silky feel to hair but the sunscreen is bogus; without an SPF it is simply a misleading, deceptive ingredient mention.

☺ **Humidity Guard Holding Spray, Maximum Hold** *($2.69 for 10.5 ounces)* is a good standard aerosol hairspray with a light hold and minimal to no stiff feel. It contains mostly alcohol, water, propellant, film former, silicone, slip agents, and fragrance.

Just for Me by Soft & Beautiful

☺ **Moisturizing Conditioning Shampoo** *($2.99 for 8 ounces)* is a basic shampoo that isn't moisturizing in the least, though it would work well for normal to slightly dry hair that is normal to fine or thin. It contains mostly water, detergent cleansing agents, lather agent, thickener, conditioning agent, detangling agent/film former, fragrance, preservatives, and coloring agents.

☺ **Creme Conditioner and Hairdress** *($2.99 for 3.4 ounces)* is greasy stuff that can build up on hair and scalp and be hard to wash off. It contains mostly water, mineral oil, thickeners, lanolin, slip agents, lanolin oil, Vaseline, detangling agent/film former, fragrance, preservatives, and coloring agents.

☺ **Leave-in Conditioner** *($2.95 for 8 ounces)* is a good leave-in conditioner that would work well for normal to dry hair that is normal to fine or thin. It contains mostly water, slip agents, detangling agents/film formers, silicones, fragrance, and preservatives. The minute amounts of vitamins and conditioning agents in this product have no benefit for hair.

☺ **Detangler** *($2.99 for 8 ounces)* is almost identical to the Leave-in Conditioner above and the same comments apply.

☺ **Oil Moisturizing Lotion** *($5.69 for 8 ounces)* is indeed oily and greasy! It contains mostly water, mineral oil, lanolin, Vaseline, lanolin oil, thickeners, fragrance, preservatives, and coloring agents. Though this can be an option for extremely dry, coarse and thick hair, it can build up and leave the hair looking greasy and slippery.

Soft Sheen

Soft Sheen has a large array of products designed for African-American hair care. The redundancy between the lines is bit shocking, but there are some good options to consider. The greasy Vaseline-, mineral oil–, and lanolin-based conditioners and styling products are definitely here, but there are also a few lighter-weight options that can work well without the typical greasy, oily appearance the former type of products can create. For more information on Soft Sheen, call (800) 621-6143.

☺ **Frizz Free Deep Conditioner** *($3.99 for 16 ounces)* contains mostly water, slip agent, detangling agents/film former, conditioning agents, more detangling agent, silicones, thickeners, fragrance, preservatives, and plant extracts. This is a good conditioner for dry hair that is normal to fine or thin. It does contain peppermint, so keep it off the scalp or you can end up with irritation.

☺ **Frizz Free Oil Moisturizer** *($3.89 for 8 ounces)* is indeed oil, and it contains mostly water, mineral oil, Vaseline, thickeners, slip agent, preservatives, plant extracts, and fragrance. This is greasy stuff and can easily build up on hair, though it can be an option for extremely dry hair that is coarse or thick. It does contain balm mint, so keep it off the scalp or you can end up with irritation.

☺ **Frizz Free Xtra Strength Moisturizing Gel Serum Especially for Coarse/Resistant Hair** *($7.99 for 2 ounces)* is a rather simple styling serum that can help in smoothing hair; it has minimal stiff or sticky feel and there's no risk of greasy buildup. It contains mostly slip agents, detangling agent/film former, thickeners, preservatives, and fragrance.

☺ **Frizz Free Leave-in Conditioning Foam** *($4.99 for 7 ounces)* is more of a styling mousse (in an aerated dispenser, not aerosol) than a conditioner. It can work for normal to slightly dry hair that is normal to fine or thin, but the film former in here adds a bit of a sticky feel. It contains mostly water, slip agents, silicones, preservatives, film former, fragrance, detangling agent, and plant extract.

☺ **Oil Sheen Spray with MRC (Moisture Retention Complex)** *($2.99 for 11.5 ounces)* is an impressively named product with exceptionally standard, greasy ingredients. It is an aerosol that mists oils over the hair. The effect is more greasy than anything else, though it can keep moisture in extremely damaged hair. It contains mostly mineral oil, propellants, plant oils, lanolin oil, silicone, conditioning agent, and fragrance.

☺ **Alternatives Conditioning Styling Gel with MRC (Moisture Retention Complex)** *($3.49 for 6 ounces)* contains mostly conditioning agent, detangling agent/film formers, slip agents, preservatives, thickeners, plant extracts, and fragrance. This is a good, basic, light- to medium-hold gel that has a somewhat sticky feel. It does contain balm mint and peppermint, which can be skin irritants, so keep it off of the scalp.

☺ **Wave Nouveau Hydra Creme Hairdress** *($3.99 for 4 ounces)* contains mostly water, thickeners, Vaseline, emollient, plant oil, silicone, film former, fragrance, preservatives, and slip agent. This is a good though somewhat greasy styling cream with a light hold. It can build up with a greasy feel, but it can work for extremely dry hair of any thickness.

☺ **Finishing Lotion** *($3.99 for 12 ounces)* is a good, very lightweight styling lotion that is more of a leave-in conditioner than it is a styling product. It can help in styling hair smooth, but with no hold and minimal control. It contains mostly water, slip agents, detangling agents, thickeners, silicones, preservatives, fragrance, and coloring agent. It would work well as a conditioner for normal to dry hair that is normal to thin or fine.

☺ **Finishing Mist** *($3.99 for 12 ounces)* is similar to the Finishing Lotion above only in spray form, and the same comments apply.

☺ **Wave Nouveau Finishing Mist** *($3.99 for 12 ounces)* is similar to the Finishing Lotion above, only in spray form, and the same comments apply.

☺ **Wave Nouveau Hydra Sette Styling Lotion** *($3.99 for 12 ounces)* is similar to the Finishing Lotion above, only in spray form, and the same comments apply.

☺ **Alternatives Firm Holding Spritz with MRC (Moisture Retention Complex)** *($3.49 for 8 ounces)* is a good standard hairspray with a medium to firm hold and a slight stiff, sticky feel. It contains mostly alcohol, water, film former, slip agents, fragrance, silicone, coloring agents, and plant extracts.

☺ **Xtra Strength Anti-Frizz Serum** *($7.99 for 2 ounces)* is just mineral oil, and it can smooth frizzies—but a silicone serum has a softer, silkier feel on hair.

☺ **Miss Cool Styling System Setting Lotion 5 Minute Fast Set** *($2.99 for 8 ounces)* is more like a simple, leave-in conditioner but it can be a good lightweight styling lotion for smoothing hair with no hold, no buildup, and no stiff or sticky feel. It contains mostly water, detangling agent, slip agents, fragrance, preservatives, and coloring agent.

The Reviews S

Baby Love by Soft Sheen

☺ **Conditioning Shampoo** *($3.79 for 11.5 ounces)* is just a gentle shampoo, and it would work well for adults or children. It contains mostly water, detergent cleansing agents, thickeners, preservatives, and fragrance.

☺ **Conditioning Detangler** *($4.19 for 8 ounces)* is, just as the name implies, a detangling conditioner that contains mostly water, detangling agents, slip agents, thickeners, fragrance, silicone, and preservatives. This would work well for normal hair of any thickness.

☺ **Moisturizing Creme Hair Dress** *($3.99 for 4 ounces)* contains mostly water, mineral oil, thickeners, Vaseline, preservatives, plant oil, conditioning agents, and fragrance. This is a fairly greasy conditioner for extremely dry hair that can easily build up and make hair look oily.

☺ **Moisturizing Hairdress Lotion** *($3.79 for 8 ounces)* is similar to the Creme Hair Dress above, only slightly more greasy, and the same comments apply.

Care Free Curl by Soft Sheen

☹ **Conditioning Shampoo** *($3.29 for 8 ounces)* uses sodium lauryl sulfate as the main detergent cleansing agent, and that makes it too potentially irritating for the scalp and drying for the hair.

☹ **Gold 3 in 1 Shampoo** *($3.10 for 8 ounces)* uses sodium C14-16 olefin sulfate and sodium lauryl sulfate as the main detergent cleansing agents, and that makes it too potentially irritating for the scalp and drying for the hair.

☺ **Instant Moisturizer Glycerin and Protein** *($3.19 for 8 ounces)* contains mostly water, slip agents, conditioning agent, detangling agent, preservatives, and fragrance. This is a good, lightweight, leave-in conditioner for normal hair of any thickness.

☺ **Keratin Conditioner, pH 5.0** *($5.99 for 16 ounces)* contains mostly water, detangling agent, thickeners, conditioning agents, preservatives, and fragrance. This is a good lightweight conditioner for normal hair of any thickness. The minute amount of keratin in here is insignificant for hair.

☺ **Curl Activator** *($3.29 for 8 ounces)* is just a lotion that adds grease to hair. It contains mostly water, slip agents, Vaseline, mineral oil, fragrance, and preservatives. It can be helpful for extremely dry hair, but it can also cause buildup and look oily on the hair.

☺ **Gold Hair and Scalp Spray** *($2.99 for 8 ounces)* contains mostly water, slip agents, conditioning agent, fragrance, and silicone. It is a good, lightweight, leave-in conditioner for normal hair.

☺ **Gold Instant Activator with Silk Moisturizers** *($2.99 for 8 ounces)* contains mostly water, slip agents, detangling agents/film former, thickeners, silicones, conditioning agents, preservatives, fragrance, and coloring agents. It is a good conditioner for normal to dry hair that is normal to fine or thin in thickness.

☺ **Snap Back Curl Restorer** *($3.29 for 8 ounces)* is just a lightweight spray that adds a bit of water and slip agents to hair, but that is more a function of the water. It contains mostly water, slip agents, preservatives, fragrance, and coloring agents.

Optimum Care by Soft Sheen

☺ **Collagen Moisture Shampoo** *($2.99 for 16 ounces)* is a standard shampoo that contains mostly water, detergent cleansing agents, lather agent, thickeners, slip agents, conditioning agents, fragrance, detangling agent/film former, preservatives, and coloring agents. The tiny amount of conditioner in here won't help really dry hair, though this can be a good shampoo for normal to slightly dry hair of any thickness.

☺ **Light Control with Aloe** *($2.99 for 3.5 ounces)* is greasy and heavy and can easily build up on hair— there's nothing light about it. This contains mostly Vaseline, mineral oil, lanolin, slip agent, silicone, castor oil, fragrance, preservatives, and coloring agents. It can have a slight stiff feel, but the grease can be a problem for a soft, smooth look. This can be an option for extremely dry hair if used minimally.

☺ **Moisture Rich with Vitamin E** *($2.99 for 3.5 ounces)* is similar to the one above and the same comments apply.

☺ **Nourishment with Lanolin and Coconut** *($2.99 for 3.5 ounces)* is similar to the Light Control above and the same comments apply.

☺ **Rich Conditioner** *($2.99 for 16 ounces)* is a good simple conditioner for normal to slightly dry hair of any thickness. It contains mostly water, thickeners, conditioning agents, detangling agent, silicone, fragrance, and preservatives.

☹ **Leave-in Conditioner with Sage and Peppermint Extracts** *($2.99 for 8 ounces)* does have peppermint in it, which can be a problem for skin, so keep it off the scalp. Other than that, this is more a styling spray for normal to slightly dry hair that is normal to fine or thin than a leave-in conditioner. It contains mostly water, slip agents, detangling agent/film formers, preservatives, and plant extracts.

☺ **Body & Shine** *($2.99 for 14.2 ounces)* is an aerosol silicone spray that can work well to add shine and a soft feel to hair. It contains mostly slip agent, propellant, silicone, and fragrance.

☺ **Setting & Wrap Lotion with Lanolin** *($4.39 for 8 ounces)* doesn't actually contain that much lanolin, which makes it better for hair. This is basically just water, preservatives, coloring agents, detangling agent/film formers, and slip agents. It has almost no hold and just minimal stiff or sticky feel, which also means it won't hold a set very well. But if you don't need much control, this can work well.

☺ **Firm Holding Spritz** *($3.59 for 8 ounces)* is standard hairspray with a medium hold and a somewhat stiff feel that can be brushed through. It contains mostly alcohol, film former, silicone, conditioning agents, and fragrance.

☺ **Soft Holding Spritz** *($2.99 for 8 ounces)* is similar to the Firm Holding Spritz above, which means it isn't soft, and the same basic comments apply.

Optimum Conditioning by Soft Sheen

OptiCleanse Neutralizing Conditioning Shampoo Step 3 *($4.39 for 16 ounces).* Because the ingredient list does not follow the FDA's legally required guidelines for listing ingredients in order from the most to the least concentration, this is a product that cannot be reviewed—there is no way to ascertain what you would be putting on your hair.

Shampoo KeraTex Conditioning Shampoo Normal *($4.29 for 16 ounces)* has the same problem as the one above and the same comment applies.

Shampoo ReparaTex Conditioning Shampoo Dry, Damaged *($4.39 for 16 ounces)* has the same problem as the one above and the same comment applies.

NutriMant Protein-Enriched Conditioner Normal *($6.29 for 16 ounces)* has the same problem as the one above and the same comment applies.

Designing Lotion Step 4 *($5.99 for 12 ounces)* has the same problem as the one above and the same comment applies.

OptiFix Extra Firm Holding Spray with Style Memory *($2.99 for 6 ounces)* has the same problem as the one above and the same comment applies.

St. Ives

St. Ives wears the contemporary disguise of being all natural, and has its herbal concoctions down solid. Yet, as with most other hair-care products of this type, the amount of plant extracts is minimal to nonexistent in comparison to the quantity of all the standard "chemical" ingredients in them. Whether the plants come from the Amazon or from Switzerland, as St. Ives would like you to believe, it is all just marketing to convince consumers that they aren't really using synthetic ingredients on their tresses. Nonetheless, all the plants in the world won't bring you the quality of hair you want. Thankfully, the plants in these products make up only a fraction of the content.

For more information on St. Ives (owned by Alberto Culver) call (818) 709-5500, (800) 333-0005, or visit its Web site at www.stives.com.

☹ **Swiss Spa Clarifying Shampoo Citrus and Ginseng for Frequently Washed Hair** *($2.79 for 20 ounces)* uses sodium lauryl sulfate as its main detergent cleansing agent, and that makes it too potentially irritating for the scalp and drying for the hair.

☹ **Swiss Spa Extra Body Shampoo Chamomile and Sunflower Volumizing for Normal/Fine Hair** *($2.79 for 20 ounces)* uses sodium lauryl sulfate as its main detergent cleansing agent and that makes it too potentially irritating for the scalp and drying for the hair.

☺ **Swiss Formula Gardenia Plus Extra Gentle Shampoo Plus Conditioner for Normal Hair** *($1.99 for 15 ounces)* contains mostly water, detergent cleansing agents, lather agent, thickeners, plant extracts, conditioning agents, silicone, detangling agent, film former, slip agent, preservatives, fragrance, and coloring agents. This would be a good shampoo for normal to dry hair that is normal to fine or thin.

☺ **Swiss Formula Papaya Plus Fortifying Shampoo Plus Conditioner for Normal Hair** *($1.99 for 15 ounces)* is almost identical to the Swiss Formula Gardenia Plus above and the same basic comments apply.

☺ **Swiss Formula Watermelon Plus, Antioxidant Shampoo + Conditioner, Extra Moisturizing for Dry, Permed or Color/Treated Hair** *($1.99 for 20 ounces)* is almost identical to the Swiss Formula Gardenia Plus above and the same basic comments apply.

☻ **Swiss Spa Extra Shine Shampoo Jojoba and Raspberry for Normal Hair** *($2.79 for 20 ounces)* uses sodium lauryl sulfate as the main detergent cleansing agent and that makes it too potentially irritating for the scalp and drying for the hair.

☻ **Swiss Spa Moisturizing Shampoo: Aloe Vera and Echinacea for Permed/ Color Treated Hair** *($2.79 for 20 ounces)* uses sodium lauryl sulfate as its main detergent cleansing agent, and that makes it too potentially irritating for the scalp and drying for the hair.

☻ **Swiss Spa Revitalizing Shampoo: Vanilla and Edelweiss for Dry/Damaged Hair** *($2.79 for 20 ounces)* uses sodium lauryl sulfate as its main detergent cleansing agent, and that makes it too potentially irritating for the scalp and drying for the hair.

☻ **Swiss Spa Strengthening Shampoo: Pear and Vitamin E for Normal/Dry Hair** *($2.79 for 20 ounces)* uses sodium lauryl sulfate as its main detergent cleansing agent, and that makes it too potentially irritating for the scalp and drying for the hair.

☺ **Swiss Spa Extra Body Conditioner Chamomile and Sunflower for Normal/Fine Hair** *($2.79 for 20 ounces)* contains mostly water, thickeners, detangling agent/film former, plant extracts, vitamins, conditioning agents, silicone, preservatives, fragrance, and coloring agents. This is a good conditioner for normal to slightly dry hair that is fine or thin.

☺ **Swiss Spa Extra Shine Conditioner: Jojoba and Raspberry for Normal Hair** *($2.79 for 20 ounces)* is similar to the Extra Body version above, only this one contains jojoba oil, which makes it better for drier hair that is fine or thin.

☺ **Swiss Spa Light Conditioner Citrus and Ginseng for Frequently Washed Hair** *($2.79 for 20 ounces)* is almost identical to the Extra Body version above and the same comments apply. This one does contain grapefruit extract, which can be irritating for the scalp.

☺ **Swiss Spa Moisturizing Conditioner: Aloe Vera and Echinacea for Permed/Color Treated Hair** *($2.79 for 20 ounces)* is almost identical to the Extra Body version above and the same comments apply.

☺ **Swiss Spa Revitalizing Conditioner: Vanilla and Edelweiss for Dry/Damaged Hair** *($2.79 for 20 ounces)* is almost identical to the Extra Body version above and the same comments apply.

☺ **Swiss Spa Strengthening Conditioner: Pear and Vitamin E for Normal/Dry Hair** *($2.79 for 20 ounces)* is almost identical to the Extra Body version above and the same comments apply.

☺ **Swiss Formula Wet Essential 2 Minute Moisture Deep Conditioning Treatment With Hydrating Liposomes** *($.99 for 2 ounces)* isn't very deep, but it is emollient for extremely dry hair of any thickness. But be careful with this one—it can build up and feel greasy and oily. It contains mostly water, detangling agent, thickeners, mineral oil, and conditioning agents.

☺ **Swiss Formula Hair Repair, Extra Moisturizing Hot Oil Treatment** *($3.79 for three 0.625-ounce treatments)* contains mostly water, detangling agents, plant extracts, conditioning agents, thickeners, preservatives, fragrance, and coloring agents. This conditioner does contain menthol, which can be a skin irritant, so keep it off the scalp. Other than that, this is a no-oil formula, though it would be a good conditioner for normal to slightly dry hair of any thickness.

☺ **Swiss Formula Hair Repair, Hair Thickening Hot Oil Treatment** *($3.79 for three 0.625-ounce treatments)* is almost identical to the Extra Moisturizing version above and the same comments apply.

☺ **Swiss Formula Hair Repair, No Frizz Retexturizing Serum** *($3.79 for 1 ounce)* is a standard but very good silicone serum that can add shine and a silky feel to the hair.

☹ **Swiss Formula Hair Repair: Split Mender, Leave in Conditioning Treatment Fusing Serum** *($3.49 for 6.8 ounces)* can't repair split ends, and for a leave-in conditioner the second ingredient shouldn't be alcohol, which can be drying to hair. It also contains mint, which can be irritating to the skin and therefore a problem for the scalp.

☺ **Professional Swiss Hair Care Styling Gel** *($1.44 for 8 ounces)* contains mostly water, slip agent, film former, thickeners, conditioning agent, plant extracts, preservatives, and fragrance. This is a good basic styling gel with a light hold and minimal stiff or sticky feel.

☺ **Swiss Formula Silk and Keratin, European Styling and Finishing Hairspray, Extra Hold** *($1.78 for 10 ounces)* is a standard hairspray with a light to medium hold and a minimal stiff, sticky feel that can easily be brushed through. It contains mostly alcohol, water, film formers, conditioning agents, slip agent, plant extracts, and fragrance.

☺ **Swiss Formula Silk and Keratin, European Styling and Finishing Hairspray, Ultimate Hold** *($1.78 for 10 ounces)* is almost identical to the Extra Hold version above and the same comments apply.

Style by Lamaur

Don't be confused; Lamaur is a company with several lines of products available at the drugstore and beauty supply stores with very similar-sounding names. Salon Style (reviewed earlier in this chapter) and this line, simply called Style, are not the same, at least not in name, though they are manufactured by the same company. For more information on Style, call (612) 571-1234 or (800) 444-0699.

☺ **Extra Body Shampoo** *($1.13 for 24 ounces)* is a good basic shampoo with a only a tiny amount of film former, so the risk of buildup is minimal. It would work well for normal hair that is normal to fine or thin. It contains mostly water, detergent cleansing agents, lather agent, thickeners, detangling agent/film former, conditioning agent, preservatives, and fragrance.

☺ **Moisturizing Shampoo** *($1.13 for 24 ounces)* is similar to the Extra Body version above, only this one contains plant oil, which makes it better for normal to dry hair that is normal to fine or thin. It contains mostly water, detergent cleansing agents, lather agent, thickeners, detangling agent/film former, conditioning agent, preservatives, and fragrance.

☺ **Moisturizing Shampoo for Dry Color-Treated/Permed Hair** *($1.99 for 12 ounces)* contains mostly water, detergent cleansing agent, lather agent, plant extracts, detangling agent/film former, thickener, preservatives, fragrance, and coloring agents. This is a good basic shampoo for normal hair that is normal to fine or thin.

☺ **Volumizing Shampoo for Fine or Thin Hair** *($1.99 for 12 ounces)* is almost identical to the Moisturizing version above and the same comments apply.

☺ **Clarifying Shampoo for Normal to Oily Hair** *($1.99 for 12 ounces)* is just shampoo without conditioning agents or film former, and that makes it great for all hair types but especially for oily hair. It contains mostly water, detergent cleansing agent, lather agent, plant extracts, thickeners, preservatives, fragrance, and coloring agents.

☺ **Pro-Vitamin Complex Shampoo Extra Body** *($1.56 for 15 ounces)* is almost identical to the Extra Body version above and the same basic comments apply. The minute amounts of vitamins in here have no effect for hair or scalp.

☺ **Regular Shampoo Fresh Apple Fragrance** *($0.99 for 13 ounces)* is just shampoo with a tiny amount of conditioning agents. It would work well for most all hair types, with minimal risk of buildup. It contains mostly water, detergent cleansing agents, lather agent, conditioning agent, thickeners, slip agent, preservatives, fragrance, and coloring agents.

☺ **Shampoo Coconut & Papaya Maintains Softness & Enhances Shine** *($1.09 for 24 ounces)* is almost identical to the Extra Body version above and the same basic comments apply.

☺ **Strawberry Formula Shampoo Fresh Strawberry Fragrance** *($0.99 for 13 ounces)* is almost identical to the Regular Shampoo Fresh Apple and the same basic comments apply.

☺ **Style Plus Extra Conditioning Shampoo and Conditioner in One** *($1.13 for 24 ounces)* contains mostly water, detergent cleansing agent, lather agent, film former, silicone, detangling agent, conditioning agents, thickeners, preservatives, and fragrance. This can be a good shampoo for dry hair that is fine or thin, but it can easily cause buildup.

☺ **Coconut & Papaya Conditioner Maintains Softness & Enhances Shine** *($1.09 for 24 ounces)* is a basic conditioner for normal hair thatis normal to fine or thin. It contains mostly water, thickeners, detangling agents, slip agents, conditioning agent, plant extracts, detangling agent/film former, preservatives, and fragrance.

☺ **Deep Conditioning Conditioner Replenishes Dry or Treated Hair** *($0.99 for 13 ounces)* isn't deep at all; rather, it is almost identical to the Coconut & Papaya version above and the same comments apply.

☺ **Extra Body Conditioner** *($0.99 for 13 ounces)* is almost identical to the Coconut & Papaya version above and the same comments apply.

☺ **Fresh Apple Regular Conditioner** *($0.99 for 13 ounces)* is almost identical to the Coconut & Papaya version above and the same comments apply.

☺ **Moisturizing Conditioner** *($0.99 for 13 ounces)* is almost identical to the Coconut & Papaya version above and the same comments apply.

☺ **Pro-Vitamin Complex Conditioner** *($0.99 for 13 ounces)* is almost identical to the Coconut & Papaya version above and the same comments apply.

☺ **Pro-Vitamin Complex Conditioner Regular Apple** *($0.99 for 13 ounces)* is almost identical to the Coconut & Papaya version above and the same comments apply.

☺ **Rainwater Conditioner Adds Softness and Shine** *($0.99 for 13 ounces)* contains mostly water, thickeners, detangling agents, conditioning agent, plant oil, plant extract, silicone, preservatives, and fragrance. This is a good simple conditioner for normal to slightly dry hair of any thickness.

☺ **Strawberry Conditioner Restores Body Rinses Clean** *($0.99 for 13 ounces)* is almost identical to the Rainwater version above and the same comments apply.

☺ **Moisturizing Conditioner for Dry Color-Treated/Permed Hair** *($1.99 for 12 ounces)* contains mostly water, thickeners, detangling agents, silicone, preservatives, and fragrance. This is not moisturizing enough for dry hair; rather, it is a good lightweight conditioner for normal hair of any thickness.

☺ **Volumizing Conditioner for Fine or Thin Hair** *($1.99 for 12 ounces)* contains mostly water, thickeners, detangling agents, plant extracts, film former, preservatives, and fragrance. This is a good lightweight conditioner for normal hair that is normal to fine or thin in thickness.

☺ **Styling Gel Mega Hold** *($0.99 for 7 ounces)* is a standard but very good styling gel with a light hold and minimal to no stiff or sticky feel, and that isn't "mega hold" by anyone's definition. It contains mostly water, film former, slip agents, silicone, preservatives, fragrance, and coloring agents.

☺ **Styling Gel Super Hold** *($0.99 for 7 ounces)* is similar to the Mega Hold above and the same comments apply.

☺ **Styling Mousse Extra Hold** *($0.99 for 5 ounces)* is a standard mousse with a light to medium hold and minimal stiff or sticky feel that contains mostly water, propellant, slip agents, film former, plant oil, silicone, thickeners, detangling agent, fragrance, and preservatives.

☺ **Hair Spray Maximum Control Mega Hold (Aerosol)** *($1.29 for 7 ounces)* is a standard aerosol hairspray that contains mostly alcohol, water, propellant, film formers, slip agents, silicone, and fragrance. It has a light hold and minimal to no stiff feel.

☺ **Hair Spray Maximum Control Mega Hold (Non-Aerosol)** *($1.29 for 7 ounces)* is almost identical to the Mega Hold (Aerosol) version above and the same comments apply.

☺ **Hair Spray Soft, Flexible Control Natural Hold (Aerosol)** *($1.29 for 7 ounces)* is almost identical to the Mega Hold (Aerosol) version above and the same comments apply.

☺ **Hair Spray Long-Lasting Control Super Hold (Aerosol) Scented and Unscented** *($1.29 for 7 ounces)* is almost identical to the Mega Hold (Aerosol) version above and the same comments apply.

☺ **Hair Spray Long-Lasting Control Super Hold Scented and Unscented (Non-Aerosol)** *($1.29 for 7 ounces)* is almost identical to the Mega Hold (Aerosol) version above only in nonaerosol form, but the same comments apply.

Suave

Suave is by far one of the least expensive lines of hair-care products you are likely to ever run into. Yet for the most part the ingredients in these products are the same ones you would find in most every hair-care product made, which gives you an idea of how overpriced everything else is. What this line means for your hair and budget is that there are some great basic products to consider. However, there are some drawbacks. The first is the smell! Some of the fragrances are just overwhelmingly sweet and cloying. Another issue is that many of Suave's shampoos use the ingredient ammonium xylenesulfonate. This fairly strong solvent tends to swell the hair shaft, making normal to fine or thin hair feel thicker. For the short term that can be great, but with repeated use it can damage the hair shaft, leading to dry, flyaway hair as well as split ends. It can also be drying and irritating for the scalp. For more information on Suave (owned by Helene Curtis), call (800) 621-3379.

☹ **Apple Essence Shampoo** *($0.78 for 15 ounces)* contains ammonium xylenesulfonate, which can be drying for the hair and drying and irritating for the scalp.

☹ **Balsam & Protein Shampoo for Normal to Dry Hair** *($0.78 for 15 ounces)* contains ammonium xylenesulfonate, which can be drying for the hair and drying and irritating for the scalp.

☹ **Daily Clarifying Shampoo** *($0.78 for 15 ounces)* contains ammonium xylenesulfonate, which can be drying for the hair and drying and irritating for the scalp.

☹ **Dandruff Control Shampoo for Fine or Oily Hair** *($1.59 for 14.5 ounces)* does contain sulfur, an ingredient that can combat dandruff, but for a shampoo, sulfur is one of the last options to consider because it can strip hair color. Another problem is that this one contains ammonium xylenesulfonate, which can be drying for the hair and drying and irritating for the scalp.

☺ **For Kids 2-1 Shampoo, Extra Conditioning, Cherry Blast** *($1.99 for 12 ounces)* is a good basic shampoo for all hair types that are normal to fine or thin, but there is nothing in here that makes it particularly better or worse for kids than adults; it would work for both if they had the same hair type. There are minimal additives in here that could cause buildup. This contains mostly water, detergent cleansing agents, lather agent, thickeners, slip agents, detangling agent/film former, preservatives, fragrances, and coloring agents.

☹ **For Kids, 2-1 Shampoo, Regular Formula, Orange Splash** *($1.99 for 12 ounces)* contains ammonium xylenesulfonate, which can be drying for the hair and drying and irritating for the scalp.

☹ **Frequent Use Shampoo** *($0.78 for 15 ounces)* contains ammonium xylenesulfonate, which can be drying for the hair and drying and irritating for the scalp.

☹ **Full Body Shampoo** *($1.74 for 22.5 ounces)* contains ammonium xylenesulfonate, which can be drying for the hair and drying and irritating for the scalp.

☹ **Moisturizing Shampoo Replenishes Moisture to Dry Hair** *($0.78 for 15 ounces)* contains ammonium xylenesulfonate, which can be drying for the hair and drying and irritating for the scalp.

☺ **Natural Care Shampoo Citrus Blend** *($0.78 for 15 ounces)* contains ammonium xylenesulfonate, which can be drying for the hair and drying and irritating for the scalp.

☺ **Natural Care Shampoo Tropical Coconut** *($0.78 for 15 ounces)* contains ammonium xylenesulfonate, which can be drying for the hair and drying and irritating for the scalp.

☺ **Peach Essence Shampoo** *($0.78 for 15 ounces)* contains ammonium xylenesulfonate, which can be drying for the hair and drying and irritating for the scalp.

☺ **Perm & Color Formula Shampoo** *($0.78 for 15 ounces)* contains ammonium xylenesulfonate, which can be drying for the hair and drying and irritating for the scalp.

☺ **Professionals AromaPure Shampoo** *($1.58 for 14.5 ounces)* contains ammonium xylenesulfonate, which can be drying for the hair and drying and irritating for the scalp.

☺ **Professionals Awapuhi Shampoo** *($1.58 for 14.5 ounces)* contains ammonium xylenesulfonate, which can be drying for the hair and drying and irritating for the scalp.

☺ **Professionals Bio Basics Shampoo** *($1.58 for 14.5 ounces)* contains ammonium xylenesulfonate, which can be drying for the hair and drying and irritating for the scalp.

☺ **Professionals Humectant Shampoo** *($1.58 for 14.5 ounces)* contains ammonium xylenesulfonate, which can be drying for the hair and drying and irritating for the scalp.

☺ **Strawberry Essence Shampoo** *($0.78 for 15 ounces)* contains ammonium xylenesulfonate, which can be drying for the hair and drying and irritating for the scalp.

☺ **Shampoo and Conditioner Dandruff Shampoo Plus Conditioner for All Hair Types** *($0.78 for 11 ounces)* uses sodium lauryl sulfate as the main detergent cleansing agent, and that makes it too potentially irritating for the scalp and drying for the hair. The sulfur in here can be problem enough for the hair; why add any more drying ingredients?

☺ **Shampoo Plus Conditioner 2-in-1 Moisturizing Formula for Dry or Damaged Hair** *($1.58 for 14.5 ounces)* is a standard, silicone-based shampoo that would work well for normal to dry hair. Like all silicone-based shampoos it can build up on hair with repeated use. It contains mostly water, detergent cleansing agents, lather agent, silicone, thickeners, slip agents, detangling agent, preservatives, and coloring agents.

☺ **Shampoo Plus Conditioner 2-in-1 Regular Formula for Normal to Dry Hair** *($1.58 for 14.5 ounces)* is almost identical to the version above for Dry or Damaged Hair and the same comments apply.

☺ **Shampoo Plus Conditioner Healthy Shine with Pro-Vitamins 2-in-1 Moisturizing Formula for Dry or Damaged Hair** *($1.58 for 14.5 ounces)* is almost identical to the version above for Dry or Damaged Hair and the same comments apply.

☺ **Shampoo Plus Conditioner Healthy Shine with Pro-Vitamins 2-in-1 Regular Formula for Normal Hair** *($1.58 for 14.5 ounces)* is almost identical to the version above for Dry or Damaged Hair and the same comments apply.

☺ **Thermal Formula Shampoo, Heat Activated for Normal to Dry Hair** *($2.54 for 14.5 ounces)* is almost identical to the version above for Dry or Damaged Hair and the same comments apply. There is nothing in this product better for styling, and it can't protect the hair from the kind of high heat produced by most blow-dryers and curling irons.

☺ **Apple Essence Conditioner** *($0.78 for 15 ounces)* is a lightweight conditioner that would work well for normal hair of any thickness to help with comb- through. It contains mostly water, thickeners, detangling agents, preservatives, fragrance, and coloring agent.

☺ **Balsam and Protein Conditioner Adds Body to Normal to Dry Hair** *($0.78 for 15 ounces)* is almost identical to the Apple Essence Conditioner above. This one does contain a teeny amount of balsam, but that shouldn't be a problem for buildup—it's basically here in name only.

☺ **Daily Clarifying Conditioner** *($0.78 for 15 ounces)* is a lightweight conditioner that would work well for normal hair that is fine or thin. It contains mostly water, thickeners, detangling agents, film former, preservatives, fragrance, and coloring agent.

☺ **For Kids Detangling Spray, Awesome Apple** *($1.99 for 10.5 ounces)* is a lightweight, leave-in conditioner that would work well for normal hair of any thickness to help with comb-through. It contains mostly water, detangling agents, slip agents, fragrance, preservatives, and coloring agent.

☺ **Frequent Use Conditioner** *($1.74 for 22.5 ounces)* is almost identical to the Apple Essence Conditioner above and the same comments apply.

☺ **Full Body Conditioner** *($1.74 for 22.5 ounces)* is almost identical to the Apple Essence Conditioner above, only this one contains film former, which would make it better for normal hair that is fine or thin.

☺ **Healthy Shine Conditioner with Pro-Vitamins Daily Treatment for Normal to Dry Hair** *($1.58 for 14.5 ounces)* contains mostly water, thickeners, detangling agents, silicone, slip agent, conditioning agents, thickeners, fragrance, and preservatives. The amount of vitamins in here is minute and has no effect on hair or scalp. This is a good conditioner for normal to dry hair of any thickness.

☺ **Moisturizing Conditioner Replenishes Moisture to Dry Hair** *($0.78 for*

15 ounces) is almost identical to the Apple Essence Conditioner above and the same comments apply. It does contain a tiny amount of film former, which makes it slightly better for normal hair that is normal to fine or thin.

☺ **Natural Care Conditioner Citrus Blend** *($0.78 for 15 ounces)* contains lemon and orange, which can be a problem for the skin, so keep it off the scalp. Other than that, it's almost identical to the Apple Essence Conditioner above, except that this one contains a tiny amount of castor oil, which can make it better for normal to dry hair that iss normal to fine or thins. It can have a slight stiff feel.

☺ **Natural Care Conditioner Tropical Coconut** *($0.78 for 15 ounces)* is almost identical to the Natural Care Conditioner Citrus Blend above and the same comments apply.

☺ **Peach Essence Conditioner** *($0.78 for 15 ounces)* is almost identical to the Apple Essence Conditioner above and the same comments apply.

☺ **Perm & Color Formula Conditioner** *($0.78 for 15 ounces)* is almost identical to the Apple Essence Conditioner above and the same comments apply.

☺ **Professionals Awapuhi Conditioner** *($1.58 for 14.5 ounces)* contains mostly water, thickeners, detangling agent, silicone, plant extracts, plant oils, slip agents, conditioning agents, preservatives, fragrance, and coloring agents. Although you may associate awapuhi with the Paul Mitchell line, that's actually irrelevant—this is just a good conditioner for normal to dry hair of any thickness.

☺ **Professionals Bio Basics Conditioner** *($1.58 for 14.5 ounces)* is similar to the Awapuhi version above but with different plant extracts, and the same basic comments apply.

☺ **Professionals Humectant Conditioner** *($1.58 for 14.5 ounces)* is similar to the Awapuhi version above but with different plant extracts, and the same basic comments apply.

☹ **Professionals Rosemary Mint Conditioner** *($1.58 for 14.5 ounces)* contains peppermint, which can be a skin irritant and cause problems for the scalp. The tingling sensation may feel good but the tingling is also a clear signal something's wrong. Keep this conditioner off the scalp.

☺ **Strawberry Essence Conditioner** *($0.78 for 15 ounces)* is an extremely simple conditioner that contains mostly water, thickeners, detangling agents, fragrance, preservatives, vitamins, plant extracts, and slip agents. This would work well for normal hair of any thickness to help with combing, though the overly sweet smell might be a bit hard to take. It does contain a tiny amount of lemon but probably not enough to be a problem for the scalp.

☺ **Thermal Formula Conditioner, Heat Activated for Normal to Dry Hair** *($1.54 to 14.5 ounces)* contains mostly water, thickeners, detangling agent, silicones, slip agent, conditioning agents, preservatives, and fragrance. This is a good conditioner for dry hair of any thickness. There is nothing in here that can protect hair from heat damage generated by the high temperatures that styling tools use.

☺ **Thermal Formula Leave-in Conditioning Mist** *($1.89 for 10.5 ounces)* is a good basic leave-in conditioner that contains mostly water, detangling agent, slip agent, conditioning agents, silicones, fragrance, and preservatives. This would work great for normal to dry hair of any thickness.

☺ **Styling Gel Natural Control** *($1.24 for 12 ounces)* is a good basic gel with a light to medium hold and a slight sticky feel that does let you brush through the hair. It contains mostly water, film formers, thickeners, slip agents, preservatives, and coloring agents.

☺ **Styling Gel Extra Control** *($1.24 for 12 ounces)* is almost identical to the Styling Gel Natural Control version above and the same comments apply.

☺ **Styling Gel Maximum Control** *($1.24 for 12 ounces)* is almost identical to the Styling Gel Natural Control version above and the same comments apply.

☺ **Styling Mousse Maximum Control** *($1.23 for 7.5 ounces)* is a standard mousse with a light to medium hold and a slight sticky feel. It contains mostly water, propellant, detangling agents/film former, fragrance, and preservatives.

☺ **Styling Mousse Extra Control** *($1.23 for 7.5 ounces)* is almost identical to the Styling Mousse Maximum Control above with slightly less hold and no stiff or sticky feel.

☺ **Hairspray Extra Hold Aerosol** *($0.78 for 7 ounces)* is a standard aerosol hairspray with a light to medium hold and a slight stiff feel that can easily be brushed through. It contains mostly alcohol, water, film formers, silicone, and fragrance.

☺ **Hairspray Extra Hold Non-Aerosol** *($0.78 for 7 ounces)* is a standard hairspray with a medium hold and a somewhat stiff feel that does let you brush through the hair. It contains mostly alcohol, water, film formers, silicone, and fragrance.

☺ **Hairspray Maximum Hold Aerosol** *($0.78 for 7 ounces)* is almost identical to the Extra Hold Non-Aerosol version above and the same basic comments apply.

☺ **Hairspray Maximum Hold Non-Aerosol** *($0.78 for 7 ounces)* is similar to the Extra Hold Non-Aerosol version above and the same basic comments apply.

Salon Formula by Suave

☹ **Salon Formula Shampoo Vitamin Enriched to Nourish All Hair Types** *($0.78 for 15 ounces)* contains ammonium xylenesulfonate, which can be drying for the hair and drying and irritating for the scalp.

☺ **Salon Formula Conditioner Vitamin Enriched to Nourish All Hair Types** *($0.78 for 15 ounces)* is an extremely simple conditioner that contains mostly water, thickeners, detangling agents, fragrance, preservatives, vitamins, plant extracts, and slip agents. This would work well for normal hair of any thickness to help with combing. The minute amounts of vitamins are here in name only; there's not enough for them to have any benefit for hair or scalp.

☺ **Salon Formula Mousse Extra Control** *($1.23 for 7.5 ounces)* is a standard mousse with a light to medium hold and minimal to no stiff or sticky feel. It contains mostly water, propellant, detangling agents/film former, fragrance, and preservatives.

☺ **Salon Formula Spray Gel Extra Control** *($0.78 for 7 ounces)* is a good basic styling spray with a light to medium hold and minimal to no stiff or sticky feel that contains mostly water, alcohol, film formers, detangling agent, fragrance, slip agent, and preservatives.

☺ **Salon Formula Hair Spray Extra Hold Aerosol** *($0.78 for 7 ounces)* is a good basic aerosol hairspray with a light hold and minimal to no stiff or sticky feel that contains mostly water, alcohol, film formers, detangling agent, fragrance, slip agent, and preservatives.

☺ **Salon Formula Hair Spray Extra Hold Non-Aerosol** *($0.78 for 7 ounces)* is similar to the Extra Hold Aerosol version above and the same basic comments apply.

☺ **Salon Formula Spritz Ultimate Control** *($0.78 for 7 ounces)* is similar to the Extra Hold Aerosol version above, but it does have a firm hold with a definite stiff feel.

☹ **Salon Formula Hot Oil Treatment** *($1.29 for three 0.5-ounce tubes)* doesn't actually contain any oil, it is just an OK conditioner for normal hair that is thin to fine. It contains mostly water, detangling agent/film former, thickeners, fragrance, preservatives, and coloring agents.

Herbal Care by Suave

☹ **Herbal Care Chamomile Shampoo** *($0.78 for 15 ounces)* contains ammonium xylenesulfonate, which can be drying for the hair and drying and irritating for the scalp.

☹ **Herbal Care Shampoo Aloe Vera, Honeysuckle, and Vitamin E** *($0.78 for 15 ounces)* contains ammonium xylenesulfonate, which can be drying for the hair and drying and irritating for the scalp.

☺ **Herbal Care Chamomile Conditioner** *($0.78 for 15 ounces)* is a lightweight conditioner that would work well for normal hair of any thickness to help with comb-through. It contains mostly water, thickeners, detangling agents, preservatives, fragrance, and coloring agent.

☺ **Herbal Care Conditioner Aloe Vera, Honeysuckle, and Vitamin E** *($0.78 for 15 ounces)* is almost identical to the Apple Essence Conditioner above and the same comments apply.

The Reviews S

☺ **Herbal Care Mousse Extra Control Rosemary, Honeysuckle & Indigo Root** *($1.39 for 6 ounces)* is a standard mousse with a light hold and minimal stiff or sticky feel. It contains mostly water, propellant, plant extracts, detangling agents/film former, fragrance, and preservatives. The plant extracts have no effect on the hair.

☺ **Herbal Care Hairspray Non-Aerosol Flexible Hold Chamomile, Arnica & White Ginger** *($1.39 for 8.5 ounces)* is a standard hairspray with a light hold and minimal to no stiff or sticky feel. It contains mostly water, propellant, plant extracts, detangling agents/film former, fragrance, and preservatives. The plant extracts have no effect on the hair.

☺ **Herbal Care Hairspray Aerosol Flexible Hold Chamomile, Arnica & White Ginger** *($1.39 for 8.5 ounces)* is similar to the Non-Aerosol Flexible Hold above and the same basic comments apply.

☺ **Herbal Care Hairspray Non-Aerosol Extra Hold Passion Flower, Goldenseal & Witch Hazel** *($1.89 for 14 ounces)* is similar to the Non-Aerosol Flexible Hold above only with slightly more hold, but only slightly, and the same basic comments apply.

Sukesha

For more information on Sukesha, call (800) 221-3496 or visit its Web site at www.sukesha.com.

☹ **Extra Body Shampoo, Mild Deep Cleansing for Added Texture** *($5.50 for 12 ounces)* uses sodium C14-16 olefin sulfate as the main cleansing agent, which can dry hair and potentially strip hair color.

☺ **Moisturizing Shampoo, Shampoo and Conditioner in One** *($5.50 for 12 ounces)* contains mostly plant water, detergent cleansing agents, lather agent, slip agents, detangling agents/film formers, thickeners, preservatives, and fragrance. This is a good shampoo for someone with normal hair that is normal to fine or thin.

☺ **Natural Balance Shampoo, Pure and Gentle for Shine and Volume Shampoo** *($5.50 for 12 ounces)* is almost identical to the Moisturizing Shampoo above and the same basic comments apply.

☺ **Conditioning Rinse** *($7.80 for 12 ounces)* contains mostly plant water, thickeners, castor oil, detangling agent, conditioning agents, silicone, slip agents, preservatives, and fragrance. This is a good conditioner for dry hair that is fine or thin. It can build up and leave a stiff, sticky feel on hair, but it can also help smooth frizzies.

☺ **Daily Hydrating Balm, Restores Vitality to Dry Damaged Hair** *($6.95 for 12 ounces)* contains mostly plant water, detangling agents, thickeners, conditioning agents, plant oil, silicone, slip agents, detangling agent/film former, preservatives, and fragrance. This is a good conditioner for dry hair that is fine or thin.

☺ **Hair Moisturizing Treatment, Intensive Formula for Elasticity and Strength** *($5.50 for 6 ounces)* contains mostly plant water, detangling agents, thickeners, conditioning agents, detangling agent/film former, preservatives, and fragrance. This is a good conditioner for normal to slightly dry hair that is fine or thin.

☺ **Shine and Body Leave-in Conditioner** *($5.95 for 8 ounces)* contains mostly plant water, film former, detangling agent, conditioning agents, slip agents, silicone, preservatives, and fragrance. This is a good leave-in conditioner that is more like a styling spray, with a light hold and minimal stiff or sticky feel. It can work well for normal to slightly dry hair that is fine or thin.

☺ **Glossing Gel, Brilliant Shine Plus Hold Formula** *($7.95 for 8 ounces)* is a good basic gel with a light to medium hold and minimal sticky feel. It also has a bit of glitter dust added, which does add a subtle shine. It contains mostly plant water, film former, silicones, conditioning agents, detangling agent/film former, thickeners, preservatives, fragrance, and coloring agents.

☺ **Styling Gel Ultimate Body and Hold Formula** *($5.95 for 6 ounces)* is similar to the one above minus the glitter, and the same basic comments apply.

☺ **Styling Mousse for Extra Control and Volume** *($6.95 for 12 ounces)* is a good standard mousse with a medium hold and a somewhat sticky feel that does let you brush through the hair. It contains mostly water, alcohol, film formers, propellant, slip agents, silicones, plant extracts, and fragrance.

☺ **Sculpting Lotion Extra Hold** *($4.95 for 12 ounces)* contains mostly plant water, film formers, conditioning agents, silicone, thickeners, preservatives, and fragrance. This styling lotion has a medium hold with minimal stiff or sticky feel and it can work well for smoothing frizzies and curls.

☺ **Freeze Frame Super Spray (Non-Aerosol)** *($5.95 for 8 ounces)* is a standard hairspray with a medium to firm hold and a somewhat stiff, sticky feel that does let hair be brushed through. It contains mostly alcohol, water, film former, silicone, conditioning agent, plant extracts, and fragrance.

☺ **Styling Hair Spray, Working Spray with Firm Control (Non-Aerosol)** *($5.95 for 8 ounces)* is almost identical to the Freeze Frame above and the same comments apply.

☺ **Maximum Hold Hair Spray, Ultimate Hold Formula (Aerosol)** *($6.95 for 10 ounces)* is a standard aerosol hairspray with a medium to firm hold and a somewhat stiff feel that does let hair be brushed through. It contains mostly alcohol, water, film former, silicone, conditioning agent, plant extracts, and fragrance.

☺ **Shaping and Styling Hair Spray, Firm Design Formula (Aerosol)** *($6.95 for 10 ounces)* is almost identical to the Maximum Hold version above and the same comments apply.

Susan Lucci Collection

Actress Susan Lucci, in her role as the multifaceted though sinister Erica Kane in the soap opera *All My Children,* has spent more years causing emotional upheaval in the lives of her family and friends than almost any other character on daytime television. And, like her alter ego Erica, she is also known for being beautifully groomed, with artfully applied makeup and every lock of hair fastidiously in place.

Of course, if Ms. Lucci is so stunningly coifed, she must therefore be incredibly knowledgeable about hair products, right? That wouldn't be my logic, but it's what the creators of the Susan Lucci line of hair-care products want you to think, and many consumers find the notion irresistible.

Considering all the lines I've reviewed, it still surprises me that the Lucci line ends up having one of the more unethical hair-care products I've run into. This is the **Sun-Hints Spray Chamomile Hair Lightening Spray** *($14.50 for two 8-ounce containers),* and it truly adds up to being one of the most deceptive hair-care products out there. The claim is that this product will lighten the hair with "extracts." Well, guess what—one of the extracts is called "albone," which the label explains is a "natural lightening agent." But it turns out that albone extract is a trade name for hydrogen peroxide, which of course will permanently lighten hair by bleaching, and will also damage hair as well. Moreover, if you did want these effects, you could get them from an 89-cent bottle of 3 percent hydrogen peroxide at the drugstore. It's not that there aren't some good products in this line, because there are, but the prices and deceptive claims are among some of the most flagrant around, and I would think twice about shopping any line with this kind of ethics.

These products are available only through QVC, the Home Shopping Channel, which does *not* ship to Canada—depending on your point of view, this is either bad or good. For more information on Susan Lucci Collection, call (800) 345-1515, or visit its Web site at www.iqvc.com.

☹ **Clarifying Shampoo with Vitamin Beads for Build-Up Removal** *($18 for two 8-ounce bottles)* uses sodium C14-16 olefin sulfate as its main cleansing agent, which can be drying for the scalp and hair and can potentially strip hair color.

☺ **Purifying Shampoo Healthy Hair Complex** *($17 for two 12-ounce bottles)* contains mostly water, detergent cleansing agents, lather agent, conditioning agents, plant extracts, detangling agent, detangling agent/film formers, preservatives, and fragrance. This shampoo won't purify anything, but it can be good for normal to dry hair that is normal to fine or thin.

☺ **Deep Conditioning Treatment Healthy Hair Complex** *($18 for two 4-ounce containers)* contains mostly water, conditioning agents, thickeners, plant extracts, preservatives, and fragrance. This is a good standard conditioner for normal to slightly dry hair of any thickness; there is nothing special in the formula that makes it more of a "treatment" for hair.

☺ **Moisture Infusion Rinse** (*$19 for two 12-ounce containers*) contains mostly water, detangling agents, conditioning agents, slip agents, thickeners, plant extracts, vitamins, preservatives, and fragrance. This is a good conditioner for normal to slightly dry hair of any thickness.

☺ **Multi-Fix Plus, Leave-in Spray Healthy Hair Complex** (*$22 for two 12-ounce containers*) is a good leave-in conditioner for normal to dry hair of any thickness. It contains mostly water, detangling agents, silicones, slip agents, conditioning agents, plant extracts, preservatives, and fragrance.

☹ **Balancing Scalp Elixir Healthy Hair Complex** (*$23 for two 4-ounce containers*) contains several ingredients that are problematic for the scalp, including menthol, balm mint, and alcohol. This irritating, toner-type product is not recommended.

☺ **$$$ Radiance** (*$19 for two 1-ounce containers*) is just an overpriced silicone serum that can add shine and leave the hair feeling silky.

☺ **$$$ Super-Lite Radiance Spray Shine Mist** (*$18 for one 4-ounce container and one 2-ounce container*) is similar to the Radiance serum above, only this one is in spray form. The same basic comments apply.

☺ **$$$ Sealer Gel-O Seal-Out Curl & Frizz Sculpt, Style & Hold** (*$25 for 4 ounces; in a set with 6 ounces of the Straight-A-Head reviewed below*) contains mostly plant water, film formers, slip agents, thickeners, preservatives, fragrance, and coloring agents. This is a good basic gel with a light to medium hold and a somewhat sticky feel that does let hair be brushed through. It does have a tiny bit of glitter but it's very subtle and hardly detectable.

☺ **$$$ Straight-A-Head Curl & Frizz Smoother** (*$25 for 6 ounces, in a set with 4 ounces of the Sealer reviewed above*) is a basic silicone serum that can add a silky feel and shine to hair.

☺ **Botanical Styling Lotion** (*$23.75 for one 12-ounce container; plus one 4-ounce container*) contains mostly water, film formers, plant extracts, conditioning agents, thickeners, silicone, preservatives, and fragrance. This lightweight styling spray has a soft hold and minimal to no sticky feel.

☺ **Pollution Shield Hairspray Healthy Hair Complex Advanced Formula** (*$12.75 for two 8-ounce containers*) is a standard hairspray with a light to medium hold and a slight stiff feel that can easily be brushed through. It contains mostly alcohol, water, film formers, slip agents, silicone, plant extracts, preservatives, and fragrance. There is nothing in here that can protect hair from pollution any more than any other hairspray that coats the hair.

The Reviews S

☺ **Climate Control Hairspray Alcohol Free** *($12.75 for two 8-ounce containers)* is almost identical to the Pollution Shield above and the same comments apply.

☹ **Sun-Hints Spray Chamomile Hair Lightening Spray** *($14.50 for two 8-ounce containers)* rates as one of the most truly deceptive hair-care products. The claim is that this product will lighten the hair with "extracts." Well, guess what? One of the extracts is called "albone," which the label explains as a "natural lightening agent." It turns out albone extract is a trade name for hydrogen peroxide, which of course will permanently lighten hair by bleaching; it will also damage hair as well. Moreover, you could get the same effect from an 89-cent bottle of 3 percent hydrogen peroxide at the drugstore.

☹ **Hair Revive System for Fine Thinning Hair Activating Shampoo with Alpha Hydroxy Acids** *($17 for two 8-ounce bottles)* contains menthol, which can be an irritant for the scalp. The cooling sensation might make some feel like their hair growth is being stimulated, but it is actually causing problems, not helping. The amount of glycolic and lactic acid in here, thankfully, isn't enough to denature the hair shaft.

☹ **Hair Revive System for Fine Thinning Hair Super-Lite Rinse** *($18 for two 8-ounce containers)* contains menthol, which can be an irritant for the scalp. It might make some feel like their hair growth is being stimulated, but it is actually causing problems, not helping.

☺ **Hair Revive System for Fine Thinning Hair Volume Tonic Hair Maximizer** *($14.50 for two 4-ounce containers)*. At least they took the menthol out of this version! This is just a good, lightweight, liquidy gel with a soft, light hold and minimal to no stiff or sticky feel. It can help with styling or as a leave-in conditioner, but it won't grow a hair on your head. It contains mostly plant water, detangling agent/film former, thickeners, conditioning agents, vitamins, silicone, slip agents, preservatives, and fragrance.

☹ **Hair Revive System for Fine Thinning Hair Root Nutrient Follicle Infusion** *($25 for two 2-ounce containers)* contains menthol, which may make the scalp tingle, but that is a signal of irritation, not of anything healthy in the least.

TCB

For hair-care products aimed at the African-American consumer, this is the classic line. For more information on TCB, call (708) 450-3000, (800) 333-6666, or visit its Web site at www.alberto-culver.com.

☹ **Apple Essence Neutralizing Shampoo** *($3.36 for 8 ounces)* uses sodium lauryl sulfate as the main detergent cleansing agent, and that makes it too potentially irritating for the scalp and drying for the hair.

☹ **Detangling Shampoo, Aloe, Henna & Kiwi, Helps Reduce Breakage** *($3.29 for 16 ounces)* uses sodium lauryl sulfate and sodium C14-17 alkyl sec sulfonate as its main detergent cleansing agents, and that makes it too potentially irritating for the scalp and drying for the hair. It also contains peppermint, which can be an irritant for the scalp.

☺ **Creme Hairdress, Aloe & Chamomile, for Moisture, Body and Shine** *($3.19 for 6 ounces)* contains mostly water, mineral oil, slip agent, thickeners, Vaseline, silicones, plant extracts, slip agents, film former, preservatives, and fragrance. This greasy conditioner has a light hold, and though it definitely can add shine to hair and help extremely dry hair, it can also look oily and feel heavy on the hair.

☺ **Hair and Scalp Conditioner, Jojoba Oil, Chamomile & Aloe** *($3.49 for 10 ounces)* contains mostly mineral oil, Vaseline, lanolin, thickeners, plant oil, plant extracts, and fragrance. This is greasy, heavy stuff that can easily build up on hair. It can be helpful for extremely dry hair, but be careful—it can look oily and slippery.

☺ **Hair Food, Sweet Almond Oil, Jojoba & Olive Oil, Moisture Rich Treatment** *($4.49 for 10 ounces)* is almost identical to the Hair and Scalp Conditioner above and the same basic comments apply.

☺ **Lite Hair and Scalp Conditioner, Kiwi, Aloe & Papaya, Replenishes Damaged Hair** *($4.39 for 10 ounces)* is definitely lighter than the versions above. This one contains mostly water, thickener, mineral oil, slip agents, silicone, plant extracts, preservatives, and fragrance. This is a good basic conditioner for dry hair of any thickness.

☺ **Lite Instant Moisturizer, Jasmine, Aloe & Lavender** *($3.59 for 8 ounces)* contains peppermint, so keep this away from the scalp. Other than that, this very simple leave-in conditioner contains mostly water, slip agents, plant extracts, preservatives, fragrance, and coloring agents. This is almost a waste of time; it can add some combing help for normal hair, but that's about it.

☺ **Protein Conditioner, Aloe, Chamomile & Yucca, Protein Therapy** *($5.29 for 16 ounces)* contains mostly water, mineral oil, slip agents, detangling agents/film formers, silicone, conditioning agents, plant extracts, more slip agents, preservatives, fragrance, and coloring agents. This is a good conditioner for very dry hair that is fine or thin, though it can easily cause buildup. It does contain peppermint, a skin irritant, so keep it away from the scalp.

☺ **Protein Conditioner Deep Penetrating Protein Therapy** *($1.79 for 12 1-ounce treatments)* is almost identical to the Aloe, Chamomile & Yucca version above and the same comments apply.

☺ **Hot Oil Treatment for Dry, Brittle, Damaged Hair, Almond & Jojoba Oils** *($3.99 for 6 ounces)* is just mineral oil with thickeners, detangling agents, fragrance, and preservatives. We checked the ingredient label twice and called the company, but there doesn't appear to be any plant oil in this product despite the name on the label. Still, this can be good for extremely dry hair, but it can also be greasy.

☺ **Oil Sheen and Conditioner Spray (Aerosol)** *($4.29 for 9 ounces)* is just a spray that places a light liquid wax over the hair. That can add shine, but it can build up and be hard to shampoo out.

☺ **Oil Sheen Spray, Sweet Almond & Jojoba Oils, Dazzling Shine (Aerosol)** *($2.99 for 11.25 ounces)* is similar to the Oil Sheen and Conditioner Spray above, only this one has plant oils added, which can add more shine and slip.

☺ **Lite Gel Activator, Aloe, Yucca & Chamomile, Moisturizes and Replenishes** *($3.49 for 10 ounces)* is just a minimal- to no-hold gel with no stiff or sticky feel; it only adds some slip and smoothing to hair when styling. It contains mostly water, slip agents, thickeners, plant extracts, preservatives, fragrance, and coloring agents. It can help when styling normal hair.

☺ **Designing Spritz, Chamomile, Almond Oil & Jojoba Oil, All Day Hold** *($3.49 for 10 ounces)* is a standard hairspray with a light to medium hold and a slight stiff feel that does let hair be brushed through. It contains mostly alcohol, water, film formers, plant oils, plant extracts, slip agents, and fragrance.

☺ **Holding Spray, Jojoba & Chamomile, Exceptional Hold (Aerosol)** *($3.29 for 11.9 ounces)* is a standard aerosol hairspray with a light hold and minimal stiff feel. It contains mostly alcohol, water, film formers, plant oils, plant extracts, slip agents, and fragrance.

Bone Strait by TCB

☹ **Shampoo** *($6.99 for 32 ounces)* uses sodium lauryl sulfate as the main detergent cleansing agent, and that makes it too potentially irritating for the scalp and drying for the hair.

☺ **Conditioner and Blow Dry Lotion** *($3.89 for 16 ounces)* is a very standard leave-in conditioner that contains mostly water, thickeners, detangling agent, slip agents, preservatives, fragrance, and coloring agents. This can be good for someone with normal hair of any thickness, but it has no effect on holding curls or making hair dry straighter.

☹ **Nutri-Shock Vitamin Enriched Leave-in Rejuvenator** *($3.49 for 16 ounces)* is a good leave-in conditioner for dry hair of any thickness. It contains mostly water, silicone, conditioning agents, vitamins, slip agent, plant oils, water-binding agents, detangling agent, detangling agent/film former, alcohol, preservatives, and fragrance. The tiny amount of sulfur in here may be a problem for dyed hair, but the tiny amount of film former is barely detectable and shouldn't cause buildup. The vitamins that are in here can't feed the scalp or hair and they offer no benefit to the health of hair over any other conditioning agent.

☺ **Wrapping Setting Lotion** *($2.69 for 12 ounces)* is a good, very standard, lightweight styling liquid that would have been far easier to use in spray form than squeezed from a bottle. It has a soft hold and a slight sticky feel, and can help hold a set just like any other light-hold styling spray. It contains mostly water, detangling agent/film former, alcohol, more detangling agent, conditioning agents, silicones, preservatives, and fragrance.

☺ **Shining Gel** *($2.99 for 4 ounces)* is just water, thickener, slip agents, mineral oil, preservatives, fragrance, and coloring agent. It has no hold, and the shine comes from the mineral oil. That can help when styling extremely dry hair with no stiff or sticky feel, though it can feel slightly greasy.

☺ **Spray Gel, Firm Hold for Slicking, Sculpting, Molding** *($2.99 for 8 ounces)* is a standard spray gel that has a light hold and minimal to no sticky feel. It contains mostly water, film former, conditioning agent, thickeners, preservatives, and fragrance.

☺ **12 Hour Holding Spritz, Lite Hold** *($1.99 for 12 ounces)* is a standard hairspray that has a light to medium hold with only a slight stiff feel that can easily be brushed through. It contains mostly alcohol, water, film former, slip agents, silicone, conditioning agent, and fragrance.

☺ **Spritz, Super Hold** *($2.29 for 8 ounces)* is almost identical to the Lite Hold above and the same comments apply.

Tegren

☹ **Advanced Formula Dandruff Shampoo** *($5.17 for 7 ounces)* uses sodium lauryl sulfate as the main detergent cleansing agent, and that makes it too potentially irritating for the scalp and drying for the hair. The coal tar in here is drying enough for the hair as it is; why add an additional ingredient unnecessarily and add to the problems?

☹ **Advanced Formula Dandruff Shampoo, Extra Conditioning** *($5.17 for 7 ounces)* is similar to the version above and the same comments apply.

☹ **Advanced Formula Dandruff Shampoo, Fresh Herbal** *($5.17 for 7 ounces)* is similar to the version above and the same comments apply.

Terax

This Italian import hair-care line has a lot of problematic formulations as well as absurd pricing for what you get. Even when a formulation doesn't have problems, it is just ordinary and basic, along the lines of Suave or White Rain hair-care products at the drugstore. That's not bad, but it makes the Italian flair embarrassing. This is a line you can easily overlook and not be missing out on anything. For more information on Terax, call (800) 213-5531 or visit its Web site at www.teraxhaircare.com.

☺ **Baby Shampoo for Children's Sensitive Skin and Hair** *($12 for 8 ounces)* is far more gentle than any of the other Terax shampoos. This one is the best option for all hair types. It contains mostly water, detergent cleansing agent, lather agent, conditioning agent, thickener, and preservative.

☹ **Original Shamp Bosco Shampoo for Oily Hair** *($14.95 for 8.4 ounces)* contains peppermint, menthol, and camphor, all skin irritants that cause problems for skin and have no effect whatsoever on oil production or in absorbing oil.

☹ **Original Shamp Delicato Shampoo for All Types of Hair** *($14.95 for 8.4 ounces)* uses sodium lauryl sulfate as the main detergent cleansing agent, and that makes it too potentially irritating for the scalp and drying for the hair.

☹ **Original Shamp Fior di Camomilla Shampoo for Blond & Delicate Hair** *($12 for 8 ounces)* uses sodium lauryl sulfate as the main detergent cleansing agent, and that makes it too potentially irritating for the scalp and drying for the hair.

☹ **Original Shamp Latte Silk Effect Shampoo** *($14.95 for 8.4 ounces)* uses sodium lauryl sulfate as the main detergent cleansing agent, and that makes it too potentially irritating for the scalp and drying for the hair.

☹ **Original Shamp Miele Shampoo for Chemically Treated or Dry Hair** *($14.95 for 8.4 ounces)* uses sodium lauryl sulfate as the main detergent cleansing agent, and that makes it too potentially irritating for the scalp and drying for the hair.

☹ **Terax Gold 3 Cereali Shampoo for Chemically Treated or Weak Hair** *($12 for 8 ounces)* uses sodium lauryl sulfate as the main detergent cleansing agent, and that makes it too potentially irritating for the scalp and drying for the hair.

☹ **Terax Gold Collagene Shampoo, Protects Dry Brittle Hair** *($12 for 8 ounces)* uses sodium lauryl sulfate as the main detergent cleansing agent, and that makes it too potentially irritating for the scalp and drying for the hair.

☹ **Terax Gold Guarana Shampoo Before-After Coloring for Color Treated Hair** *($12 for 8.4 ounces)* uses sodium lauryl sulfate as the main detergent cleansing agent, and that makes it too potentially irritating for the scalp and drying for the hair.

☹ **Terax Gold Nodandr Shampoo Anti-Dandruff Shampoo** *($20 for 8.4 ounces)* uses sodium lauryl sulfate as the main detergent cleansing agent, and that makes it too potentially irritating for the scalp and drying for the hair.

☹ **Terax Gold Ortica Shampoo for Oily Hair** *($12 for 8 ounces)* uses sodium lauryl sulfate as the main detergent cleansing agent, and that makes it too potentially irritating for the scalp and drying for the hair.

☹ **Terax Gold Perla Shampoo Gentle Cleansing for All Hair Types** *($12 for 8.4 ounces)* uses sodium lauryl sulfate as the main detergent cleansing agent, and that makes it too potentially irritating for the scalp and drying for the hair.

☺ **$$$ Life Drops Leave-in Vegetable Protein Lotion for Normal and Damaged Hair** *($30 for 6.7 ounces)* gives hair no life whatsoever. This is a standard, very ordinary leave-in conditioner that can be OK for normal hair that is fine or thin, but it can build up and the alcohol in here can be a problem with repeated use. It contains mostly water, alcohol, detangling agent, slip agent, conditioning agent, fragrance, castor oil, preservatives, and coloring agents.

☺ **$$$ Novo Terax Plus 2 Lotion for Brittle or Dry Hair** *($18 for 2 ounces)* is OK for normal hair but that's about it. Conditioners don't get much more boring than this one. This contains mostly water, slip agent, thickeners, detangling agent, fragrance, and preservatives.

☹ **$$$ Original Crema Hair Treatment** *($19 for 5 ounces)* is similar to the Novo Terax version above, only in cream form, and the same basic comments apply.

☹ **$$$ Terax Gold Shine Conditioner Leave-in Protein Conditioner for Extra Shine and Volume to Hair** *($16 for 6 ounces)* is similar to the Novo Terax version above and the same basic comments apply.

☹ **$$$ Rigene Herbage Tonic for the Sheen of the Hair, Special Care for Permed and Tinted Hair** *($15 for 8.4 ounces)* is similar to the Novo Terax version above, only in spray form, and the same basic comments apply. There is nothing in here that is helpful for dry hair.

☺ **$$$ Tera Gloss Instant Restorer for Damaged Hair** *($12 for 1 ounce)* is as standard a silicone serum as they come, and completely overpriced, but it does work well for adding shine and a silky-soft feel to hair.

☺ **Terax Gold Mousse** *($14.50 for 8.4 ounces)* is a standard (and overpriced) mousse that has a light to medium hold and a somewhat sticky feel that can be brushed through. It contains mostly water, film former, propellant, thickeners, fragrance, detangling agent, castor oil, and preservatives.

☺ **Luxcent Hair Pomade** *($14 for 2.5 ounces)* is a very boring pomade that is just thickening agents, preservatives, and fragrance. This can look heavy and thick, but it can help smooth out frizzies. There are far better pomades than this version.

☺ **Terax Gold Gomma Gel, Moulding Gel** *($10 for 5 ounces)* is an exceptionally standard gel that just contains water, slip agent, thickeners, film former, fragrance, and preservative. It has a light to medium hold and a slight sticky feel that can be brushed through.

☺ **Aria Pura Volumizing Ecological Spray, Forte** *($14 for 8.4 ounces)* is a standard hairspray with a light hold and minimal to no stiff feel that contains mostly alcohol, film formers, slip agent, silicone, and fragrance.

☺ **Aria Pura Volumizing Ecological Spray** *($14 for 8.4 ounces)* is almost identical to the Spray Forte above and the same comments apply.

Theorie

For more information on Theorie, call (888) 794-6123.

☺ **Moisturizing Shampoo for Normal to Dry, Damaged, or Coarse Hair** *($4.99 for 12.5 ounces)* contains mostly water, detergent cleansing agents, lather agent, conditioning agents, water-binding agent, fragrance, film former, preservatives, and coloring agents. This would work well for normal to dry hair that is normal to fine or thin. The film former in here would add unnecessary thickness for hair that is already coarse.

☺ **Shampoo for Normal to Dry Hair** *($4.99 for 12.5 ounces)* is almost identical to the Moisturizing version above and the same comments apply.

☺ **Volumizing Shampoo for Normal to Thin or Fine Hair** *($4.99 for 12.5 ounces)* is almost identical to the Moisturizing version above and the same comments apply.

☺ **Conditioner for Normal to Fine Hair** *($4.99 for 12.5 ounces)* contains mostly water, thickeners, detangling agents, slip agents, fragrance, silicones, preservatives, and coloring agents. This would be a good conditioner for normal to dry hair of any thickness.

☺ **Moisturizing Conditioner for Normal to Dry Hair** *($4.99 for 12.5 ounces)* is almost identical to the Conditioner for Normal to Fine Hair above and the same comments apply.

☺ **Volumizing Conditioner for Normal to Thin or Fine Hair** *($4.99 for 12.5 ounces)* is almost identical to the Conditioner for Normal to Fine Hair above and the same comments apply.

☺ **SpecifiCurl Styling Mist for Curls and Waves** *($4.13 for 8 ounces)* is a standard styling spray with a light to medium hold and minimal stiff or sticky feel. It contains mostly water, alcohol, detangling agent/film formers, slip agents, conditioning agents, silicone, fragrance, preservatives, and coloring agents.

☺ **HydroFy Hydrating Mist for Moisture and Heat Protection** *($4.99 for 8 ounces)* is standard styling spray with a light hold and minimal to no stiff or sticky feel. It contains mostly water, detangling agent/film formers, silicones, conditioning agents, slip agents, preservatives, and coloring agents. There is nothing in here that can protect hair from the heat generated by styling tools.

☺ **Up Root Hydragel for Volume and Lift at the Roots** *($5.13 for 4 ounces)* is a basic styling gel with minimal to no hold and no stiff or sticky feel at all. It can help when styling hair that doesn't need much control or hold. It contains mostly water, film former, thickeners, conditioning agents, silicone, plant extracts, slip agents, preservatives, and coloring agents.

☺ **VersaHold Multi-Use Styling Gel for Control and Versatility** *($4.13 for 6 ounces)* is a basic styling gel with light to medium hold and a slight sticky feel. It contains mostly water, film former, thickeners, conditioning agents, silicone, plant extracts, slip agents, preservatives, and coloring agents.

☺ **Volume All-Over Clear Foam for Body and Control** *($6.17 for 7 ounces)* is an aerated mousse that contains mostly water, film formers, slip agents, fragrance, preservatives, and coloring agents. This has a medium to firm hold and a somewhat sticky feel that does let hair be brushed through.

☺ **Volume All-Over Volumizing Foam** *($6.17 for 7 ounces)* is almost identical to the Body and Control version above and the same comments apply.

☺ **Smooth Styles Styling Creme for Definition and Smoothness** *($6.17 for 5.5 ounces)* is a good styling cream for straightening hair. It has a light hold with minimal sticky feel. It can feel and look heavy, so use it sparingly. It contains mostly water, thickeners, detangling agents, silicones, film former, slip agents, fragrance, Vaseline, more slip agents, preservatives, and coloring agents.

ThermaSilk

The good news is that I found most of the new ThermaSilk hair-care products to be excellent and inexpensive. I would recommend most of them quite enthusiastically. The bad news is that the claims these products make about releasing conditioning benefits under heat don't hold up, at least not all the way on high heat. First, not all of the ThermaSilk products are meant to ever get near heat. And what good are conditioning ingredients, even those supposedly meant to be activated with heat, when they're in a shampoo, which is mostly rinsed down the drain? Or when they are added to finishing hairsprays and mousses, which are applied after the heat has been turned off? What's even more significant is that none of the conditioning agents in this line are unique—they are the same ones that show up in countless other hair products.

What is true is that heat can help all conditioning agents penetrate the hair cuticle, and that indirect heat is better than heat applied directly to the hair. Indirect heat is the type you get when you're sitting under a dryer bonnet and the heat is at least 6 inches away from the hair. When a conditioner is left on your hair and the warmth circulates around it, the cuticle can open up and the conditioning agents can form a better bond with the hair shaft. But that's not what happens with blow-dryers and curling irons, which can heat up to over 200 degrees Fahrenheit in direct contact with the hair, much like a hot iron on a blouse! This kind of direct heat is so intense that it literally smokes the hair, burning off the protective cuticle layer. No matter how it's formulated or how good it is, no conditioner can protect hair from that kind of heat damage, any more than it could protect skin from heat damage caused by touching a burner on the stove. For more information on ThermaSilk, call (800) 621-3379.

☺ **Heat Activated Shampoo for Normal Hair** *($3.42 for 13 ounces)* is a standard, detergent-based shampoo that contains mostly water, detergent cleansing agents, lather agent, silicone, thickeners, fragrance, detangling agent, and preservatives. It would work well for normal to dry hair of any thickness but, like any silicone-based shampoo, it can cause buildup with repeated use.

☺ **Heat Activated Shampoo for Colored or Permed Hair** *($3.42 for 13 ounces)* is almost identical to the version for Normal Hair above and the same basic comments apply.

☺ **Heat Activated Shampoo for Dry or Damaged Hair** *($3.24 for 13 ounces)* is almost identical to the version above for Normal Hair and the same comments apply.

☺ **Heat Activated Shampoo Volumizing for Fine or Thin Hair** *($3.42 for 13 ounces)* is almost identical to the Normal Hair version and the same comments apply.

☺ **Heat Activated Conditioner for Dry or Damaged Hair** *($3.24 for 13 ounces)* contains mostly water, thickeners, silicone, conditioning agents, more thickeners, fragrance, slip agents, detangling agents, and preservatives. This is a good conditioner for normal to dry hair of any thickness.

☺ **Heat Activated Conditioner Regular for Normal Hair** *($3.42 for 13 ounces)* is almost identical to the version above for Dry or Damaged Hair and the same comments apply.

☺ **Heat Activated Conditioner for Colored or Permed Hair** *($3.42 for 13 ounces)* is almost identical to the Dry or Damaged Hair version above and the same comments apply.

☺ **Heat Activated Conditioner Volumizing for Fine or Thin Hair** *($3.42 for 13 ounces)* is almost identical to the Dry or Damaged Hair version above and the same comments apply.

☺ **Heat Activated Light Conditioning Mist** *($2.99 for 10.3 ounces)* is a very lightweight, leave-in conditioner that would be very good for someone with normal hair of any thickness. It contains mostly water, detangling agent, slip agents, conditioning agents, preservatives, fragrance, and silicone.

☺ **Heat Activated Shine & Hold Gel Extra Control** *($2.99 for 8 ounces)* is a standard gel with a medium hold and minimal to no stiff or sticky feel. The one twist is that this one has glitter. Glitter doesn't cling well to hair and ends up getting all over clothing. This contains mostly water, film formers, conditioning agents, silicone, thickeners, slip agent, fragrance, and preservatives.

☺ **Heat Activated Styling Gel Extra Control** *($2.99 for 7 ounces)* is almost identical to the Shine & Hold version above, minus the glitter, but the other comments apply.

☺ **Heat Activated Conditioning Mousse Extra Control** *($2.99 for 7 ounces)* is a standard mousse with a light hold and a slight sticky feel that does let hair be brushed through. It contains mostly water, alcohol, propellant, detangling agent, silicone, conditioning agents, preservatives, and fragrance.

☺ **Heat Activated Volumizing Mousse Maximum Control** *($2.99 for 7 ounces)* is a standard mousse with a light to medium hold and a somewhat sticky feel that does let hair be brushed through. It contains mostly water, alcohol, propellant, detangling agent, mineral oil, conditioning agents, preservatives, and fragrance.

☺ **Heat Activated Shape & Hold Spray Firm Hold (Aerosol)** *($2.99 for 7 ounces)* is a standard aerosol hairspray with a soft, light hold and minimal to no stiff feel. It contains mostly alcohol, propellant, film formers, conditioning agents, silicones, and fragrance.

☺ **Heat Activated Shape & Hold Spray Firm Hold (Non-Aerosol)** *($2.99 for 10.5 ounces)* is almost identical to the Aerosol version above, only this one is in nonaerosol form, and the same comments apply.

☺ **Heat Activated Shape & Hold Spray Flexible Hold Aerosol** *($2.99 for 7 ounces)* is almost identical to the Aerosol version above and the same comments apply.

☺ **Heat Activated Shape & Hold Spray Flexible Hold Non-Aerosol** *($2.99 for 10.5 ounces)* is almost identical to the Aerosol version above, only this one is in nonaerosol form, and the same comments apply.

Thicker Fuller Hair

Thicker Fuller Hair is a line of shampoos, conditioners, styling products, and thickening treatments aimed at seducing the vast number of women who long for—well, "thicker, fuller hair." You're supposed to believe that the secret ingredient that will deliver your dream of model-like tresses is something called Cell-U-Plex. It's in there, but the tiny amount of conditioning agents and plant extracts it represents may not do much, considering what is present in far greater quantity in many of these products—skin irritants such as menthol and eucalyptus, and ingredients that can be drying to the hair such as sodium lauryl sulfate and ammonium xylenesulfonate. In short, there is absolutely nothing special in these products that can add fullness or thickness to hair, at least not any more than any other hair product with film-forming ingredients that coat the hair, which with repeated use tend to build up. Overall, this line needs to go back to the drawing board.

For more information about Thicker, Fuller Hair, call (714) 556-1028, (800) 966-6960, or visit its Web site at www.advreslab.com.

☹ **Moisturizing Shampoo for Dry or Damaged Hair** *($4.99 for 12 ounces)* contains menthol and eucalyptus, which can be drying and irritating for the scalp.

The Reviews T

☻ **Perm, Color Treated Shampoo for Chemically Treated Hair** *($4.99 for 15 ounces)* contains menthol and eucalyptus, which can be drying and irritating for the scalp.

☻ **Revitalizing Shampoo for All Hair Types** *($4.99 for 15 ounces)* contains menthol and eucalyptus, which can be drying and irritating for the scalp.

☻ **Therapeutic Anti-Dandruff Shampoo Medicated Formula** *($5.59 for 8 ounces)* has so many irritating ingredientsthat just listing them makes me itch. It contains sodium lauryl sulfate as the main detergent cleansing agent, and that makes it too potentially irritating for the scalp and drying for the hair. It also contains menthol, eucalyptus, and ammonium xylenesulfonate, which just add to already existing scalp problems without any benefit whatsoever.

☺ **Intensive Conditioning Treatment Bodifying Reconstructor for Dry or Damaged Hair** *($1.99 for two 0.375-ounce packets)* contains menthol and eucalyptus, which can be drying and irritating for the skin, so keep it far away from the scalp. Other than that, it is a good conditioner for normal to dry hair of any thickness. It contains mostly water, thickeners, detangling agents, silicones, slip agents, plant extracts, vitamins, conditioning agents, plant oil, preservatives, and fragrance.

☺ **Perm, Color Treated Conditioning Rinse** *($3.99 for 12 ounces)* contains menthol and eucalyptus, which can be drying and irritating for the skin, so keep it far away from the scalp. Other than that, it is a good conditioner for normal to dry hair of any thickness. It contains mostly water, thickeners, detangling agents, silicones, slip agents, plant extracts, vitamins, conditioning agents, plant oil, preservatives, and fragrance.

☻ **Weightless Conditioning Rinse for All Hair Types** *($4.99 for 15 ounces)* is almost identical to the Perm, Color Treated version above and the same comments apply.

☻ **Therapeutic Scalp Treatment with Concentrated Cell-u-plex** *($8.99 for six 0.23-ounce treatments)* contains menthol, eucalyptus, and alcohol, all of which can be drying and irritating for the scalp.

☻ **Ultra-Light Styling Gel Extra Hold Formula** *($4.99 for 3.5 ounces)* contains menthol, eucalyptus, and alcohol, which can be drying and irritating for the scalp. Other than that, this is just a medium- to firm-hold gel that has a slight stiff, sticky feel. It contains mostly water, film formers, plant extracts, conditioning agents, plant oil, thickeners, silicone, preservatives, and fragrance.

☻ **Ultra-Light Styling Gel Volume & Style** *($3.99 for 5 ounces)* is almost identical to the Extra Hold version above and the same comments apply.

☻ **Thickening Styling Mousse** *($3.99 for 6 ounces)* is almost identical to the Extra Hold gel above, only this one is in mousse form, but the same basic comments apply.

☺ **Instant Thickening Serum Volume & Texture** *($5.59 for 4 ounces)* is a standard styling gel that contains mostly water, film former, plant extracts, thickeners, silicones, conditioning agents, plant oil, preservatives, and fragrance. This is a good standard gel that has a light to medium hold and minimal stiff or sticky feel.

☺ **Instant Thickening Spray** *($5.59 for 4.2 ounces)* is a standard styling spray that has a medium to firm hold and a stiff, sticky feel. It would work well for normal to dry hair that is fine or thin. It contains mostly alcohol, water, film formers, castor oil, plant extracts, conditioning agents, plant oil, and fragrance. It also contains menthol and eucalyptus, which can be drying and irritating for the skin, so keep it far away from the scalp.

☺ **Volumizing Finishing Spray Volume & Style** *($3.99 for 8 ounces)* is a standard hairspray that has a medium hold and a slight stiff, sticky feel. It contains mostly alcohol, water, film former, plant extracts, silicone, conditioning agents, plant oil, and fragrance. It also contains menthol and eucalyptus, which can be drying and irritating for the skin, so keep it far away from the scalp.

☺ **Volumizing Finishing Styler, Maximum Hold Hair Spray** *($3.91 for 8 ounces)* is similar to the Finishing Spray above and the same comments apply.

TIGI

For giving great product names to standard ingredients, TIGI leads the pack. But its claims about sun and environmental protection are bogus; neither is possible, or at least not any more likely than what's provided by any other hair-care product, and that's negligible at best. This line is a salon favorite, and the products are hard to resist, but look carefully and you'll find that its élan is mostly in the packaging and not in the product. For more information on TIGI, call (214) 931-1567, (800) 256-9391, (888) 795 HAIR, or visit its Web site at www.tigihaircare.com.

☹ **Gentle Cleansing Shampoo** *($7.50 for 8 ounces)* uses TEA-lauryl sulfate as the main cleansing agent, which is too drying for the hair and scalp.

☺ **Moisturizing Shampoo** *($6.95 for 8 ounces)* isn't all that moisturizing, though it is a good basic shampoo for all hair types with minimal chance of buildup. It contains mostly water, detergent cleansing agents, lather agent, thickeners, conditioning agent, detangling agent, plant extracts, slip agent, preservatives, fragrance, and coloring agents.

☹ **Treatment Shampoo** *($7.95 for 8 ounces)* uses TEA-lauryl sulfate as one of the main cleansing agents, which is too drying for the hair and scalp.

☺ **Deep Reconstruct Conditioner** *($10.96 for 8 ounces)* isn't deep—if anything, it is extremely lightweight and would work for someone with normal hair of any thickness. It contains mostly water, detangling agent, conditioning agent, thickeners, preservatives, fragrance, and coloring agents.

☺ **Instant Conditioner** *($7.96 for 8 ounces)* is a good conditioner for normal to slightly dry hair of any thickness. It contains mostly water, thickeners, conditioning agents, detangling agents, preservatives, plant oil, silicone, fragrance, detangling agent/film former, and coloring agents. The film former is here in such a minute amount that it can't add much if any thickness to hair. There's also some henna in here, but this too is such a minute amount that it has minimal effect on hair.

☹ **Peppermint Treatment Conditioner** *($9.50 for 8 ounces)* contains peppermint and menthol, which are both skin irritants that cause problems for the scalp.

☺ **Protein Protective Spray** *($8.50 for 8 ounces)* isn't all that protective, it is just a very lightweight, leave-in conditioner that would work well for normal hair of any thickness. It contains mostly water, conditioning agents, detangling agent/film former, preservatives, and fragrance.

☺ **Gel Gloss** *($8.96 for 8 ounces)* is a standard gel with a light to medium hold and minimal stiff or sticky feel. It contains mostly plant water, film former, alcohol, slip agents, thickeners, conditioning agent, silicone, preservatives, and fragrance.

☺ **Molding Gel** *($6.96 for 8 ounces)* is almost identical to the Gel Gloss above and the same basic comments apply.

☺ **Strong Mousse for Fine to Medium Hair** *($8.95 for 6 ounces)* is a standard mousse with a medium hold and a sticky feel but that can be brushed through. It contains mostly water, propellant, film former, slip agents, silicone, and fragrance.

☺ **Extra Strong Mousse for Medium to Thick Hair** *($8.95 for 6 ounces)* is similar to the Strong Mousse above, only it really has more hold and a more sticky feel.

☺ **Spray Mousse** *($11.50 for 8 ounces)* isn't a mousse at all, rather it is a standard hairspray with a light hold and minimal to no stiff or sticky feel. It contains mostly alcohol, water, film formers, thickeners, fragrance, and conditioning agent.

☺ **EnviroShape Firm Hold Hairspray** *($11.50 for 10 ounces)* is a very standard aerosol hairspray with a medium to firm hold and a somewhat stiff feel that does let hair be brushed through. It contains mostly alcohol, propellant, film formers, conditioning agent, slip agents, and fragrance.

☺ **Hold & Gloss Spray** *($11.50 for 8 ounces)* is similar to the EnviroShape above, only this one includes silicone, which can add more shine.

☺ **Non-Aerosol Finishing Spray** *($10.50 for 8 ounces)* is similar to the Hold & Gloss above and the same comments apply.

☺ **Hair Glaze** *($9.95 for 1 ounce)* is just Vaseline, wax, and fragrance, and it works the same as any pomade. It can add shine and help control stubborn frizzies or coarse hair but it can also add a greasy, heavy feel to hair, so use it sparingly.

☺ **Enviro-Fixx** *($9.95 for 8 ounces)* is just a very lightweight styling spray that can also be used as a leave-in conditioner, it's that light. It has minimal hold and minimal to no stiff or sticky feel, and contains mostly plant water, film formers, castor oil, conditioning agent, silicone, preservatives, fragrance, and coloring agent.

☺ **Styling Pure Gloss** *($15.50 for 2 ounces)* is a standard silicone serum that can add a silky feel and shine to hair.

Bed Head by TIGI

☺ **Moisture Maniac Shampoo** *($7.96 for 12 ounces)* has a great name, but there is nothing in this product that will help fix the effect that sleeping on a pillow all night can have on the way hair looks any more than any other shampoo that would just wash out "the bends" a pillow would make. Still, this is a good, basic shampoo for normal hair that is fine or thin. It contains mostly water, detergent cleansing agents, lather agent, detangling agent/film former, thickeners, preservatives, coloring agents, and fragrance.

☺ **Moisture Maniac Conditioner** *($11.95 for 8.5 ounces)* is a lightweight conditioner that contains mostly water, detangling agents, thickeners, slip agents, preservatives, coloring agent, and fragrance. It would work fine for normal hair of any thickness to help with combing.

☺ **Power Trip Hair Gel** *($12 for 7 ounces)* is an extremely standard hair gel with medium hold and a slight stiff, sticky feel that does let hair be brushed through. It contains mostly water, film formers, thickeners, preservatives, slip agent, coloring agents, and fragrance.

☺ **Control Freak Frizz Control & Straightener** *($15.95 for 9 ounces)* contains mostly water, detangling agent/film former, slip agents, silicone, thickeners, plant extracts, preservatives, and coloring agents. This standard gel has a light hold with minimal to no stiff or sticky feel. It can help with styling but it isn't as intense as the name implies. It also contains a small amount of glitter that does add subtle shine.

☺ **A Hair Stick for Cool People** *($17.96 for 2.7 ounces)* is just castor oil, thickeners, fragrance, and preservatives. This is just a greasy, sticky wax that works well as a pomade to smooth out stubborn curls and frizzies, but it can also have a stiff, sticky feel, so use it sparingly.

☺ **Hard Head Hard Hold Hairspray (Aerosol)** *($11.95 for 10 ounces)* is a standard hairspray with a light to medium hold and a slight stiff feel that does let hair be brushed through. It contains mostly alcohol, propellant, film formers, silicones, slip agents, and fragrance.

Blue by TIGI

☺ **Thickening Shampoo for Fuller Hair** *($7.96 for 12 ounces)* contains mostly water, detergent cleansing agents, detangling agent/film former, lather agent, conditioning agents, thickeners, silicone, more conditioning agents, fragrance, preservatives, and coloring agents. This is a good shampoo for normal to slightly dry hair that is fine or thin. As is true with all shampoos of this type that contains film formers, it can cause buildup with repeated use.

☺ **Fast-Fix for Unruly Morning Hair** *($8.95 for 8 ounces)* contains mostly water, silicones, detangling agents, slip agents, film former, conditioning agents, plant extracts, fragrance, preservatives, and coloring agents. This is more of very light-hold styling spray than a leave-in conditioner. It would work well for normal to dry hair that is normal to fine or thin.

☺ **Catwalk Root Boost Foam-Lotion Spray for Texture & Lift** *($11.50 for 8 ounces)* is a unique name for a standard mousse with a light hold and minimal to no sticky feel. It contains mostly water, alcohol, detangling agent, film formers, thickeners, conditioning agent, propellant, slip agents, and fragrance.

☺ **Texturing Pomade with Essential Oils** *($9.96 for 2 ounces)* is a standard pomade that contains mostly plant water, safflower oil, castor oil, slip agents, thickeners, fragrant oils, fragrance, and preservatives. It has a minimal hold and a slight sticky feel. This can help when smoothing out frizzies or stubborn curls, but it can also leave a greasy, thick feel on hair, so use it sparingly.

☺ **Thickening Cream with Essential Oils** *($15.95 for 3.4 ounces)* contains mostly plant water, thickeners, conditioning agent, slip agent, fragrant oils, film former, fragrance, and more film former. This styling-gel-like cream has a light hold and a slight sticky feel. It can help when smoothing hair and frizzies but it can also feel heavy and greasy, so use it sparingly.

☺ **Catwalk Medium Hold Working Hairspray** *($11.95 for 8 ounces)* is a standard light- to medium-hold aerosol hairspray with a slight stiff feel that can be brushed through. It contains mostly alcohol, propellants, film formers, slip agents, silicones, conditioning agent, plant extracts, and fragrance.

Essensuals by TIGI

☺ **Hair & Body Wash** *($4 for 2 ounces)* contains mostly detergent cleansing agents, plant water, plant oil, fragrance oils, detangling agent/film former, vitamins, conditioning agent, lather agent, fragrance, and coloring agents. There is no reason to wash the body with a product that contains film former, though this one can be good for normal to dry hair that is normal to fine or thin.

☹ **Spa Shampoo** *($9.50 for 8.5 ounces)* uses TEA-lauryl sulfate as one of the main cleansing agents, and that makes it too drying for the scalp and hair.

☺ **Thickening Conditioner** *($12.96 for 8 ounces)* contains mostly water, thickener, detangling agents, conditioning agents, detangling agent/film former, plant extracts, preservatives, and fragrance. This can work well for normal to dry hair that has normal to fine or thin thickness.

☺ **Leave-in Conditioner** *($11.95 for 8.5 ounces)* contains mostly water, detangling agents/film former, silicones, slip agents, fragrant oils, conditioning agents, preservatives, fragrance, and coloring agents. This is more a styling spray than a conditioner. It has a light hold and minimal sticky feel, and it can work well for normal to dry hair that is fine or thin.

☺ **Spray Gel** *($11.95 for 8.5 ounces)* is a good spray gel that has a light to medium hold with minimal stiff or sticky feel. It contains mostly plant water, film former, fragrant oils, silicone, slip agents, thickener, and fragrance.

☺ **Spray Shine** *($14.50 for 4.4 ounces)* is a standard spray silicone serum that can add shine and a silky feel to hair. There are far less expensive (though identical) versions at the drugstore.

Tresemme

For more information on Tresemme, call (708) 450-3000, (800) 333-666, or visit its Web site at www.alberto-culver.com.

☹ **European Anti-Fatigue Shampoo, Revitalizing/Shine for Dry/Damaged Hair** *($2.49 for 24 ounces)* uses sodium lauryl sulfate as the main detergent cleansing agent, and that makes it too potentially irritating for the scalp and drying for the hair.

☹ **European Anti-Fatigue Shampoo, Volumizing for Fine or Thin Hair** *($2.49 for 24 ounces)* uses sodium lauryl sulfate as the main detergent cleansing agent, and that makes it too potentially irritating for the scalp and drying for the hair.

☹ **European Body-Building Shampoo** *($2.49 for 32 ounces)* uses sodium lauryl sulfate as the main detergent cleansing agent, and that makes it too potentially irritating for the scalp and drying for the hair.

☺ **European Color Treated & Permed Shampoo** *($2.49 for 32 ounces)* contains mostly water, detergent cleansing agents, lather agent, detangling agents/film formers, preservatives, and fragrance. This can work well for normal hair that is fine or thin. The film formers in here can cause buildup.

☹ **European Deep Cleansing Shampoo** *($2.49 for 32 ounces)* uses sodium lauryl sulfate as the main detergent cleansing agent, and that makes it too potentially irritating for the scalp and drying for the hair.

☹ **European Moisturizing Body Shampoo for Fine/Thin Hair** *($7.99 for 33.8 ounces)* uses sodium lauryl sulfate as one of the main detergent cleansing agents, and that makes it too potentially irritating for the scalp and drying for the hair.

☹ **European Natural Shampoo with Vitamins A, C, and E** *($2.49 for 32 ounces)* uses sodium lauryl sulfate as the main detergent cleansing agent, and that makes it too potentially irritating for the scalp and drying for the hair.

☺ **European Vitamin E Moisture Rich Shampoo for Dry or Damaged Hair** *($2.49 for 24 ounces)* contains mostly water, detergent cleansing agent, lather agent, detangling agents/film formers, conditioning agent, slip agents, plant extracts, detangling agent, preservatives, and fragrance. This isn't very moisturizing, especially for dry hair, though it would work well for normal to dry hair that is fine or thin.

☺ **European Anti-Fatigue Conditioner, Revitalizing/Shine for Dry or Damaged Hair** *($2.49 for 24 ounces)* contains mostly water, thickeners, detangling agents, plant extract, silicones, conditioning agents, plant oils, film former, preservatives, and fragrance. This is a good conditioner for normal to dry hair that is fine or thin. It does contain a tiny amount of sulfur, which may dry hair and strip hair color with repeated use.

☺ **European Anti-Fatigue Conditioner, Volumizing for Fine or Thin Hair** *($2.49 for 24 ounces)* is almost identical to the Anti-Fatigue version above and the same comments apply.

☺ **European Body-Building Conditioner** *($2.49 for 32 ounces)* contains mostly water, thickeners, detangling agents, film former, conditioning agents, plant oils, silicone, detangling agent/film former, preservatives, and fragrance. This is a good conditioner for normal to dry hair that is fine or thin. This conditioner can have a slight stiff, sticky feel on hair. It also contains a tiny amount of sulfur, which may dry hair and strip hair color with repeated use.

☺ **European Color-Treated and Permed Conditioner** *($2.49 for 32 ounces)* contains mostly water, thickeners, detangling agents/film formers, conditioning agents, slip agents, film former, silicones, preservatives, and fragrance. This is a good conditioner for normal to dry hair that is fine or thin.

☺ **European Natural Conditioner with Vitamins A, C, and E** *($2.49 for 32 ounces)* is a lightweight conditioner for normal hair of any thickness, to help with combing. It contains mostly water, detangling agent, thickeners, plant extracts, conditioning agent, vitamins, plant oils, more conditioning agents, preservatives, coloring agents, and fragrance. The minute amounts of conditioning agents, plant oil, and vitamins have minimal effect on hair.

☺ **European Remoisturizing Conditioner** *($2.40 for 32 ounces)* is similar to the Natural Conditioner above and the same comments apply.

☺ **European Vitamin E Moisture Rich Conditioner** *($2.49 for 32 ounces)* contains mostly water, thickeners, detangling agent, silicones, conditioning agents, plant oil, plant extracts, slip agents, preservatives, and fragrance. This is a good conditioner for normal to dry hair of any thickness. It does contain a tiny amount of sulfur, and that has a minor risk of becoming drying or stripping hair color with repeated use.

☺ **Tres Mend, European Natural Silk Protein Hair Reconstructor** *($0.67 for 1 ounce)* won't mend one hair on anyone's head. It's just a good basic conditioner for normal to slightly dry hair that is normal to fine or thin. It contains mostly water, thickeners, detangling agent/film former, more thickeners, detangling agent, mineral oil, conditioning agent, silicone, preservatives, and fragrance.

☺ **European Natural Leave-in Conditioner with Vitamins A, C, and E, Lightweight Formula** *($2.49 for 32 ounces)* is a good leave-in conditioner for dry hair that is normal to fine or thin. It contains mostly water, silicones, detangling agent/film former, alcohol, detangling agent, slip agent, conditioning agents, water-binding agents, plant oils, vitamins, plant extracts, preservatives, and fragrance. The vitamins here are window dressing and have minimal effect on hair or scalp.

☺ **Tres Pac, Deeply Penetrating Protein Treatment** *($3 for 2 ounces)* isn't all that penetrating, it's just a good basic conditioner for dry hair of any thickness. It contains mostly water, thickeners, conditioning agent, detangling agents, mineral oil, preservatives, and fragrance.

☺ **European Extra Body Hot Oil Treatment** *($2.49 for three 1-ounce tubes)* contains minimal oil, and is less a treatment than just a good basic conditioner for normal to dry hair of any thickness. It does penetrate hair better when it's warm and left on for a few minutes, just like any conditioner would. This contains mostly water, detangling agent, slip agent, thickeners, preservatives, conditioning agents, plant oils, fragrance, and coloring agents. It also contains a tiny amount of sulfur, and that has a minor risk of becoming drying or stripping hair color with repeated use.

☹ **Instant Hot Oil Treatment for Color Treated and Permed Hair** *($2.49 for three 1-ounce tubes)* is a version that contains no oil, and it isn't all that conditioning. It contains mostly thickeners, alcohol, detangling agents, film former, slip agents, fragrance, and coloring agents.

☺ **European Tres Shine Anti-Frizz Shine Mist** *($5.49 for 4 ounces)* is a lightweight silicone spray that can add a soft, silky feel and shine to hair.

☺ **European Tres Gel Spray Extra Hold** *(2.76 for 10 ounces)* is a good standard spray gel with a medium hold and a slight sticky feel that does let hair be brushed through. It contains mostly water, film formers, thickeners, detangling agent, silicone, preservatives, and fragrance.

☺ **European Tres Gelee Styling Gel, Flexible Hold** *($2.76 for 9 ounces)* is a good standard gel with a light hold and minimal to no sticky feel. It contains mostly water, film formers, thickeners, detangling agent, silicone, preservatives, and fragrance.

☺ **European Tres Gelee Styling Gel, Extra Hold** *($2.76 for 9 ounces)* is a good standard gel with a light to medium hold and minimal sticky feel that does let hair be brushed through. It contains mostly water, film formers, thickeners, detangling agent, silicone, preservatives, and fragrance.

☹ **European Tres Gelee Styling Gel, Mega Hold** *($2.76 for 9 ounces)* is similar to the Extra Hold version above, only it has more hold and a more sticky feel. This is more sticky than most hair styles would ever need.

☺ **European Tres Foam, Volumizing** *($2.76 for 7 ounces)* is an aerated foam that has a light to medium hold and a somewhat sticky feel that can still be brushed through. It contains mostly water, film former, detangling agent/film former, thickener, detangling agents, silicone, slip agent, preservatives, and fragrance.

☺ **European Tres Mousse Styling Mousse, Extra Hold** *($3.69 for 10.5 ounces)* is a standard mousse with a light to medium hold and a slight sticky feel that does brush out. It contains mostly water, propellants, film formers, detangling agents/film formers, thickeners, alcohol, fragrance, detangling agents, silicones, conditioning agents, and coloring agents.

☺ **European Tres Mousse Styling Mousse, Super Hold** *($2.39 for 10.5 ounces)* is almost identical to the Extra Hold version above and the same comments apply.

☺ **European Tres Mousse Thickening Styling Mousse** *($2.39 for 10.5 ounces)* is similar to the Extra Hold version above, only with a more sticky feel that still lets hair be brushed through.

☺ **European Tres Hold Fixative Spray** *($2.97 for 8.1 ounces)* is a standard aerosol hairspray with a medium to firm hold and a slight stiff feel that can be brushed through. It contains mostly alcohol, propellants, film formers, fragrance, and silicone.

☺ **Tresemme Two Extra Hold Working Hair Spray (Aerosol)** *($2.97 for 13 ounces)* is almost identical to the Fixative Spray above and the same comments apply.

☺ **Tresemme Two Ultra Fine Mist Hair Spray** *($2.97 for 11.2 ounces)* is almost identical to the Super Hold version above and the same comments apply.

☺ **European Tres Spray Styling Spritz, Super Hold** *($3.69 for 10.5 ounces)* is a medium- to firm-hold hairspray with a slight stiff, sticky feel. It contains mostly alcohol, water, film formers, slip agents, conditioning agents, fragrance, and preservatives.

☺ **4+4 Styling Gel Fixative** *($3.99 for 9 ounces)* is a standard styling gel with a light to medium hold and minimal stiff or sticky feel. It contains mostly water, alcohol, film formers, slip agents, thickeners, detangling agents, silicones, fragrance, preservatives, and conditioning agents. The amount of conditioning agents in here is so minute that it is strictly window dressing and has no real impact on hair.

☺ **4+4 Super Hold Styling Glaze** *($4.79 for 8 ounces)* is a standard styling liquid with a medium hold and a somewhat sticky feel that still lets hair be brushed through. It contains mostly water, alcohol, film formers, thickeners, detangling agents, fragrance, preservatives, slip agents, silicones, conditioning agents, and coloring agents. The amount of conditioning agents in here is so minute that it is strictly window dressing and has no real impact on hair.

☺ **4+4 Extra Hold Styling Mousse** *($3.99 for 13.5 ounces)* is a standard mousse with a medium hold and a slight sticky feel that does let hair be brushed through. It contains mostly water, propellant, alcohol, film formers, fragrance, thickeners, detangling agents, silicones, preservatives, conditioning agents, and coloring agents.

☺ **4+4 Special Solutions Split Ends Styling Mousse** *($4.99 for 13.5 ounces)* is almost identical to the Extra Hold Styling Mousse above, only with slightly less hold and a less sticky feel, and the same comments apply.

☺ **4+4 Hair Straightener & Polisher** *($7.99 for 9 ounces)* contains mostly water, slip agents, silicones, film formers, thickeners, plant extracts, conditioning agents, preservatives, and fragrance. This is a silicone serum with a slight amount of hold. It can work well for smoothing stubborn curls and frizzies with no stiff or sticky feel.

☺ **4+4 Contour Hair Creme** *($7.99 for 9 ounces)* is a good basic styling cream with a medium hold and a sticky feel that does let you brush through hair. It can work well for smoothing out stubborn curls and frizzies, but it can also easily feel heavy and look greasy, so use it sparingly. It contains mostly water, film formers, mineral oil, plant extracts, plant oil, conditioning agents, slip agents, preservatives, and fragrance.

☺ **4+4 Extra Hold Brush Out Shaping Spray** *($4.99 for 12.9 ounces)* is a standard, medium- to firm-hold aerosol hairspray with a somewhat stiff feel that does let hair be brushed though. It contains mostly alcohol, propellant, film formers, fragrance, conditioning agents, and preservatives.

☺ **4+4 Extra Hold Formula Hair Spray** *($1.99 for 12.2 ounces)* is almost identical to the Brush Out version above and the same comments apply.

☺ **4+4 Super Hold Styling Spritz** *($3.99 for 12 ounces)* is almost identical to the Brush Out version above, only in nonaerosol form, and the same basic comments apply.

☺ **4+4 Ultra Fine Mist Control Extra Hold Hair Spray** *($1.99 for 12.2 ounces)* is almost identical to the Brush Out version above and the same comments apply.

Tressa

For more information on Tressa, call (800) 879-8737.

☺ **Colourage Shampoo, Gentle Cleansing for Color-Treated Hair** *($8.49 for 12 ounces)* is a standard shampoo that contains just water, detergent cleansing agents, lather agent, fragrance, preservatives, and detangling agent. It would work great for all hair types and it can't create buildup.

☺ **Perm Care Shampoo, Moisturizing Shampoo for Permed Hair** *($8.49 for 12 ounces)* is similar to the Colourage Shampoo above, only this one contains a tiny amount of film former, not really enough to affect the performance of this all-around basic shampoo.

The Reviews T

☹ **Pliance Shampoo, Moisturizing Shampoo for Normal to Dry Hair** *($8.49 for 12 ounces)* uses sodium C14-16 olefin sulfate and TEA-dodecylbenzenesulfonate as its detergent cleansing agents, which are both too drying for the hair and scalp.

☹ **Remove All Plus Shampoo, Purifying Treatment for Use Prior to Perming** *($8.49 for 12 ounces)* uses TEA-lauryl sulfate as its main detergent cleansing agent, which is too drying for the hair and scalp.

☺ **Clear Intervals** *($13.56 for 9 ounces)* is a gentle standard shampoo, made with just water, detergent cleansing agent, lather agent, detangling agent, thickener, fragrance, and preservatives. It would work great for all hair types and it can't create buildup.

☺ **Watercolors Crimson Splash** *($13.56 for 9 ounces)* is identical to the Clear Intervals shampoo above, only with temporary dye agents that can minimally enhance hair color.

☺ **Watercolors Fluid Fire** *($13.56 for 9 ounces)* is identical to the Crimson Splash Wash above and the same comments apply.

☺ **Watercolors Golden Mist** *($13.56 for 9 ounces)* is identical to the Crimson Splash Wash above and the same comments apply.

☺ **Watercolors Liquid Copper** *($13.56 for 9 ounces)* is identical to the Crimson Splash Wash above and the same comments apply.

☺ **Watercolors Mocha Drench** *($13.56 for 9 ounces)* is identical to the Crimson Splash Wash above and the same comments apply.

☺ **Watercolors Molten Bronze** *($13.56 for 9 ounces)* is identical to the Crimson Splash Wash above and the same comments apply.

☺ **Watercolors Violet Wash** *($13.56 for 9 ounces)* is identical to the Crimson Splash Wash above and the same comments apply.

☺ **Watercolors Wet Brick** *($13.56 for 9 ounces)* is identical to the Crimson Splash Wash above and the same comments apply.

☺ **Watercolors Wet Sand** *($13.56 for 9 ounces)* is identical to the Crimson Splash Wash above and the same comments apply.

☺ **FortipHy Deep Conditioner, Nourishes Weak Links in Permed Hair** *($7.99 for 4 ounces)* isn't deep or nourishing, it's just a good conditioner for dry hair of any thickness. It contains mostly water, thickeners, mineral oil, conditioning agents, silicone, slip agents, preservatives, detangling agent/film former, preservatives, and fragrance. The amount of film former in here isn't enough to be a problem for thicker hair types.

☺ **Infuse Deep Conditioner, Replenishing Moisturizer for Color-Treated Hair** *($7.99 for 4 ounces)* is almost identical to the FortipHy above and the same basic comments apply.

☺ **Quench Deep Conditioner, Deep Conditioning for All Hair Types** *($9.99 for 6 ounces)* is almost identical to the FortipHy above and the same basic comments apply.

☺ **ModipHy Normalizer Conditioner, Light Conditioning for Permed Hair** *($7.99 for 12 ounces)* is a lightweight conditioner that would work well for normal to slightly dry hair of any thickness. It contains mostly water, thickeners, detangling agents, conditioning agent, silicone, slip agent, preservatives, fragrance, and coloring agent.

☺ **Immedia Leave-in Conditioner, UV Protection for Color-Treated Hair** *($8.99 for 8 ounces)* is a good leave-in conditioner for normal to dry hair that is normal to fine or thin. It contains mostly water, conditioning agent, silicone, detangling agent, film former, preservatives, fragrance, and castor oil. It can have a slight sticky feel on hair.

☺ **Smoothing Gloss Protective Shiner** *($8 for 2 ounces)* is a standard silicone serum that can add a soft, silky feel to hair as well as shine.

☺ **Aglaze Forming Lotion, Light to Medium Hold for All Hair Types** *($7.49 for 8 ounces)* is a light- to medium-hold styling lotion (like a very liquidy gel) with minimal stiff or sticky feel. It contains mostly water, film formers, detangling agent, conditioning agent, slip agent, preservatives, fragrance, and coloring agents.

☺ **Supplex Styling Lotion, Medium Hold for All Hair Types** *($6.99 for 8 ounces)* is a light-hold styling spray that has minimal stiff or sticky feel. It contains mostly water, film formers, detangling agent, conditioning agent, slip agent, preservatives, fragrance, and coloring agents.

☺ **Perk-it Curl Revitalizer** *($8 for 8 ounces)* contains mostly water, detangling agent/film former, slip agents, castor oil, preservatives, and fragrance. This is a lightweight styling spray that has a soft hold and minimal to no stiff or sticky feel. It can work for any styling need, not just forming curls.

☺ **Brace Styling Gel Maximum Hold for All Hair Types** *($6.49 for 4 ounces)* is a good basic styling gel with a light to medium hold. It has a slight sticky feel that can easily be brushed through. It contains mostly water, film formers, slip agents, conditioning agent, thickeners, preservatives, and fragrance.

☺ **Sustain Design Spray, Maximum Hold for All Hair Types (Aerosol)** *($9.99 for 10 ounces)* is a standard aerosol hairspray with a firm hold and a somewhat stiff feel that can still let hair be brushed through.

☺ **Hair Spray Working and Finishing Spray (Aerosol)** *($8.99 for 10 ounces)* is similar to the Sustain version above, only this one is in aerosol form.

☺ **Sculpting Spray Flexible Holding Spray (Non-Aerosol)** *($7.99 for 8 ounces)* is similar to the Sustain version above, and the same basic comments apply.

The Reviews T

☺ **Aliquis Design Spray, Firm Hold for All Hair Types** *($8.99 for 8 ounces)* is a standard hairspray with a medium to firm hold and a somewhat stiff feel that does let hair be brushed through. It contains mostly alcohol, water, film former, slip agents, silicone, and fragrance.

☺ **Boost Spray Glaze with Bold Control** *($7.99 for 8 ounces)* is a light-hold hairspray with minimal stiff or sticky feel. It contains mostly water, alcohol, film former, castor oil, detangling agent/film former, fragrance, and preservatives.

Vertu by Tressa

☺ **Hydra Swash Hydrating Shampoo** *($11 for 14 ounces)* contains mostly water, detergent cleansing agents, lather agent, plant extracts, preservatives, detangling agent/film former, fragrance, thickeners, and slip agent. This is a good basic shampoo for all hair types with minimal chance of buildup from the minute amount of film former in here.

☹ **Ultra Swash Clarifying Shampoo** *($11 for 14 ounces)* uses TEA-lauryl sulfate as one of the main cleansing agents, which is too drying for the hair and scalp.

☺ **Day Splash Moisturizing Conditioner** *($10 for 14 ounces)* is a simple, ordinary conditioner that would be good for normal hair of any thickness to help with combing. It contains mostly water, thickeners, plant extracts, detangling agent, conditioning agent, silicone, slip agent, preservatives, and fragrance.

☺ **$$$ Super Splash Therapeutic Conditioner** *($18 for 10 ounces)* is an exceptionally standard conditioner with an absurd price. It would be good for dry hair of any thickness. It contains mostly water, thickeners, mineral oil, plant extracts, conditioning agent, slip agent, silicone, preservatives, fragrance, and coloring agents.

☺ **Shine Aire** *($12 for 8 ounces)* is just a silicone spray; it has no hold, it just leaves a soft shine and a silky feel on hair.

☺ **Gelatin Bodifying Gel** *($11 for 10 ounces)* is a standard gel with a medium to firm hold and a somewhat sticky feel that does let hair be brushed through. It contains mostly water, film former, plant extracts, thickener, silicone, slip agent, fragrance, and preservatives.

☺ **Trans Foam Shaping Lotion** *($16.50 for 7 ounces)* is more of a liquidy gel that has a bit of foaming action. Other than the odd dispensing system, it is a good styling gel that has a light to medium hold with minimal to no stiff or sticky feel. It contains mostly water, film former, propellants, slip agents, plant extracts, conditioning agents, silicone, thickener, preservatives, and fragrance.

☺ **Air Form Finishing Mist** *($15 for 14 ounces)* is a standard hairspray with a medium to firm hold and a stiff feel that can be brushed through. It contains mostly alcohol, water, film former, more alcohol, plant extracts, silicone, and slip agents.

Trevor Sorbie

Trevor Sorbie is one of the many hair designers who has launched his own hair-care product lines. As in every designer line I've reviewed, there are some good products to consider here, along with some to avoid. For more information on Trevor Sorbie, call (905) 825-5800, (800) 322-8738, or visit its Web site at www.trevorsorbie.com.

☹ **Cleane Shampoo for All Hair Types** *($6.58 for 8.5 ounces)* contains ammonium xylenesulfonate, which can be drying for the hair and drying and irritating for the scalp.

☹ **Cleane Shampoo for Chemically Treated Hair** *($6.33 for 8.5 ounces)* contains ammonium xylenesulfonate which can be drying for the hair, drying and irritating for the scalp, and really bad for chemically treated hair.

☹ **Cleane/Forme Energizing Shampoo** *($7.49 for 8 ounces)* contains ammonium xylenesulfonate, which can be drying for the hair and drying and irritating for the scalp.

☺ **Deep Conditioner Intensive Moisturizing Creme Treatment** *($8.40 for 5 ounces)* contains mostly water, thickeners, detangling agents, fragrance, conditioning agents, plant oil, detangling agent/film former, and preservatives. This is a good basic conditioner for normal hair of any thickness. The minute amount of conditioning agents and film former in here can have minimal to no effect on the hair.

☺ **Riche Conditioner** *($9.38 for 8.5 ounces)* isn't all that rich; it is similar to the Deep Conditioner above, only with the addition of silicone. It's still just a good basic conditioner for normal hair of any thickness.

☺ **Riche Leave-in Conditioner** *($7.40 for 10 ounces)* isn't all that rich; it is just a good, basic, leave-in conditioner for normal to dry hair that is fine or thin. It contains mostly water, slip agents, detangling agents, castor oil, conditioning agent, detangling agents/film formers, silicone, fragrance, and preservatives.

☺ **Sculpte Jel Super Firm Support** *($8.21 for 5 ounces)* is a standard gel with a light to medium hold and a slight sticky feel that does let hair be brushed through. It contains mostly water, film former, thickeners, alcohol, slip agents, and preservatives.

☺ **Sliquid Styling Gel** *($5.99 for 8.5 ounces)* is almost identical to the Sculpte Jel above and the same comments apply.

☺ **Design Forme Conditioning Styler Mousse for Soft Hold and Body** *($9.95 for 7 ounces)* is a standard mousse with a light to medium hold and minimal stiff or sticky feel. It contains mostly water, propellant, film former, conditioning agent, detangling agent, thickeners, silicone, fragrance, and preservatives.

☺ **Shaping Mousse for Volume and Control** *($8.05 for 6 ounces)* is a standard mousse with a medium hold and a somewhat sticky feel. It contains mostly water, propellant, film formers, alcohol, thickeners, conditioning agent, fragrance, and preservatives.

☺ **Glossaire** *($9.49 for 2.6 ounces)* is a no-hold, gel-like pomade with no stiff or sticky feel for smoothing hair and frizzies. It contains mostly water, slip agents, plant extracts, fragrance, and preservatives. There are better products for adding shine to hair than this overpriced version.

☺ **Texturecreme Styler with Jojoba Oil** *($9.99 for 5 ounces)* is a styling cream with no hold and minimal to no stiff or sticky feel, though it can feel heavy on hair, so use it sparingly. This works well to smooth stubborn curls and frizzies. It contains mostly water, plant oil, thickeners, film former, conditioning agent, preservatives, and fragrance.

☺ **Curl Forme Energizer** *($9.95 for 8 ounces)* contains mostly water, slip agents, detangling agent, detangling agent/film former, conditioning agents, preservatives, and fragrance. This is a lightweight styling spray or leave-in conditioner that has minimal hold and no stiff or sticky feel.

☺ **Lift-it Volumizer, Hair Thickening Spray for Root Lift and Volume** *($8.21 for 8.5 ounces)* is a standard styling spray with a light hold and a minimally stiff feel that does brush out. It contains mostly water, film former, alcohol, detangling agent/ film former, slip agent, fragrance, castor oil, and preservatives.

☺ **Lift-It Bodifier Medium Hold Spray Gel** *($8.21 for 10 ounces)* is a styling spray with a light to medium hold and a slight sticky feel that does let hair be brushed through. It contains mostly water, film former, silicone, detangling agent/film former, conditioning agents, thickeners, castor oil, fragrance, and preservatives.

☺ **Affix Hair Spray for Extra Firm Hold** *($8.55 for 10 ounces)* is a standard hairspray with a light to medium hold and a slight stiff feel that can be brushed through. It contains mostly alcohol, film former, slip agent, conditioning agent, silicone, and fragrance.

☺ **Finishe Forme Energizing Hair Spray** *($7.91 for 10 ounces)* is similar to the Affix above and the same comments apply.

☺ **Spraye** *($7.91 for 10 ounces)* is similar to the Affix above, only in aerosol form, but the same comments apply.

☺ **Hot Shapes Thermo-Protective Spray for Heat Styling** *($6.53 for 5 ounces)* is a light- to medium-hold hairspray that can be used as a styling spray, but it does leave a bit of a stiff feel on hair. There is nothing in here that can protect the hair from the heat of styling tools.

TRI

For more information about TRI, call (800) 458-8874 or visit its Web site at www.trihaircare.com.

☹ **Ecollogen Shampoo Treatment** *($5.99 for 8 ounces)* uses TEA-lauryl sulfate as the main cleansing agent, which can be too drying for the hair and scalp.

☺ **Jojoba Shampoo Treatment** *($6.99 for 8 ounces)* contains mostly water, detergent cleansing agents, lather agent, plant oil, henna, conditioning agent, fragrance, and coloring agents. This is a good basic shampoo for normal to dry hair that is normal to fine or thin. Henna can build up on hair with repeated use and make it feel stiff.

☹ **Safe Strip Shampoo** *($7.50 for 16 ounces)* uses sodium C14-16 olefin sulfate as the main cleansing agent, which does make it rather stripping and unsafe for most hair types.

☹ **Whole Wheat Shampoo Treatment** *($9.49 for 8 ounces)* uses sodium C14-16 olefin sulfate as one of the main cleansing agents, which can be too drying for the scalp and hair and potentially strip hair color.

☺ **Chamomile pH Rectifier** *($6.20 for 8 ounces)* is an almost do-nothing, leave-in conditioner that contains mostly water, slip agent, plant extracts, preservatives, apple cider vinegar, and detangling agent. It can lower pH, but so can most hair-care products with a low pH. This can minimally help with combing if you have normal hair.

☺ **Electri-Therm Control Treatment** *($5.49 for 8 ounces)* contains menthol and lime oil, which can be skin irritants, so keep it off the scalp. Other than that, this is a lightweight, leave-in conditioner that is mostly water, slip agents, detangling agent, conditioning agent, fragrance, preservatives, and coloring agents. It would be OK for someone with normal hair of any thickness.

☺ **Express Conditioning Detangler** *($8.49 for 8 ounces)* contains mostly water, conditioning agents, detangling agent/film former, silicones, slip agents, fragrance, and preservatives. This is a good, leave-in conditioner for dry hair that is normal to fine or thin.

☹ **Jojoba Hair and Scalp Conditioner** *($7.49 for 4 ounces)* has TEA-dodecylbenzene sulfonate as its second ingredient, and that can be drying for the scalp and hair and potentially strip hair color with repeated use.

☺ **Protein Bodifier Treatment** *($7.99 for 8 ounces)* is just a styling spray with a light hold and minimal stiff or sticky feel; it contains mostly water, alcohol, conditioning agents, film former, preservatives, and fragrance.

☹ **Unific Energy Moisturizing Treatment** *($10.99 for 6 ounces)* contains peppermint, a skin irritant that can cause problems for the scalp. This is a treatment you would have to avoid using near the roots, but the basic formulation is so boring it's best to just avoid this one altogether.

☺ **Whole Wheat Conditioning Rinse** *($6.49 for 4 ounces)* is just a good, leave-in conditioner for normal to dry hair of any thickness. It contains mostly water, thickeners, conditioning agents, detangling agent, plant oil, preservatives, and fragrance.

The Reviews T

☹ **Unific Energy Protein Pac** *($8 for 4 ounces)* has TEA-dodecylbenzene sulfonate as its second ingredient, which can be drying for the scalp and hair and potentially strip hair color with repeated use.

☺ **$$$ Tri Lights** *($9.49 for 1 ounce)* is just an overpriced silicone serum that can make hair feel silky soft and also add shine.

☺ **Body Infusion** *($9.99 for 9 ounces)* is a styling spray that has a light to medium hold and a slight sticky feel, and that does let hair be brushed through. It can help when styling to make hair feel fuller. It contains mostly water, alcohol, propellant, film former, conditioning agents, and fragrance.

☺ **Bodyfusion Designing Gel** *($9.99 for 8 ounces)* is a standard styling gel with a medium hold and a slight stiff, sticky feel. It contains mostly water, film formers, slip agent, conditioning agents, thickeners, silicone, fragrance, preservatives, and coloring agents.

☺ **Gel Spray** *($7 for 8 ounces)* is a standard spray gel with a light hold and minimal to no stiff or sticky feel. It contains mostly water, detangling agent/film former, film former, thickeners, plant extracts, preservatives, and fragrance. It does contain balm mint, a skin irritant, so keep it off the scalp.

☺ **Sculpture Styling Gel** *($5.99 for 5 ounces)* is a standard styling gel with a light to medium hold and minimal to no stiff or sticky feel. It contains mostly water, film former, conditioning agent, thickeners, silicone, preservatives, fragrance, and coloring agents.

☺ **Fashion Styling Mousse** *($7.49 for 5.5 ounces)* is a standard mousse with a light to medium hold and a slight sticky feel that does let hair be brushed through. It contains mostly water, film former, alcohol, propellant, detangling agent/film former, silicone, slip agents, thickeners, and fragrance.

☺ **Control and Finishing Mist** *($6.99 for 8 ounces)* is a standard hairspray with a medium hold and a slight stiff feel that does let hair be brushed through. It contains mostly alcohol, film former, water, fragrance, slip agents, and coloring agents.

☺ **Covert Control Holding Spray** *($8.49 for 9 ounces)* is a standard aerosol hairspray that has a light to medium hold and minimal stiff feel. It contains mostly alcohol, propellant, film former, silicones, slip agents, and fragrance.

☺ **Prego Extra Extra Firm Hair Spray** *($6.75 for 8 ounces)* is just alcohol, shellac, water, slip agent, and fragrance. This definitely has a firm hold and a stiff, sticky feel, though it can be brushed through.

☺ **Aerogel (Aerosol)** *($8.99 for 6 ounces)* is a standard aerosol hairspray that has a light to medium hold and a slight stiff feel that does let hair be brushed through. It contains mostly alcohol, propellant, film former, slip agent, silicones, more slip agent, conditioning agent, and fragrance.

☺ **Aerogel (Non-Aerosol)** *($10.99 for 8 ounces)* is a standard hairspray that can be used as a styling spray too. It has a light hold and minimal to no stiff or sticky feel. It contains mostly alcohol, propellant, film former, slip agent, silicones, more slip agent, conditioning agent, and fragrance.

Tricomin
(see Folligen)

Ultra Swim

For more information on Ultra Swim, call (800) 745-2429 or in Canada (800) 268-3949.

☺ **Chlorine Removal Hair Treatment Shampoo** *($6.84 for 15 ounces)* contains a few problematic ingredients for hair, including urea and sodium thiosulfate. Both of those can denature the hair shaft with repeated use. I suspect they can be effective in preventing minerals from binding to hair, but the risk to the hair probably isn't worth it.

☺ **Chlorine Removal Shampoo Plus** *($6.84 for 15 ounces)* is similar to the version above and the same comments apply.

☺ **Chlorine Damaged Hair Treatment, Conditioner for All Hair Types** *($6.84 for 15 ounces)* is just a standard conditioner that would work well for dry hair of any thickness. It contains mostly water, detangling agent, slip agent, thickeners, mineral oil, conditioning agents, preservatives, and fragrance. There's nothing that makes this better for chlorine-damaged hair.

☺ **Ultra Repair Conditioner** *($6.84 for 15 ounces)* can't repair anything, it's just a good basic conditioner for normal to dry hair of any thickness. It contains mostly water, detangling agent, thickeners, conditioning agents, slip agents, fragrance, and preservatives.

Vibrance Organic Care

For more information on Vibrance Organic Care, call (800) 621-3379.

☹ **Nourishing Shampoo + Conditioner with Vitamins & Keratin** *($2.84 for 15 ounces)* uses sodium lauryl sulfate as the main detergent cleansing agent, and that makes it too potentially irritating for the scalp and drying for the hair.

☹ **Nourishing Shampoo with Vitamins & Keratin Body Building for Fine/ Thin Hair** *($2.84 for 15 ounces)* contains ammonium xylenesulfonate, which can be drying for the hair and drying and irritating for the scalp.

The Reviews T

☹ **Nourishing Shampoo with Vitamins & Keratin Moisture Rich for Dry/ Damaged Hair** *($2.84 for 15 ounces)* contains ammonium xylenesulfonate, which can be drying for the hair and drying and irritating for the scalp.

☹ **Nourishing Shampoo with Vitamins & Keratin Revitalizing for Permed/ Colored Hair** *($2.84 for 15 ounces)* contains TEA-dodecylphenyl sulfonate, which can be drying for the hair and scalp and can potentially strip hair color with repeated use.

☺ **Nourishing Conditioner with Vitamins & Keratin Body Building for Fine/Thin Hair** *($3.79 for 15 ounces)* contains mostly water, thickeners, silicone, detangling agent, conditioning agents, slip agent, preservatives, fragrance, and vitamins. This is a good conditioner for normal to dry hair of any thickness. The minute amount of vitamins in here can't affect the hair.

☺ **Nourishing Conditioner with Vitamins & Keratin Moisture Rich for Dry/Damaged Hair** *($2.84 for 15 ounces)* is similar to the Body Building version above, only this one has slightly more silicone, which makes it better for dry hair of any thickness.

☺ **Nourishing Conditioner with Vitamins & Keratin Revitalizing Conditioner for Permed/Colored Hair** *($2.84 for 15 ounces)* is almost identical to the Moisture Rich version above and the same comments apply.

Victoria Jackson

For more information on Victoria Jackson, call (800) VMAKEUP, or visit its Web site at www.vmakeup.com. In the listings that follow, the first price is retail; the second price is for this line's club members.

☹ **Body Giving Shampoo** *($14.95, $9.95 for 8 ounces)* uses TEA-lauryl sulfate as the main cleansing agent, which can be too drying for the hair and irritating for the scalp.

☺ **Time Activated Hair Conditioner** *($14.95, $9.95 for 8 ounces)* contains mostly water, detangling agent, thickeners, conditioning agents, preservatives, plant extracts, fragrance, and coloring agent. This is a good lightweight conditioner for normal to slightly dry hair of any thickness. Perhaps by "time activated" they mean what I've been saying all along—this conditioner works better when left on hair for a while.

☺ **$$$ Brilliant Shine** *($26, $15.95 for 1 ounce)* is just an overpriced silicone serum that can add shine and a silky feel to hair. There are identical versions at the drugstore for a fraction of the price.

☺ **Accelerated Styling Mist** *($14.95, $9.95 for 8 ounces)* is a lightweight styling spray with a very light hold and minimal to no stiff or sticky feel. It contains mostly water, alcohol, slip agents, conditioning agent, silicone, preservatives, film former, and fragrance.

☺ **Anti-Elements Holding Spray** (*$14.95 for $9.95 for 8 ounces*) is a standard hairspray with a light hold and minimal to no stiff, sticky feel. It contains mostly alcohol, water, film former, slip agents, silicone, and fragrance.

Vidal Sassoon

At one time, Vidal Sassoon's name was equivalent to the leading edge in hair fashion. Sassoon set the standard for designer style and training, and was one of the first designers to open a sort of graduate school where stylists could obtain advanced training and skills. Given the quality of training taking place in "beauty schools," this was and still is a much-needed essential. Quality cutting and styling were Sassoon's hallmarks, but so were his products. In creating them, he was at the forefront of the present trend, followed by all designers who want their reputation—and talent—represented in a product line. Sassoon's products were long ago bought by Procter & Gamble, and these products now bear that trademark and have nothing to do with the kinds of products more typical of a more fashion-minded hair-care line. There are some good products to consider here, but some are a far cry from what I think Sassoon would ever have wanted. For more information on Vidal Sassoon, call (800) 723-9569 or in Canada (800) 668-0151. You can also visit its Web site at www.vssassoon.com.

☹ **Clarifying Shampoo, Removes Residue for Better Styling** (*$2.79 for 13 ounces*) contains ammonium xylenesulfonate, which can be drying for the hair and drying and irritating for the scalp.

☹ **Stylist Choice Shampoo A, Extra Body for Fine or Thin Hair** (*$2.79 for 13 ounces*) contains ammonium xylenesulfonate, which can be drying for the hair and drying and irritating for the scalp.

☹ **Stylist Choice Shampoo B, Body Building Texture for Normal Hair** (*$2.79 for 13 ounces*) contains ammonium xylenesulfonate, which can be drying for the hair and drying and irritating for the scalp.

☹ **Stylist Choice Shampoo C, Revitalizing for Permed or Color Treated Hair** (*$2.79 for 13 ounces*) contains ammonium xylenesulfonate, which can be drying for the hair and drying and irritating for the scalp.

☹ **Stylist Choice Shampoo D, Rich Moisturizing Texture for Dry or Damaged Hair** (*$2.79 for 13 ounces*) contains ammonium xylenesulfonate, which can be drying for the hair and drying and irritating for the scalp.

☹ **Ultra Care Shampoo, Conditioner and Protective Finishing Rinse All in One, Body Building Texture for Normal Hair** (*$2.79 for 13 ounces*) contains ammonium xylenesulfonate, which can be drying for the hair and drying and irritating for the scalp.

☹ **Ultra Care Shampoo, Conditioner and Protective Finishing Rinse All in One, Extra Body for Fine or Thin Hair** *($2.79 for 13 ounces)* contains ammonium xylenesulfonate, which can be drying for the hair and drying and irritating for the scalp.

☹ **Ultra Care Shampoo, Conditioner and Protective Finishing Rinse All in One, Moisturizing for Dry, Permed or Color-Treated Hair** *($2.79 for 13 ounces)* contains ammonium xylenesulfonate, which can be drying for the hair and drying and irritating for the scalp.

☺ **Stylist Choice Conditioner #1, Extra Body for Fine or Thin Hair** *($2.79 for 13 ounces)* contains mostly water, silicones, thickeners, detangling agent/film former, conditioning agents, alcohol, fragrance, and preservatives. This is a good basic conditioner for normal to dry hair that is fine or thin.

☺ **Stylist Choice Conditioner #2, Balanced for Normal Hair** *($2.79 for 13 ounces)* is almost identical to the Extra Body version above and the same comments apply.

☺ **Stylist Choice Conditioner #3, Revitalizing for Permed or Color-Treated Hair, Heat Defense Formula** *($2.79 for 13 ounces)* is almost identical to the Extra Body version above and the same comments apply.

☺ **Stylist Choice Conditioner #3, Revitalizing for Permed or Color-Treated Hair, Texturizing Formula** *($2.79 for 13 ounces)* is almost identical to the Extra Body version above, only minus the film former, which makes this a good basic conditioner for dry hair of any thickness.

☺ **Stylist Choice Conditioner #4, Moisture Rich for Dry or Damaged Hair** *($2.79 for 13 ounces)* is almost identical to the Extra Body version above and the same comments apply.

☺ **Treatments Deep Moisturizing Conditioner** *($2.93 for 6.7 ounces)* is almost identical to the Extra Body version above and the same comments apply.

☺ **Heat Defense, Styling Heat Protectant** *($2.79 for 10.2 ounces)* contains nothing that can protect hair from the heat of styling tools, though it is a good lightweight, leave-in conditioner for normal to dry hair that is fine or thin. This has a slight amount of hold that can be used for styling. It contains mostly water, detangling agent/film former, slip agents, conditioning agents, film former, silicone, preservatives, and fragrance.

☺ **Alcohol-Free Spray-on Gel Extra Hold** *($2.99 for 8.5 ounces)* is a very standard, simple spray gel that has a light to medium hold and minimal stiff or sticky feel. It contains mostly water, film former, preservatives, fragrance, and slip agents.

☺ **Spray-on Gel Extra Hold** *($2.99 for 8.5 ounces)* is a basic styling spray that has a light hold and minimal to no stiff or sticky feel. It contains mostly water, film former, preservatives, fragrance, and slip agents.

☺ **Alcohol-Free Styling Gel Extra Hold** *($2.99 for 7.1 ounces)* is a very liquid gel with a light hold and minimal to no stiff or sticky feel. It contains mostly water, detangling agent/film former, conditioning agent, thickeners, slip agent, preservatives, and fragrance.

☺ **Alcohol-Free Styling Mousse Extra Body for Volume** *($2.99 for 8 ounces)* is a standard mousse with a light hold and minimal sticky feel that does let hair be brushed through. It contains mostly water, propellant, detangling agent/film former, slip agents, preservatives, fragrance, and conditioning agents.

☺ **Alcohol-Free Styling Mousse Extra Hold for Control** *($2.99 for 8 ounces)* is a standard mousse with a light to medium hold and minimal sticky feel that can be brushed through. It contains mostly water, propellant, detangling agent/film former, slip agents, preservatives, fragrance, and conditioning agents.

☺ **Flexible Hold Hair Spray for Fine Hair with Formesilk (Aerosol)** *($2.99 for 8.25 ounces)* is a standard aerosol hairspray with a medium to firm hold and a somewhat stiff feel. It can be brushed through, but I wouldn't call this flexible. It contains mostly alcohol, water, propellant, film former, silicone, slip agents, and fragrance.

☺ **Flexible Hold Hair Spray for Fine Hair with Formesilk (Non-Aerosol)** *($2.99 for 8.5 ounces)* is similar to the Aerosol version above, only in nonaerosol form, and the same basic comments apply.

☺ **Flexible Hold Hair Spray with Formesilk (Aerosol)** *($2.99 for 8.25 ounces)* is almost identical to the Aerosol version above and the same comments apply.

☺ **Flexible Hold Hair Spray with Formesilk (Non-Aerosol) Scented and Unscented** *($2.99 for 8.5 ounces)* is similar to the Aerosol version above, only in nonaerosol form, and the same basic comments apply. The unscented version still has a masking fragrance.

☺ **Finishing Hair Spray, Extra Hold (Aerosol)** *($3.59 for 8.5 ounces)* is a standard, medium-hold hairspray with a slight stiff feel that can be brushed through. It contains mostly alcohol, water, film formers, silicone, conditioning agents, more silicone, slip agents, and fragrance.

☺ **Non-Aerosol Finishing Hairspray Extra Hold Unscented** *($2.99 for 10.2 ounces)* is almost identical to the Finishing Hair Spray above and the same comments apply. This does have a masking fragrance.

☺ **Styling Freeze, Maximum Hold (Non-Aerosol)** *($2.24 for 8.5 ounces)* is almost identical to the Finishing Hair Spray above and the same comments apply.

☺ **Ultra Firm Hold Hair Spray (Aerosol)** *($2.99 for 8.25 ounces)* is a standard aerosol hairspray with a firm hold and a somewhat stiff feel that does let hair be brushed through. It contains mostly alcohol, propellant, water, film formers, silicones, slip agent, and fragrance.

☺ **Ultra Firm Hold Hair Spray (Non-Aerosol) Scented and Unscented** *($2.99 for 10.2 ounces)* is almost identical to the Ultra Firm Aerosol version above and the same comments apply. The unscented version does contain a masking fragrance.

Wanakee

If you could see the picture on the brochure for the Wanakee hair care products of the gorgeous African-American women with bountiful, long, perfectly straight hair, you too might be seduced by their claims. They are supposed to contain something called Verifen, a complex that can make straight-hair dreams come true. But such a wonder doesn't exist. The ingredients in the Wanakee products are just the same as those found in hundreds and hundreds of products made by other lines. What this line does have that makes it different from many African-American hair-care lines are far fewer greasy, oily products. To that extent, it is far better for African-American hair. While that is impressive, nothing in these products makes them better than many other products for extremely dry, fine, or thin hair, or for problems that result from hair straightening and styling—the main concerns for many African Americans. The one main drawback for this line is that it doesn't take more advantage of silicone technology. This ingredient works wonders on many hair types, especially to add shine and a silky feel, and would make this line far more current and interesting for any woman with dry or extremely dry hair. There are some good products to consider here, but Wanakee is not the final miracle for African-American hair-care needs.

For more information on Wanakee, call (800) HAIR OI, or visit its Web site at www.wanakee.com.

☺ **Beneficial Phase Shampoo** *($8.95 for 8 ounces)* is a standard, detergent-based shampoo, just like a thousand other shampoos. Even if the minuscule amounts of vitamins and plant extracts at the end of the ingredient listing could affect the hair (which they can't), they would be washed away before they could do anything. This contains mostly water, detergent cleansing agents, lather agent, detangling agent/ film former, thickeners, preservatives, detangling agent, plant oil, plant extracts, and fragrance. It is a good basic shampoo for normal hair that is fine or thin.

☺ **Moisture Emphasis Shampoo** *($10.95 for 8 ounces)* is almost identical to the Beneficial version above and the same comments apply.

☺ **Advanced Conditioning Treatment** *($12.95 for 8 ounces)* isn't all that advanced, but it is a good, though heavy, conditioner for someone with extremely dry hair. It contains mostly water, thickener, slip agent, detangling agent/film former, preservatives, Vaseline, mineral oil, fragrance, and conditioning agents.

☺ **Moisture Emphasis Conditioner** *($15.95 for 8 ounces)* is more thick and heavy than moisturizing. It is just a very standard conditioner that would work well for extremely dry hair of any thickness. It contains mostly water, detangling agents, thickeners, castor oil, preservatives, vitamins, slip agents, and fragrance.

☺ **Constant Care for Ends** *($15 for 4 ounces)* is just thickeners and Vaseline. This greasy wax can help extremely dry hair, though be careful—it can look and feel greasy. Plus, this is a lot of money for Vaseline and wax.

☺ **Detangling Spray Conditioner** *($8.95 for 8 ounces)* is a lightweight, leave-in conditioner that can also work as a soft-hold styling spray with no stiff or sticky feel. It would work for normal to slightly dry hair that is normal to thin or fine. It contains mostly water, conditioning agent, film former, detangling agent, preservatives, slip agent, silicone, and fragrance.

☺ **$$$ Oil for the Hair** *($29.95 for 8 ounces)* doesn't actually contain any oil! It's just an extremely overpriced group of thickeners and slip agents. That can help when styling, and it is less greasy than other "oil"-type products, but this formula doesn't add up to more than 10 cents' worth of ingredients.

☺ **$$$ Penetrating Nourishment for Braids** *($21.95 for 8 ounces)* is almost identical to the Oil for the Hair above, only in spray form.

☺ **Hairline Essential Creme** *($8.95 for 4 ounces)* is just a standard styling cream that has a light to medium hold with minimal stiffness, though it does have a somewhat greasy feel. It contains mostly water, conditioning agent, film former, thickeners, preservatives, Vaseline, mineral oil, vitamins, and fragrance.

Wash 'N Curl

These products can't help curl hair, but you already knew that, right? For more information on Wash 'N Curl, call (201) 935-3232 or visit its Web site at www. CCAindustries.com.

☹ **Curling Shampoo for Normal Hair** *($3.29 for 8 ounces)* uses TEA-lauryl sulfate as the main cleansing agent, which makes it too drying for the hair and too drying and irritating for the scalp.

☹ **Curling Shampoo for Dry, Treated, or Damaged Hair** *($3.29 for 8 ounces)* uses TEA-lauryl sulfate as the main cleansing agent, which makes it too drying for the hair and too drying and irritating for the scalp.

☺ **Extra Strength Curling Shampoo for Dry, Damaged, Color-Treated Hair** *($3.29 for 8 ounces)* contains mostly water, detergent cleansing agents, lather agent, film former, fragrance, preservatives, and coloring agents. The film former in here can add a feel of thickness to fine or thin hair, but that's about it—it has no effect on making hair curl, unless you help style it that way.

☺ **Extra Strength Curling Shampoo for Fine, Limp, Dry Hair** *($3.29 for 8 ounces)* is virtually identical to the Extra Strength Dry Damaged version above and the same comments apply.

Wella

For more information on Wella, call (800) 843-2656, (800) 565-2588 or visit its Web site at www.wellacorp.com.

Elan Plus by Wella

☺ **Alcohol Free Extra-Hold Styling Foam** *($2.99 for 10.6 ounces)* contains mostly water, film former, propellant, more film formers, castor oil, slip agent, detangling agent, and fragrance. This is a standard mousse that has a light hold and minimal to no stiff or sticky feel.

☺ **Conditioning Setting Lotion Extra Hold** *($6.99 for 16 ounces)* is a rather ordinary styling liquid that would be far easier to use in a spray container than this squeeze bottle. It has minimal hold and minimal to no stiff or sticky feel, and it can help when styling if you need only minimal control. It contains mostly water, alcohol, detangling agent/film former, film formers, thickeners, fragrance, and coloring agents.

☺ **Conditioning Setting Lotion Regular Hold** *($6.99 for 16 ounces)* is almost identical to the Extra Hold version above and the same comments apply.

☹ **Finishing Spray (Aerosol)** *($2.99 for 10 ounces)* is a standard aerosol hairspray that has an extremely firm hold (one of the strongest I've come across) and a definite stiff feel that is not easy to brush through. It contains mostly alcohol, film former, propellant, water, and fragrance.

Liquid Hair by Wella

☺ **Clarifying Shampoo for All Hair Types** *($7.50 for 12 ounces)* has a great name, but the product is completely routine. This is a standard shampoo with minimal conditioning agents. That makes it great for most all hair types except an oily scalp or hair. The fact that the conditioning agent is keratin, the substance hair is made out of, doesn't mean it can merge with or reinforce hair in the least, any more than putting "skin" in a skin-care product can add more skin to your own. It contains mostly water, detergent cleansing agents, lather agent, thickeners, conditioning agents, fragrance, and preservatives.

☺ **Color Preserver Daily Shampoo for Color-Treated Hair** *($7.50 for 12 ounces)* contains mostly water, detergent cleansing agents, thickeners, lather agent, detangling agents, film formers, conditioning agents, fragrance, and preservatives.

This is a good shampoo for normal to slightly dry hair that is fine or thin. The film formers in here can easily build up on hair with repeated use.

☺ **Moisturizing Shampoo for Dry or Chemically Treated Hair** *($7.50 for 12 ounces)* contains mostly water, detergent cleansing agents, lather agent, thickeners, detangling agents, conditioning agents, castor oil, detangling agent/film former, preservatives, fragrance, and coloring agent. This is a good shampoo for normal to dry hair that is fine or thin.

☺ **Volumizing Shampoo for Fine or Normal Hair** *($7.50 for 12 ounces)* is almost identical to the Moisturizing version above and the same basic comments apply.

☺ **Color Preserver Daily Conditioner for Color-Treated Hair** *($8.50 for 12 ounces)* contains mostly water, thickeners, detangling agent, silicone, conditioning agent, preservative, film former, and fragrance. This is a good basic conditioner for normal to dry hair that is normal to fine or thin.

☺ **Moisture Rinse Daily Conditioner for All Hair Types** *($8.50 for 12 ounces)* contains mostly water, thickeners, detangling agent, conditioning agents, film former, silicone, preservative, and fragrance. This is a good basic conditioner for normal to slightly dry hair that is fine or thin. The film former in here can easily build up on hair with repeated use.

☺ **Vital Signs Intensive Moisturizing Treatment for Dry, Chemically Treated Hair** *($13 for 6 ounces)* contains mostly water, thickeners, detangling agent, lanolin, detangling agent/film former, conditioning agents, slip agents, plant extracts, fragrant oil, coloring agents, preservative, and fragrance. This is a good basic conditioner for dry to very dry hair that is normal to fine or thin.

☺ **Restructurizer Leave-in Treatment** *($15 for 6.8 ounces)* contains mostly water, conditioning agents, detangling agent, preservative, film former, and fragrance. This is a good, basic, leave-in conditioner for normal to dry hair that is normal to fine or thin.

☺ **Physical Therapy, Wearable Volumizer Treatment for All Hair Types** *($13 for 6 ounces)* contains mostly water, conditioning agents, detangling agents, plant oils, film former, preservatives, silicone, and fragrance. This is a good leave-in conditioner for dry hair that is normal to fine or thin.

☺ **Hair Polish** *($10 for 3.4 ounces)* is a standard silicone gel that has castor oil in it, which adds a very slight sticky hold that can help when styling hair smooth.

☹ **Crystal Styler Creme-Gel, Extra Strong Hold for All Hair Types** *($10 for 6 ounces)* is gel with a light to medium hold and minimal stiff or sticky feel that also has glitter added. The sparkle part is just a soft dusting and nothing like sequins in the least. It contains mostly water, thickeners, slip agents, film former, castor oil, preservatives, and fragrance.

☺ **Brilliant Spray Gel** *($10 for 6 ounces)* is a standard spray gel with a light hold and minimal stiff or sticky feel that contains mostly water, thickeners, slip agent, conditioning agent, detangling agent/film former, castor oil, preservatives, and fragrance. It can help when styling hair smooth, with little to no hold or stiffness.

☺ **Fast Finish Fixing Spritz** *($8 for 6.8 ounces)* is a standard hairspray with a medium to firm hold and a slight stiff feel that does let hair be brushed through. It contains mostly alcohol, water, film formers, conditioning agent, silicone, and fragrance.

Wella Balsam

☺ **Conditioning Shampoo for Normal Hair** *($2.99 for 32 ounces)* contains mostly water, detergent cleansing agent, thickeners, detangling agents/film former, slip agents, lather agent, preservatives, and coloring agents. This is a good shampoo for normal hair that is fine or thin. The film formers in here can easily build up on hair.

☺ **Instant Conditioner, Extra Body, Excellent for Fine, Limp, and/or Damaged Hair** *($3.29 for 32 ounces)* is a very ordinary but good conditioner for dry hair that is thick or coarse. It contains mostly water, thickeners, Vaseline, detangling agent, fragrance, preservatives, and coloring agents. It can have a greasy feel on hair.

☺ **Instant Conditioner, Regular** *($3.49 for 24 ounces)* is almost identical to the Extra Body version above and the same comments apply.

☺ **Kolestral Concentrate** *($4.29 for 6 ounces)* is similar to the Extra Body version above, only minus the detangling agent. This is emollient, but it can be heavy on hair.

☺ **Kolestral Professional Treatment for Hair and Scalp** *($3.49 for 6 ounces)* contains mostly water, thickeners, lanolin, Vaseline, preservatives, and fragrance. This is best kept off the scalp; it's very heavy and greasy and would only be appropriate for extremely dry hair. On the scalp it can clog pores.

☺ **In-Depth Treatment for Problem Hair** *($4.99 for 16 ounces)* contains mostly water, thickeners, conditioning agents, mineral oil, fragrance, and preservatives. This ordinary conditioner isn't "in-depth," it's just good for dry hair of any thickness.

☺ **pH-D Diagnosis In-Depth Treatment** *($5.29 for 16 ounces)* is almost identical to the In-Depth version above and the same basic comments apply.

☺ **pH-D Diagnosis Regenal Instant Normalizer** *($4.99 for 16 ounces)* is just water, thickener, Vaseline, detangling agent, preservatives, and fragrance. That makes this a good but very ordinary conditioner for extremely dry hair of any thickness.

White Rain

Hair care doesn't get much less expensive than this. There are definitely some options here to consider, and some—as in every line—to avoid. For basic products, such as shampoos for cleaning the hair with no conditioning or volumizing additives so you don't have to worry about buildup, or conditioners that work just for detangling, there are some good choices. Even the hairsprays and gel are light and effective. Don't be a price snob; if a product works, it works—let go of the myth that price is the way to judge the quality of any cosmetic. One word of warning: some of the fruit scents are hard to take, but when those aren't present, the herb and regular fragrances are rather standard and pleasant. For more information on White Rain call (800) 872-7202.

Collections by White Rain

☺ **Baby Shampoo Classic Care Tear Free Formula Gentle Cleansing** *($1.09 for 15 ounces)* contains mostly water, detergent cleansing agents, lather agent, thickener, fragrance, preservatives, and coloring agents. This is a gentle shampoo that would work for any normal hair type and it wouldn't cause buildup!

☺ **Plus for Kids Classic Care Shampoo & Detangler in One Tear Free** *($1.09 for 15 ounces)* contains mostly water, detergent cleansing agents, thickener, detangling agent/film former, fragrance, preservatives, and lather agent. This is a good basic shampoo that would work for normal to slightly dry hair that is normal to fine or thin in thickness. There is nothing in this product that makes it better for kids.

☺ **Classic Care Shampoo Extra Body** *($1.09 for 15 ounces)* contains mostly water, detergent cleansing agents, lather agent, thickener, slip agent, fragrance, and preservatives. This is a good shampoo that would work for all hair types and it wouldn't cause buildup!

☺ **Classic Care Shampoo Regular** *($0.99 for 15 ounces)* is almost identical to the Extra Body version above and the same comments apply.

☺ **Classic Care Shampoo Revitalizing Formula** *($0.99 for 15 ounces)* contains mostly water, detergent cleansing agents, lather agent, thickeners, conditioning agents, fragrance, and preservatives. This isn't revitalizing in the least, it's just a good basic shampoo for someone with normal to slightly dry hair of any thickness. There is minimal risk of buildup.

☺ **Shampoo Moisturizing** *($0.97 for 15 ounces)* contains mostly water, detergent cleansing agents, lather agent, thickeners, detangling agent, fragrance, preservatives, and coloring agents. This isn't moisturizing in the least, though it is a good basic shampoo for all hair types.

☺ **Shampoo Salon Formula** *($0.97 for 15 ounces)* is virtually identical to the Extra Body version above and the same comments apply.

☹ **Two in One: Shampoo + Conditioner in One Extra Body for All Hair Types** *($1.07 for 16.8 ounces)* uses sodium lauryl sulfate as one of the main detergent cleansing agents, and that makes it too potentially irritating for the scalp and drying for the hair. It also contains ammonium xylenesulfonate, which can be drying for hair as well.

☹ **Two in One: Shampoo + Conditioner in One Replenishing for Dry Hair** *($1.07 for 16.8 ounces)* uses sodium lauryl sulfate as one of the main detergent cleansing agents, and that makes it too potentially irritating for the scalp and drying for the hair. It also contains ammonium xylenesulfonate, which can be drying for hair as well.

☹ **Two in One: Shampoo + Conditioner in One Revitalizing with Pro-Vitamin B5** *($1.07 for 16.8 ounces)* uses sodium lauryl sulfate as one of the main detergent cleansing agents, and that makes it too potentially irritating for the scalp and drying for the hair. It also contains ammonium xylenesulfonate, which can be drying for hair as well.

☺ **Classic Care Conditioner Extra Body** *($1.09 for 15 ounces)* contains mostly water, thickeners, detangling agent, preservatives, and fragrance. This is a very ordinary but good conditioner for normal hair only, to help with combing.

☺ **Classic Care Conditioner Regular** *($0.99 for 15 ounces)* is almost identical to the Conditioner Extra Body above and the same comments apply.

☺ **Classic Care Conditioner Revitalizing Formula** *($0.99 for 15 ounces)* is almost identical to the Conditioner Extra Body above and the same comments apply.

☺ **Conditioner Moisturizing** *($0.97 for 15 ounces)* is almost identical to the Conditioner Extra Body above and the same comments apply.

☺ **Conditioner Salon Formula** *($0.97 for 15 ounces)* is almost identical to the Conditioner Extra Body above and the same comments apply.

☺ **Leave-in Conditioner E for Daily Nourishment with Vitamin E Aloe Extracts & UV Filter** *($0.99 for 7 ounces)* is a good, basic, leave-in conditioner for normal to slightly dry hair of any thickness. It contains mostly water, conditioning agents, thickeners, preservatives, detangling agent, slip agent, detangling agents/film formers, and fragrance. The minute amount of sunscreen in here can't protect one hair from sun damage.

☺ **Extra Hold Styling Gel with Pro-Vitamin B5** *($0.99 for 4 ounces)* is a good styling gel with a light hold and minimal to no stiff or sticky feel. It contains mostly water, film former, thickeners, preservatives, conditioning agents, and fragrance.

☺ **Maximum Hold Styling Gel with Chamomile & Rosemary Extracts** *($0.99 for 4 ounces)* is a good styling gel with a light to medium hold and a slight stiff, sticky feel that does let hair be brushed through. It contains mostly water, film former, thickeners, preservatives, conditioning agents, and fragrance.

☺ **Maximum Hold Spray Gel with Chamomile & Rosemary Extracts** *($0.99 for 7 ounces)* is a good spray gel with a light to medium hold and minimal to no stiff or sticky feel. It contains mostly water, film formers, conditioning agent, silicone, detangling agent, fragrance, slip agents, and plant extracts.

☺ **Extra Body Mousse with Pro-Vitamin B5 & Conditioner** *($1.59 for 5 ounces)* is a standard mousse with a medium hold and a slight sticky feel that can be brushed through. It contains mostly water, alcohol, propellant, film formers, thickeners, conditioning agent, silicone, preservatives, fragrance, detangling agent, and slip agents.

☺ **Maximum Hold Styling Mousse with Chamomile & Rosemary Extracts** *($0.99 for 5 ounces)* is virtually identical to the Extra Body version above, only this one does contain a small amount of silicone and that can help add shine.

☺ **Extra Hold Styling Mousse with Pro-Vitamin B5** *($1.59 for 5 ounces)* is virtually identical the Extra Body version above, only this one does contain a small amount of silicone and that can help add shine.

☺ **Firm Hold Hair Spray Aerosol** *($1.59 for 7 ounces)* is a standard but good aerosol hairspray with a light hold and a minimally stiff feel that can easily be brushed through. It contains mostly alcohol, water, propellant, film former, slip agent, fragrance, and silicone.

☺ **Extra Hold Hair Spray Aerosol Scented and Unscented** *($1.59 for 7 ounces)* is almost identical to the Firm Hold above and the same comments apply. The unscented version has a masking fragrance.

☺ **Extra Hold Hair Spray for Extra Long Lasting Hold Non-Aerosol Scented and Unscented** *($1.59 for 7 ounces)* is almost identical to the Extra Hold Aerosol version above, only with slightly more hold and slightly stiffer feel, but it still can be brushed through.

☺ **Extra Hold Hair Spray with Pro-Vitamin B5 Non-Aerosol** *($0.86 for 8.75 ounces)* is almost identical to the Extra Long Lasting version above and the same comments apply.

☺ **Extra Hold Styling Spritz with Pro-Vitamin B5** *($0.99 for 7 ounces)* is a standard but good hairspray with a light to medium hold and a slight stiff feel that can easily be brushed through. It contains mostly alcohol, water, propellant, film former, slip agent, fragrance, and silicone.

☺ **Hair Spray Maximum Hold Aerosol** *($1.59 for 7 ounces)* is almost identical to the Extra Hold Styling Spritz above and the same comments apply.

☺ **Maximum Hold Hair Spray with Chamomile & Rosemary Extracts Non-Aerosol** *($0.99 for 7 ounces)* is virtually identical to the Extra Hold Styling Spritz above and the same comments apply.

Essential by White Rain

☹ **Apple Essence Shampoo** *($1.09 for 16.8 ounces)* contains ammonium xylenesulfonate, which can be drying for the hair and drying and irritating for the scalp.

☹ **Coconut Essence Shampoo** *($1.09 for 13.5 ounces)* contains ammonium xylenesulfonate, which can be drying for the hair and drying and irritating for the scalp.

☹ **Strawberry Essence Shampoo** *($1.07 for 16.8 ounces)* contains ammonium xylenesulfonate, which can be drying for the hair and drying and irritating for the scalp.

☺ **Apple Essence Conditioner** *($1.09 for 13.5 ounces)* contains mostly water, thickeners, detangling agent, preservatives, fragrance, slip agent, and coloring agent. This is strictly for detangling normal hair.

☺ **Coconut Essence Conditioner** *($1.07 for 16.8 ounces)* is virtually identical to the Apple Essence above and the same comments apply.

☺ **Strawberry Essence Conditioner** *($1.07 for 16.8 ounces)* is virtually identical to the Apple Essence above and the same comments apply.

Exotics by White Rain

☺ **Hibiscus Petals Shampoo, for Shine** *($1.09 for 13.5 ounces)* is just a good basic shampoo that would work well for all hair types without any buildup. It contains mostly water, detergent cleansing agents, lather agent, thickener, fragrance, conditioning agent, preservatives, slip agent, plant extracts, and coloring agents.

☺ **Lotus Petals Shampoo, for sShine** *($1.09 for 13.5 ounces)* is a good basic shampoo that would work well for all hair types without any buildup. It contains mostly water, detergent cleansing agents, lather agent, thickeners, fragrance, detangling agents, preservatives, slip agent, plant extracts, and coloring agents.

☺ **Orchid Petals Shampoo, for Shine** *($1.09 for 13.5 ounces)* is almost identical to the Hibiscus Petals Shampoo above and the same comments apply.

☺ **Hibiscus Petals Conditioner** *($1.07 for 16.8 ounces)* contains mostly water, thickeners, detangling agent, preservatives, fragrance, conditioning agent, slip agent, and coloring agent. This is strictly for detangling normal hair.

☺ **Lotus Petals Conditioner, for Shine** *($1.07 for 16.8 ounces)* is almost identical to the Hibiscus Petals Conditioner above and the same comments apply.

☺ **Orchid Petals Conditioner, for Shine** *($1.07 for 16.8 ounces)* is almost identical to the Hibiscus Petals Conditioner above and the same comments apply.

Herbs & Blossoms by White Rain

☺ **Ginger Lily Shampoo Moisturizing** *($1.07 for 13.5 ounces)* is just a good basic shampoo that would work well for all hair types without any buildup. It contains mostly water, detergent cleansing agents, lather agent, thickener, fragrance, detangling agent, conditioning agent, slip agent, preservatives, plant extracts, and coloring agents. The teeny amount of conditioner in here has minimal to no impact on the hair.

☺ **Jasmine Shampoo, Extra Body** *($1.07 for 13.5 ounces)* is virtually identical to the Ginger Lily Shampoo above and the same basic comments apply.

☺ **Passionflower Shampoo Revitalizing** *($1.07 for 13.5 ounces)* is virtually identical to the Ginger Lily Shampoo above and the same basic comments apply.

☺ **Ginger Lily Conditioner Moisturizing** *($1.07 for 13.5 ounces)* contains mostly water, thickeners, detangling agents, preservatives, conditioning agents, fragrance, slip agent, plant extracts, and coloring agent. This is strictly for detangling normal hair; the amount of conditioning agents in here is negligible and has minimal to no effect on hair.

☺ **Jasmine Conditioner Extra Body** *($1.07 for 13.5 ounces)* is almost identical to the Ginger Lily Conditioner above and the same comments apply.

☺ **Passionflower Conditioner Revitalizing** *($1.07 for 13.5 ounces)* is almost identical to the Ginger Lily Conditioner above and the same comments apply.

☺ **Angelica Hairspray Maximum Hold** *($1.07 for 7 ounces)* is a standard medium- to firm-hold hairspray with a stiff feel that does let hair be brushed through. It contains mostly alcohol, water, film former, slip agents, fragrance, plant extracts, and coloring agents.

☺ **Chamomile Hairspray Extra Hold** *($1.07 for 7 ounces)* is a standard, light-hold hairspray with minimal stiff feel that does let hair be brushed through. It contains mostly alcohol, water, film former, slip agents, fragrance, plant extracts, and coloring agents.

Solutions by White Rain

☹ **Solutions C Shampoo Super Shine** *($1.09 for 13.5 ounces)* contains ammonium xylenesulfonate, which can be drying for the hair and drying and irritating for the scalp.

☺ **Solutions E Shampoo Super Nourishing** *($1.09 for 13.5 ounces)* is just a good basic shampoo that would work well for all hair types without any buildup. It contains mostly water, detergent cleansing agents, lather agent, thickeners, fragrance, detangling agents, conditioning agent, preservatives, and slip agents. The teeny amount of conditioner in here has minimal to no impact on the hair.

☹ **Solutions B5 Conditioner Super Volume** *($1.09 for 13.5 ounces)* contains mostly water, thickeners, detangling agents, preservatives, fragrance, conditioning agents, detangling agent/film former, and slip agent. This conditioner is mostly for detangling normal hair. The teeny amount of film former won't add much thickness and the conditioning agents are barely present. This conditioner does contain peppermint, a skin irritant, so keep it off the scalp.

☹ **Solutions C Conditioner Super Shine** *($1.09 for 13.5 ounces)* is almost identical to the Solutions B5 above, only this one contains a small amount of silicone, which can make it good for normal to slightly dry hair of any thickness, but the peppermint in here is a problem.

☺ **Solutions E Conditioner Super Nourishing** *($1.09 for 13.5 ounces)* is almost identical to the Solutions B5 above, only this one doesn't contain peppermint. All the other comments apply.

Willow Lake

For more information on Willow Lake, call (612) 571-1234 or (800) 444-0699.

☺ **Cherry Bark & Irish Moss Conditioning Shampoo** *($3.59 for 16 ounces)* is a standard, silicone-based shampoo that contains mostly water, detergent cleansing agent, lather agent, film former, silicone, plant extracts, thickeners, slip agents, preservatives, fragrance, and coloring agents. It would work well for normal to slightly dry hair that is fine or thin. The film former in here can cause buildup with repeated use.

☹ **Citrus & Rosemary Shampoo** *($3.59 for 16 ounces)* includes grapefruit extract, and that can be an irritant for the scalp.

☹ **Lavender & Mint Shampoo** *($2.59 for 16 ounces)* contains peppermint, a skin irritant that can cause problems for the scalp.

☹ **Witch Hazel & Honeysuckle Shampoo** *($3.59 for 16 ounces)* contains mostly water, detergent cleansing agent, lather agent, plant extracts, detangling agent, thickener, preservatives, fragrance, and coloring agents. The witch hazel can be drying for the scalp and hair.

☺ **Hops, Apricot & Almond Conditioner** *($3.10 for 16 ounces)* contains mostly water, thickeners, detangling agent/film former, detangling agents, slip agents, plant extracts, preservatives, fragrance, and coloring agents. This is a good conditioner for normal hair that is fine or thin.

☺ **Sunflower, Honey & Hibiscus Conditioner** *($3.10 for 16 ounces)* contains mostly water, thickeners, detangling agents, detangling agent/film former, plant extracts, conditioning agent, mineral oil, preservatives, fragrance, and coloring agents. This is a good conditioner for normal to slightly dry hair that is fine or thin.

☺ **Vitamin E, Carrot Extract & Milk Protein Conditioner** *($3.10 for 16 ounces)* is almost identical to the Sunflower version above and the same comments apply.

☺ **Rosehips & Ivy Spray Gel, Natural Hold** *($2.91 for 8 ounces)* is a standard styling spray with a medium hold and a slight stiff, sticky feel that can be brushed through. It contains mostly water, film former, plant extracts, detangling agent/film former, slip agents, silicone, preservatives, and fragrance.

☺ **Aloe and Clover Blossom Mousse, Extra Hold** *($3.76 for 8.5 ounces)* is a standard mousse with a light to medium hold and minimal to no stiff or sticky feel.

It contains mostly water, propellants, detangling agents/film formers, plant extract, conditioning agent, silicone, preservatives, and fragrance.

☺ **White Lily and Jasmine Hair Spray, Extra Hold Aerosol** *($3.76 for 8.5 ounces)* is a standard, medium-hold aerosol hairspray that has a slight stiff feel that can be brushed through. It contains mostly alcohol, propellant, film formers, plant extracts, slip agent, silicone, and fragrance.

☺ **Raspberry Leaf & Vitamin E Non-Aerosol Hair Spray, Extra Hold** *($2.91 for 8 ounces)* is a standard, light- to medium-hold hairspray that has a slight stiff feel that does let hair be brushed through. It contains mostly alcohol, film formers, water, slip agents, silicone, coloring agent, and fragrance. The red coloring agent may make this hairspray look like raspberry, but the negligible amount of raspberry leaf extract in this product has no effect on hair whatsoever.

☺ **Orange Blossom & Clove Spritz, Maximum Hold** *($2.91 for 8 ounces)* is almost identical to the Raspberry Leaf version above and the same basic comments apply.

Zero Frizz

Zero Frizz is a great name for products meant to help fight the endless battle some women fight to prevent their hair from the frizzies. It turns out this small group of products does offer some good styling options for smoothing hair and getting rid of frizzies, at least temporarily, but zero frizz is not realistic with just these products. For more information on Zero Frizz, call (714) 556-1028, (800) 966-6960, or visit its Web site at www.advreslab.com.

☹ **Hydrating Shampoo** *($4.99 for 12 ounces)* contains ammonium xylenesulfonate, which can be drying for the hair and drying and irritating for the scalp.

☺ **Instant Conditioner** *($4.99 for 12 ounces)* contains mostly water, thickeners, silicones, detangling agent, conditioning agents, preservatives, and fragrance. This would be a very good conditioner for dry hair of any thickness.

☺ **Anti-Frizz Hair Serum** *($6.99 for 4 ounces)* is standard silicone serum that can add shine and a soft, silky feel to hair.

☺ **Anti-Frizz Glistening Mist** *($6.99 for 4 ounces)* is almost identical to the serum above, only this one is in spray form.

☺ **Anti-Frizz Styling Gel** *($4.99 for 6 ounces)* is just a basic gel with a light to medium hold and a slight sticky feel that does let hair be brushed through. It contains mostly water, film former, slip agents, silicone, thickeners, preservatives, and fragrance.

☺ **Anti-Frizz Styling Mousse** *($4.99 for 6 ounces)* is just a basic mousse with a light to medium hold and minimal stiff or sticky feel. It contains mostly water, propellant, film formers, silicones, thickeners, detangling agent, preservatives, and fragrance.

CHAPTER TEN

The Best Products

Too Many Choices?

I know some of you will be angry with me for creating such a cumbersome list of recommended products. I almost wish there were fewer good products, to help narrow your choices, but the truth is, there is little difference in quality between lines and many of the products are of equally good value. I know it seems shocking to realize how similar—if not identical—most shampoos, hairsprays, mousses, and gels are across product lines. But if you were a hair-care chemist, you wouldn't be surprised in the least because you would know that the technology for hair-care products is limited. As I've mentioned throughout this book, there are only so many ingredients that clean hair, make it feel soft and combable, keep it in place, and help with styling (making hair straight, smooth, or form better curls).

Some women have suggested that I reduce the listings to only my absolute favorites or even a top-ten list. I understand the frustration, but if there isn't a hierarchy out there, or if it only reflects my own preferences, that still won't help you achieve how you want your hair to be. Most of you know I have a preference for superior formulations for the least amount of money, but the list in this chapter concentrates simply on performance.

If so many products are recommended, you may be wondering why it seems that so many women are disappointed with the hair-care products they buy, and are endlessly switching to find the right one. Disappointment can be due to a poor formulation with problematic ingredients, but more often it is the misleading marketing language and the erroneous claims that lead a woman to expect something the product can't deliver, or the fact that the products don't explain why you need to be aware of possible problems with buildup.

The best I can do is tell you what my research and experience have found to be true, and allow you, as the consumer, to take it from there. I should mention that one of the purposes of my newsletter, *Cosmetics Counter Update,* is to narrow the range of options, in more detail and with more explanation. In the "Dear Paula" section of the newsletter, where readers write to me with their particular concerns and needs, I address those in detail and make specific recommendations depending on the individual situation and history. In this book, the goal is to provide more general information, giving consumers enough room to find what works best for them among all the products with great, reliable formulations.

The following product lists summarize the individual reviews in Chapter Nine. Be sure to read those more-detailed product evaluations before making any final decisions. I sincerely hope that all of these recommendations will make you feel informed and confident when shopping for hair-care products.

Misleading Product Names

Keep in mind that a hair-care company's name for a product does not always correspond with my recommendations. Just because a product label says it "can repair hair," is recommended for damaged hair or a sensitive, itchy scalp, or can make hair feel fuller and thicker doesn't mean the formulation itself supports that label or claim. Further, the hair-care industry's inane and meaningless use of terms like Mega, Super, Firm, Super Firm, Flexible, Ultra Firm, Freeze Spritz, Soft, or Natural hold are used at random and vary wildly. Often there is no difference between products with these arbitrary descriptive ratings, and I often found that the Mega hold products had a softer hold than the Flexible hold ones. This was especially true for gels and mousses.

Additionally, you will find many selections in the following list of recommended products with names that sound like they should be in the dry-hair group, but that I have included in the normal or slightly dry hair group—and vice versa. What counts is how the product is formulated, not what the companies want you to believe about their products. There are lots of products labeled as being good for one type of hair when they are really best for another type.

Hair Note: Please keep in mind as you read the following recommendations that the descriptions of how to combine products for the varying hair problems are listed in Chapter Four, *Hair Type.*

Also, keep in mind that a company's description of what its product is for more often than not does not agree with my assessment of how that product performs.

The Best Shampoos that Won't Cause Buildup

None of these shampoos contain conditioning agents or film formers, which are the ingredients that can cause buildup. All of these truly work great for all hair types if used in conjunction with the appropriate conditioner. **General guidelines for use:** These are reliable, well-formulated shampoos that can be used on their own on a daily or regular basis, or they can be alternated with a conditioning or volumizing shampoo from "The Best Shampoos for Adding Volume or Conditioning" list below. Depending on your hair type, after rinsing you would follow with the appropriate conditioner for your hair type.

All Ways Natural Neutralizing Conditioning Shampoo with Color Action *($3.99 for 12 ounces);* **American Crew** Shampoo Concentrate *($4.99 for 15.5 ounces);* **Apple Pectin by Lamaur** Shampoo Concentrate *($4.99 for 15.5 ounces)* and Naturals Witch Hazel & Honeysuckle Shampoo *($4.99 for 16 ounces);* **Aveda** Pure-Fume Brilliant Shampoo for Treated, Dry or Textured Hair *($10 for 8 ounces)* and Madder Root Pure Plant Shampoo *($6.50 for 8 ounces);* **Avon** Techniques Tri-Nutriv Formula Fortifying Shampoo Plus Conditioner in One *($3.99 for 11 ounces),* Techniques Tri-Nutriv Formula Hydrating Shampoo for Dry/Damaged Hair *($3.99 for 11 ounces),* and Techniques Tri-Nutriv Formula Replenishing Shampoo for Normal Hair *($3.99 for 11 ounces);* **Back to Basics** Wild Berry Volumizing Shampoo, for All Hair Types *($7.50 for 12 ounces);* **Beauty Without Cruelty** Daily Benefits Shampoo, Benefits All Hair Types *($6.95 for 16 ounces);* **The Body Shop** Banana Shampoo for Normal to Dry Hair *($9.50 for 16.9 ounces),* Chamomile Shampoo for Dry or Blonde Hair *($9.50 for 16.9 ounces),* Seaweed & Peony Shampoo for Normal Hair *($9.50 for 16.9 ounces),* and Tangerine Beer Shampoo for Normal Hair *($6 for 5 ounces);* **Bumble and Bumble** Clarifying Shampoo *($9 for 8 ounces)* and Seaweed Shampoo *($9 for 8 ounces);* **Clinique** Daily Wash Shampoo *($10 for 6 ounces);* **Focus 21** Hair Toys Shampoo *($3.82 for 8 ounces);* **SeaPlasma by Focus 21** SeaPlasma Shampoo *($3.99 for 12 ounces);* **Framesi Biogenol** Clarifying Shampoo *($5.99 for 8 ounces);* **Garden Botanika** Chamomile Moisture & Shine Shampoo *($8 for 12 ounces)* and Tri Wheat Hair Repair Shampoo *($8.50 for 12 ounces);* **Definition by Goldwell** Definition Coated & Oily Shampoo *($7.90 for 12 ounces)* and Definition Demineralizing Shampoo for Coated and Oily Hair *($7.95 for 12 ounces);* **Exclusives by Goldwell** Exclusives Body-Building Shampoo *($5.90 for 8 ounces)* and Exclusives Deep Cleansing Shampoo *($5.90 for 8 ounces);* **Halsa Highlights** Herbal Swedish Formula Daily Shampoo, Marigold and Orange Blossom *($2.57 for 20 ounces);* **System 911 by Hayashi** Shampoo Emergency Repair for Dry Damaged Hair *($6 for 8.4 ounces);* **ISO** Purifying Shampoo, Clarifies and Renews *($6.49 for 10 ounces);* **Jheri Redding** Citrus Shampoo for All Hair Types *($1.90 for 24 ounces),* Honey Wheatgerm Shampoo for All Hair Types *($1.90 for 24 ounces),* Strawberry Shampoo for All Hair Types *($1.90 for 24 ounces),* and Vanilla Shampoo for All Hair Types *($1.90 for 24 ounces);* **KMS** Ultra Volume Shampoo, Extra Body for Fine, Lifeless Hair *($6.50 for 8 ounces);* **Puritives by KMS** Shampoo *($8.25 for 8.45 ounces);* **Healthy Alternative by KMS** Healthy Alternative Totally Clean Shampoo *($10 for 12 ounces);* **ColorVive by L'Oreal** ColorVive Daily Care for Color-Treated Hair Gentle Shampoo plus UV Filter, Regular Colored or Highlighted *($2.99 for 13 ounces),* and ColorVive Daily Care for Color-

Treated Hair Gentle Shampoo plus UV Filter, for Dry Hair Colored or Highlighted (*$3.79 for 13 ounces*); **BodyVive by L'Oreal** BodyVive Daily Body for Fine Hair, Thickening Shampoo plus Ceramide-R & Protein, Thin/Extra Fine (*$3.79 for 13 ounces*); **VitaVive by L'Oreal** VitaVive Daily Care for Normal Hair, Multi-Vitamin Clear Shampoo (*$3.79 for 13 ounces*); **L'Oreal Kids** Extra Gentle 2-in-1 Shampoo, Extra Conditioning, Burst of Cherry-Almond (*$3.49 for 9 ounces*), Extra Gentle 2-in-1 Shampoo, Extra Manageability, Burst of Tropical Punch (*$3.49 for 9 ounces*), Extra Gentle 2-in-1 Shampoo, Fine Hair, Burst of Banana-Melon (*$3.49 for 9 ounces*), Extra Gentle 2-in-1 Shampoo, Normal Hair, Burst of Fruity Apricot (*$3.49 for 9 ounces*), and Extra Gentle 2-in-1 Shampoo, Thick or Curly or Wavy Hair, Burst of Watermelon (*$3.49 for 9 ounces*); **M.A.C.** Clarifying Shampoo (*$7 for 8 ounces*), Maintain Shampoo (*$7 for 8 ounces*), and Retain Shampoo (*$7 for 8 ounces*); **Mastey** Clarte Normalizing Creme Shampoo (*$9 for 10.2 ounces*), Enove Volumizing Creme Shampoo (*$9 for 10.2 ounces*), Traite Moisturizing Creme Shampoo Nutrient Rich Cleansing Complex (*$9 for 10.2 ounces*), and Le Remouver Deep Cleansing Clarifier (*$9 for 10.2 ounces*); **Essentials by Matrix** Essential Color Therapy Shampoo (*$12.95 for 16 ounces*); **Neutrogena** Anti-Residue Shampoo (*$5.29 for 6 ounces*) and Moisturizing Shampoo for Permed or Color Treated Hair (*$5.29 for 6 ounces*); **Paul Mitchell** Baby Don't Cry Shampoo (*$7.50 for 16 ounces*), Shampoo Two (*$7.50 for 16 ounces*), and Shampoo Three (*$11.50 for 16 ounces*); **Queen Helene** Placenta Acid-Balanced Conditioning Shampoo Concentrate with Panthenol, Pearlescent Formula (*$3.99 for 16 ounces*), Rum Scented Shampoo Concentrate Plus Egg, Triple Lathering Formula Conditioning Shampoo for Dry and Brittle Hair (*$3.19 for 16 ounces*), Garlic Shampoo Unscented (*$3 for 21 ounces*), Mint Julep Shampoo with Protein, Concentrated (*$2.99 for 16 ounces*), and RX-18 Shampoo, Removes Build-Up and Residue (*$3.19 for 16 ounces*); **CAT by Redken** CAT Revitalizing Shampoo (*$5.50 for 10.1 ounces*); **Bonacure by Schwarzkopf** Extra Rich Repair Shampoo, Repair Formula (*$8.40 for 8.5 ounces*); **Natural Styling by Schwarzkopf** Conditioning Shampoo (*$5.90 for 6.8 ounces*); **Baby Love by Soft Sheen** Conditioning Shampoo (*$3.79 for 11.5 ounces*); **Style by Lamaur** Clarifying Shampoo for Normal to Oily Hair (*$1.99 for 12 ounces*), Regular Shampoo Fresh Apple Fragrance (*$0.99 for 13 ounces*), Shampoo Coconut & Papaya Maintains Softness & Enhances Shine (*$1.09 for 24 ounces*), and Strawberry Formula Shampoo Fresh Strawberry Fragrance (*$0.99 for 13 ounces*); **Terax** Baby Shampoo for Children's Sensitive Skin and Hair (*$12 for 8 ounces*); **Tressa** Colourage Shampoo, Gentle Cleansing for Color-Treated Hair (*$8.49 for 12 ounces*), Perm Care Shampoo, Moisturizing Shampoo for Permed Hair (*$8.49 for 12 ounces*), and Clear Intervals (*$13.56 for 9 ounces*); **Vertu by Tressa** Hydra Swash Hydrating Shampoo (*$11 for 14 ounces*); **TIGI** Moisturizing Shampoo (*$6.95 for 8 ounces*); **Collections by White Rain** Baby Shampoo Classic Care Tear

Free Formula Gentle Cleansing *($1.09 for 15 ounces)*, Classic Care Shampoo Extra Body *($1.09 for 15 ounces)*, Classic Care Shampoo Regular *($0.99 for 15 ounces)*, Shampoo Salon Formula *($0.97 for 15 ounces)*, and Shampoo Moisturizing *($0.97 for 15 ounces)*; **Exotics by White Rain** Hibiscus Petals Shampoo, for shine *($1.09 for 13.5 ounces)*, Lotus Petals Shampoo *($1.09 for 13.5 ounces)*, and Orchid Petals Shampoo *($1.09 for 13.5 ounces)*; **Herbs & Blossoms by White Rain** Ginger Lily Shampoo Moisturizing *($1.07 for 13.5 ounces)*, Jasmine Shampoo, Extra Body *($1.07 for 13.5 ounces)*, and Passionflower Shampoo Revitalizing *($1.07 for 13.5 ounces)*; and **Solutions by White Rain** E Shampoo Super Nourishing *($1.09 for 13.5 ounces)*.

The Best Shampoos for Adding Volume or Conditioning or Both

All of the following shampoos contain some type of film-forming (hairspray-type) or conditioning ingredients, which means they can all contribute to buildup on hair. **In the individual reviews for these products, I occasionally did not mention that they may cause buildup (it just became so repetitive), but as long as film-former or conditioning ingredients are listed in the product description, it should be assumed that buildup can be an eventual problem with repeated use.**

Shampoos with conditioning agents are never recommended for oily scalp or hair because they deposit emollients (conditioning agents that coat the hair shaft), which can add to the problem. Also, because film-forming ingredients can feel "heavy" or "thick" on the hair and scalp, hair thickening or volumizing products can be problematic for those with oily hair and scalp. If you do want to use a hair-thickening product, it is best to use a conditioner or leave-in conditioner that can perform that function, because these allow you to keep the potentially problematic ingredients off of the scalp, and let you prevent any buildup there.

General guidelines for use: All of the following shampoos are best used alternately with one of the above "Shampoos for All Hair Types that Won't Cause Buildup." How often to alternate these depends on many factors, including how many styling products you use, how often you wash your hair, and what kind of look you are trying to create. It takes experimenting to find the right frequency of use for these two types of shampoos (those with conditioning and thickening agents and those that are just shampoo).

NORMAL TO DRY SCALP AND HAIR THAT IS NORMAL TO FINE OR THIN: **American Crew** Daily Moisturizing Shampoo for Normal to Dry Hair & Scalp *($5.95 for 8 ounces)*; **Apple Pectin by Lamaur** Naturals Irish Moss & Wild Cherry Bark Shampoo *($4.99 for 16 ounces)*; **Avon Hair Care Techniques** Tri-Nutriv Formula Restructuring Shampoo for Permed/Color Treated Hair *($3.99 for 11 ounces)* and Tri-Nutriv Formula Volumizing Shampoo for Fine/Thin Hair *($3.99 for 11 ounces)*; **Back to Basics** Beer Shampoo Honey Wheat Pilsner for All Hair Types *($7.95 for 10 ounces)*, Beer Shampoo Peach Amber Ale for Volumizing Fine Hair *($7.95 for 10 ounces)*, and Sunflower Moisture Infusing Shampoo, for All Hair Types *($6.95 for 12 ounces)*; **Bain de Terre** Recovery Complex Repairative Shampoo *($10 for 16.9 ounces)*; **Citre Shine** Volumizing Shampoo for Fine to Normal Hair *($3.42 for 16 ounces)*; **Dark & Lovely** 3-in-1 Plus Detangling/Conditioning Shampoo *($2.49 for 16 ounces)*, Beautiful Beginnings Vitamin E & Aloe Conditioning Shampoo Plus Detangler *($2.19 for 8 ounces)*, and Color Care Shampoo *($2.29 for 8 ounces)*; **Aromatherapy by Freeman** Aromatherapy Calming Shampoo for Normal to Dry Hair *($4.11 for 16 ounces)*, and Aromatherapy Energizing 2-in-1 Shampoo *($4.11 for 16 ounces)*; **Botanicals by Freeman** Kiwi Fruit Therapy Shampoo for Dry or Damaged Hair *($3.49 for 16 ounces)*; **Fudge** Oomf Shampoo *($8 for 10.1 ounces)*; **Exclusives by Goldwell** Exclusives Color Care Shampoo *($5.90 for 8 ounces)*; **Kerasilk by Goldwell** Kerasilk Care & Smoothness Conditioning Shampoo for Dry, Damaged, or Curly Hair *($5.90 for 8 ounces)* and Kerasilk Care & Volumizing Shampoo *($6.50 for 8 ounces)*; **Classic Line by Graham Webb** Cleanse Stick Straight High Gloss Smoothing Shampoo *($8 for 8.5 ounces)*; **Hayashi** Daily Shampoo for Frequent Shampooers, Normal to Oily Hair *($6.90 for 10.6 ounces)*; **J. F. Lazartigue** Cereal Shampoo Volumizing Treatments Shampoo *($19 for 5.1 ounces)*; **Jheri Redding** Balsam Shampoo for All Hair Types *($1.90 for 24 ounces)*; **Jhirmack** Gelave Strengthening Shampoo for Normal Hair *($3.69 for 20 ounces)*; **Johnson & Johnson** Kids 2-in-1 Shampoo *($2.99 for 9 ounces)*, Kids No More Tangles Shampoo *($2.99 for 9 ounces)*, Kids Xtreme Clean Shampoo *($2.99 for 9 ounces)*, No More Tears Baby Shampoo *($3.49 for 20 ounces)*, No More Tears Baby Shampoo 2-in-1 Detangler *($3.49 for 20 ounces)*, No More Tears Baby Shampoo Moisturizing Formula with Honey and Vitamin E *($2.89 for 15 ounces)*, and Ultra Sensitive Baby Shampoo *($2.73 for 6.75 ounces)*; **Blue Line by Joico** Biojoba Treatment Shampoo *($8.60 for 8.45 ounces)*, Kerapro Conditioning Shampoo for Normal to Dry & Chemically Treated Hair *($5.40 for 8.45 ounces)*, Lavei Extra Body Shampoo for Fine/Limp Oily Hair *($4.90 for 8.45 ounces)*, Triage Moisture Balancing Shampoo for Normal Hair *($5.80 for 8.45 ounces)*, and Volissima Volumizing Shampoo *($6.95 for 8.45 ounces)*; **KMS** Moisturizing Shampoo, Extra Body for Dry, Damaged Hair *($5.95 for 8 ounces)*; **Curl Up by KMS** Curl Up Shampoo *($10 for 8.3 ounces)*; **Rebalance by L'anza** Strait-Line Curl Relaxing Shampoo *($8.96 for 8.5 ounces)*; **HydraVive by L'Oreal** HydraVive Daily Care for Dry Hair, Moisture Shampoo plus Hydra-Protein, Dry/Damaged *($3.79 for 13 ounces)*; **L'Oreal Kids** Extra Gentle 2-in-1 Shampoo, Extra Conditioning, Burst of Cherry-Almond *($3.49 for 9 ounces)*, Extra Gentle 2-in-1 Shampoo, Extra Manageability, Burst of Tropical Punch *($3.49 for 9 ounces)*, Extra

Gentle 2-in-1 Shampoo, Fine Hair, Burst of Banana-Melon *($3.49 for 9 ounces)*, Extra Gentle 2-in-1 Shampoo, Normal Hair, Burst of Fruity Apricot *($3.49 for 9 ounces)*, and Extra Gentle 2-in-1 Shampoo, Thick or Curly or Wavy Hair, Burst of Watermelon *($3.49 for 9 ounces)*; **M Professional** Abuse Shampoo Tormented, Permed or Color Treated Hair *($4.60 for 13 ounces)*, Big Shampoo *($4.60 for 13 ounces)*, and Just Shampoo Regular, Dry or Just Dirty Hair *($4.60 for 13 ounces)*; **Biolage by Matrix** Color Care Shampoo *($12.99 for 16 ounces)*; **PRO-V Color by Pantene** Pro-V Color Gentle Cleansing Shampoo for Color Treated and Highlighted Hair *($5.49 for 13 ounces)*; **Paul Mitchell** Awapuhi Shampoo *($8.50 for 16 ounces)*; **Pert Plus** Shampoo Plus Conditioner in One, Dry or Damaged Hair *($3.71 for 15 ounces)*, Extra Body for Fine Hair *($3.71 for 15 ounces)*, Oily Hair *($3.71 for 15 ounces)*, Normal Hair *($3.71 for 15 ounces)*, Tear-Free Pert Plus for Kids, Light Conditioning *($3.49 for 15 ounces)* and Tear-Free Pert Plus for Kids, Normal Conditioning *($3.71 for 15 ounces)*; **Phytotherathrie** Phytojoba Gentle, Regulating Milk Shampoo for Dry Hair with Jojoba Oil (1%) *($15 for 6.8 ounces)*, Phytolactum Scalp-Cleansing Shampoo for Normal Hair/Sensitive Scalp with Phytolactine and Almond Milk Extract *($15 for 3.3 ounces)*, Phytorhum Fortifying Shampoo for Lifeless Hair with Egg Yolk and Rum *($15 for 6.8 ounces)* and Phytovolume Volumizer Shampoo for Fine Limp Hair with Yarrow Extract *($15 for 6.8 ounces)*; **Professional** Luxury Shampoo *($3.62 for 16 ounces)* and Uniquely for Normal to Fine Hair *($3.62 for 16 ounces)*; **Pro-Vitamin** Special Effects Fat Hair Thickening Shampoo *($4.19 for 12.5 ounces)*; **Quantum** Moisturizing Shampoo for Permed, Color-Treated and Dry Hair *($4.49 for 15 ounces)* and Volumizing Shampoo for Fine, Limp, and Lazy Hair *($8.99 for 33.8 ounces)*; **Outrageous by Revlon** Two-in-One Shampoo Plus Conditioner Extra Body *($2.99 for 15 ounces)* and Two-in-One Shampoo Plus Conditioner Moisturizing *($2.34 for 15 ounces)*; **Rusk** Look Gentle Cleanse for Normal Hair *($5 for 8 ounces)*, Moist Wash Luxurious Moisturizing Cleanse *($5 for 8 ounces)*, Sensories Full Green Tea & Alfalfa Shampoo *($8.80 for 13 ounces)*, Sensories Moist Sunflower & Apricot Shampoo *($8.50 for 13 ounces)*, and Sensories Smoother Passionflower & Aloe Shampoo *($8.80 for 13 ounces)*; **Salon Style by Lamaur** Conditioning Shampoo, Hydration with Detangling Silks *($2.22 for 15 ounces)*, Moisture Potion Shampoo *($2.22 for 15 ounces)*, Nutrishine Shampoo *($2.22 for 15 ounces)*, Strengthening Shampoo *($2.22 for 15 ounces)*, and Therapy Shampoo *($2.22 for 15 ounces)*; **Bonacure by Schwarzkopf** Basic Beauty Shampoo for Frequent Use, Basic Formula *($7.60 for 8.5 ounces)* and Volume Shampoo for Fine Hair, Volume Formula *($7.90 for 8.5 ounces)*; **Silhouette Styling System by Schwarzkopf** Style Care Shampoo #1 *($6 for 6.8 ounces)*; **Scruples** Renewal Shampoo for Color Treated Hair *($3.50 for 4 ounces)*; **Collectives by Sebastian** Cello Shampoo Extraordinary Shine for Normal to Slightly Oily Hair *($6.30 for 10.2 ounces)*, Cello Shampoo for Normal to Dry

Hair *($6.30 for 10 ounces)*, and Potion 5 Shampoo Revitalizing Treatment Shampoo for Hair and Scalp *($4.25 for 8.5 ounces)*; **Performance Active by Sebastian** Cleanser: A Hair and Body Wash *($8.30 for 8.5 ounces)*; **Botanicals by Soft & Beautiful** Color Code Neutralizing Decalcifying Shampoo *($3.50 for 16 ounces)* and Moisturizing Shampoo, Pro-Vitamin Formula *($3.95 for 16 ounces)*; **Just for Me by Soft & Beautiful** Moisturizing Conditioning Shampoo *($2.99 for 8 ounces)*; **St. Ives Swiss Formula** Gardenia Plus Extra Gentle Shampoo Plus Conditioner for Normal Hair *($1.99 for 15 ounces)*, Papaya Plus Fortifying Shampoo Plus Conditioner for Normal Hair *($1.99 for 15 ounces)*, and Watermelon Plus, Antioxidant Shampoo + Conditioner, Extra Moisturizing for Dry, Permed or Color/Treated Hair *($1.99 for 20 ounces)*; **Style by Lamaur** Extra Body Shampoo *($1.13 for 24 ounces)*, Moisturizing Shampoo *($1.13 for 24 ounces)*, Moisturizing Shampoo for Dry Color-Treated/Permed Hair *($1.99 for 12 ounces)*, Volumizing Shampoo for Fine or Thin Hair *($1.99 for 12 ounces)*, Pro-Vitamin Complex Shampoo Extra Body *($1.56 for 15 ounces)*, and Style Plus Extra Conditioning Shampoo and Conditioner in One *($1.13 for 24 ounces)*; **Sukesha** Moisturizing Shampoo, Shampoo and Conditioner in One *($5.50 for 12 ounces)* and Natural Balance Shampoo, Pure and Gentle for Shine and Volume Shampoo *($5.50 for 12 ounces)*; **Susan Lucci Collection** Purifying Shampoo Healthy Hair Complex *($17 for two 12-ounce bottles)*; **Theorie** Moisturizing Shampoo for Normal to Dry, Damaged, or Coarse Hair *($4.99 for 12.5 ounces)*, Shampoo for Normal to Dry Hair *($4.99 for 12.5 ounces)*, and Volumizing Shampoo for Normal to Thin or Fine Hair *($4.99 for 12.5 ounces)*; **Bed Head by TIGI** Moisture Maniac Shampoo *($7.96 for 12 ounces)*; **Blue by TIGI** Thickening Shampoo for Fuller Hair *($7.96 for 12 ounces)*; **Essensuals by TIGI** Hair & Body Wash *($4 for 2 ounces)*; **Tresemme** European Color Treated & Permed Shampoo *($2.49 for 32 ounces)* and European Vitamin E Moisture Rich Shampoo for Dry or Damaged Hair *($2.49 for 24 ounces)*; **TRI** Jojoba Shampoo Treatment *($6.99 for 8 ounces)*; **Wanakee** Beneficial Phase Shampoo *($8.95 for 8 ounces)* and Moisture Emphasis Shampoo *($10.95 for 8 ounces)*; **Wash 'N Curl** Extra Strength Curling Shampoo for Dry, Damaged, Color-Treated Hair *($3.29 for 8 ounces)* and Extra Strength Curling Shampoo for Fine, Limp, Dry Hair *($3.29 for 8 ounces)*; **Liquid Hair by Wella** Color Preserver Daily Shampoo for Color-Treated Hair *($7.50 for 12 ounces)*, Moisturizing Shampoo for Dry or Chemically-Treated Hair *($7.50 for 12 ounces)*, and Volumizing Shampoo for Fine or Normal Hair *($7.50 for 12 ounces)*; **Wella Balsam** Conditioning Shampoo for Normal Hair *($2.99 for 32 ounces)*; **White Rain Collections** Plus for Kids Classic Care Shampoo & Detangler in One Tear Free *($1.09 for 15 ounces)*; and **Willow Lake** Cherry Bark & Irish Moss Conditioning Shampoo *($3.59 for 16 ounces)*.

DRY TO VERY DRY SCALP AND HAIR THAT IS NORMAL TO FINE OR THIN: **Texture Line by ARTec** Smoothing Shampoo *($9.40 for 12 ounces)* and

Volume Shampoo *($9.40 for 12 ounces)*; **Back to Basics** Beer Shampoo Black Cherry Stout for Dry, Damaged Hair *($7.95 for 10 ounces)*, Honey Hydrating Shampoo, for Overworked Hair *($6.95 for 12 ounces)*, and Milk Shampoo *($7.95 for 12 ounces)*; **Basic Texture by Back to Basics** Be Thick Thickening Shampoo *($7.95 for 12 ounces)*; **The Body Shop** Brazil Nut Rich Shampoo for Dry, Damaged & Chemically Treated Hair *($9.50 for 16.9 ounces)*; **Bumble and Bumble** Thickening Shampoo *($11 for 8 ounces)*; **Finesse Bodifying** Shampoo for Fine or Thin Hair *($2.58 for 15 ounces)* and Enhancing Shampoo for Normal, Healthy Hair *($2.58 for 15 ounces)*; **Framesi Biogenol** Ultra Body Shampoo *($5.95 for 8 ounces)*; **Papaya Provita by Freeman** Papaya Provita Miracle Shampoo for Ultra Body *($2.99 for 16 ounces)* and Papaya Silk Miracle Shampoo with Ginseng, Extra Nourishing Formula for Normal Hair *($1.99 for 16 ounces)*; **Bodacious by Graham Webb** Bodacious Moisturizing Shampoo *($6.95 for 8.5 ounces)*; **Ion** Anti-Frizz Smoothing Shampoo *($3.99 for 12 ounces)*; **Frizz-Ease by John Frieda** Corrective Shampoo and Shiner, Conditioning and Glossing Formula *($4.14 for 12.7 ounces)*; **Ready to Wear by John Frieda** Custom Cleansing and Glistening Shampoo, Tailored for Dry/Chemically Treated Hair *($4.59 for 11 ounces)* and Custom Cleansing and Thickening Shampoo, Tailored to Thicken and Shine Fine/Limp Hair *($4.59 for 11 ounces)*; **Flat Out by KMS** Flat Out Shampoo, Smoothing Shampoo for All Hair Types *($7.95 for 8.28 ounces)*; **Essentials by Matrix** Nourishing Shampoo *($12.95 for 16 ounces)*; **Motions at Home** After Shampoo Moisture Plus Conditioner *($2.99 for 6 ounces)*; **Neutrogena** Clean Balancing Shampoo for Normal Hair *($4.99 for 10.1 ounces)*, Clean Replenishing Shampoo for Dry, Damaged Hair *($4.99 for 10.1 ounces)*, and Clean Volumizing Shampoo for Fine, Thin Hair *($4.99 for 10.1 ounces)*; **Nexxus** Rejuv-a-Perm Vitalizing Shampoo *($11.50 for 16.9 ounces)*; **PhytoSpecific by Phytotherathrie** Hydra-Repairing Shampoo with Shea Butter *($18 for 5.07 ounces)*; and **Queen Helene** Cocoa Butter Shampoo *($3.59 for 21 ounces)*.

NORMAL TO DRY SCALP AND HAIR OF ANY THICKNESS: **African Pride** Shampoo and Conditioner 2-in-1 Formula *($3.99 for 12 ounces)*; **African Royale** Soft As Me Herbal Shampoo *($3.49 for 8 ounces)*; **Apple Pectin by Lamaur** Plus Shampoo/Conditioner System in One *($5.49 for 15.5 ounces)*; **Back to Basics** Aloe Vera Daily Shampoo for All Hair Types *($5.95 for 10 ounces)* and Get Curly Curl Enhancing Shampoo *($7.95 for 12 ounces)*; **Bain de Terre** Aloe Bath Moisturizing Shampoo *($8.95 for 16.9 ounces)*; **Conditions 3-in-1 by Clairol** Shampoo Plus, Clean and Light, Shampoo/Sheer Conditioner/Protectant *($1.75 for 12 ounces)*; **Finesse Revitalizing** Shampoo for Permed, Color-Treated or Overstyled Hair *($2.58 for 15 ounces)*, Plus Shampoo Plus Conditioner Enhancing for Normal Hair *($2.58 for 15 ounces)*, and Plus Shampoo Plus Conditioner Moisturizing for Dry or Coarse

Hair *($2.58 for 15 ounces)*; **Aromatherapy by Freeman** Aromatherapy Calming 2-in-1 Shampoo Cleansing Plus Conditioning for Normal to Dry Hair *($4.11 for 16 ounces)*; **Beautiful Hair by Freeman** Beautiful Hair Wild Cherry Extra Humectant Moisturizing Shampoo *($2.88 for 16 ounces)*; **Botanicals by Freeman** Hawaiian Ginger Shampoo Ultra Body and Shine *($3.49 for 16 ounces)*; **Papaya Provita by Freeman** Papaya Provita Shampoo plus Conditioner in One for Normal to Dry Hair *($1.99 for 16 ounces)*; **Fudge** The Shampoo for Normal to Dry Hair *($8 for 10.1 ounces)*; **Classic Line by Graham Webb** Cleanse Infusion Shampoo for Fine, Thin & Limp Hair *($9.95 for 8 ounces)* and Cleanse Thermal Care Shampoo for Dry, Damaged and Chemically Treated Hair *($8.26 for 8.5 ounces)*; **Hayashi** Protect Shampoo Moisturizing Formula for Color Treated Hair *($7 for 10.6 ounces)*; **System 911 by Hayashi** Shampoo Emergency Repair for Dry Damaged Hair *($6 for 8.4 ounces)*; **System Hinoki by Hayashi** Shampoo Volumizing Cleaner for Fine and Thinning Hair *($6.60 for 8.4 ounces)*; **Infusium 23 Shampoo** UV Protection Formula for Damaged Hair *($3.44 for 16 ounces)*; **Jason Natural Cosmetics** Color-Treated, Frizzy, Dry Hair Therapy All Natural Damage Control Creme Shampoo *($11.79 for 16 ounces)*, Extra Rich Natural E.F.A. Shampoo, Hair Nourishing Formula for Normal to Dry Hair *($5.50 for 17.5 ounces)*, For Kids Only! Extra Mild Shampoo *($7.50 for 17.5 ounces)*, Forest Essence Conditioning Shampoo *($7.09 for 17.5 ounces)*, Hemp Enriched Shampoo for All Hair Types *($7.50 for 17.5 ounces)*, Natural Aloe Vera 84% Shampoo, Hair Nourishing Formula *($5.50 for 17.5 ounces)*, Natural Apricot Keratin Shampoo *($2.30 for 17.5 ounces)*, Natural Jojoba Shampoo, UV protection, Extra Body, Super Shine *($5.50 for 17.5 ounces)*, Natural Vitamin A, C & E Shampoo *($5.50 for 17.5 ounces)*, and Rich Natural Sea Kelp Shampoo, Concentrated Extra Gentle, Super Shine *($3.10 for 17.5 ounces)*; **J. F. Lazartigue** Essentials for Curly or Frizzy Hair Nourishing Shampoo, Straightened Hair *($18 for 6.8 ounces)*; Milk Shampoo for Dry Hair, Dry Hair Care Shampoo *($29 for 8.4 ounces)*, Shampoo for Frequent Use Combination Hair Care *($25 for 8.4 ounces)*, and Treatment Cream Shampoo with Collagen, Dry Hair Care *($33 for 6.8 ounces)*; **Professional Prescription by Jheri Redding** Biotin Shampoo for Fine, Thin, or Weak Hair *($4.99 for 15 ounces)*; **Jhirmack** Shine Shampoo for All Hair Types *($3.69 for 20 ounces)*; **KMS** Color Response Shampoo Nutritive Shampoo for Colored or Color-Highlighted Hair *($6.95 for 8 ounces)*; **AMP: Amino-Magnesium-Panthenol by KMS** Volume Shampoo for All Hair Types *($6.67 for 8 ounces)*; **Silker by KMS** Silker Shampoo *($8.50 for 12 ounces)*; **Color Vitality Shampoo by KMS** Color Vitality Shampoo *($10 for 8.5 ounces)*; **Lange** Baby Shampoo and Bath *($8.10 for 10 ounces)* and Panthenol C3 Shampoo for Clarifying and Chelating *($7.49 for 8 ounces)*; **Colors & Curls by L'anza** Protein Plus Shampoo, Shampoo for Bleached and Permed Hair *($7.50 for*

10.1 ounces); **Rebalance by L'anza** Deep Cleansing Shampoo, Shampoo for Fine Hair and Oily Scalp *($7 for 10.1 ounces)* and Remedy Shampoo, Shampoo for Problem Scalps and Dry Hair *($8.60 for 8.5 ounces);* **Volume Formula by L'anza** Bodifying Shampoo *($7.96 for 12.6 ounces);* **BodyVive by L'Oreal** BodyVive Daily Body for Fine Hair, Volumizing Shampoo plus Ceramide-R & Protein, Regular *($3.79 for 13 ounces);* **VitaVive by L'Oreal** VitaVive Daily Care for Normal Hair 2-in-1, Multi-Vitamin Shampoo + Conditioner *($4.29 for 13 ounces);* **Essentials by Matrix** Simply Clean Shampoo *($11.75 for 16 ounces);* **Nexxus Diametress** Hair Thickening Shampoo *($9.50 for 8.4 ounces)* and Exoil Deep Cleansing Shampoo *($4.50 for 8.4 ounces);* **Nexxus** Vita Tress Biotin Shampoo *($13 for 16.9 ounces);* **Nick Chavez Perfect Plus** Shampoo 1, Clarifier, For Normal to Oily Hair *($8 for 8 ounces);* **Paul Mitchell** Shampoo Two *($7.50 for 16 ounces)* and The Wash Moisture Balancing Shampoo *($13 for 16 ounces);* **Phytotherathrie** Phytomiel "Le Petit Phyto" Hypoallergenic Plant Based Shampoo for Baby's Hair with Honey Absolute and Apricot *($15 for 2.5 ounces)* and Phytosteine Sebum Cleansing Shampoo for Oily Hair/Sensitive Scalp with Plant Extracts Enriched with a Derivative of Cysteine 2.3% and Phytolactine 1% *($16.50 for 6.8 ounces);* **PhytoPlage by Phytotherathrie** Sun Shampoo for Hair and Body with Bancoulier Oil *($15 for 3.3 ounces);* **Principal Secret** Gentle Daily Shampoo *($11, $7.75 for 10 ounces)* and Deep Cleansing Shampoo *($11, $7.75 for 6 ounces);* **Professional** Hawaiian Ginger Shampoo *($3.62 for 16 ounces)* and Shine Extraordinaire *($3.62 for 16 ounces);* **Fat CAT by Redken** Body Booster Shampoo for Fine Hair *($6.50 for 10.1 ounces);* **One 2 One by Redken** One 2 One Moisturizing Shampoo *($8.75 for 10.1 ounces)* and One 2 One Volumizing Shampoo *($8.75 for 10.1 ounces);* **Outrageous by Revlon** Daily Beautifying Shampoo for Normal Hair *($2.34 for 15 ounces);* **Collectives by Sebastian** Misty Rose Shampoo for Dry Hair *($6.30 for 10.2 ounces)* Green Apple Shampoo for Normal Hair *($5.80 for 10.2 ounces),* and Moisture Shampoo for Normal to Dry Hair *($7.30 for 10.2 ounces);* **Laminates by Sebastian** Shampoo Polishing Shampoo *($8.50 for 8.5 ounces);* **Shaper Slipline by Sebastian** Shampoo, Conditioning Shampoo for All Hair Types *($5.80 for 10.2 ounces);* **Senscience** Energy Shampoo for Dry Hair *($8.63 for 16.9 ounces)* and Energy Shampoo for Normal Hair *($8.63 for 16.9 ounces);* **Optimum Care by Soft Sheen** Collagen Moisture Shampoo *($2.99 for 16 ounces);* **Suave** Shampoo Plus Conditioner 2-in-1 Moisturizing Formula for Dry or Damaged Hair *($1.58 for 14.5 ounces),* Shampoo Plus Conditioner 2-in-1 Regular Formula for Normal to Dry Hair *($1.58 for 14.5 ounces),* Shampoo Plus Conditioner Healthy Shine with Pro-Vitamins 2-in-1 Moisturizing Formula for Dry or Damaged Hair *($1.58 for 14.5 ounces),* Shampoo Plus Conditioner Healthy Shine with Pro-Vitamins 2-in-1 Regular Formula for Normal Hair *($1.58 for 14.5 ounces),* Thermal Formula Shampoo, Heat

Activated for Normal to Dry Hair *($2.54 for 14.5 ounces)*, ThermaSilk Heat Activated Shampoo for Normal Hair *($3.42 for 13 ounces)*, Heat Activated Shampoo for Colored or Permed Hair *($3.42 for 13 ounces)*, Heat Activated Shampoo for Dry or Damaged Hair *($3.24 for 13 ounces)*, and Heat Activated Shampoo Volumizing for Fine or Thin Hair *($3.42 for 13 ounces)*; **Liquid Hair by Wella** Clarifying Shampoo for All Hair Types *($7.50 for 12 ounces)*; and **White Rain Collections** Classic Care Shampoo Revitalizing Formula *($0.99 for 15 ounces)*.

   DRY TO VERY DRY SCALP AND HAIR OF ANY THICKNESS: All Ways Natural by African Pride Shampoo Moisturizing Formula *($3.19 for 12 ounces)*; **Aura** Pure Organic Shampoo Enriched Cleansing for All Hair Types *($4.99 for 16 ounces)*; **Aveda** Shampure, Above and Beyond Shampoo *($9.84 for 8.4 ounces)*; **All Sensitive by Aveda** All Sensitive Shampoo *($9.50 for 5.7 ounces)*; **Back to Basics** Raspberry Almond Intensive Shampoo *($7.95 for 12 ounces)*; **Beauty Without Cruelty (BWC)** Moisture Plus Shampoo, Benefits Dry/Treated Hair *($6.95 for 16 ounces)*; **Focus 21** Jojoba Sebum Emulsifier Shampoo *($2.29 for 8 ounces)*; **Framesi Biogenol** Bathe Moisturizing Shampoo *($3.96 for 4 ounces)*; **Salon Textures by Freeman** Salon Textures Volumizing Aire Shampoo *($4.99 for 16.9 ounces)*; **Super Straight Hair by Freeman** Super Straight Hair Shampoo, Honeydew & Lilac *($3.42 for 12 ounces)*; **Garden Botanika** Hair Care Chamomile Moisture & Shine Shampoo *($8 for 12 ounces)* and Hair CareTri Wheat Hair Repair Shampoo *($8.50 for 12 ounces)*; **Definition by Goldwell** Definition Permed & Curly Shampoo *($7.95 for 12 ounces)*; **KMS** Cleanse-pHree Shampoo, Gentle Cleansing for Normal, Healthy Hair *($5.95 for 8 ounces)*; **Moisture Replace by KMS** Moisture Replace Shampoo *($10 for 12 ounces)*; **Healthy Alternative by KMS** Healthy Alternative Everyday Shampoo *($10 for 12 ounces)*; **FortaVive by L'Oreal** FortaVive Daily Care for Damaged Hair, Repairing Shampoo plus Ceramide-R *($3.79 for 13 ounces)*; **HydraVive by L'Oreal** HydraVive Daily Care for Dry Hair, Shampoo + Conditioner plus Hydra-Protein Two-in-One *($3.79 for 13 ounces)*; **Nick Chavez Perfect Plus** Shampoo 2, Moisture Booster, Colored and Chemically Treated Hair *($8 for 8 ounces)*; **All Soft by Redken** All Soft Shampoo *($7.50 for 10.1 ounces)*; **Climatress by Redken** Climatress Shampoo Normal to Dry Hair *($7.50 for 10.1 ounces)*; **Color Extend Redken** Color Extend Shampoo *($7.50 for 10.1 ounces)*; and **Sheenique Silk** Neutralizing Shampoo *($4.49 for 16 ounces)*.

   DRY TO VERY DRY SCALP AND HAIR THAT IS THICK TO COARSE: Goldwell Shampoo 5 Turbocharged Shampoo for Dry and Damaged Hair *($5.90 for 8.4 ounces)*; **Definition by Goldwell** Definition Dry & Porous Shampoo *($7.90 for 12 ounces)*; **Intensives by Graham Webb** Intensives Super Silk Shampoo Reconstructive Shampoo for Dry, Brittle, & Chemically Treated Hair *($7.80 for 6 ounces)*;

Jhirmack EFA Moisturizing Shampoo for Dry/Color Treated or Permed Hair *($3.69 for 20 ounces)*; **KMS** NEFA Natural Essence Reconstructive Shampoo for Chemically Treated Hair *($6.50 for 8 ounces)*; **Essentials by Matrix** Perm Fresh Shampoo *($12.95 for 16 ounces)*; **Phytotherathrie** Phytocadamia Restoring Shampoo for Very Dry Hair with Macadamia Oil and Illipe Butter *($15 for 6.8 ounces)*; **Igora Color Care by Schwarzkopf** Shampoo *($8.10 for 10.1 ounces)*; and **Senscience** Inner Conditioner for Coarse Hair *($12.39 for 16.9 ounces)*.

The Best Lines with Temporary Color-Enhancing Shampoos

These include shades designed for gray hair to reduce yellow tones. **General guidelines for use:** Color-enhancing shampoos make the most difference for lighter hair shades rather than darker shades. These shampoos do not cover gray. The longer they are left on, the more likely the dye agent can cling to the hair; however, the longer they are left on, the more drying they can also be for hair. These can be used for everyday washing but they can eventually add too much color to lighter hair shades or make hair feel dry. It can be helpful to alternate with one of the shampoos listed above in "The Best Shampoos for All Hair Types that Won't Cause Buildup."

ALL HAIR TYPES: ARTec, Aveda, Complements by Clairol, Garden Botanika, Hayashi, Jason Natural Cosmetics, Mastey, Paul Mitchell, Redken Shades EQ, ColorStay by Revlon, and **Tressa.**

The Best Color-Enhancing Shampoos or Conditioners Just for Gray Hair

The following are not included in the sections Color-Enhancing Shampoos or Color-Enhancing Conditioners because these lines offer only the selection for gray hair. **General guidelines for use:** Color-enhancing shampoos of any kind make the most difference for lighter hair shades rather than darker shades. Though they do not cover gray, the blue or violet dye agents in these kinds of products subtly camouflage the yellow or brassy color of gray hair. If you choose a shampoo version, remember that the longer these are left on, the more likely the dye agent can cling to the hair; however, that can also make them more drying for the hair. Still, for conditioners of this type, the longer they are left on the more conditioning they can be. Both the shampoo and conditioner can be used for everyday washing but they can eventually add too much color, making hair look violet or blue. It can be helpful to alternate with one of the shampoos above in "The Best Shampoos for All Hair Types that

Won't Cause Buildup," or one of the conditioners later in this chapter suitable for your hair type.

Alberto Conditioning Hairdressing, Gray, White & Silver Blonde Hair *($2.99 for 1.5 ounces)*; **Sparkling Silver Hair by Freeman** Sparkling Silver Hair Shampoo for Gray or Blond Hair, Violet & Gardenia *($3.29 for 12 ounces)*; **Jhirmack** Silver Brightening Shampoo for Gray, Bleached, or Highlighted Hair *($3.69 for 20 ounces)* and Silver Brightening Conditioner for Gray, Bleached, or Highlighted Hair *($3.69 for 20 ounces)*; **KMS** Classic Silver for Gray or Blonde Hair *($6.95 for 8 ounces)*; **Matrix** SoSilver Shampoo *($12.95 for 16 ounces)*; **Nexxus** Simply Silver Toning Shampoo *($6.50 for 8.4 ounces)*; and **Phytotherathrie** Phytargent Whitening Shampoo for Grey and White Hair with Azulene from Camomile *($15 for 6.8 ounces)*.

The Best Dandruff Shampoos

General guidelines for use: Dandruff products work best when they are allowed to stay in contact with the scalp for several minutes. Because these tend to be drying, it can be helpful to alternate a dandruff shampoo with a shampoo listed above in "Shampoos for All Hair Types that Won't Cause Buildup."

FOR ALL HAIR TYPES: Aveda Scalp Remedy Anti-Dandruff Styling Tonic *($12.60 for 3.7 ounces)*; **Avon** Techniques Tri-Nutriv Formula Controlling Dandruff Shampoo Plus Conditioner in One *($4.99 for 11 ounces)*; **Bain de Terre** Alpine Mist Dandruff Shampoo *($6.50 for 8.5 ounces)*; **Head & Shoulders** Dandruff Shampoo for Fine or Oily Hair *($3.39 for 15.2 ounces)*, Dandruff Shampoo for Normal Hair *($3.39 for 15.2 ounces)*, Dandruff Shampoo Plus Conditioner, 2 in 1, for Fine or Oily Hair *($3.39 for 15.2 ounces)*, Dry Scalp Dandruff Shampoo Conditioner, 2 in 1, for Normal to Dry Hair *($3.28 for 15.2 ounces)*, Dry Scalp Dandruff Shampoo for Normal or Dry Hair *($4.50 for 25.4 ounces)*, Dry Scalp Dandruff Shampoo Plus Conditioner, 2 in 1, for Normal to Dry Hair *($3.39 for 25.4 ounces)*, and Refresh Pyrithione Zinc Dandruff Shampoo for All Hair Types *($5.78 for 25.4 ounces)*; **Jason Natural Cosmetics** Tea Tree Oil Hair and Scalp Therapy Shampoo *($5.99 for 17.5 ounces)*; **J. F. Lazartigue** Anti Dandruff Cream Anti Dandruff Treatments After Shampoo *($28 for 3.4 ounces)*; **Kenra** Dandruff Shampoo *($10.95 for 10.1 ounces)*; **KMS** CliniDan the Dandruff Solution *($7.95 for 8 ounces)* and Healthy Alternative Dandruff Shampoo *($10 for 12 ounces)*; **Nexxus** Dandarrest Dandruff Shampoo *($11.50 for 16.9 ounces)*; **Nizoral** *($9.99 for 4 ounces)*; **Pantene** Pro-Vitamin Pyrithione Zinc Anti-Dandruff Shampoo *($3.39 for 13 ounces)*; **Phytotherathrie** Phytocoltar Dandruff Cream Shampoo for Dandruff *($16.50 for 3.3 ounces)*; **Redken** Solve, Anti-Dandruff Shampoo *($9.90 for 8.5 ounces)*; and **Selsun Blue** 2-in-1 Treatment Dandruff Shampoo and Conditioner in One *($6.64 for 11 ounces)*.

FOR ANY SCALP DERMATITIS: Cortaid *($4.29 for 1 ounce),* **Lanacort** *($2.99 for 0.5 ounce),* and **Neutrogena** T/Scalp Antipruritic Anti-Itch Liquid *($6.36 for 2 ounces)* are all 1% hydrocortisone and would work well to calm an itchy scalp.

The Best Coal-Tar Shampoos (for dandruff, psoriasis, seborrhea, or other scalp dermatitis)

General guidelines for use: Products for scalp dermatitis work best when they are allowed to stay in contact with the scalp for several minutes. Because these tend to be drying, it can be helpful to alternate a dandruff shampoo with a shampoo listed above in "Shampoos for All Hair Types that Won't Cause Buildup."

FOR ALL HAIR TYPES: Good Sense T+ Plus Gel Shampoo *($2.99 for 8.5 ounces)* [not reviewed in Chapter Nine]; **Ionil** T Therapeutic Coal Tar Shampoo *($7.99 for 4 ounces)* [not reviewed in Chapter Nine]; **Neutrogena** Therapeutic T/ Gel Shampoo Extra Strength Formula *($8.49 for 6 ounces)* and Therapeutic T/Gel Shampoo Original Formula *($4.50 4.4 ounces);* and **Zetar** Medicated Antiseborrheic Shampoo *($16.39 for 6 ounces)* [not reviewed in Chapter Nine].

The Best Products for Preventing Mineral Buildup from Swimming or Hard Water

Shampoos, conditioners, or treatment products that make claims about preventing damage caused by minerals or chemicals from pools, ocean water, or hard water clinging to hair need to contain ingredients that help prevent that from happening. Chelating ingredients can perform that function. **General guidelines for use:** These types of products can be used on a daily basis with no negative impact on hair, followed with the appropriate styling products (particularly silicone serums or gels to add softness and a silky feel to hair that may be overly dry from exposure to hard water, pool water, or ocean water).

Hair Note: I wish there were more of these types of products to recommend, but there just aren't that many available. I suspect the reason for that is due to the kinds of ingredients that prevent minerals from binding to hair. The more effective the demineralizing ingredients are, the less likely it is that the shampoo will lather. Most consumers expect their shampoos to lather, and relate that to clean hair.

FOR ALL HAIR TYPES: Aveda Hair Detoxifier *($9 for 8.45 ounces);* **Ion Crystal Clarifying Treatment** *($1.99 for 0.18 ounce);* **Jason Natural Cosmetics** Swimmers & Sports Hair and Scalp Reconditioning Shampoo *($7.09 for 17.5 ounces)* and Swimmers & Sports Hair and Scalp Reconditioning Conditioner *($6.69 for 8* *ounces);* **Blue Line by Joico** Resolve Deep Cleansing Chelating Shampoo *($6.30 for 8.45 ounces)* and Phine Conditioning Chelating Treatment *($6 for 4.4 ounces);* **KMS** pHirst Active Clarifier Shampoo for All Hair Types *($7.45 for 8 ounces);* **Healthy Alternative by KMS** Healthy Alternative Clarifying Shampoo *($10 for 12 ounces);* **Nexxus** Aloe Rid Clarifying Treatment *($5.50 for 5 ounces).*

The Best Conditioners

Conditioners are products that allow hair to feel soft, smooth, and combable and—when film-forming ingredients are included—can add a feeling of thickness to hair. All conditioners work best when they are left on hair for as long as possible, or you can apply *indirect* heat to help them penetrate better. None of that requires a special product, which is why all conditioners, even so-called specialty treatments, are included in this section.

Whether or not to use a rinse-off or leave-in conditioner is a matter of personal preference. There is no particular advantage in choosing one over the other for any hair type. As is true for any hair-care product, the performance you get depends on the formulation. Because leave-in conditioners are almost exclusively liquids, they generally do not contain enough conditioning agents to coat hair, these are usually not recommended for very dry or coarse hair. The exception to that is when the leave-in conditioner contains a good amount of oils or silicone, which are a great way to smooth and moisturize dry hair. Keep in mind, though, that a good many leave-in conditioners tend to be aimed at those with normal to slightly dry hair that is normal to fine or thin and that these tend to contain film formers.

One of the challenges in compiling the following lists is that there is a fine line between the different ways you might experience a conditioner. **Sometimes all it takes is using less of one that is really better for dry hair to make it work for slightly dry or normal hair.** Likewise, you may only need to leave a conditioner meant for normal to slightly dry hair on a little longer to have it work better for your hair.

Hair Note: In the individual reviews for these products, I occasionally did not mention that they may cause buildup (it just became so repetitive), but as long as film-forming or conditioning ingredients are listed in the product description, it should be assumed that buildup can be an eventual problem with repeated use, especially when these are used with a shampoo that contains similar conditioning or film-forming agents.

General guidelines for use: Only use conditioner where needed. Do not apply it on the scalp unless that area is dry or the roots are dry. If you have an oily scalp, do not apply conditioner near the scalp at all. It is fine to apply conditioner only on the ends of hair, and that also prevents the hair from becoming limp or heavy with conditioning agents. Conditioners that contain film formers or heavy oils are harder to wash out of hair than other types of conditioner. If you have dry or coarse hair try to leave the conditioner on for as long as possible. If you have more normal hair, rinse it off quickly or use a lightweight, detangling, nonconditioning product, and rinse it off quickly or use a leave-in version. You may find that it helps to select a shampoo listed above in "Shampoos for All Hair Types that Won't Cause Buildup" to use in conjunction with conditioners to be sure you are not depositing too many conditioning agents or film formers on the hair, which would make buildup more of a problem.

NORMAL HAIR REGARDLESS OF THICKNESS: Alberto Clarifying Formula Conditioner, Daily Light Conditioning *($0.99 for 15 ounces)*, Naturals Conditioner, Tropical Dreams (awapuhi, papaya, aloe) *($1.49 for 15 ounces)*, Normal Daily Light Conditioning Conditioner *($0.99 for 13 ounces)*, Salon Formula Conditioner *($1.49 for 15 ounces)*, Split Ends Treatment Conditioner *($0.99 for 15 ounces)*, and Strawberry 'n Creme Conditioner, Essence of Wild Strawberry *($1.49 for 15 ounces)*; **Aussie** Slip Detangler *($3.99 for 12 ounces)*; **Avon** Techniques Tri-Nutriv Formula Replenishing Conditioner for Normal Hair *($3.99 for 11 ounces)*; **Bain de Terre** White Clover Daily Detangling Conditioner *($8.95 for 16.9 ounces)*; **SeaPlasma by Focus 21** SeaPlasma All Purpose Skin and Hair Moisturizer *($6.29 for 16 ounces)*; **Splash by Focus 21** Splash Detangler *($5.99 for 12 ounces)*; **Papaya Provita by Freeman** Papaya Silk 1-Minute Miracle Treatment Conditioner with Ginseng, Ultra Body *($2.39 for 16 ounces)*; **Hayashi** Spaah Skin and Hair Fitness Spray Mist Rehydrante *($3.80 for 2 ounces)*; **Johnson & Johnson** Kids No More Bed-Head Spray *($2.99 for 10 ounces)*, No More Tangles Spray Detangler *($2.99 for 10 ounces)*, and No More Tears Baby Gentle Detangler *($2.49 for 20 ounces)*; **Healthy Alternative by KMS** Healthy Alternative Clarifying Treatment *($10 for 8.1 ounces)*; **Ouidad** Balancing Rinse *($9 for 8 ounces)*; **Paul Mitchell** Botanical Body-Building Treatment **Phytotherathrie** Phyto 7 Plant Based Treatment Cream for Dry Hair with Extracts of Plants *($15 for 1.7 ounces)*; **Rave** Frizz Taming Spray Ultra Smoothness *($1.89 for 9 ounces)*; **Silhouette Styling System by Schwarzkopf** Style Care Conditioner #2 *($7.90 for 6.8 ounces)* and Intensive Treatment #3 *($9.30 for 4.1 ounces)*; **Care Free Curl by Soft Sheen** Snap Back Curl Restorer *($3.29 for 8 ounces)*; **Baby Love by Soft Sheen** Conditioning Detangler *($4.19 for 8 ounces)*; **Style by Lamaur** Moisturizing Conditioner for Dry Color-Treated/Permed Hair *($1.99 for 12 ounces)*; **Suave** For Kids Detangling Spray, Awesome Apple *($1.99 for 10.5 ounces)*, Frequent Use Conditioner *($1.74 for 22.5 ounces)*, Apple Essence Conditioner *($0.78 for 15 ounces)*, Balsam and Protein Conditioner Adds Body to Normal to Dry Hair *($0.78 for 15 ounces)*, and Strawberry Essence Conditioner *($0.78 for 15 ounces)*; **Salon Formula by Suave** Salon Formula Conditioner Vitamin Enriched to Nourish

All Hair Types *($0.78 for 15 ounces)*; **Herbal Care by Suave** Herbal Care Chamomile Conditioner *($0.78 for 15 ounces)* and Herbal Care Conditioner Aloe Vera, Honeysuckle, and Vitamin E *($0.78 for 15 ounces)*; **TCB** Lite Instant Moisturizer, Jasmine, Aloe & Lavender *($3.59 for 8 ounces)*; **Bone Strait by TCB** Conditioner and Blow Dry Lotion *($3.89 for 16 ounces)*; **TIGI** Deep Reconstruct Conditioner *($10.96 for 8 ounces)*; Protein Protective Spray *($8.50 for 8 ounces)*; **Bed Head by TIGI** Moisture Maniac Conditioner *($11.95 for 8.5 ounces)*; **Vertu by Tressa** Day Splash Moisturizing Conditioner *($10 for 14 ounces)*; **Trevor Sorbie** Deep Conditioner Intensive Moisturizing Creme Treatment *($8.40 for 5 ounces)* and Riche Conditioner *($9.38 for 8.5 ounces)*; **TRI** Electri-Therm Control Treatment *($5.49 for 8 ounces)*; **Collections by White Rain** Classic Care Conditioner Extra Body *($1.09 for 15 ounces)*, Classic Care Conditioner Regular *($0.99 for 15 ounces)*, Classic Care Conditioner Revitalizing Formula *($0.99 for 15 ounces)*, Conditioner Moisturizing *($0.97 for 15 ounces)*, and Conditioner Salon Formula *($0.97 for 15 ounces)*; **Essential by White Rain** Apple Essence Conditioner *($1.09 for 13.5 ounces)*, Coconut Essence Conditioner *($1.07 for 16.8 ounces)*, Strawberry Essence Conditioner *($1.07 for 16.8 ounces)*, and Hibiscus Petals Conditioner *($1.07 for 16.8 ounces)*; **Exotics by White Rain** Lotus Petals Conditioner, for shine *($1.07 for 16.8 ounces)* and Orchid Petals Conditioner, for shine *($1.07 for 16.8 ounces)*; and **Herbs & Blossoms by White Rain** Ginger Lily Conditioner Moisturizing *($1.07 for 13.5 ounces)*, Jasmine Conditioner Extra Body *($1.07 for 13.5 ounces)*, and Passionflower Conditioner Revitalizing *($1.07 for 13.5 ounces)*.

   NORMAL TO DRY HAIR THAT IS NORMAL TO FINE OR THIN: Afri-can Pride Leave-in Conditioner *($3.99 for 12 ounces)*; **All Ways Natural by African Pride** 911 Leave-in Conditioner, Extra Dry Formula *($4.59 for 16 ounces)*, 911 Leave-in Hair Conditioner, Original Formula *($3.62 for 8 ounces)*, 911 Leave-in Hair Treatment *($4.39 for 16 ounces)*, and 911 Leave-in Hair Treatment, Extra Dry Formula *($4.39 for 16 ounces)*; **Alberto** Extra Body Conditioner, Maximum Fullness with Collagen *($0.99 for 15 ounces)*, Extra Body Permed/Color Treated Conditioner, Maximum Fullness *($1.49 for 15 ounces)*, Hair Therapy Revitalizing Daily Conditioner *($2.59 for 8 ounces)*, Henna Conditioner, Enhances Shine *($0.99 for 15 ounces)*, Jojoba Conditioner, Revives Overworked Hair *($0.99 for 15 ounces)*, Moisturizing Conditioner, Moisture and Softness *($0.99 for 15 ounces)*, Naturals Conditioner, Fruitsation (melon, wild berry, wheat germ extract) *($0.99 for 15 ounces)*, VO Fine Thickening Conditioner, Dry, Color Treated, Permed *($3.09 for 13 ounces)*, VO Fine Thickening Conditioner, Regular *($3.09 for 13 ounces)*, Hot Creme One Minute Intensive Hair Treatment Hydrating with Vitamin E *($2.99 for two 0.50-ounce tubes)*, Hot Oil Aromatherapy Hair Treatment, Chamomile & Ylang Ylang *($2.99 for two 0.50-ounce tubes)*, Hot Oil Hair Treatment, Moisturizing, for Permed or Color Treated

Hair *($2.99 for two 0.50-ounce tubes)*, Hot Oil Hair Treatment, Strengthening *($2.99 for two 0.50-ounce tubes)*, Hot Oil Shower Works Hair Treatment, Moisturizing *($4.66 for 2 ounces)*, and Hot Oil Treatment, Split Ends Control *($2.99 for two 0.50-ounce tubes)*; **ARTec** Kiwi Leave-in Bodifying Detangler *($10 for 8.4 ounces)*; **Texture Line by ARTec** Volume Conditioner *($9.98 for 8 ounces)*; **Aubrey Organics** White Camellia Shine Conditioner Spray *($6.95 for 4 ounces)*; **Aura** Elixir Leave-on Conditioner for Hair Rejuvenation *($4.69 for 8 ounces)* and Jojoba Hot Oil Treatment, Heat Activated Conditioning that Helps Repair and Revitalize Hair *($1.59 for 1 ounce)*; **Aussie** Hair Salad Conditioner for Fine, Flyaway Hair *($3.59 for 12 ounces)* and Real Volume Leave-in Volumizer *($5.99 for 8 ounces)*; **Aveda** Rosemary/Mint Equalizer, Hair Conditioning Rinse *($8.40 for 8.45 ounces)*, Elixir Daily Leave-on Hair Conditioner *($9.60 for 8.45 ounces)*, Styling Curessence Hair Renewal for Strength and Control *($14 for 8.4 ounces)*, and Volumizing Tonic for All Hair Types *($10.50 for 3.7 ounces)*; **Avon** Techniques Tri-Nutriv Formula Volumizing Conditioner for Fine/Thin Hair *($3.99 for 11 ounces)*, and Techniques Tri-Nutriv Formula Hot Oil Treatment for Hair *($5.99 for two 1-ounce tubes)*; **Back to Basics** Wild Berry Volumizing Conditioner for All Hair Types *($8.95 for 12 ounces)*; **Basic Texture by Back to Basics** Get Curly Curl Enhancing Conditioner *($8.95 for 12 ounces)*; **Bain de Terre** Herbal Reconstructing Pac *($8.50 for 4 ounces)*; **Bumble and Bumble** Deep Conditioner *($15.20 for 5 ounces)*, Leave In Conditioner *($12.40 for 8 ounces)*, and Seaweed Conditioner *($9.20 for 8 ounces)*; **Citre Shine** Perm Color Treated Conditioner for Chemically Treated Hair *($3.99 for 16 ounces)*; Reconstructing Conditioner for Dry or Damaged Hair *($3.99 for 16 ounces)*; **Herbal Essences by Clairol** Conditioner, Clean-Rinsing for Normal to Oily Hair *($3.48 for 12 ounces)*, Conditioner, Intensive Conditioning Balm for Dry/Damaged/Overstressed Hair *($3.48 for 10.2 ounces)*, Conditioner, Protects Colored/Permed/Dry/Damaged Hair *($3.48 for 12 ounces)*, and Conditioner, Light Conditioning for Fine/Limp Hair *($3.48 for 12 ounces)*; **Clinique** Extra Benefits Conditioner *($10 for 4 ounces)*; **Dark & Lovely** Beautiful Beginnings Vitamin E & Aloe Leave-in Conditioner Plus Detangler *($2.59 for 8 ounces)*; **SeaPlasma by Focus 21** SeaPlasma Intensified Hair Booster Plus *($3.29 for 8 ounces)* and Hair Remoisturizing Treatment *($3.29 for 4 ounces)*; **Framesi Biogenol** Moisture Rinse *($6.95 for 8 ounces)*; **Beautiful Hair by Freeman** Beautiful Hair Hawaiian Ginger Supremely Silk Texturizing Conditioner *($3.49 for 16 ounces)*; **Real Shiny Hair by Freeman** Real Shiny Hair Conditioner, Orange & Lemon *($3.42 for 12 ounces)*; **Definition by Goldwell** Definition Balance & Vitality Conditioner *($11.95 for 12 ounces)* and Definition Color & Highlights Conditioning Treatment *($11.95 for 12 ounces)*; **Hayashi** Daily Conditioner Detangling Rinse, All Hair Types *($7.90 for 8.4 ounces)*, Color Sealing Conditioner Liquid Diamonds *($10.50 for 8.4 ounces)*, Protect Conditioner Moisture Lock for Color Treated Hair *($7.90 for 8.4* *ounces)*, and No Rinse Leave-in Conditioner for Volume and Shine *($6 for 8.4 ounces)*; **Infusium 23** Pro-Vitamin Hair Treatment Moisturizing Treatment *($5.43 for 16 ounces)*, Maximum Body Formula Leave-in Treatment for Fine/Thin Hair *($4.19 for 8 ounces)*, Moisturizing Formula Leave-in Treatment for Normal to Dry Hair *($3.44 for 8 ounces)*, Original Formula Leave-in Treatment for Damaged Hair *($3.44 for 8 ounces)*, and UV Protection Formula Leave-in Treatment for Damaged Hair *($3.44 for 8 ounces)*; **Jheri Redding** Aloe Vera Conditioner for All Hair Types *($1.90 for 24 ounces)*, Balsam Conditioner for All Hair Types *($1.90 for 24 ounces)*, Repairers Detangler *($2.79 for 14 ounces)*, and Porofill Conditioner Porosity Equalizer *($2.99 for 16.5 ounces)*; **Professional Prescription by Jheri Redding** Enforce Conditioner for Normal to Slightly Damaged Hair *($8.49 for 33.8 ounces)* and Biotin Leave-in Treatment for Fine, Thin, Weak Hair *($4.99 for 8 ounces)*; **Jhirmack** EFA Moisturizing Conditioner for Dry, Permed and Color Treated Hair *($3.69 for 20 ounces)*, Nutri-Body Volumizing Conditioner for All Hair Types *($2.70 for 11 ounces)*, and Shine Conditioner for All Hair Types *($2.70 for 11 ounces)*; **Ready to Wear by John Frieda** Wear and Tear Repair, Instant Conditioner and Shiner *($4.59 for 11 ounces)*; **Blue Line by Joico** Lite Instant Detangler and Conditioner *($5.50 for 8.45 ounces)*; **Kenra** Hair Re-Moisturizer *($10.50 for 10.1 ounces)*, Max Conditioner *($10.50 for 10.1 ounces)*, Max Revitalisant Volumizing Protein-Enriched Conditioner *($24.95 for 33.8 ounces)*, and Daily Provision Lightweight Leave-in Conditioner *($9.95 for 10.1 ounces)*; **KMS** Color Response Color Last Color Protector and Detangling Spray for Colored or Color-Highlighted Hair *($7.95 for 8 ounces)*, Color Response Detangling Reconstructor, Advanced Reconstructor and Detangler for Colored or Color-Highlighted Hair *($8.95 for 8.11 ounces)*, pHinish Reconstructor, Active Clarifier for All Hair Types *($6.50 for 4 ounces)*, and Trilogy Leave-in Reconstructor for All Hair Types *($7.95 for 8 ounces)*; **AMP: Amino-Magnesium-Panthenol by KMS** Volume Reconstructor for All Hair Types *($8.95 for 8.11 ounces)*; **Silker by KMS** Silker Detangler for All Hair Types *($8.50 for 8.11 ounces)* and Silker Leave In Treatment *($9.50 for 8.5 ounces)*; **Lange** CVS: Conditioner Volumizer Styler Leave-in Conditioner *($14.50 for 8 ounces)*; **Colors & Curls by L'anza** Moisture Treatment Super Hydrating Treatment *($28 for 16.1 ounces)*; **Volume Formula by L'anza** Weightless Rinse *($8.96 for 12.6 ounces)*; **BodyVive by L'Oreal** BodyVive Daily Body for Fine Hair, No Weight Conditioner plus Ceramide-R & Protein, All Fine Hair *($3.79 for 13 ounces)*; **FortaVive by L'Oreal** FortaVive Daily Care for Damaged Hair, Repairing Conditioner plus Ceramide-R *($3.79 for 13 ounces)*; **HydraVive by L'Oreal** HydraVive Daily Care for Dry Hair, Moisture Conditioner plus Hydra-Protein, Dry/Damaged *($3.79 for 13 ounces)*; **M Professional Hair** Just Conditioner Regular, Dry or Just Needy Hair *($4.60 for 13 ounces)*; **Mastey** Basic Superpac Protein Complex Reconstructor *($16.20 for 10.2 ounces)*, Liquid Pac Revitalizing Reconstructor

($5.90 for 5.1 ounces), Moisturee Revitalizing Hydrating Complex *($13.80 for 10.2 ounces)*, and Activateur Curl Enhancer with Sunscreen *($5.50 for 5.1 ounces)*; **Logics by Matrix** Colorsure Conditioner *($14.95 for 13.5 ounces)* and Leave-In Protector *($13.95 for 13.5 ounces)*; **Essentials by Matrix** Perm Fresh Leave-in Treatment *($11.75 for 12 ounces)* and 5 + Protopak Restructurizing Treatment *($4.75 for 1 ounce)*; **Biolage by Matrix** Conditioning Balm *($10.95 for 4 ounces)* and Daily Leave-in Tonic *($12.75 for 13.5 ounces)*; **Nick Chavez Perfect Plus** Daily Detangler *($12 for 8 ounces)*; **Pantene** Progressive Treatment Creme Conditioner, for Dry Hair, Moisture Replenishing Formula *($3.47 for 7 ounces)*, Progressive Treatment Creme Conditioner, Extra Body for Fine or Normal Hair *($3.47 for 7 ounces)*, Progressive Treatment Creme Conditioner for Permed or Color Treated Hair, Revitalizing Formula *($3.47 for 7 ounces)*, Progressive Treatment Creme Conditioner, Vitamin Therapy *($3.47 for 7 ounces)*, Pro-Vitamin Daily Treatment Conditioner, Extra Body for Fine Hair *($3.39 for 13 ounces)*, Pro-Vitamin Daily Treatment Conditioner, Moisturizing for Dry or Damaged Hair *($3.39 for 13 ounces)*, Pro-Vitamin Daily Treatment Regular Conditioning for Normal Hair *($3.39 for 13 ounces)*, Pro-Vitamin Daily Treatment Conditioner, Revitalizing for Permed or Color Treated Hair *($3.39 for 13 ounces)*, Pro-Vitamin Daily Light Spray Conditioner *($3.39 for 10.2 ounces)*, and Pro-Vitamin Hair Strengthening Complex *($9.64 for 3.4 ounces)*; **Paul Mitchell** Awapuhi Moisture Mist *($7 for 8 ounces)*, Hair Repair Treatment *($9 for 6 ounces)* and The Rinse Balancing Conditioner *($12.95 for 16 ounces)*; **Phytotherathrie** Phyyto Men Revitalizing Hair Lotion with Alcoholic Extract of Burdock *($17 for 6.76 ounces)*; **Prell** Conditioner Moisturizing Formula for Dry/Damaged Hair *($2.60 for 15.2 ounces)*; **Principal Secret** No-Rinse Condition With Sun Protection *($13, $9 for 6 ounces)*; **Professional** Polymeric Reconstructor *($4.60 for 16 ounces)*; **Queen Helene** Cocoa Butter Hair Conditioner *($3.59 for 21 ounces)* and Cholesterol Instant Leave-In Hair Conditioner *($3 for 16 ounces)*; **CAT by Redken** CAT Protein Reconstructing Treatment *($11.95 for 5 ounces)*; **Color Extend Redken** Color Extend Conditioner *($8 for 8.5 ounces)*; **Extreme Redken** Extreme Treatment *($12.95 for 5 ounces)*; **Robert Craig** Conditioning Spray 3-in-1 Formulation *($12 for 8 ounces)*; **Salon Style by Lamaur** Botanical Reconstructor Conditioner *($2.22 for 20 ounces)*, Moisture Potion Conditioner *($2.22 for 20 ounces)*, and Deep Conditioner, Hydrobalance Hair Masque *($2.22 for 15 ounces)*; **Natural Styling by Schwarzkopf** Conditioning Rinse *($6.40 for 6.8 ounces)*; **Scruples** Reconstruct Leave-in Protein Spray *($9.95 for 8.5 ounces)*; **Collectives by Sebastian** Cello-Primer Detangler Build-Up Remover *($5.50 for 5.1 ounces)*, Formulating Creme Deep Conditioner 5-Minute Conditioning Treatment *($17.50 for 10.2 ounces)*, Moisture Base Moisturizing Conditioner *($7.75 for 5.1 ounces)*, Sheen Instant Conditioner *($11.30 for 10.2 ounces)*, and Cello-Fix Leave On Conditioner Spray for Damaged Hair *($12 for 10.2 ounces)*; **Performance Ac-**

tive by Sebastian Conditioner: A One Minute Conditioning Masque for Hair *($20 for 8.5 ounces)* and Gelee *($17.50 for 5.1 ounces)*; **Just for Me by Soft & Beautiful** Leave-in Conditioner *($2.95 for 8 ounces)* and Detangler *($2.99 for 8 ounces)*; **Care Free Curl by Soft Sheen** Gold Instant Activator with Silk Moisturizers *($2.99 for 8 ounces)* and Gold Instant Activator with Silk Moisturizers *($2.99 for 8 ounces)*; **St. Ives** Swiss Spa Extra Body Conditioner Chamomile and Sunflower for Normal/Fine Hair *($2.79 for 20 ounces)*, Swiss Spa Extra Shine Conditioner: Jojoba and Raspberry for Normal Hair *($2.79 for 20 ounces)*, Swiss Spa Moisturizing Conditioner: Aloe Vera and Echinacea for Permed/Color Treated Hair *($2.79 for 20 ounces)*, Swiss Spa Revitalizing Conditioner: Vanilla and Edelweiss for Dry/Damaged Hair *($2.79 for 20 ounces)*, and Swiss Spa Strengthening Conditioner: Pear and Vitamin E for Normal/Dry Hair *($2.79 for 20 ounces)*; **Style by Lamaur** Coconut & Papaya Conditioner Maintains Softness & Enhances Shine *($1.09 for 24 ounces)*, Deep Conditioning Conditioner Replenishes Dry or Treated Hair *($0.99 for 13 ounces)*, Extra Body Conditioner *($0.99 for 13 ounces)*, Fresh Apple Regular Conditioner *($0.99 for 13 ounces)*, Moisturizing Conditioner *($0.99 for 13 ounces)*, Pro-Vitamin Complex Conditioner *($0.99 for 13 ounces)*, Pro-Vitamin Complex Conditioner Regular Apple *($0.99 for 13 ounces)*, and Volumizing Conditioner for Fine or Thin Hair *($1.99 for 12 ounces)*; **Suave** Daily Clarifying Conditioner *($0.78 for 15 ounces)*, Full Body Conditioner *($1.74 for 22.5 ounces)*, Moisturizing Conditioner Replenishes Moisture to Dry Hair *($0.78 for 15 ounces)*, Natural Care Conditioner Citrus Blend *($0.78 for 15 ounces)*, Natural Care Conditioner Tropical Coconut *($0.78 for 15 ounces)*, Peach Essence Conditioner *($0.78 for 15 ounces)*, and Perm & Color Formula Conditioner *($0.78 for 15 ounces)*; **Sukesha** Daily Hydrating Balm, Restores Vitality to Dry Damaged Hair *($6.95 for 12 ounces)*, Hair Moisturizing Treatment, Intensive Formula for Elasticity and Strength *($5.50 for 6 ounces)*, and Shine and Body Leave-in Conditioner *($5.95 for 8 ounces)*; **Essensuals by TIGI** Thickening Conditioner *($12.96 for 8 ounces)* and Leave-in Conditioner *($11.95 for 8.5 ounces)*; **Tressa** Immedia Leave-in Conditioner, UV Protection for Color-Treated Hair *($8.99 for 8 ounces)*; **Tresemme** European Color-Treated and Permed Conditioner *($2.49 for 32 ounces)* and Tres Mend, European Natural Silk Protein Hair Reconstructor *($0.67 for 1 ounce)*, and European Natural Leave-in Conditioner with Vitamins A, C, and E, Lightweight Formula *($2.49 for 32 ounces)*; **Trevor Sorbie** Riche Leave-in Conditioner *($7.40 for 10 ounces)*; **TRI** Express Conditioning Detangler *($8.49 for 8 ounces)*; **Vidal Sassoon** Stylist Choice Conditioner #1, Extra Body for Fine or Thin Hair *($2.79 for 13 ounces)*, Stylist Choice Conditioner #2, Balanced for Normal Hair *($2.79 for 13 ounces)*, Stylist Choice Conditioner #3, Revitalizing for Permed or Color-Treated Hair, Heat Defense Formula *($2.79 for 13 ounces)*, Stylist Choice Conditioner #4, Moisture Rich for Dry or Damaged Hair *($2.79 for 13 ounces)*, Treatments Deep Moisturizing

Conditioner *($2.93 for 6.7 ounces)*, and Heat Defense, Styling Heat Protectant *($2.79 for 10.2 ounces)*; **Wanakee** Detangling Spray Conditioner *($8.95 for 8 ounces)*; **Liquid Hair by Wella** Color Preserver Daily Conditioner for Color-Treated Hair *($8.50 for 12 ounces)*, Moisture Rinse Daily Conditioner for All Hair Types *($8.50 for 12 ounces)*, Restructurizer Leave-in Treatment *($15 for 6.8 ounces)*, and Physical Therapy, Wearable Volumizer Treatment for All Hair Types *($13 for 6 ounces)*; and **Willow Lake** Hops, Apricot & Almond Conditioner *($3.10 for 16 ounces)*, Sunflower, Honey & Hibiscus Conditioner *($3.10 for 16 ounces)*, and Vitamin E, Carrot Extract & Milk Protein Conditioner *($3.10 for 16 ounces)*.

    DRY TO VERY DRY HAIR THAT IS NORMAL TO FINE OR THIN: **African Pride** Instant Oil Moisturizing Hair Lotion *($5.49 for 12 ounces)*; **Basic Texture by Back to Basics** Be Thick Thickening Conditioning Rinse *($8.95 for 12 ounces)*; **Herbal Essences by Clairol** Leave-in Conditioner, Lightweight Formula for All Hair Types *($3.48 for 10.2 ounces)*; **Daily Defense by Clairol** Fortifying Leave-in Conditioning Spray *($3.48 for 10.2 ounces)*; **Dark & Lovely** Color Care Conditioner *($2.29 for 8 ounces)*; **Salon Textures by Freeman** Salon Textures Leave-in Aire Conditioner *($3.99 for 5.3 ounces)*; **Kerasilk by Goldwell** Kerasilk Volumizing Leave-in Conditioner *($8.90 for 6 ounces)*; **Classic Line by Graham Webb** 24 Karat, Leave-in Conditioner, Reconstructor and Shine *($10.95 for 8 ounces)*, 30 Second Sheer Conditioner for Daily Use *($9.96 for 8.5 ounces)*, and Condition Stick Straight High Gloss Smoothing Conditioner *($8 for 8.5 ounces)*; **Jheri Redding** Extra Protein Pac for Extremely Damaged Hair *($0.99 for 1 ounce)*; **Kiehl's** Lecithin and Coconut Enriched Hair Masque with Panthenol *($21.50 for 14 ounces)*; **Essentials by Matrix** Essential Color Therapy Revitalizing Conditioner *($10.25 for 4 ounces)*; **Motions at Home** After Shampoo Moisture Plus Conditioner *($2.99 for 6 ounces)*; and **Liquid Hair by Wella** Vital Signs Intensive Moisturizing Treatment for Dry, Chemically Treated Hair *($13 for 6 ounces)*.

    NORMAL TO DRY HAIR OF ANY THICKNESS: **African Pride** African Miracle Hair & Scalp Spray *($5.49 for 12 ounces)*; **African Royale** Daily Doctor Leave-in Conditioner *($3.49 for 12 ounces)*; **Alberto** Naturals Conditioner, Vanilla Blossom (vanilla, honeysuckle, chamomile) *($0.99 for 15 ounces)*, Normal Conditioner, Superb Manageability *($0.99 for 15 ounces)*, Pear Mango Passion Herbal Conditioner, Dry, Color-Treated or Permed, Aloe and Passion Flower Extracts *($0.99 for 15 ounces)*, and Sun Kissed Raspberry Herbal Conditioner, Normal, Juniper and Chamomile Extracts *($0.99 for 15 ounces)*; **Apple Pectin by Lamaur** Creme Conditioner *($4.99 for 15.5 ounces)*, Deep Moisturizing Treatment for Dry/Damaged Hair *($3.99 for 4 ounces)*, Naturals Hops, Apricot & Almonds Conditioner *($4.99 for 16 ounces)*, and Naturals Sunflower, Honey & Hibiscus Conditioner *($4.99 for 16 ounces)*; **ARTec** Kiwi Coloreflector Weightless Conditioner *($23 for 16 ounces)*; **Aubrey**

Organics Biotin Hair Repair *($14.80 for 4 ounces)* and Blue Green Algae Hair Rescue Conditioning Mask *($13.50 for 4 ounces)*; **Aveda** Cherry/Almond Bark, Reconstructive Hair Conditioner *($21.50 for 7.9 ounces)*; **Back to Basics** Sunflower Detangling and Conditioning Spray *($6.95 for 8 ounces)* and Sunflower Moisture Infusing Conditioner for All Hair Types *($7.95 for 12 ounces)*; **Beauty Without Cruelty** Daily Benefits Conditioner, Benefits All Hair Types *($6.95 for 16 ounces)*, Moisture Plus Conditioner, Benefits Dry/Treated Hair *($6.95 for 16 ounces)*, and Revitalize Leave-in Conditioner, Benefits Dry/Treated Hair *($6.95 for 8.5 ounces)*; **BioSilk** Conditioner Moisturizer *($8 for 10 ounces)*, Sealer Plus Finishing Rinse *($8.80 for 10 ounces)*, and Silk Filler Leave-in Repairative Treatment *($11 for 10 ounces)*; **The Body Shop** Amlika Leave-in Conditioner All Hair Types *($10.50 for 16.9 ounces)*, Brazil Nut Damage Care Conditioner for Dry, Damaged & Chemically Treated Hair *($10.50 for 16.9 ounces)*, Brazil Nut Conditioner, Dry, Damaged & Chemically Treated Hair Extra Rich and Moisturizing *($10.50 for 16.9 ounces)*, Light Conditioner for Normal to Oily Hair *($4.50 for 5 ounces)*, and Seaweed & Peony Strengthening Conditioner Normal Hair *($6 for 8.4 ounces)*; **Bumble and Bumble** Prep *($10 for 8 ounces)*; **Citre Shine** Instant Conditioner for All Hair Types *($3.42 for 16 ounces)* Leave-in Volumizing Treatment Conditioner for Normal to Fine/Limp Hair *($3.42 for 12 ounces)*, Self-Heating Hot Oil Treatment for Dry or Damaged Hair *($3.42 for three 1-ounce treatments)*, and Vitamin C Citrus Hot Oil *($3.99 for three 1-ounce treatments)*; **Herbal Essences by Clairol** Conditioner, Moisturizing for Normal Hair *($3.48 for 12 ounces)*; **Daily Defense by Clairol** Conditioner Defense 1 for Fine Hair *($3.48 for 13.5 ounces)*, Conditioner Defense 2 for Normal Hair *($3.48 for 13.5 ounces)*, Conditioner Defense 3 for Color-Treated/Permed Hair *($3.48 for 13.5 ounces)*, Conditioner Defense 4 for Dry/Damaged Hair *($3.48 for 13.5 ounces)*, and Conditioner, Extra Defense for Damaged/Overstressed Hair *($3.29 for 10.2 ounces)*; **Conditions 3-in-1 by Clairol** Detangler Plus *($1.75 for 8 ounces)*, Protein Enriched Beauty Pack Treatment, Extra Body Formula *($5.62 for 4 ounces)*, andCurl Refresher *($1.75 for 8 ounces)*; **Finesse** Enhancing Conditioner for Normal, Healthy Hair *($2.58 for 15 ounces)* and Light Conditioning Spray for All Hair Types *($2.58 for 10.5 ounces)*; **Enviro-Tek by Focus 21** Enviro-Tek Antioxidant Moisturizing Spray *($5.51 for 12 ounces)*, Enviro-Tek Antioxidant Reconstructor Conditioner *($6.04 for 12 ounces)*, and Enviro-Tek Antioxidant Leave-in Conditioner Spray *($6.14 for 12 ounces)*; **Splash by Focus 21** Splash Leave-in Conditioner Spray *($3.99 for 12 ounces)*; **Framesi Biogenol** Reconditor for Dry, Damaged Hair *($8.50 for 5 ounces)* and Ultra Deep Conditioner *($16.96 for 8 ounces)*; **Aromatherapy by Freeman** Aromatherapy Calming Conditioner for Normal to Dry Hair *($4.11 for 16 ounces)* and Aromatherapy Energizing Conditioner for Normal to Dry Hair *($4.11 for 16 ounces)*; **Beautiful Hair by Freeman** Beautiful Hair Kiwi Fruit Ultra Therapy Treatment Conditioner *($2.88 for 16 ounces)* and Hawaiian Mango Conditioner for Normal Hair *($2.99 for*

16 ounces); **Salon Textures by Freeman** Salon Textures Intense Aire Conditioner *($3.99 for 5.3 ounces);* **Super Straight Hair by Freeman** Super Straight Hair Conditioner, Honeydew & Lilac *($3.42 for 12 ounces);* **Garden Botanika Hair Care** Fruit Complex Daily Conditioner *($9 for 12 ounces),* Kelp & Nettle Leave-in Conditioner *($9 for 12 ounces),* and Panthenol Remoisturizing Conditioner *($9 for 12 ounces);* **Exclusives by Goldwell** Exclusives Body-Building Conditioner *($8.50 for 8 ounces)* and Exclusives Revitalizing Conditioner Spray *($11.90 for 8 ounces);* **Classic Line by Graham Webb** The Untangler Leave-In Detangling Spray *($11 for 8.5 ounces);* **Bodacious by Graham Webb** Bodacious Moisturizing Conditioner Renew & Revitalize *($9 for 10 ounces);* **Hayashi** Moisture Balancer Hair Mask for Healthier Hair *($19.50 for 16 ounces);* **System 911 by Hayashi** Emergency Pak Reconstructor for Damaged Hair *($29 for 16 ounces),* Protein Mist Leave-in Conditioner Detangler, Body Building *($7.90 for 8.4 ounces),* and Hair Thickener Leave-in Body Booster for Fine and Thinning Hair *($9 for 4 ounces);* **Infusium 23** Pro-Vitamin Hair Treatment Original Hair Treatment for Damaged/Unmanageable Hair *($5.43 for 16 ounces)* and Re-Vitalizing Conditioner for Normal to Dry Hair *($5.43 for 16 ounces);* **Ion** Anti-Frizz Leave-in Conditioner *($4.29 for 12 ounces),* Conditioning Miracle Microwavable Treatment Pac *($1.99 for 1 ounce),* Effective Care Intensive Therapy Treatment *($3.99 for 4 ounces),* Finishing Rinse with Electro-Bond Proteins *($4.99 for 16 ounces),* Moisturizing Treatment *($4.99 for 4 ounces),* Reconstructor Treatment *($8.99 for 16 ounces),* Finishing Detangler *($4.99 for 16 ounces),* and Hot Oil Deep Penetrating Treatment *($1.69 for 1 ounce);* **ISO** Nourishing Daily Conditioner *($17.49 for 33.8 ounces),* Recovery Treatment Intensive Moisturizing Conditioner *($7.49 for 5 ounces),* Stress Defense Conditioner Leave-in Protection *($7.49 for 10 ounces),* and SportMist Leave-in Conditioner *($7.49 for 10 ounces);* **Jason Natural Cosmetics** Color Sealant Conditioner for All Shades of Hair, Enhances Shine as It Conditions *($6.69 for 8 ounces),* Extra Rich Natural E.F.A. Conditioner, Hair Nourishing Formula for Normal to Dry Hair *($5.50 for 17.5 ounces);* For Kids Only! Extra Gentle Conditioner *($7 for 8 ounces),* Forest Essence Vital Conditioner *($6.69 for 8 ounces),* Hemp Enriched Conditioner for All Hair Types, Especially Dry/Damaged Hair *($7 for 8 ounces),* Natural Aloe Vera 84% Conditioner, Hair Nourishing Formula *($5.50 for 17.5 ounces),* Natural Apricot Keratin Conditioner *($3.10 for 17.5 ounces),* Natural Biotin Conditioner *($5.50 for 17.5 ounces),* Natural Jojoba Conditioner *($5.50 for 17.5 ounces),* Natural Vitamin A, C & E Conditioner *($5.50 for 17.5 ounces),* Rich Natural Sea Kelp Conditioner; Concentrated Extra Gentle, Super Shine *($2.30 for 17.5 ounces),* Tall Grass Hi-Protein Conditioner *($6.69 for 8 ounces),* and Thin-to-Thick Hair and Scalp Therapy Hair Thickening Conditioner *($7.59 for 8 ounces);* **J. F. Lazartigue** Essentials for Curly or Frizzy Hair Conditioner Detangling and Nourishing *($18 for 6.8 ounces),* Hair-Body Emulsion Volumizing

Treatments After-Shampoo Treatment *($19 for 5.1 ounces)*, Vita-Cream with Milk Proteins Dry Hair Care After Shampoo Treatment *($43 for 6.8 ounces)*, Vita-Cream with Milk-Proteins for Fine Hair, Dry Hair Care *($43 for 6.8 ounces)*, Volume Hair Conditioner without Rinse, Volumizing Treatments After Shampoo Treatment *($22 for 2.54 ounces)*, Disentangling Instant Silk Protein Spray *($18 for 3.4 ounces)*, and Cereal Hair Mask, Volumizing Treatment After Shampoo Treatment *($26 for 2.54 ounces)*; **Jheri Redding** Extra Humidicon Humidifying Conditioner *($5.99 for 8 ounces)*, Extra Bio-Body Biotin Leave-in Treatment for Fine, Weak and Thin Hair *($5.99 for 8 ounces)*, and Natural Protein 100% Natural Conditioner *($8.49 for 15 ounces)*; **Professional Prescription by Jheri Redding** Curative Body Building Conditioner for Fine, Limp Hair *($5.99 for 12.5 ounces)*, Curative Daily Strengthening Conditioner for Fine, Weak, or Chemically-Treated Hair *($5.99 for 12.5 ounces)*, and Keratin Reconstructor for Severely Damaged Hair *($8.49 for 33.8 ounces)*; **Blue Line by Joico** Volissima Volumizing Reconditioner *($7.95 for 8.45 ounces)*, Altima Protective Leave-in Reconditioner *($8.60 for 8.45 ounces)*, Integrity Leave-in Reconditioning Treatment *($8.60 for 8.45 ounces)*, H.K.P. Liquid Protein Hair Reconstructor *($10 for 8.45 ounces)*, K-Pak Deep Penetrating Creme Hair Reconstructor *($15.95 for 6.6 ounces)*, Nucleic Pak Moisturizing Creme Hair Reconstructor *($12.20 for 4.4 ounces)*, Shade Endurance Color Sealant with Antioxidants and UVA-UVB Protection *($7.95 for 8.45 ounces)*, and Jojoba Oil *($12.50 for 2 ounces)*; **Kiehl's** Hair Conditioning & Grooming Aid Formula 133 *($14.95 for 8 ounces)*, Leave-in Hair Conditioner *($26.50 for 8 ounces)*, and Panthenol Protein Hair Conditioner *($14.95 for 8 ounces)*; **KMS** Prolimin Gold, the Ultimate Reconstructive Treatment *($4 for 1 ounce)*, Strategy Reconstructor, Nutrient-Enriched for Chemically Treated Hair *($9.95 for 8.11 ounces)*, and Ultra-Pak Reconstructor, Extra Body for Fine, Lifeless Hair *($9.95 for 4 ounces)*; **Puritives by KMS** Reconstructor *($8.95 for 8.79 ounces)*; **Silker by KMS** Silk Reconstructor *($10 for 8.1 ounces)*; **Color Vitality Shampoo by KMS** Color Vitality Reconstructor *($10.95 for 8.1 ounces)* and Color Vitality Color Last Treatment *($12.95 for 8.5 ounces)*; **Lange** Panthenol Protein Hair Moisturizer for Dehydrated Hair *($8.50 for 4 ounces)*, Panthenol 5% Treatment Hair and Skin Fixative *($11.49 for 8 ounces)*, and Elastin Panthenol Protein Pak *($32 for 8 ounces)*; **Colors & Curls by L'anza** Detangler Weightless Rinse Out Conditioner *($5.95 for 8.5 ounces)*, Reconstructor Intensive Hair Repair Treatment *($12.90 for 4.2 ounces)*, Leave-in Protector, Daily Color and Perm Protector *($6.50 for 4.2 ounces)*, and Hair Polish *($9.99 for 3.3 ounces)*; **Long Hair Formula by L'anza** Condition *($12.95 for 13.5 ounces)* and Strengthen *($12.95 for 5.07 ounces)*; **ColorVive by L'Oreal** ColorVive Weekly Protective Conditioning, Dry Defense Plus UV Filter 5-Minute Treatment *($1.59 for 1 ounce)*, ColorVive Daily Care for Color-Treated Hair, Creme Conditioner plus UV Filter, Regular Colored or Highlighted *($2.99 for 13 ounces)*, ColorVive

Daily Care for Color-Treated Hair, Creme Conditioner plus UV Filter, for Dry Hair Colored or Highlighted *($3.79 for 13 ounces)*; **HydraVive by L'Oreal** HydraVive Weekly Protein Conditioning Moisture Solution with Hydra-Protein 5-Minute Treatment *($1.59 for 1 ounce)*; **VitaVive by L'Oreal** VitaVive Daily Care for Normal Hair, Multi-Vitamin Conditioner *($3.79 for 13 ounces)*; **L'Oreal Kids** Extra Gentle Conditioner Plus Detangler, Hard to Manage Hair, Burst of Juicy Grape *($3.49 for 9 ounces)*; **M.A.C.** Intensive Conditioner *($8 for 5 ounces)*, Moisture Rinse *($10 for 8 ounces)*, and Protective Spray *($8 for 8 ounces)*; **M Professional** Abuse Conditioner, Extra-Dry, Permed, or Chemically-Treated Hair *($4.60 for 13 ounces)*; **Mastey** Frehair Finishing Creme Rinse *($9 for 10.2 ounces)* and HC Formula +B5 Hair & Scalp Mender *($9 for 10.2 ounces)*; **Amplify Volumizing System by Matrix** Conditioner *($13.75 for 13.5 ounces)*; **Essentials by Matrix** Essential Body & Strength Reconstructor *($14 for 8 ounces)*, Nutrient Rich Conditioner *($10.95 for 4 ounces)*, Perm Fresh Moisture Supply *($10.95 for 4 ounces)*, Simply Silk Detangling Rinse *($8.99 for 13.5 ounces)*, Essential Color Therapy Leave-in Conditioner *($14.95 for 12 ounces)*, and Instacure Leave-in Treatment *($18.95 for 12 ounces)*; **Biolage by Matrix** Detangling Solution *($12.75 for 13.5 ounces)*; **Vavoom by Matrix** Conditioning *($11.95 for 16 ounces)* and Styling Conditioner *($11.95 for 16 ounces)*; **Vital Nutrients by Matrix** BodyFusion Extra Volume Conditioner *($12.75 for 13.5 ounces)* and MoistureRich Fusion Conditioner *($12.75 for 13.5 ounces)*; **Motions at Home** Critical Protection and Repair Treatment *($6.99 for 15 ounces)*; **Neutrogena** Clean Balancing Conditioner for Normal Hair *($4.99 for 10.1 ounces)*, Clean Replenishing Conditioner for Dry, Damaged Hair *($4.99 for 10.1 ounces)*, Clean Volumizing Conditioner for Fine Hair *($4.99 for 10.1 ounces)*; Conditioner Detangling Formula *($5.29 for 6 ounces)*, Conditioner Revitalizing Formula for Permed or Color Treated Hair *($5.29 for 6 ounces)*, and HeatSafe Instant Heat-Activated Hair Treatment for Dry or Damaged Hair, Regular Formula *($8.49 for 6 ounces)*; **Nexxus** Vita Tress Biotin Creme *($11.50 for 2.1 ounces)*, VitaTress Hair Volumizer *($10 for 10.1 ounces)*, and Headress Leave-in Conditioner *($22 for 16.9 ounces)*; **Nick Chavez Perfect Plus** Conditioner, Adds Body and Shine While It Detangles *($10 for 8 ounces)*; **Ouidad** Deep Treatment *($30 for 4 ounces)* and Botanical Boost *($10 for 8 ounces)*; **Pantene** Pro-Vitamin Deep Fortifying Hair Treatment *($3.39 for 13 ounces)*; **PRO-V Color by Pantene** Pro-V Color Vitalizing Care Conditioner for Color Treated and Highlighted Hair *($5.49 for 12 ounces)*, and PRO-V Color Pro-V Color Intensive Care Masque for Color Treated and Highlighted Hair *($7.59 for 5.1 ounces)*; **Paul Mitchell** The Detangler Instant Condition and Shine *($7.95 for 8 ounces)*, Lite Detangler *($9 for 8 ounces)*, and Super Charged Conditioner *($8.50 for 4 ounces)*; **philosophy** the big blow off liquid protein hair conditioner *($12 for 6 ounces)*, entangled daily conditioner *($12 for 8 ounces)*, and the breaking point overnight intensive hair conditioner

($12 for 2 ounces); **Phytotherathrie** Phyto 9 Vegetal Hydrating Cream for Very Dry Hair with Macadamia Oil *($18 for 1.7 ounces);* **Principal Secret** Tangle-Free Moisturizing Conditioner *($13, $9 for 10 ounces);* **Pro-Vitamin** Anti-Frizz Hydrating Conditioner *($3.99 for 10 ounces);* **Quantum** Daily Moisturizer Leave-in Detangler and Conditioner *($4.29 for 12 ounces);* **Queen Helene** Cholesterol Creamy Hair Conditioner *($2.99 for 16 ounces);* **All Soft by Redken** All Soft Concentrate *($13.95 for 5 ounces),* All Soft Conditioner *($8 for 8.5 ounces),* and All Soft Hair Masque *($9.95 for 5 ounces);* **CAT by Redken** CAT Replenishing Conditioner *($6.25 for 6 ounces)* and Fat CAT Body Booster Detangler *($7.25 for 6 ounces);* **Extreme Redken** Extreme Conditioner for Damaged Hair *($7.50 for 8.5 ounces);* **Glypro by Redken** Glypro+ Conditioner for Fine/Delicate Hair *($7.95 for 8.5 ounces);* **One 2 One by Redken Daily Recovery Conditioner** *($8.75 for 10.1 ounces);* **Shades EQ by Redken** Shades EQ, Color Care Protector, Leave-in *(6.407 for 5 ounces);* **Flex by Revlon** Fresh Scent Extra Body Flex Light and Free Conditioner Maximizes *($2.09 for 15 ounces),* Fresh Scent Moisturizing Flex Light and Free Conditioner *($2.09 for 15 ounces),* and Fresh Scent Normal Flex Light and Free Conditioner *($2.09 for 15 ounces);* **Outrageous by Revlon** Outrageous Daily Beautifying Conditioner for Normal Hair *($2.34 for 15 ounces),* Moisture-Rich Conditioner for Dry, Permed or Color-Treated Hair *($2.34 for 15 ounces),* and Volumizing Conditioner for Fine Hair *($3.19 for 15 ounces);* **Rusk** ResQ Intensive Hair Treatment *($10.96 for 6 ounces),* ResQ Restorative Conditioner Normal to Dry Hair *($9 for 12 ounces),* Sensories Calm Guarana & Ginger 60 Second Hair Revive *($8.95 for 13 ounces),* Sensories Invisible Hibiscus & Kukui Foaming Detangler *($9.90 for 13 ounces),* Treatment Ultra Rich Conditioner *($11 for 5 ounces),* and Sensories Brilliance Grapefruit & Honey Leave-in Color Protector *($9.90 for 8 ounces);* **Salon Selectives** Botanical Blends Conditioner Strengthening with Melon Rose *($1.96 for 15 ounces),* Conditioner Type M Moisturizing *($1.96 for 15 ounces),* and Conditioner Type L Light Conditioning Spray *($1.67 for 7 ounces);* **Laminates by Sebastian** Conditioner *($12 for 8.5 ounces);* **Igora Color Care by Schwarzkopf** Conditioner *($9.90 for 10.1 ounces),* Intensive Treatment *($14.90 for 5.1 ounces),* and Rinse for Color-Treated Hair *($9.50 for 8.45 ounces);* **Scruples** ER Emergency Repair for Damaged Hair *($9.95 for 6 ounces),* and Renewal Hair Conditioner for Color Treated Hair *($5.95 for 4 ounces);* **Performance Active by Sebastian** Gelee and Conditioner *($22 for 8.5 ounces);* **Shaper Slipline by Sebastian** Conditioner, Body Building Conditioner for All Hair Types *($8.50 for 10.2 ounces);* **Senscience** Inner Conditioner for Fine Hair *($12.39 for 16.9 ounces)* and Inner Conditioner for Medium Hair *($12.39 for 16.9 ounces);* **Sheenique** Nubian Results Moisturizing Conditioner *($5.99 for 16 ounces);* **Care Free Curl by Soft Sheen** Instant Moisturizer Glycerin and Protein *($3.19 for 8 ounces),* Keratin Conditioner, pH 5.0 *($5.99 for 16 ounces)* and Gold Hair and Scalp

Spray *($2.99 for 8 ounces)*; **Optimum Care by Soft Sheen** Rich Conditioner *($2.99 for 16 ounces)*; **Style by Lamaur** Rainwater Conditioner Adds Softness and Shine *($0.99 for 13 ounces)* and Strawberry Conditioner Restores Body Rinses Clean *($0.99 for 13 ounces)*; **Suave** Healthy Shine Conditioner with Pro-Vitamins Daily Treatment for Normal to Dry Hair *($1.58 for 14.5 ounces)*, Professionals Awapuhi Conditioner *($1.58 for 14.5 ounces)*, Professionals Bio Basics Conditioner *($1.58 for 14.5 ounces)*, Professionals Humectant Conditioner *($1.58 for 14.5 ounces)*, Thermal Formula Conditioner, Heat Activated for Normal to Dry Hair *($1.54 to 14.5 ounces)*, and Thermal Formula Leave-in Conditioning Mist *($1.89 for 10.5 ounces)*; **Susan Lucci Collection** Deep Conditioning Treatment Healthy Hair Complex *($18 for two 4-ounce containers)*, Moisture Infusion Rinse *($19 for two 12-ounce containers)*, and Multi-Fix Plus, Leave-in Spray Healthy Hair Complex *($22 for two 12-ounce containers)*; **TCB** Lite Hair and Scalp Conditioner, Kiwi, Aloe & Papaya, Replenishes Damaged Hair *($4.39 for 10 ounces)*; **Theorie** Conditioner for Normal to Fine Hair *($4.99 for 12.5 ounces)*, Moisturizing Conditioner for Normal to Dry Hair *($4.99 for 12.5 ounces)*, and Volumizing Conditioner for Normal to Thin or Fine Hair *($4.99 for 12.5 ounces)*; **ThermaSilk** Heat Activated Conditioner for Dry or Damaged Hair *($3.24 for 13 ounces)*, Heat Activated Conditioner Regular for Normal Hair *($3.42 for 13 ounces)*, Heat Activated Conditioner for Colored or Permed Hair *($3.42 for 13 ounces)*, Heat Activated Conditioner Volumizing for Fine or Thin Hair *($3.42 for 13 ounces)*, and Heat Activated Light Conditioning Mist *($2.99 for 10.3 ounces)*; **TIGI** Instant Conditioner *($7.96 for 8 ounces)*; **Tressa** FortipHy Deep Conditioner, Nourishes Weak Links in Permed Hair *($7.99 for 4 ounces)*, Infuse Deep Conditioner, Replenishing Moisturizer for Color-Treated Hair *($7.99 for 4 ounces)*, Quench Deep Conditioner Deep Conditioning for All Hair Types *($9.99 for 6 ounces)*, and ModipHy Normalizer Conditioner, Light Conditioning for Permed Hair *($7.99 for 12 ounces)*; **Vertu by Tressa** Super Splash Therapeutic Conditioner *($18 for 10 ounces)*; **Tresemme** European Natural Conditioner with Vitamins A, C, and E *($2.49 for 32 ounces)*, European Remoisturizing Conditioner *($2.40 for 32 ounces)*, and Tres Pac, Deeply Penetrating Protein Treatment *($3 for 2 ounces)*; **TRI** Whole Wheat Conditioning Rinse *($6.49 for 4 ounces)*; **Ultra Swim** Chlorine Damaged Hair Treatment, Conditioner for All Hair Types *($6.84 for 15 ounces)* and Ultra Repair Conditioner *($6.84 for 15 ounces)*; **Vibrance Organic** Care Nourishing Conditioner with Vitamins & Keratin Body Building for Fine/Thin Hair *($3.79 for 15 ounces)*, Nourishing Conditioner with Vitamins & Keratin Moisture Rich for Dry/Damaged Hair *($2.84 for 15 ounces)*, and Nourishing Conditioner with Vitamins & Keratin Revitalizing Conditioner for Permed/Colored Hair *($2.84 for 15 ounces)*; **Victoria Jackson** Time Activated Hair Conditioner *($14.95, $9.95 for 8 ounces)*; **Vidal Sassoon** Stylist Choice Conditioner #3, Revitalizing for Permed or Color-

Treated Hair, Texturizing Formula *($2.79 for 13 ounces)*; **Wella Balsam** In-Depth Treatment for Problem Hair *($4.99 for 16 ounces)* and pH-D Diagnosis In-Depth Treatment *($5.29 for 16 ounces)*; **Collections by White Rain** Leave-in Conditioner E for Daily Nourishment with Vitamin E Aloe Extracts & UV Filter *($0.99 for 7 ounces)*; and **Zero Frizz** Instant Conditioner *($4.99 for 12 ounces)*.

DRY TO VERY DRY HAIR THAT IS NORMAL TO COARSE: African Pride Hair, Scalp & Skin Oil *($3.99 for 8 ounces)*; Magical GRO Magical Herbal Recipe *($4.99 for 5.5 ounces)*, Magical GRO Magical Oil Recipe *($3.99 for 5.5 ounces)*, Magical GRO Maximum Herbal Strength *($4.99 for 5.5 ounces)*, and Miracle Creme *($3.99 for 5.5 ounces)*; **All Ways Natural by African Pride** 100% Natural Indian Hemp Herbal Hair and Scalp Treatment Conditioner *($4.79 for 4 ounces)*, 100% Natural Indian Hemp Super Lite Herbal Hair and Scalp Treatment Conditioner *($3.09 for 4 ounces)*, Castor Oil Conditioning Hair Dress *($2.29 for 5.5 ounces)*, Conditioner Moisturizing Formula *($3.99 for 12 ounces)*, Indian Hemp Conditioning Hair Dress *($3.99 for 5.5 ounces)*, Super GRO Conditioning Hair Dress *($3.49 for 5.5 ounces)*, Super Lite Indian Hemp Conditioning Hair Dress *($3.99 for 5.5 ounces)*, Super Lite Super GRO Conditioning Hair Dress *($3.99 for 5.5 ounces)*, 911 Leave-in Conditioner, Feather Light Creme Formula, Extra Dry *($3.19 for 18 ounces)*, 911 Leave-in Creme Conditioner, Original Formula *($3.19 for 8 ounces)*, Instant Oil Moisturizer Leave-in Conditioner *($4.19 for 12 ounces)*, and Break No More Creme Hair Dressing *($3.39 for 4 ounces)*; **African Royale** Extra Light Creme of Ginseng *($3.49 for 6 ounces)*, Extra Light Super G.R.O. with Ginseng *($5.19 for 6 ounces)*, Maximum Strength Super G.R.O. *($5.19 for 6 ounces)*, M.O.M. Miracle Oil Moisturizer *($3.59 for 8 ounces)*, and Mink Oil Gel for Hair and Scalp *($3.49 for 6 ounces)*; **Texture Line by ARTec** Smoothing Conditioner *($10.46 for 8 ounces)*; **Aubrey Organics** Blue Green Algae Hair Rescue Vegetal Protein Cream Rinse *($12 for 8 ounces)*, Green Tea Herbal Cream Rinse *($9.65 for 8 ounces)*, Honeysuckle Rose Hair & Scalp Conditioner *($8.75 for 4 ounces)*, Island Naturals Island Spice Cream Rinse *($7.75 for 8 ounces)*, Jojoba & Aloe Hair Rejuvenator & Conditioner *($12.85 for 4 ounces)*, Polynatural 60/80 Conditioner *($9 for 8 ounces)*, Rose Mosqueta Rose Hips Conditioning Hair Cream *($9.35 for 4 ounces)*, and Swimmers Conditioner *($8.15 for 8 ounces)*; **Aura** Cherry Almond Bark Revitalizing Conditioner for Dry, Damaged Hair *($6.99 for 8.75 ounces)*; **Aussie** 3 Minute Miracle Reconstructor Deep Conditioning for Damaged Hair *($6.39 for 16 ounces)*, Hair Insurance Leave-in Conditioner Vitamin Enriched *($3.99 for 8 ounces)*, and Instant Daily Conditioner for Daily Conditioning, High Protein Conditioner *($5.39 for 12 ounces)*; **Aveda** Curessence Intensive Repair Treatment for Damaged Hair *($25.44 for 18.4 ounces)* and Deep-Penetrating Hair Revitalizer, Intensive Hair Conditioner *($23.88 for 7.9 ounces)*; **Pure-Fume by Aveda** Pure-Fume Brilliant Conditioner for Treated, Dry, or Textured Hair *($18 for*

7.9 ounces); **All Sensitive by Aveda** All Sensitive Conditioner *($9.50 for 5.5 ounces);* **Avon** Techniques Tri-Nutriv Formula Hydrating Conditioner for Dry/Damaged Hair *($3.99 for 11 ounces);* **Back to Basics** Honey Hydrating Conditioner for Overworked Hair *($8.95 for 12 ounces),* Milk Conditioner *($8.95 for 12 ounces),* and Raspberry Almond Intensive Conditioner *($8.95 for 12 ounces);* **Basic Texture by Back to Basics** So Straight Smoothing Anti-Frizz Conditioner *($8.95 for 12 ounces);* **Bain de Terre** Botanical Boost Fortifying Conditioner *($8 for 10.2 ounces),* Herbal Conditioning Seal *($5.95 for 8 ounces),* and Marithyme Moisture-Rich Conditioner *($7.50 for 5 ounces);* **BioSilk** Fruit Cocktail Reconstructing Treatment *($11 for 10 ounces);* **The Body Shop** Intensive Treatment for Normal to Dry Damaged & Chemically Treated *($8 for 5 ounces);* **Citre Shine** Instant Repair Miracle Creme Conditioner for Dry or Damaged Hair *($3.99 for 5 ounces)* and Volumizing Conditioner for Fine to Normal Hair *($3.42 for 16 ounces);* **Frizz Control by Clairol** Taming Conditioner *($3.78 for 12 ounces);* **Dark & Lovely** 24-Hr. Therapy Moisture & Shine Replenisher *($4.99 for 8 ounces),* Beautiful Beginnings Vitamin E & Aloe Natural Oil Moisturizer Plus Detangler *($3.59 for 8 ounces),* Ultra Cholesterol Super Moisturizing & Conditioning Treatment *($2.49 for 15 ounces),* Ultra Cholesterol Plus Super Moisturizing/Conditioning Treatment *($2.49 for 15 ounces),* Corrective Leave-in Condition Therapy *($4.29 for 8 ounces),* Deep Penetrating Conditioner for Relaxed and Color-Treated Hair *($1.19 for 0.75 ounce),* Pro Therapy Protein Intensive Conditioner *($2.99 for 16 ounces),* Restore & Repair Reconstructive Hair Therapy *($2.59 for 4 ounces),* Rich & Natural Hair Dress Conditioner *($2.79 for 4 ounces),* and The Restorer Super Strengthening Hot Oil *($4.99 for 8 ounces);* **Finesse** Bodifying Conditioner for Fine or Thin Hair *($2.58 for 15 ounces),* Deep Fortifying Conditioner for Weak or Damaged Hair *($3.49 for 15 ounces),* Moisturizing Conditioner for Dry or Coarse Hair *($2.58 for 15 ounces),* and Revitalizing Conditioner for Permed, Colored or Overstyled Hair *($2.58 for 15 ounces);* **Focus 21** Hair Toys Moisturizing Spray *($5.62 for 8 ounces)* and Reconditioning Formula *($3.29 for 8 ounces);* **Framesi Biogenol** Biogenol Color Care System Ultra-Deep Masque Deep Conditioner *($11.95 for 4 ounces);* **Botanicals by Freeman** Cherry Humectant Conditioner for Dry or Damaged Hair *($3.49 for 16 ounces),* Hair Rescue Conditioner *($3.49 for 8 ounces),* Split-End Mender *($1.99 for 5 ounces),* and Instant Infusion Treatment, Sunflower Oil, Gardenia and Pennyroyal *($3.49 for 16 ounces);* **Salon Textures by Freeman** Salon Textures Daily Aire Conditioner *($3.99 for 7 ounces);* **Fudge** 1 Shot *($5.50 for 0.88 ounce),* The Conditioner *($8 for 10.14 ounces),* Dynamite Hair Rebuilder *($16 for 5.2 ounces),* and Oomf Conditioner Extra Gutz for Fine Limp Hair *($12 for 6.76 ounces);* **Goldwell** Care 5 Turbocharged Intensive Conditioner for Dry and Damaged Hair *($11.90 for 8.4 ounces)* and Care R Leave In Revitalizer *($11.90 for 7.6 ounces);* **Definition by Goldwell** Definition Dry & Porous Conditioner *($11.90 for*

12 ounces), Definition Dry & Porous Intensive Treatment *($25.95 for 16 ounces)*, and Definition Permed & Curly Conditioning Treatment *($11.90 for 12 ounces)*; **Exclusives by Goldwell** Exclusives Color Care Conditioner *($8.50 for 8 ounces)*, Exclusives Conditioner Moisturizing *($14 for 16 ounces)*, and Exclusives Turbo-Hydrating Conditioner *($9 for 12 ounces)*; **Kerasilk by Goldwell** Kerasilk Care & Gloss Shining Conditioner for All Hair Types *($9.50 for 5 ounces)*, Kerasilk Care & Smoothness Conditioning Treatment for Dry, Damaged, or Curly Hair *($7 for 3.4 ounces)*, and Kerasilk Conditioner *($7.25 for 3.3 ounces)*; **Intensives by Graham Webb** Intensives Pure Gold Conditioner Intense Moisturizer *($9.95 for 6 ounces)*, Intensives ThermaSilk Therapy Advanced Hair Recovery Treatment *($4 for 1 ounce)*, Intensives Vivid Color Moisturizing Conditioner *($11 for 8.5 ounces)*, and Intensives Silk Protein Leave In Conditioner and Reconstructor *($15 for 8.5 ounces)*; **Halsa Highlights** Herbal Swedish Formula Daily Conditioner, Chamomile and Rose Hips *($2.57 for 20 ounces)* and Herbal Swedish Formula Daily Conditioner, Marigold and Orange Blossom *($2.57 for 20 ounces)*; **Infusium** 23 Pro-Vitamin Hair Treatment Maximum Body Treatment for Fine/Thin Hair *($5.43 for 16 ounces)*, Maximum Body Revitalizing Conditioner for Fine/Thin Hair *($5.43 for 16 ounces)*, and Power Pac Treatment 5 Minute Formula *($3.44 for 1 ounce)*; **Jason Natural Cosmetics** Color-Treated Frizzy, Dry Hair Therapy Creme Conditioner *($9.49 for 8 ounces)*; **J. F. Lazartigue** Especially for Curly or Frizzy Hair Treatment Oil *($39 for 3.5 ounces)*; **Professional Prescription by Jheri Redding** Humectin Humidifier for Dry, Dull, Damaged Hair *($3.99 for 8 ounces)*, Super Protein Pac for Extremely Damaged Hair, pH Balanced Formula *($4.99 for 8 ounces)*, and Hot Oil Treatment for Dry, Brittle, and Dull Hair *($5.49 for 4 ounces)*; **Frizz-Ease by John Frieda** Glistening Creme Conditioner *($4.50 for 8 ounces)* and Prescription Oils, Hot Oil Treatment, with Natural Oils and Vitamin E *($4.99 for 1.8 ounces)*; **Ready to Wear by John Frieda** Miracle Mend, Deep Penetrating Conditioner *($4.99 for 4 ounces)* and Miraculous Recovery Conditioning Treatment, Professional Strength *($6.37 for 4 ounces)*; **Blue Line by Joico** Moisturizer Moisture Balancer *($7.25 for 4.4 ounces)*; **Kiehl's** Extra-Strength Conditioning Rinse for Dry Hair *($17.50 for 8 ounces)*, Extra-Strength Conditioning Rinse with Added Coconut *($10.95 for 4 ounces)*, High-Gloss Conditioning and Styling Oil for Hair *($19.95 for 1.5 ounces)*, and Deep Conditioning Protein Pak *($22.50 for 4 ounces)*; **KMS** RePlace Reconstructor, Moisture-Enriched for Dry, Damaged Hair *($6.95 for 4 ounces)*; **Flat Out by KMS** Flat Out Hair Repair Curl Control Reconstructor for All Hair Types *($10.50 for 8.11 ounces)*; **Moisture Replace by KMS** Moisture Replace Constructor *($10 for 8.1 ounces)* and Moisture Replace Deep Therapy *($8.95 for 3.4 ounces)*; **Rebalance by L'anza** Power Treatment, Active Conditioning Formula *($12.40 for 4.2 ounces)* and Strait-Line Curl Relaxing Conditioner *($9.96 for 6.7 ounces)*; **FortaVive by L'Oreal** FortaVive Weekly

Ceramide Replacement, Pure Strength with Ceramide-R 5-Minute Treatment *($1.59 for 1 ounce)*; **Motions at Home** Hair and Scalp Daily Moisturizing Hair Dressing *($4.62 for 6 ounces)*; **Nexxus** Humectress Moisturizing Conditioner *($16 for 16.9 ounces)* and Keraphix Creme Reconstructor *($22 for 16.9 ounces)*; **philosophy** shear splendor daily conditioner for chemically treated hair *($13 for 8 ounces)*; **Phytotherathrie** Phytherose Revitalizing Treatment for Dry Hair with Abyssinian Rose Tea (20%) *($18 for 5 ounces)*, Phytolait Beauty Milk for Hair *($15 for 1.3 ounces)*, and Phytomoelle Restorative and Rehydrating Mask for Very Dry Hair with Vegetal Marrow *($29 for 3.3 ounces)*; **PhytoSpecific by Phytotherathrie** Multi-Regenerating Creme Bath with Jojoba Oil, Deep-Down Treatment for Very Dry, Brittle and Damaged Hair *($19 for 6.75 ounces)*; **PhytoSpecific by Phytotherathrie** Revitalizing Treatment with Vegetal Oils for Dry Hair and Scalp *($19 for 3.35 ounces)*; **PhytoPlage by Phytotherathrie** After-Sun Repair Dual Usage Cream or Mask with Bancoulier Oil and Marsh Mallow *($17 for 2.5 ounces)*; **Professional** Detangling Conditioner *($4.60 for 16 ounces)*, Moisture Potion *($4.60 for 16 ounces)*, Special Treatment *($4.60 for 16 ounces)*, and Ultimate Reconstructor *($4.60 for 4 ounces)*; **Pro-Vitamin** Instant Repair Corrective Conditioner *($3.29 for 16 ounces)*, Maximum Body Conditioner *($3.99 for 10 ounces)*, MegaShine Conditioner *($3.99 for 10 ounces)*, Perm and Color Corrective Conditioner *($4.19 for 12.5 ounces)*, Special Effects Fat Hair Thickening Conditioner *($4.19 for 12.5 ounces)*, and Special Effects Straighten Out Straightening Conditioner *($4.19 for 12.5 ounces)*; **Queen Helene** Cholesterol Hair Conditioning Cream *($2.59 for 15 ounces)*, Cholesterol with Ginseng Conditioning/Strengthening Cream *($2.92 for 15 ounces)*, Placenta Cream Hair Conditioner with Panthenol *($3.49 for 15 ounces)*, Super Cholesterol Hair Conditioning Cream for Extremely Damaged Hair *($6.29 for 32 ounces)*, Jojoba Hot Oil Treatment *($5.49 for 8 ounces)*, Cholesterol Hot Oil Treatment *($5.49 for 8 ounces)*, and Placenta Hot Oil Treatment *($5.49 for 8 ounces)*; **Climatress by Redken** Climatress Conditioner for Normal to Dry Hair *($8 for 8.5 ounces)* and Climatress Treatment *($9.95 for 5 ounces)*; **St. Ives** Swiss Formula Wet Essential 2 Minute Moisture Deep Conditioning Treatment With Hydrating Liposomes *($.99 for 2 ounces)*; **Scruples** Cohesion Intercellular Hair Binder *($5.95 for 4 ounces)*, Moisturex Intensive Moisturizing Hair Treatment *($5.95 for 4 ounces)*, and Quickseal Fortifying Creme Conditioner *($5.95 for 4 ounces)*; **Senscience** Inner Conditioner for Coarse Hair *($12.39 for 16.9 ounces)*; **Sheenique** Silk Reforming Complex, Stops Breakage *($7.99 for 16 ounces)*, Nubian Silk Oil Treatment *($2.99 for 2 ounces)*, and Silk Braid Oil *($2.99 for 8 ounces)*; **Botanicals by Soft & Beautiful** Creme Moisturizer, Extra Light *($3.59 for 4 ounces)*, Hair Moisturizing Complex *($3.95 for 16 ounces)*, Oil Moisturizing Lotion *($3.72 for 8 ounces)*, Herbal Aloe Therapy Creme *($4.95 for 4 ounces)*, and Botanical Oil *($4.95 for 4 ounces)*; **Just for Me by Soft & Beautiful** Oil Moisturizing Lotion *($5.69 for 8 ounces)*; **Soft Sheen** Frizz Free Oil Moisturizer *($3.89 for 8 ounces)*; **Care Free Curl by Soft Sheen** Curl Activator *($3.29 for 8 ounces)*; **Optimum Care by Soft Sheen** Light Control with Aloe *($2.99 for 3.5 ounces)*, Moisture Rich with Vitamin E *($2.99 for 3.5 ounces)*, and Nourishment with Lanolin and Coconut *($2.99 for 3.5 ounces)*; **Baby Love by Soft Sheen** Moisturizing Creme Hair Dress *($3.99 for 4 ounces)* and Moisturizing Hairdress Lotion *($3.79 for 8 ounces)*; **TCB** Creme Hairdress, Aloe & Chamomile, for Moisture, Body and Shine *($3.19 for 6 ounces)*, Hair and Scalp Conditioner, Jojoba Oil, Chamomile & Aloe *($3.49 for 10 ounces)*, and Hair Food, Sweet Almond Oil, Jojoba & Olive Oil, Moisture Rich Treatment *($4.49 for 10 ounces)*; **Wanakee** Advanced Conditioning Treatment *($12.95 for 8 ounces)*, Moisture Emphasis Conditioner *($15.95 for 8 ounces)*, and Constant Care for Ends *($15 for 4 ounces)*; and **Wella Balsam** Instant Conditioner, Extra Body, Excellent for Fine, Limp, and/or Damaged Hair *($3.29 for 32 ounces)*, Instant Conditioner, Regular *($3.49 for 24 ounces)*, Kolestral Concentrate *($4.29 for 6 ounces)*, Kolestral Professional Treatment for Hair and Scalp *($3.49 for 6 ounces)*, and pH-D Diagnosis Regenal Instant Normalizer *($4.99 for 16 ounces)*.

The Best Lines with Temporary Color-Enhancing Conditioners

These include shades designed for gray hair to reduce yellow tones. **General guidelines for use:** Color-enhancing conditioners make the most difference for lighter hair shades rather than darker shades. They do not cover gray. The longer they are left on, the more likely the dye agent can cling to the hair. Unlike color-enhancing shampoos, the longer these conditioners are left on, the more conditioning they can be and the more the dye agents will cling to the hair. These can be used for everyday washing but they can eventually add too much color to lighter hair shades. It can be helpful to alternate with a different conditioner, from those listed above, that is suitable for your hair type and that does not contain dye agents.

<u>ALL HAIR TYPES:</u> **ARTec, Aveda, BioSilk, Colorance by Goldwell, John Frieda Sheer Blonde, Matrix, Paul Mitchell,** and **ColorStay by Revlon.**

The Best Silicone-Based Serums, Sprays, and Gels

These help make dry, coarse, or frizzy hair smoother. They can also help straighten hair, depending on the styling method. Use them sparingly or they can make hair look greasy. A handful of silicone serums also contain a small amount of film form- ers. These add shine and a silky feel but also help provide light to medium hold. The difference between this group of silicone-based sprays and gels and other types is that the overall performance of these products is that of a pure silicone product that is silky and slippery, while the gels and styling sprays in the next section are more about hold and forming hair. **General guidelines for use:** These are best used after sham- pooing and conditioning, but before applying other styling products such as gels or styling sprays.

<u>NO HOLD TO LIGHT HOLD:</u> **African Pride** Braid Sheen Spray *($3.99 for 12 ounces)*, Braid Sheen Spray Extra Conditioning Formula *($4.99 for 8 ounces)*, and Wonder Weave Intensive Shine Glosser *($3.99 for 2 ounces)*; **African Royale** Dia- mond Drops *($3.99 for 2 ounces)*; **Texture Line by ARTec** Shine & Frizz Repair *($12 for 2 ounces)*; **Aussie** Gloss *($5.44 for 2.02 ounces)*; **Aveda** Pure-Fume Brilliant Emol- lient for Hair *($14 for 3 ounces)* and Pure-Fume Brilliant Spray On for Hair *($14 for 3 ounces)*; **Avon** Techniques Tri-Nutriv Formula Leave-In Treatment for Lightweight Conditioning *($5.99 for 11 ounces)*, Techniques Tri-Nutriv Formula Dry End Serum *($5.99 for 1 ounce)*, Techniques Tri-Nutriv Formula Frizz Treatment Capsules *($5.99 for 18 capsules, 0.58 ounce total)*, and Techniques Tri-Nutriv Formula Heat Guard Blow Dry Treatment for Hair *($5.99 for 6.7 ounces)*; **Bain de Terre** Recovery Com- plex Spa Therapy *($22 for 4 ounces)*; **BioSilk** Shine On Brilliant Finish *($19.50 for 5 ounces)* and Silk Therapy *($40 for 4 ounces)*; **Bumble and Bumble** BB Straight *($18.40 for 5 ounces)*, Defrizz *($18.40 for 4 ounces)*, and Gloss *($11.20 for 4 ounces)*; **Citre Shine** Shine Miracle Anti-Frizz Polisher for All Hair Types *($5.91 for 4 ounces)*, Shine Miracle Laminator: An Extraordinary Shine Treatment for All Hair Types *($3.42 for 1 ounce)*, and Shine Mist Spray Laminator for All Hair Types *($3.42 for 3 ounces)*; **Frizz Control by Clairol** Defrizz Refresher & Shiner *($3.78 for 5 ounces)* and High Gloss Hair Serum *($4.79 for 2 ounces)*; **Focus 21** Liposheen Hair Restorer *($16.79 for 4 ounces)*; **BIO2 Tanicals by Focus 21** Shine In Polishing Spray *($9.50 for 2 ounces)* and Shine In Polishing Stick *($16 for 2.5 ounces)*; **Definition by Goldwell** Definition Finish & Shine Hair Shiner *($7.50 for 3.6 ounces)*; **Classic Line by Gra- ham Webb** Stick Straight High Gloss Shine and Anti-Frizz Serum *($16 for 2 ounces)*; **Bodacious by Graham Webb** Bodacious Silky and Soft Spray Shine *($8.75 for 4 ounces)*; **System Design by Hayashi** Hi-Shine Polishing Drops *($11.50 for 1 ounce)* and Spray & Shine Polishing Spray *($11.50 for 4 ounces)*; **Infusium 23** Hair Treat- ment Capsules *($5.43 for 18 0.034-ounce capsules)*; **Ion** Hot 'N' Moist Intensive Hair and Scalp Treatment *($1.99 for 1 ounce)*, Anti Frizz Oil Free Anhydrous Gloss *($7.99 for 1.8 ounces)*, and Anti Frizz Glossing Mist *($6.99 for 4 ounces)*; **Jason Natural Cosmetics** All Natural Hi-Shine Plus for Maximum Shine and UV Protection *($7.09 for 4 ounces)* and All Natural Frizz Control, Repairs Damage and Restores Shine for

Smooth, Soft Hair *($7.09 for 2 ounces);* **Jheri Redding** Frizz Out Hair Serum *($2.53 for 1.5 ounces);* **Professional Prescription by Jheri Redding** Replenishing Hair Shiner for All Hair Types *($7.49 for 4 ounces)* and Replenishing Mica Spray Polish for Normal, Dry, Damaged, or Chemically Treated Hair *($4.99 for 4 ounces);* **Jhirmack** HeatCare Styling Protectant *($2.99 for 7.7 ounces);* **Frizz-Ease by John Frieda** Hair Serum *($13.09 for 3 ounces)* and Instant Touch-up, Serum Spray *($6.30 for 3 ounces);* **Blue Line by Joico** Transformations Spray Glace *($14.95 for 4 ounces);* **KMS** Shine Complex Glossifier for Finishing *($11.95 for 2 ounces)* and Shine Complex Spray Glossifier, Shines, Smooths, Protects for Finishing *($10.50 for 4.23 ounces);* **Flat Out by KMS** Flat Out Weightless Shine Spray *($9 for 1.5 ounces)* and Flat Out Shine Serum *($8 for 1 ounce);* **Kenra** Reflect Shine Alcohol-Free Spray Shine *($11.95 for 2.2 ounces);* **Long Hair Formula by L'anza** ProtecShine *($14.95 for 1.7 ounces);* **Lange** Spray Shine for Hair *($11.99 for 4 ounces);* **Rebalance by L'anza** Shine Gel Controls and Softens Frizzy Hair *($13.49 for 3.3 ounces);* **Studio Line by L'Oreal** Studio Senses The Shiny Look Liquid Shine & Hold *($6.31 for 6 ounces)* and Studio Senses The Feel for Better Hair Texture *($3.99 for 8 ounces);* **Mastey** Lumineux Hair Shine Mist *($10 for 5.1 ounces);* **Logics by Matrix** Smooth FX *($12.50 for 1.7 ounces);* **Biolage by Matrix** Shine Renewal *($12 for 3.9 ounces);* **Vavoom by Matrix** Liquid Shine *($17.95 for 1.25 ounces)* and Spray Shine *($14.75 for 4 ounces);* **Motions at Home** Salon Sheen *($7.69 for 4 ounces);* **M Professional** Shine On Laminate Brilliant Shine Finish *($4.60 for 2 ounces)* and Defrizzer Elixer, Makes Hair Behave, *($4.60 for 2 ounces);* **Nexxus** Headress Design Shine *($14 for 1 ounce)* and Headress Hair Glow *($14 for 3.3 ounces);* **Nick Chavez Perfect Plus** Shine *($16 for 2 ounces);* **Ouidad** Shine Hair Glaze *($20 for 1 ounce);* **Paul Mitchell** Gloss *($20 for 5.1 ounces)* and The Shine *($13.50 for 4.2 ounces);* **philosophy** curly head silicone hair serum for frizzy hair *($11 for 2 ounces);* **Pro-Vitamin** Pro-Vitamin C Anti-Frizz Hair Serum *($5.99 for 2.75 ounces),* Pro-Vitamin E Instant Repair Hair Serum *($5.99 for 2.75 ounces),* Special Effects ColorShield, Color Extender/UV Protector *($5.99 for 5 ounces),* Special Effects Extreme Shine, Weightless Shine and Anti-Frizz Treatment *($5.99 for 5 ounces),* and Special Effects Straighten Out Hair Straightener and Anti-Frizz Serum *($5.99 for 5 ounces);* **Quantum** Lustre Finish for Instant Shine *($5.99 for 6.25 ounces);* **Redken** Glass Smoothing Complex 1 *($12 for 2 ounces);* **CAT by Redken** CAT Polishing Shine *($7.95 for 2 ounces);* **Robert Craig** Spray Shine 3-in-1 Formulation *($18 for 8 ounces);* **Rusk** Sheer Brilliance Polisher for Smooth, Refining & Shining *($13 for 4 ounces)* and Shining Sheen & Movement Mist *($12.10 for 4 ounces);* **Bonacure by Schwarzkopf** Gloss Tonic, Specific Formula *($8 for 5.1 ounces);* **Silhouette Styling System by Schwarzkopf** Gloss Creme Control & Shine *($11.90 for 1.8 ounces);* **Scruples** Renewal Hair Therapy Polish *($19.95 for 4 ounces);* **Laminates by Sebastian** Hi Gloss Spray *($9.50 for 1.7 ounces),* Gel *($17.80 for 5.1 ounces),* and Drops *($9.50 for 1.7 ounces)*; **Senscience** Simply Shine Lustre *($14.99 for 3.4 ounces)*, VitalRich Moisturizing Hairdress *($7.99 for 3.55 ounces)*, and VitalEsse Repair and Shine *($11.99 for 1.8 ounces)*; **Sheenique** Silk Sheen Spray On Hair Polish *($4.99 for 4 ounces)*; **Botanicals by Soft & Beautiful** Vitamin Enriched Oil Sheen with Sunscreen *($4.19 for 17.2 ounces)* and Oil Sheen with Sunscreen (Aerosol) *($3.19 for 10 ounces)*; **Optimum Care by Soft Sheen** Body & Shine *($2.99 for 14.2 ounces)*; **Rusk** Radical Sheen Texturizing Polishing Gel *($15.35 for 3 ounces)*; **St. Ives** Swiss Formula Hair Repair, No Frizz Retexturizing Serum *($3.79 for 1 ounce)*; **Susan Lucci Collection** Radiance *($19 for two 1-ounce containers)*, Super-Lite Radiance Spray Shine Mist *($18 for one 4-ounce container and one 2-ounce container)*, and Straight-A-Head Curl & Frizz Smoother *($15 for 6 ounces)*; **Terax** Tera Gloss Instant Restorer for Damaged Hair *($12 for 1 ounce)*; **TIGI** Styling Pure Gloss *($15.50 for 2 ounces)*; **Essensuals by TIGI** Spray Shine *($14.50 for 4.4 ounces)*; **Tresemme** European Tres Shine Anti-Frizz Shine Mist *($5.49 for 4 ounces)*; **Tressa** Smoothing Gloss Protective Shiner *($8 for 2 ounces)*; **Vertu by Tressa** Shine Aire *($12 for 8 ounces)*; **TRI** Tri Lights *($9.49 for 1 ounce)*; **Victoria Jackson** Brilliant Shine *($26, $15.95 for 1 ounce)*; **Liquid Hair by Wella** Hair Polish *($10 for 3.4 ounces)*; and **Zero Frizz** Anti-Frizz Hair Serum *($6.99 for 4 ounces)* and Anti-Frizz Glistening Mist *($6.99 for 4 ounces)*.

LIGHT TO MEDIUM HOLD: Texture Line by ARTec Texture Shine Spray (Non-Aerosol) *($12.56 for 4 ounces)*; **Citre Shine** Shine Miracle Volumizing Polisher for Normal to Fine Hair *($4.29 for 5 ounces)*, Straightening Balm *($3.42 for 3.3 ounces)*, Volumizing Shine Miracle Hair Polisher for Normal to Fine Hair *($5.91 for 4 ounces)*, and Straightening Balm *($3.42 for 3.3 ounces)*; **Framesi Biogenol** Color Care System One Tip Slip Ends Repair and Shiner *($9.90 for 2 ounces)*; **Fudge** Erekt Cold Turkey for Curly Hair *($17 for 4 ounces)* and Head Polish Silicone Shine *($14 for 1.4 ounces)*; **I.C.E. by Joico** Slicker Defining Lotion Supple Definition *($8 for 5 ounces)*; **J. F. Lazartigue** Root Volumizer for Hair, Volumizing Treatments After Shampoo Treatment *($18 for 2.54 ounces)*; **M.A.C.** Hair Gloss *($8 for 2.5 ounces)*; **Pro-Vitamin** Special Effects Fat Hair Thickening and Strengthening Serum *($5.99 for 5 ounces)*; and **Tresemme 4+4 Hair Straightener & Polisher** *($7.99 for 9 ounces)*.

The Best Styling Sprays (including Spray Gels)

These products help for all general styling needs ranging from holding curls to styling hair straight, but how they work all depends on your styling method. **General guidelines for use:** Apply in a thin layer over damp hair before styling. These can be applied over silicone serums or silicone sprays. A pomade, balm, cream, or wax can be used over more stubborn areas once hair is dry and styling is done, but before you use a hairspray.

LIGHT HOLD: All Ways Natural by African Pride 911 Heat Protector Heat Styling Protection *($3.29 for 8 ounces)*; **Aussie** MiraCurls Curls & Curves *($2.83 for 8 ounces)* and Spray Gel *($2.83 for 12 ounces)*; **Aveda** Flax Seed/Aloe Strong Hold Spray On Styling Gel *($10 for 8.45 ounces)*; **Dark & Lovely** Conditioning Setting Lotion for Relaxed & Color-Treated Hair *($2.79 for 8 ounces)*, Conditioning Set & Wrap All-Day Hold *($2.79 for 8 ounces)*, and Silky Set Conditioning Set & Wrap Lotion All-Day Hold *($3.69 for 8 ounces)*; **Garden Botanika** Protein Protective Spray Gel *($9.50 for 12 ounces)*; **Classic Line by Graham Webb** Styling VHS Volumizing & Thickening Spray *($10.96 for 8.5 ounces)*; **Hayashi** Spray and Curl Revitalizer for Natural and Permed Hair *($5.95 for 8.4 ounces)*; **Ion** Anti-Frizz Gel Styling Mist *($3.99 for 11.5 ounces)*; **ISO** Defining Lotion, Liquid Texturizer *($8.49 for 10 ounces)*; **Focus 21** Art Form Sculpting Spray (Non-Aerosol) *($3.99 for 8 ounces)*; **Enviro-Tek by Focus 21** Enviro-Tek Antioxidant Styling Spray *($6.25 for 12 ounces)*; **Framesi Biogenol** Color Care System Bodifying Spray *($8.96 for 10 ounces)*, Biogenol Pro-Form Thermal Setting Lotion *($8.99 for 10 ounces)*, and Biogenol Snapp Curl Rejuvenator *($8.99 for 10 ounces)*; **Beautiful Hair by Freeman** Beautiful Hair Botanicals Apple, Pear, and Peach Shaping Curl Control *($2.48 for 8.5 ounces)*, Beautiful Hair Botanicals Kiwi Fruit No Frizz Styling Gel Ultimate Hold *($3.49 for 8.5 ounces)*, and Beautiful Hair Botanicals Wild Cherry Shaping Shine Gel *($2.99 for 8.5 ounces)*; **Papaya Provita by Freeman** Papaya Silk Miracle Anti-Frizz Curling Spray with Ginseng *($1.99 for 10.1 ounces)*; **Jheri Redding** Blow-Dry Activated Thickening Spray *($2.24 for 6 ounces)*, Curl Energizer Frizz Control *($2.24 for 14 ounces)*, and Alcohol-Free Spray Gel *($2.24 for 14 ounces)*; **Frizz-Ease by John Frieda** 5-Minute Manager, Blow-Dry Lotion *($3.14 for 6.7 ounces)*; **Ready to Wear by John Frieda** Thickening Lotion, Instant Makeover for Fine/Limp Hair *($6.89 for 4.2 ounces)*; **Blue Line by Joico** Perm Endurance Perm Revitalizer and Styling Spray *($7.25 for 8.45 ounces)* and Travallo Design and Finishing Spray *($7.95 for 8.45 ounces)*; **Kenra** Thickening Spray Light Hold for Volume, Body and Shine 4 *($11.95 for 8 ounces)*; **Kiehl's** Hair Thickening Spray for Dry or Hard-to-Manage Hair (Non-Aerosol) *($10.95 for 4 ounces)* and Panthenol Protein Hair Conditioner Softener & Grooming Aid *($14.95 for 8 ounces)*; **AMP: Amino-Magnesium-Panthenol by KMS** Volume Amplifying Spray for All Hair Types *($9.95 for 8 ounces)*; **Lange** Panthenol Thermal Styling Spray *($6.49 for 8 ounces)* and Elastin Configuration 1, Fine, Limp Hair Thickener *($14.50 for 8 ounces)*; **Rebalance by L'anza** Gel Mist, Light Control Gel *($9.70 for 10.1 ounces)*; **Studio Line by L'Oreal** Studio Line Pumping Curls *($2.99 for 8 ounces)*; **Mastey** Enplace Hair Sculpting Liquid Gel Alcohol-Free *($9 for 10.2 ounces)* and Enplace Sculpting Lotion with Sunscreen *($5.90 for 5.1 ounces)*; **Logics by Matrix** Shine FX *($17.50 for 3.1 ounces)*; **Biolage by Matrix** Glaze *($12.75 for 13.5 ounces)*; **Nexxus** Styling and Finishing Hair Spray Natural Hold *($7.50 for 10.1* *ounces);* **Nick Chavez Perfect Plus** Volumizing Mist for Fine, Thin and Thinning Hair *($14 for 8 ounces)* and Plus Spray Gel, for Lift and Volume, Locks in Curl, Smoothes Frizzies *($12 for 8 ounces);* **Pantene** Pro-Vitamin Daily Heat Activated Conditioner *($3.39 for 10.2 ounces)* and Pro-Vitamin Styling Spray Gel, Extra Hold *($2.79 for 8.5 ounces);* **Paul Mitchell** The Heat Humidity Resistant Styling Spray *($11 for 8.5 ounces)* and Soft Sculpting Spray Gel *($7 for 8 ounces);* **Phytotherathrie** Phyto Style Heat-Protective Spray with Wheat Amino-Acids (Non-Aerosol) *($15 for 5 ounces);* **Quantum** Perm Revitalizer to Revive and Moisturize Curls *($3.99 for 8 ounces);* **Queen Helene** Designing Lotion, Maximum Hold *($3.29 for 16 ounces);* **Rave** Bodifying Gel Spray Ultra Hold Alcohol Free *($1.79 for 7.1 ounces);* **Redken** Airset Heat Styling Protectant Soft Control 3 *($6.95 for 8.5 ounces)* and Hot Sets Thermal Setting Mist 22 *($6.95 for 5 ounces);* **CAT by Redken** Fat CAT Body Booster Treatment for Fine Hair *($8.95 for 5 ounces);* **Robert Craig** Spray Gel 3-in-1 Formulation *($10 for 8 ounces);* **Rusk** Thick Body and Texture Amplifier *($10.90 for 6 ounces);* **Salon Selectives** Spray Gel Max Control Level 15 *($1.67 for 7 ounces);* **Salon Style by Lamaur** Design Elements Spray-on Styling Gel, Extra Hold *($2.27 for 10 ounces)* and Shaping Elixxer Alcohol-Free Spray Gel, Natural Hold *($2.29 for 8 ounces);* **Natural Styling by Schwarzkopf** Curl Revitalizer *($7.50 for 8.45 ounces);* **XTAH by Sebastian** XTAH Primer Pre-Fixxer *($15.96 for 8.5 ounces);* **Senscience** Inner Repair Leave-In Conditioner *($7.20 for 8 ounces);* **Natural Styling by Schwarzkopf** Setting Lotion *($8.20 for 8.45 ounces);* **Sheenique** Botanical Potion Wearable Treatment Highly Concentrated Botanical Leave-in Conditioner and Style Finisher *($5.99 for 5.1 ounces),* Stayz-N Leave-on Treatment *($2.99 for 8 ounces),* and Silk Braid Sheen Spray *($3.69 for 8 ounces);* **Botanicals by Soft & Beautiful** Perm Repair Leave-in Conditioner *($2.95 for 2 ounces);* **Soft Sheen** Wave Nouveau Finishing Mist *($3.99 for 12 ounces),* Finishing Mist *($3.99 for 12 ounces),* and Miss Cool Styling System Setting Lotion 5 Minute Fast Set *($2.99 for 8 ounces);* **Bone Strait by TCB** Spray Gel, Firm Hold for Slicking, Sculpting, Molding *($2.99 for 8 ounces);* **Theorie** HydroFy Hydrating Mist for Moisture and Heat Protection *($4.99 for 8 ounces);* **TIGI** Enviro-Fixx *($9.95 for 8 ounces);* **Tressa** Supplex Styling Lotion, Medium Hold for All Hair Types *($6.99 for 8 ounces)* and Perk-it Curl Revitalizer *($8 for 8 ounces);* **Trevor Sorbie** Lift-it Volumizer, Hair Thickening Spray for Root Lift and Volume *($8.21 for 8.5 ounces);* **TRI** Gel Spray *($7 for 8 ounces)* and Protein Bodifier Treatment *($7.99 for 8 ounces);* **Victoria Jackson** Accelerated Styling Mist *($14.95, $9.95 for 8 ounces);* **Vidal Sassoon** Spray-on Gel Extra Hold *($2.99 for 8.5 ounces);* and **Liquid Hair by Wella** Brilliant Spray Gel *($10 for 6 ounces).*

　　LIGHT TO MEDIUM HOLD: Apple Pectin by Lamaur Scentsates Apple Raspberry Spray Gel Medium Hold *($4.49 for 8 ounces);* **Basic Texture by Back to Basics** Be Thick Thickening & Texturizing Spray Gel *($8.95 for 8.5 ounces);* **Citre**

Shine Ultra-Hold Design Spritz Styler for Wet or Dry Application *($3.27 for 12 ounces)*; **Herbal Essences by Clairol** Spray Gel, Extra Hold for Targeted Control *($3.48 for 8.5 ounces)*; **Botanicals by Freeman** Peach Kernel, Butter Rose and Kola Nut Shaping Curl Control *($2.48 for 8.5 ounces)* and Botanical Hair Thickening Spritz *($3.99 for 6 ounces)*; **Goldwell Exclusives** Designing Super Shine Spray Gel *($9.50 for 8 ounces)*; **System Design by Hayashi** Volume + Firm Texture Design Mist *($7.90 for 8.4 ounces)*; **Infusium 23** Fortifying Spray Gel Extra Firm Hold Formula *($3.44 for 8 ounces)* and Fortifying Spray Gel Firm Hold Formula *($3.44 for 8 ounces)*; **Jhirmack** Spray Styling Gel *($2.72 for 8.4 ounces)*; **Blue Line by Joico** Spray Gel Liquid Styling Gel *($6.70 for 8.45 ounces)*; **Kenra** Thermal Styling Spray Firm Hold Heat Activated Styling Spray 19 *($10.95 for 8.5 ounces)*; **KMS** ThermaStat Thermal Styling Spray (Non-Aerosol) *($7.95 for 8 ounces)*; **Moisture Replace by KMS** Moisture Replace 2-in-1 Styling Spray *($8.95 for 8.5 ounces)*; **Lange** Texturizing Spray with Marine Collagen *($8.49 for 8 ounces)*; **Volume Formula by L'anza** Root Effects *($9.72 for 7.1 ounces)*; **Mastey** Designer Firm Hold Volumizing Liquid Mousse with Sunscreen *($5.90 for 5.1 ounces)* and Designer Soft Hold Volumizing Liquid Mousse with Sunscreen *($5.50 for 5.1 ounces)*; **Amplify Volumizing System by Matrix** Root Lifter *($13.75 for 8.5 ounces)*; **Biolage by Matrix** Hydro-Glaze Soft Styling Spray *($14.95 for 8.5 ounces)* and Thermal-Active Setting Spray *($14.50 for 8 ounces)*; **Vavoom by Matrix** Sculpting Spray Gel *($12.75 for 12 ounces)*; **Essentials by Matrix** Sculpting Glaze *($10.95 for 13.5 ounces)*; **Ouidad** Styling Mist *($9 for 8 ounces)*; **Paul Mitchell** Volumizing Spray *($11 for 8 ounces)*; **Phytotherathrie** Phytovolume Actif Volumizer Spray for Fine and Limp Hair, Enriched with Hair Protein *($16 for 3.3 ounces)*; **CAT by Redken** Fat CAT Body Booster Volumist for Fine Hair *($8.95 for 6 ounces)*; **Salon Formula by Suave** Salon Formula Spray Gel Extra Control *($0.78 for 7 ounces)*; **Theorie** SpecifiCurl Styling Mist for Curls and Waves *($4.13 for 8 ounces)*; **Essensuals by TIGI** Spray Gel *($11.95 for 8.5 ounces)*; **Trevor Sorbie** Lift-It Bodifier Medium Hold Spray Gel *($8.21 for 10 ounces)*; **TRI** Body Infusion *($9.99 for 9 ounces)*; **Senscience** Swing Thermal Setting Spray *($8.10 for 7.6 ounces)*; **Tresemme** European Tres Gel Spray Extra Hold *(2.76 for 10 ounces)*; **Vidal Sassoon** Alcohol-Free Spray-on Gel Extra Hold *($2.99 for 8.5 ounces)*; **Collections by White Rain** Maximum Hold Spray Gel with Chamomile & Rosemary Extracts *($0.99 for 7 ounces)*; and **Willow Lake** Rosehips & Ivy Spray Gel, Natural Hold *($2.91 for 8 ounces)*.

MEDIUM TO FIRM HOLD: Dep Level 6 Volumizing Spray Gel Extra Hold *($2.40 for 8 ounces)*; **Classic Line by Graham Webb** Styling Voltage High Gloss Sculpting Spray *($10.96 for 8.5 ounces)*; and **Kenra** Empower Spray Gel Medium to Firm Hold Styling Fixative 15 *($8.95 for 10.1 ounces)*.

The Best Gels (including Liquid Gels)

These gels are helpful for all general styling needs, from holding curls to styling hair straight, and how they work all depends on your styling method. **General guidelines for use:** Apply in a thin layer over damp hair before styling. These can be applied over silicone serums or silicone sprays. A pomade, balm, cream, or wax can then be used over more stubborn areas once styling is done but before you use a hairspray.

NO HOLD TO LIGHT HOLD: **African Pride** Wonder Weave Moisturizing Styling Gel *($3.99 for 8.5 ounces)*; **Alberto** Hairdressing Gel for Men, Extra Hold *($2.39 for 4.5 ounces)*; **Apple Pectin by Lamaur** Naturals Orange Flower & Clove Styling Gel *($4.49 for 8 ounces)*; **Texture Line by ARTec** Texture Gel *($10.46 for 8 ounces)*, Volume Gel *($10.46 for 8 ounces)*, and Smoothing Serum *($12.56 for 8 ounces)*; **Aubrey Organics** B-5 Design Gel *($10.55 for 8 ounces)* and Mandarin Magic Gingko Leaf & Ginseng Root Hair Moisturizing Jelly *($10.55 for 8 ounces)*; **Aura** Flax Seed Aloe Sculpting Gel *($5.49 for 8 ounces)*; **Aussie** Gelloteen Smoothing Gel *($2.89 for 8 ounces)* and Natural Gel *($2.83 for 7 ounces)*; **Avon Hair Care** Techniques Tri-Nutriv Formula Sculpting Gel for Shape & Control *($3.99 for 6 ounces)* and Techniques Tri-Nutriv Formula Hair Volumizer *($5.99 for 7.6 ounces)*; **Basic Texture by Back to Basics** Get Curly Curl Enhancing Gel *($9.95 for 6.8 ounces)*; **BioSilk** Glazing Gel Medium Hold *($8 for 10 ounces)*, Rock Hard Gelee Hard Hold Gel *($10 for 4 ounces)* and Silk Strate Temporary Straightener *($5 for 5 ounces)*; **Citre Shine** Style & Shine Gel, Clear Shine *($3.42 for 12 ounces)*, Style & Shine Gel, Frizz Control *($3.42 for 12 ounces)*, Style & Shine Gel, Mega Hold *($2.99 for 16 ounces)*, Style & Shine Gel, Super Hold *($3.42 for 12 ounces)*, and Styler Texture Style Potion *($3.42 for 5 ounces)*; **Clinique** Hair Shaper Gel Alcohol-Free *($10 for 4 ounces)*; **Dark & Lovely** Quick Styling Regular Hold Gel *($2.29 for ounces)* and Quick Styling Super Hold Gel *($2.29 for 4.5 ounces)*; **Dep** Level 2 Water-Based Gel Extra Shine with Light Control *($2.99 for 12 ounces)*, Level 3 Shine Gel Natural Hold *($1.99 for 4 ounces)*, Level 4 Water-Based Gel Super Control with Moisturizers *($2.99 for 12 ounces)*, Level 4 Shine Gel Natural Hold Non-Sticky *($2.99 for 12 ounces)*, Level 5 Volumizing Gel Flexible Hold *($2.99 for 12 ounces)*, Level 5 Water-Based Gel Extra Super Control *($2.40 for 12 ounces)*, and Level 5 Straightening Cream Flexible Hold *($3.19 for 5 ounces)*; **Focus 21** Hair Toys Gel *($3.82 for 8 ounces)* and Thikk Protective Hair Thickener *($3.46 for 4 ounces)*; **SeaPlasma by Focus 21** SeaPlasma Designing Gel *($3.99 for 12 ounces)* and SeaPlasma Moisture Mousse *($5.44 for 8 ounces)*; **Framesi Biogenol** Shine In Prep-It Style Start *($19.98 for 4 ounces)*; **Beautiful Hair by Freeman** Beautiful Hair Botanicals Kiwi Fruit No Frizz Styling Gel Ultimate Hold *($3.49 for 8.5 ounces)*; **Botanicals by Freeman** Hair Thickening Serum *($3.99* *for 4 ounces);* **Fudge** Hair Gum Hair Controller Hold Factor 1 *($14 for 5.2 ounces)* and Oomf Booster Styling Muscle for Fine Limp Hair *($12 for 6.76 ounces);* **Definition by Goldwell** Definition Style & Shine Creative Pomade *($7.90 for 3.4 ounces);* **Exclusives by Goldwell** Exclusives Designing Body-Building Styling Gel *($7.90 for 6 ounces)* and Exclusives Body-Building Designing Glaze *($7 for 8 ounces);* **Classic Line by Graham Webb** Styling Exothermic Styling Gel *($9.96 for 8.5 ounces)* and Styling Root Infusion Root Volumizing Serum *($10 for 4 ounces);* **System 911 by Hayashi** Gelplus Fixative Styling Gel with Natural Gums *($8 for 8.4 ounces);* **Infusium 23** Split End Repair, Repair Formula *($5.43 for 3 ounces);* **One 2 One Redken** One 2 One Straight Hair Straightening Balm *($12.50 for 5 ounces);* **J. F. Lazartigue** Hair Styling Gel *($20 for 3.4 ounces)* and Hair Volume Tonic, Root Volumizing Treatments After Shampoo Treatment *($32 for 3.4 ounces);* **Jheri Redding** Alcohol-Free Shine Gel *($2.79 for 20 ounces);* **Jhirmack** Alcohol-Free Sculpting Gel *($2.99 for 4 ounces);* **Blue Line by Joico** JoiGel Styling Gel *($7.95 for 8.8 ounces);* **I.C.E. by Joico** I.C.E. Sculpting Lotion *($6.60 for 8.45 ounces);* **Kenra** Texture-ize Light Hold Texturing Gel 6 *($6.95 for 4.2 ounces),* Styling Lotion Light Hold for Texture, Body and Shine 8 *($13.95 for 8 ounces),* and Straightening Serum, Smoothing and Conditioning Curl Relaxant *($12.95 for 10.1 ounces);* **Kiehl's** Extra Strength Styling Gel *($14.50 for 4 ounces);* **Puritives by KMS** Pure Gel Medium Hold *($8.95 for 8.79 ounces);* **L.A. Looks** Styling Gel, Body Building (Level 2) *($2.29 for 16 ounces),* Styling Gel, Frizz Control (Level 2) *($2.29 for 16 ounces),* Styling Gel, Shine Enhancing (Level 2) *($2.29 for 16 ounces),* and Styling Gel, Extra Super Hold (Level 3) *($2.29 for 16 ounces);* **Rebalance by L'anza** Mega Gel, Flexible Style Control Gel *($9.90 for 8.5 ounces)* and Anti-Oxidant Replenisher *($14.96 for 8.5 ounces);* **Studio Line by L'Oreal** Studio Line Anti-Frizz Alcohol-Free *($2.99 for 6 ounces);* **L'Oreal Kids** Extra Gentle Styling Gel Plus Manager, All Hair Types, Burst of Cherry-Almond, No Alcohol *($3.49 for 9 ounces);* **M.A.C.** Styling Gel *($7.60 for 5 ounces);* **M Professional** Serious Memory Gel *($4.60 for 9.5 ounces)* and Shaping Memory Gel Any Kind of Hair Don't Lose Control *($4.60 for 9.5 ounces);* **Mastey** Shine Naturel Wet & Shine with Sunscreen *($5.90 for 5.1 ounces);* **Amplify Volumizing System by Matrix** Liquid Gel *($12.75 for 5.1 ounces);* **Vavoom by Matrix** Forming Gel *($10.95 for 12 ounces)* and Smoothing Gel *($14 for 9.75 ounces);* **Ouidad** Tress F/X *($8 for 8 ounces);* **Pantene** Pro-Vitamin Sculpting Gel, Extra Hold, Alcohol Free *($2.79 for 7.1 ounces);* **Paul Mitchell** Extra-Body Sculpting Gel *($6.95 for 6 ounces),* Super Clean Sculpting Gel *($6.50 for 6 ounces),* and Hair Sculpting Lotion *($5.50 for 8 ounces);* **philosophy** memory styling gel *($12 for 4 ounces)* and let's get something straight straightening balm for humid climates *($12 for 4 ounces);* **Phytotherathrie** PhytoFix Setting Gel for All Hair Types *($15 for 3.3 ounces);* **Professional** Wearable Treatment *($4.60 for 16 ounces);* **Quantum** Smoothing Gel Thermal Activated *($5.99 for 7 ounces);* **Queen Helene Cholesterol Conditioning Styling Gel** *($3.29 for 16 ounces);* **Rave** Sculpting Gel Mega Hold Alcohol Free *($1.49 for 4 ounces);* **Redken One 2 One** Groom Brushing Gloss *($12.50 for 3.4 ounces);* **Silhouette Styling System by Schwarzkopf** Moulding Creme Ultra Control *($13 for 5.3 ounces);* **Scruples** Smooth Out Non-Chemical Straightening Gel *($11.95 for 8.5 ounces);* **Sebastian** Potion 7 Restructure and Reconditioning Treatment *($17.50 for 5.1 ounces),* Potion 9 Wearable Treatment to Restore and Restyle, Super Concentrated *($13.50 for 5.1 ounces),* and Wet Liquid Sculpting Gel *($7.80 for 10.2 ounces);* **Collectives by Sebastian** Thick-Ends: An Ends Conditioner *($11.30 for 5.1 ounces);* **Laminates by Sebastian** Get It Straitt *($17 for 8.5 ounces);* **Senscience** Straighten Out Smoothing Gel *($9.99 for 6.8 ounces);* **Sheenique** Silk Styling Gel Ultimate Hold *($3.99 for 16 ounces)* and Soft 'N' Clear Styling Gel *($3.99 for 16 ounces);* **Soft & Beautiful** Sculpting Gel *($4.95 for 8 ounces);* **Soft Sheen** Frizz Free Xtra Strength Moisturizing Gel Serum Especially for Coarse/Resistant Hair *($7.99 for 2 ounces);* **St. Ives** Professional Swiss Hair Care Styling Gel *($1.44 for 8 ounces);* **Style by Lamaur** Styling Gel Mega Hold *($0.99 for 7 ounces)* and Styling Gel Super Hold *($0.99 for 7 ounces);* **TCB Bone Strait** Lite Gel Activator, Aloe, Yucca & Chamomile, Moisturizes and Replenishes *($3.49 for 10 ounces)* and Shining Gel *($2.99 for 4 ounces);* **Theorie** Up Root Hydragel for Volume and Lift at the Roots *($5.13 for 4 ounces);* **ThermaSilk** Heat Activated Styling Gel Extra Control *($2.99 for 7 ounces);* **Tresemme** European Tres Gelee Styling Gel, Flexible Hold *($2.76 for 9 ounces);* **Vidal Sassoon** Alcohol-Free Styling Gel Extra Hold *($2.99 for 7.1 ounces);* and **Collections by White Rain** Extra Hold Styling Gel with Pro-vitamin B5 *($0.99 for 4 ounces).*

LIGHT TO MEDIUM HOLD: Aussie Styling Gel *($3.89 for 8 ounces);* **Pure-Fume by Aveda** Pure-Fume Brilliant Forming Gel *($10.50 for 4 ounces)* and Pure-Fume Brilliant Retexturing Gel *($15 for 7.9 ounces);* **Back to Basics** Vanilla Bean Forming Gel *($8.50 for 12 ounces)* and Wild Berry Firm Holding Styling Gel *($8.95 for 8.5 ounces);* **Bain de Terre** Flax Seed Styling Gel *($7.50 for 5 ounces);* **Citre Shine** Style & Shine Gel, Extra Body *($3.42 for 12 ounces);* **Herbal Essences by Clairol** Styling Gel, Extra Hold for Shape & Control *($3.48 for 8.5 ounces);* **Daily Defense by Clairol** Gel, Extra Hold for Styling Control *($3.18 for 7 ounces);* **Conditions 3-in-1 by Clairol** Gel, Extra Hold *($1.75 for 4 ounces),* Gel, Maximum Hold *($1.75 for 4 ounces),* Gel, Moisturizing *($1.75 for 4 ounces),* and Gel, Natural Hold *($1.75 for 4 ounces);* **Dep** Level 6 Moisturizing Gel Extra Hold *($2.40 for 12 ounces),* Level 7 Shaping Gel Extra Super Hold *($2.99 for 12 ounces),* and Level 8 Texturizing Gel Ultimate Hold *($2.99 for 12 ounces);* **Focus 21** Panasea Gel *($10.90 for 4 ounces);* **Splash by Focus 21** Splash Sculpting Gel Extra Firm *($8.39 for 16 ounces)* and Splash Sculpting Gel Firm Alcohol Free *($2.97 for 12 ounces);* **Framesi**

Biogenol Biogenol Color Care System Forming Glaze Strong Hold *($6.49 for 8 ounces)*, Framesi Biogenol Brash Hard Gel *($5.99 for 5 ounces)*, and Biogenol Definition Conditioning Cream Gel *($15.99 for 8 ounces)*; **Beautiful Hair by Freeman** Beautiful Hair Botanicals Wild Cherry Shaping Shine Gel *($2.99 for 8.5 ounces)*; **Botanicals by Freeman** Shaping Styling Gel Mega Hold Limeflower, Pineapple and Nettle *($2.85 for 8.5 ounces)* and Shaping Styling Gel Mega Hold Factor 30 *($2.85 for 8.5 ounces)*; **Fudge** Skrewd Gives Hair That Unexpected Twist Heat Responsive *($17 for 4.2 ounces)*; **Exclusives by Goldwell** Exclusives Designing Firm Holding Forming Lotion *($7.90 for 8 ounces)*; **System Design by Hayashi** Instant Replay Gel *($7.50 for 6 ounces)* and Uncurl Smoothing Glaze Keeps Hair Straight *($11.90 for 6.8 ounces)*; **Infusium 23** Pro-Vitamin Styling Gel Extra Firm Hold Formula *($3.44 for 4 ounces)*; **Ion** Anti-Frizz Styling Gelle for Textured and Maximum Hold Styling *($4.19 for 6 ounces)*; **ISO** Smoothie Gel, Texture Tamer *($8 for 5 ounces)*, Intensifying Gel, Brilliant Hold and Shine *($8.49 for 5 ounces)*, and SportStyler Firm, Flexible Gel *($8.49 for 5.1 ounces)*; **Jheri Redding** 3 in 1 Professional Gel *($1.89 for 16 ounces)*, Alcohol-Free Straightening Gel *($2.59 for 16 ounces)*, Alcohol-Free Volumizing Gel *($2.59 for 16 ounces)*, Alcohol-Free Frizz Out Gel *($2.79 for 20 ounces)*, Alcohol-Free Mega Hold Gel *($2.79 for 20 ounces)*, and Alcohol-Free Styling Gel Firm Hold *($2.24 for 8 ounces)*; **Professional Prescription by Jheri Redding** Styling Gel for All Hair Types *($4.49 for 6 ounces)*; **Frizz-Ease by John Frieda** Corrective Styling Gel with Encapsulated Silicone *($3.14 for 4 ounces)*; **Blue Line by Joico** Volissima Volumizing Gel *($9.50 for 8.45 ounces)*; **ICE by Joico** Controller Gel Full Effect *($7 for 5 ounces)*; **Kenra** Capture Glaze Medium Hold Styling Fixative 14 *($8.95 for 10.1 ounces)* and Root Volumizing Serum Volumizer for Root Lift and Style Support 20 *($11.95 for 6 ounces)*; **KMS** Styling & Setting Gel, Maximum Hold Gel for Finishing *($9.95 for 8.11 ounces)* and Sculpturing Lotion Styling Liquid, Light Hold Liquid for Finishing *($5.95 for 8 ounces)*; **Hair Play by KMS** Hair Play Tacky Gel *($12 for 4 ounces)*; **L.A. Looks** Styling Gel, Mega Hold (Level 4) *($2.29 for 16 ounces)* and Styling Gel, Mega Mega Hold (Level 5) *($2.29 for 16 ounces)*; **Lange** Designing Gelee Form Styler *($6.99 for 8 ounces)* and Super Shaper Gel Extra Firm Hold *($7.49 for 3 ounces)*; **Colors & Curls by L'anza** Liquid Gel *($8.90 for 6.7 ounces)*; **Studio Line by L'Oreal Studio** Line Anti-Sticky Invisi-Gel Alcohol-Free Extra Body *($2.99 for 6.8 ounces)*, Studio Line Anti-Sticky Invisi-Gel Alcohol-Free Mega Body *($2.99 for 6.8 ounces)*, Studio Line Total Control Clean Gel Alcohol Free Multi-Vitamin Formula Extra Hold *($2.99 for 6.8 ounces)*, Studio Line Mega Gel Multi-Vitamin Formula Mega Hold *($2.99 for 6.8 ounces)*, and Studio Line Lasting Curls Gel *($2.99 for 6 ounces)*; **Mastey** Le Gel Firm Hold Styling Gel Alcohol Free *($5.90 for 5.1 ounces)* and Le Gel Soft Hold Hair Styling Gel with Sunscreen *($5.90 for 5 ounces)*; **Vavoom by Matrix** Glazing *($10.95 for 4 ounces)*;

Logics by Matrix Designing Glissage Gel *($9.95 for 4.5 ounces)*; **Essentials by Matrix** Styling Gel *($9.95 for 4 ounces)*; **Biolage by Matrix** Defining Elixir Texturizing Jelly *($11 for 4 ounces)* and Gelee *($12.75 for 13.5 ounces)*; **Vital Nutrients by Matrix** BodyFusion Designing Gel *($9.99 for 8 ounces)*; **Nexxus** Versastyler Designing Lotion *($10 for 16.9 ounces)* and Fluid Styling Potion Liquid Gel *($8 for 8.4 ounces)*; **Phytotherathrie** Phyto Style Finishing Gel *($13.50 for 3.3 ounces)*; **Principal Secret** Perfect Styling Gel *($11, $7.75 for 6 ounces)*; **Professional** Forming Gel Coiffure *($3.29 for 12 ounces)* and Gel with Awapuhi *($3.29 for 12 ounces)*; **Quantum** Styling Gel Natural Hold for Sculpt, Style or Set *($4.99 for 7 ounces)*; **Queen Helene** Crystalene Clear Moisturizing Styling Gel for All Types of Hair Design *($3 for 16 ounces)*, Designing Gel for Maximum Hold and Extra Volume *($2.99 for 16 ounces)*, Styling Gel Normal *($3 for 16 ounces)*, Styling Gel Superhold *($3.19 for 16 ounces)*, Styling Gel Hard to Hold *($3.19 for 16 ounces)*, Sculpturing Gel & Glaze *($3 for 12 ounces)*, Liquid Styling Gel for Extra Control, Contouring and Shaping *($2.89 for 12 ounces)*, Pro-Rich Protein Conditioning and Styling Gel *($3 for 16 ounces)*, and Super Protein 4 in 1 Hair Conditioner and Styling Gel *($3.20 for 16 ounces)*; **Rave** Bodifying Gel Ultra Hold *($1.99 for 10 ounces)*; **Redken** Centigrade Thermactive Gel 4 *($11 for 8.5 ounces)* and Outline Fixing Gel 12 *($6.95 for 8.5 ounces)*; **CAT by Redken** Styling Gel *($7.50 for 6 ounces)* and Fat CAT Body Booster Fine Hair Thickening Lotion *($8.95 for 6 ounces)*; **Rusk** Jel Fx *($5.84 for 5 ounces)* and Jele Gloss Bodifying Lotion *($8.80 for 12 ounces)*; **Salon Selectives** Smoothing Gel Flexible Control Gel Level 10 *($1.67 for 7 ounces)*; Texturizing Gel Max Control Level 15 Alcohol-Free *($1.67 for 7 ounces)*, Sculpting Gel Ultra Control Level 20 Alcohol Free *($1.67 for 7 ounces)*, and Botanical Blends Texturizing Gel Extra Control Kiwi Jasmine Blend Alcohol-Free *($1.67 for 7 ounces)*; **Natural Styling by Schwarzkopf** Shaping Gel *($7.90 for 8.11 ounces)*; **Silhouette Styling System by Schwarzkopf** Styling Gel Super Hold *($7.90 for 8.75 ounces)*; **Scruples** Tea Tree Sculpting Glaze Concentrate *($7.95 for 8.5 ounces)*, Enforce Sculpting Glaze Concentrate *($5.95 for 4 ounces)*, and Renewal Forming Gel for Color Treated Hair *($6.50 for 6 ounces)*; **Performance Active by Sebastian** Texturizer & Body Builder *($16.50 for 8.5 ounces)*; **Shaper Slipline by Sebastian** Clean Gel *($10.50 for 10.2 ounces)*; **XTAH by Sebastian** XTAH Vinyl Fabricator *($18.86 for 4.4 ounces)*; **Sheenique** Silk Freez Style Gel *($3.99 for 16 ounces)*; **Soft Sheen** Alternatives Conditioning Styling Gel with MRC (Moisture Retention Complex) *($3.49 for 6 ounces)*; **Suave** Styling Gel Natural Control *($1.24 for 12 ounces)*, Styling Gel Extra Control *($1.24 for 12 ounces)*, and Styling Gel Maximum Control *($1.24 for 12 ounces)*; **Sukesha** Glossing Gel, Brilliant Shine Plus Hold Formula *($7.95 for 8 ounces)* and Styling Gel Ultimate Body and Hold Formula *($5.95 for 6 ounces)*; **Susan Lucci Collection** Sealer Gel-O Seal-Out Curl & Frizz Sculpt, Style & Hold *($25 for 4 ounces)*; **Terax** Gold Gomma Gel, Moulding

Gel *($10 for 5 ounces)*; **Theorie** VersaHold Multi-Use Styling Gel for Control and Versatility *($4.13 for 6 ounces)*; **Thicker, Fuller Hair** Instant Thickening Serum Volume & Texture *($5.59 for 4 ounces)*; **TIGI** Gel Gloss *($8.96 for 8 ounces)* and Molding Gel *($6.96 for 8 ounces)*; **Bed Head by TIGI** Power Trip Hair Gel *($12 for 7 ounces)*; **Tressa** Aglaze Forming Lotion, Light to Medium Hold for All Hair Types *($7.49 for 8 ounces)* and Brace Styling Gel Maximum Hold for All Hair Types *($6.49 for 4 ounces)*; **Tresemme** European Tres Gelee Styling Gel, Extra Hold *($2.76 for 9 ounces)* and 4+4 Styling Gel Fixative *($3.99 for 9 ounces)*; **Trevor Sorbie** Sculpte Jel Super Firm Support *($8.21 for 5 ounces)* and Sliquid Styling Gel *($5.99 for 8.5 ounces)*; **TRI** Bodyfusion Designing Gel *($9.99 for 8 ounces)* and Sculpture Styling Gel *($5.99 for 5 ounces)*; **Vertu by Tressa** Trans Foam Shaping Lotion *($16.50 for 7 ounces)*; **Collections by White Rain** Maximum Hold Styling Gel with Chamomile & Rosemary Extracts *($0.99 for 4 ounces)*; and **Zero Frizz** Anti-Frizz Styling Gel *($4.99 for 6 ounces)*.

   <u>**MEDIUM TO FIRM HOLD:**</u> **Intensives by Graham Webb** Intensives Power Gel Maximum Hold Styling & Setting Gel *($13.16 for 8 ounces)*, Intensives Vivid Color Firm Hold Foaming Gel, Color Locking Foaming Gel for Color Treated Hair *($10.50 for 6 ounces)*, and Intensives Making Waves Curl Defining Texturizer *($13.16 for 8.5 ounces)*; **I.C.E. by Joico** I.C.E. Gel Super Hold Styling Gel *($7.95 for 8.8 ounces)* and Thermal I.C.E. Heat-Activated Volumizer *($7.95 for 8.45 ounces)*; **Kenra** Endurance Gel Extra Firm-Hold Styling Fixative 21 *($9.95 for 10.1 ounces)* and Outcome Extra Gel Firm Hold Styling Fixative 17 *($8.95 for 10.1 ounces)*; **Flat Out by KMS** Flat Out Styling Shine Gel *($8 for 7 ounces)*; **Hair Stay by KMS** Hair Stay Styling Gel *($12.95 for 8.1 ounces)*; **Redken** Contour Shaping Lotion 8 *($6.95 for 8.5 ounces)*, Creatif Contour Shaping Lotion 8L *($13 for 16.9 ounces)*, and Hardwear Super Strong Gel 16 *($10 for 8.5 ounces)*; **Laminates by Sebastian** Get a Grip Liquid Texture *($16 for 5.1 ounces)*; and **Vertu by Tressa** Gelatin Bodifying Gel *($11 for 10 ounces)*.

The Best Mousses

   Mousses are helpful for all general styling needs ranging from holding curls to styling hair straight, and how they work depends completely on your styling method. Most typically mousses are used to hold curls or the natural shape of hair in place with minimal use of styling tools. **General guidelines for use:** Apply in a thin layer over damp hair before styling. These can be applied over silicone serums or silicone sprays. A pomade, balm, cream, or wax can then be used over more stubborn areas once styling is done but before you use a hairspray.

NO HOLD TO LIGHT HOLD: Alberto Alcohol-Free Styling Mousse, Conditioning Extra Hold *($2.29 for 7 ounces)* and Alcohol-Free Styling Mousse, Extra Body Extra Hold *($2.59 for 7 ounces);* **Apple Pectin by Lamaur** Naturals Chamomile & Sage Mousse *($4.49 for 8 ounces)* and Ultra Hold Styling Mousse *($4.99 for 8 ounces);* **Aura** Lemongrass Mousse Alcohol-Free Formula *($4.99 for 9 ounces);* **Aussie** Maximum Hold Mousse *($2.83 for 6.5 ounces);* **Aveda** Phomollient *($13.20 for 7 ounces);* **Avon Hair Care** Techniques Tri-Nutriv Formula Styling Mousse for Volume and Control *($3.99 for 6 ounces);* **Back to Basics** Sunflower Whipped Creme Mousse *($8.95 for 8 ounces);* **BioSilk** Silk Mousse Medium Hold *($9 for 10 ounces);* **Citre Shine** Super-Hold Styling Mousse Styler, for Wet or Dry Application *($3.42 for 8 ounces)* and Volumizing Mousse *($3.42 for 8.5 ounces);* **Classic Line by Graham Webb** Style Magnitude Mousse for Volume & Condition *($5.94 for 3 ounces);* **Infusium 23** Fortifying Mousse Extra Firm Hold Formula *($3.44 for 6 ounces)* and Fortifying Mousse Firm Hold Formula *($3.44 for 6 ounces);* **Kenra Artformation** Mousse Firm Hold Bodifying Formula 17 *($9.95 for 8 ounces)* and Volume Styling Mousse Medium Hold Conditioning Formula 12 *($9.95 for 8 ounces);* **Studio Line by L'Oreal** Studio Line Mega Mousse Mega Body *($2.99 for 6.9 ounces)* and Studio Line Springing Curls Mousse *($2.99 for 6 ounces);* **Logics by Matrix** Forming Foam *($12.95 for 10 ounces);* **Pantene** Pro-Vitamin Styling Mousse, Extra Hold for Control *($2.79 for 8 ounces);* **Phytotherathrie** Phyto Style Volumizing Mousse *($15 for 5 ounces);* **Robert Craig** Mousse 3-in-1 Formulation *($12 for 7 ounces);* **Salon Selectives** Botanical Blends Bodifying Mousse Extra Control Kiwi Jasmine Alcohol-Free *($1.67 for 7 ounces)* and Volumizing Mousse Flexible Control Level 10 Alcohol-Free *($1.67 for 7 ounces);* **Silhouette Styling System by Schwarzkopf** Non-Aerosol Styling Mousse Natural Hold *($13.90 for 6.8 ounces);* **Senscience** Effervesse Soft Styling Foam *($9.99 for 7.7 ounces);* **Soft Sheen** Frizz Free Leave-in Conditioning Foam *($4.99 for 7 ounces);* **Herbal Care by Suave** Herbal Care Mousse Extra Control Rosemary, Honeysuckle & Indigo Root *($1.39 for 6 ounces);* **ThermaSilk** Heat Activated Conditioning Mousse Extra Control *($2.99 for 7 ounces);* **Blue by TIGI** Catwalk Root Boost Foam-Lotion Spray for Texture & Lift *($11.50 for 8 ounces);* **Vidal Sassoon** Alcohol-Free Styling Mousse Extra Body for Volume *($2.99 for 8 ounces);* and **Elan Plus by Wella** Alcohol Free Extra-Hold Styling Foam *($2.99 for 10.6 ounces).*

LIGHT TO MEDIUM HOLD: Alberto Moisturizing Styling Mousse, Extra Control *($2.69 for 8 ounces);* **Texture Line by ARTec** Aeromousse (Aerosol) *($12.96 for 10 ounces)* and Texture Mousse *($11.96 for 8.5 ounces);* **Basic Texture by Back to Basics** Get Control Volumizing Mousse *($8.95 for 8.5 ounces);* **Bain de Terre** Botanical Boost Uplifting Root Foam *($8.95 for 8 ounces)* and Herbal Styling Mousse *($6.95 for 6.5 ounces);* **Frizz Control by Clairol** Restructurizing Mousse *($2.99 for 8 ounces);* **Herbal Essences by Clairol** Styling Mousse, Extra Hold, for Volume and

Manageability *($3.12 for 8 ounces)* and Styling Mousse, Maximum Hold, for Volume and Manageability *($3.11 for 8 ounces)*; **Daily Defense by Clairol** Mousse, Extra Hold for Body and Volume *($3.18 for 8 ounces)*; **Conditions 3-in-1 by Clairol** Mousse, Extra Hold *($1.75 for 6 ounces)*, Mousse, Moisturizing *($1.75 for 6 ounces)*, and Mousse, Natural Hold *($1.75 for 6 ounces)*; **Finesse** Touchables Mousse Extra Control Alcohol Free *($2.08 for 7 ounces)*, Touchables Mousse Moisturizing, Alcohol Free *($2.08 for 7 ounces)*, and Touchables Volumizing Foamer *($2.08 for 7 ounces)*; **Focus 21** Hair Candy Designing Mousse, Extra Body *($3.99 for 8 ounces)*; **Framesi Biogenol** Biogenol Color Care System Bodifying Foam Strong Hold *($9.96 for 9 ounces)*; **Salon Textures by Freeman** Salon Textures Volumizing Aire Mousse *($4.99 for 8 ounces)*; **Fudge** Pump Up *($20 for 7.1 ounces)*; **Exclusives by Goldwell** Exclusives Designing Firm Holding Mousse *($9.50 for 10.2 ounces)*; **Bodacious by Graham Webb** Bodacious Sculpting Foam *($8.95 for 8 ounces)*; **System Design by Hayashi** Triple Play Volumizing Mousse Strong Hold *($9.90 for 7 ounces)*, **Ion** Anti-Frizz Liquid Mousse Styling Spray *($3.99 for 12 ounces)*; **Ion** Styling Mousse Alcohol-Free *($4.49 for 10 ounces)*; **ISO** Transforming Foam Volumizing Mousse *($8.49 for 8 ounces)*; **Jason Natural Cosmetics** All Natural Mousse, All Hair Types *($7.09 for 7 ounces)*; **Jheri Redding** 3 in 1 Professional Mousse, Extra Control *($2.24 for 8 ounces)* and Alcohol-Free Mousse, Volumizing Ultra Control (Scented and Unscented) *($2.24 for 8 ounces)*; **Professional Prescription by Jheri Redding** Replenishing Polishing Mousse for Normal to Dry Hair *($4.49 for 9 ounces)*; **Frizz-Ease by John Frieda** Corrective Styling Mousse *($4.14 for 6 ounces)*; **Ready to Wear by John Frieda** Quick Coif, Thickening and Conditioning Mousse *($4.59 for 7.5 ounces)*; **I.C.E. by Joico** I.C.E. Whip Designing Foam *($11.95 for 10 ounces)*; **KMS** Mousse Styling Foam, Medium Hold Foam for Finishing *($8.45 for 6.17 ounces)*; **AMP: Amino-Magnesium-Panthenol by KMS** Volume Styling Foam, Firm Hold for All Hair Types *($9.50 for 6.17 ounces)*; **Hair Stay by KMS** Hair Stay Styling Foam *($14.95 for 8 ounces)*; **L.A. Looks** Gel 2 Mousse, Extra Super Hold & Body *($2.29 for 7.5 ounces)*, Gel 2 Mousse, Mega Hold & Body *($2.29 for 7.5 ounces)*, and Styling Mousse, Extra Super Body *($2.29 for 7 ounces)*; **Colors & Curls by L'anza** Bodifying Foam, Moisturizing Setting Foam *($8.95 for 7.1 ounces)* and Bodifying Foam, Super Hold and Shine *($9.40 for 7 ounces)*; **Biolage by Matrix** Hydro-Foaming Styler *($13.99 for 9 ounces)*; **Vavoom by Matrix** Pomousse *($20 for 3.75 ounces)* and Volumizing Foam *($13.50 for 9 ounces)*; **Nexxus** Mousse Plus Alcohol Free *($11.50 for 10.6 ounces)*; **Nick Chavez Perfect Plus** Aloe Mousse *($12 for 6 ounces)*; **Paul Mitchell** Extra Body Sculpting Foam *($9 for 6 ounces)* and Sculpting Foam *($8.50 for 6 ounces)*; **Quantum** Volumizing Foam for Instant Volume and Body *($5.49 for 9 ounces)*; **Rave** Bodifying Mousse Ultra Hold for Control *($1.99 for 13 ounces)* and Volumizing Mousse + Gel Volume & Lasting Control *($1.89 for 6 ounces)*; **Redken** Touch Control Texture Whip Styling 5 *($9.95 for 6.7 ounces);* **Rusk** Blofoam Spray-on Texturizing Foam *($11 for 10 ounces)* and Mousse Volumizing Foam *($12.10 for 8 ounces);* **Salon Selectives** Styling Foam Flexible Control Level 10 Air Infused Alcohol-Free *($1.67 for 7 ounces)* and Shaping Mousse Maximum Control Level 15 Alcohol-Free *($1.67 for 7 ounces);* **Salon Style by Lamaur** Body Boost Alcohol-Free Mousse with Botanicals, Extra Hold *($2.22 for 7 ounces);* **Silhouette Styling System by Schwarzkopf** Non-Aerosol Styling Mousse Super Hold *($13.90 for 6.8 ounces),* Styling Mousse Natural Hold *($8.50 for 6.5 ounces),* and Styling Mousse Super Hold *($8.50 for 6.5 ounces);* **Scruples** Creme Parfait Ultra Thick Styling Mousse *($9.95 for 10.6 ounces),* Emphasis Texturizing Styling Mousse *($5.95 for 6 ounces),* and More Emphasis Extra Body Styling Mousse *($5.95 for 6 ounces);* **Collectives by Sebastian** Fizz Styling Foam *($12.80 for 8 ounces)* and Fizz Extra Extra Firm Styling Foam *($13.40 for 8 ounces);* **Senscience** Volumesse Body Building Foam *($9.95 for 7 ounces);* **Style by Lamaur** Styling Mousse Extra Hold *($0.99 for 5 ounces);* **Suave** Styling Mousse Maximum Control *($1.23 for 7.5 ounces)* and Styling Mousse Extra Control *($1.23 for 7.5 ounces);* **Salon Formula by Suave** Salon Formula Mousse Extra Control *($1.23 for 7.5 ounces);* **Sukesha** Styling Mousse for Extra Control and Volume *($6.95 for 12 ounces);* **Terax** Terax Gold Mousse *($14.50 for 8.4 ounces);* **ThermaSilk** Heat Activated Volumizing Mousse Maximum Control *($2.99 for 7 ounces);* **TIGI** Strong Mousse for Fine to Medium Hair *($8.95 for 6 ounces);* **Tresemme** European Tres Foam, Volumizing *($2.76 for 7 ounces),* European Tres Mousse Styling Mousse, Extra Hold *($3.69 for 10.5 ounces),* European Tres Mousse Styling Mousse, Super Hold *($2.39 for 10.5 ounces)* and European Tres Mousse Thickening Styling Mousse *($2.39 for 10.5 ounces);* **Tresemme 4+4** Extra Hold Styling Mousse *($3.99 for 13.5 ounces)* and Special Solutions Split Ends Styling Mousse *($4.99 for 13.5 ounces);* **Trevor Sorbie** Design Forme Conditioning Styler Mousse for Soft Hold and Body *($9.95 for 7 ounces)* and Shaping Mousse for Volume and Control *($8.05 for 6 ounces);* and **TRI** Fashion Styling Mousse *($7.49 for 5.5 ounces);* **Vidal Sassoon** Alcohol-Free Styling Mousse Extra Hold for Control *($2.99 for 8 ounces);* **Collections by White Rain** Extra Body Mousse with Pro-Vitamin B5 & Conditioner *($1.59 for 5 ounces),* Maximum Hold Styling Mousse with Chamomile & Rosemary Extracts *($0.99 for 5 ounces),* and Extra Hold Styling Mousse with Pro-Vitamin B5 *($1.59 for 5 ounces);* **Willow Lake** Aloe and Clover Blossom Mousse, Extra Hold *($3.76 for 8.5 ounces);* and **Zero Frizz** Anti-Frizz Styling Mousse *($4.99 for 6 ounces).*

MEDIUM TO FIRM HOLD: Conditions 3-in-1 by Clairol Mousse, Maximum Hold *($1.89 for 6 ounces);* **Intensives by Graham Webb** Intensives Vivid Color Firm Hold Foaming Gel, Color Locking Foaming Gel for Color Treated Hair *($10.50 for 6 ounces);* **ICE by Joico** Amplifier Mousse *($13 for 8.8 ounces);* **Essentials by Matrix** Moussette Styling Foam *($12.95 for 9 ounces);* **Redken** Guts Volume Boosting Spray Foam 10 *($9.95 for 10.58 ounces)*; **CAT by Redken** CAT Sculpting Mousse *($9.50 for 7 ounces)*; **Theorie** Volume All-Over Clear Foam for Body and Control *($6.17 for 7 ounces)* and Volume All-Over Volumizing Foam *($6.17 for 7 ounces)*; and **TIGI** Extra Strong Mousse for Medium to Thick Hair *($8.95 for 6 ounces)*.

The Best Pomades, Balms, Creams, Lotions, Greases, and Waxes

The products in this group are the best for making coarse, frizzy, or curly hair smoother or straight, depending on your styling method. There is no advantage to using one version over another, other than personal preference. They all work the same by placing wax or rich emollients on hair to help gain control in styling. What all of these have in common is that they can make hair look and feel greasy, heavy, and flat, so use them sparingly and only where the most control is needed. **General guidelines for use:** These are best used in conjunction with other styling products such as gels or styling sprays, but only over stubborn frizzies or curls that need smoothing.

NO HOLD TO LIGHT HOLD: **Alberto** Conditioning Hairdressing, Extra Body for Fine Hair *($2.99 for 1.5 ounces)*, Conditioning Hairdressing, Normal/Dry Hair *($2.99 for 1.5 ounces)*, and Conditioning Hairdressing, Unscented *($2.99 for 1.5 ounces)*; **American Crew** Grooming Cream for Hold and Shine *($12.50 for 3.53 ounces)*, Pomade for Hold & Shine *($12.50 for 4 ounces)*, and Texture Creme for Control and Shine *($10 for 4 ounces)*; **Texture Line by ARTec** Texture Creme *($15.70 for 8.4 ounces)*; **Pure-Fume by Aveda** Pure-Fume Brilliant Anti-Humectant Pomade *($14 for 2 ounces)*, Pure-Fume Brilliant Humectant Pomade *($12.60 for 2 ounces)*; **Back to Basics** Sunflower Texturizing Creme *($9.98 for 4 ounces)* and So Straight Anti-Frizz Straightening Balm *($9.95 for 6.8 ounces)*; **Bain de Terre** Beezwax Styling Stick *($8.95 for 1.9 ounces)*; **BioSilk** Silk Pomade Designing Finish *($10 for 4 ounces)* and Silk Polish Shining Paste *($10 for 4 ounces)*; **The Body Shop** Coconut Oil Hair Shine *($5.45 for 1.7 ounces)* and Define & No Frizz Cream Texturizer, with Rose Hips Oil & Ginseng *($7.95 for 5.3 ounces)*; **Bumble and Bumble** Grooming Creme *($19 for 5 ounces)*, Styling Creme *($17 for 8 ounces)*, Styling Wax *($10.40 for 1.25 ounces)*, and Brilliantine *($12.40 for 2 ounces)*; **Citre Shine** Styler Glossing Wax *($4.29 for 1.4 ounces)*; **Frizz Control by Clairol** Taming Balm *($3.78 for 2 ounces)*; **Dark & Lovely** Vitamin E & Oil Scalp Conditioner and Hair Dress *($3.19 for 4 ounces)*; **BIO2 Tanicals by Focus 21** Shine In Polishing Cream *($16 for 5 ounces)*; **Framesi Biogenol** Shine In Polishing Cream *($16 for 5 ounces)*, and Stop-Frizz Anti-Humectant *($12.99 for 2 ounces)*; **Fudge** Hair Putty Hold Factor 3 *($14 for 3.5 ounces)*, Hair Licorice Hold Factor 5 *($14 for 3.5 ounces)*, and Hair Varnish Hold Factor 4 *($14 for*

3.17 ounces); **Exclusives by Goldwell** Exclusives Designing Gel Polish *($10 for 2 ounces);* **Classic Line by Graham Webb** Stick Straight Curl Relaxer Straightens & Smoothes *($13.16 for 6 ounces);* **System Design by Hayashi** Hi-Gloss Brilliantine *($7.80 for 2 ounces);* **Sheer Blonde by John Frieda** Golden Opportunity Glossing and Grooming Creme *($5.83 for 4.4 ounces);* **Frizz-Ease by John Frieda** Secret Weapon Styling Creme with 24-Hour Conditioning Action *($4.99 for 4 ounces);* **Blue Line by Joico** Brilliantine Shine Enhancing Pomade *($8.65 for 2 ounces)* and Straight Edge Heat-Activated Straightener *($11.80 for 8.45 ounces);* **I.C.E. by Joico** Waxer Water Soluble Wax *($15.50 for 4.2 ounces);* **Jheri Redding** Blow-Dry Acti-vated Straightening Lotion *($2.24 for 6 ounces);* **Kenra** Artform Pomade *($7.95 for 2 ounces);* **Kiehl's** Creme de la Creme Groom Repairateur with Silk *($13.50 for 2 ounces),* Creme with Silk Groom *($15.50 for 4 ounces),* Shine 'N Lite Groom for Dull or Thick Hair *($10.95 for 4 ounces),* and "Wet Look" Groom *($11.50 for 4 ounces);* **KMS** Configure Molding Creme for Shine, Control and Definition *($14.50 for 4.06 ounces);* **Flat Out by KMS** Flat Out Lite Relaxing Creme, Non-Chemical Curl Re-laxer and Defrizzant *($17.95 for 6 ounces)* and Flat Out Relaxing Balm, Non-Chemical Curl Relaxer and Defrizzant *($16.95 for 6 ounces);* **Curl Up by KMS** Curl Up Curl-ing Balm, Non-Chemical Curl Intensifier *($12.95 for 5 ounces);* **Hair Play by KMS** Hair Play Configure Creme *($10 for 4 ounces);* **Silker by KMS** Silker 2-in-1 Shaping Cream *($10 for 4 ounces);* **Rebalance by L'anza** Strait-Line Temporary Curl Relaxer and Smoother *($11 for 6.7 ounces);* **Volume Formula by L'anza** Body Styling Cream *($8.96 for 8.5 ounces);* **Studio Line by L'Oreal** Studio Senses The Touch Define & Shine Pomade *($4.49 for 2 ounces);* **M.A.C.** Curl Enhancer *($8 for 8.4 ounces);* **Icon for Men by Matrix** Grooming Cream *($7.99 for 4 ounces);* **Essentials by Matrix** Glossifier Hair Polish *($9.95 for 4 ounces);* **Vital Nutrients by Matrix** MoistureRich Fusion Defining Cream *($9.99 for 4 ounces);* **Nexxus** Retexxtur Transforming Po-made *($14 for 4 ounces);* **Nick Chavez Perfect Plus** Straightening Pomade *($14 for 8 ounces);* **Ouidad** Clear Control *($15 for 2 ounces);* **Paul Mitchell** Foaming Pomade *($10 for 5.1 ounces)* and Slick Works Definition with Shine *($12 for 5.1 ounces);* **Phytotherathrie** Phytobaume Untangling Balm for All Hair Types with Mallow *($15 for 6.8 ounces)* and Phytodefrisant Plant Based Relaxing Balm for All Hair Types *($15 for 3.3 ounces);* **PhytoSpecific by Phytotherathrie** Beauty Styling Creme for Normal to Dry Hair with Shea Butter *($13 for 3.38 ounces)* and Restructuring Milk with Canola Oil for Normal to Dry Hair *($17 for 5.07 ounces);* **Professional** Balm Revitalisant *($4.60 for 16 ounces);* **Pro-Vitamin** Special Effects Hair Control Hair Glossing and Styling Stick *($5.45 for 2.5 ounces);* **Redken** Details Conditioning Styling Complex 2 *($10 for 5 ounces),* Shine Design Weightless Finishing Gel 2L *($9 for 2.85 ounces),* Undone Weightless Finishing Creme 2 *($14.95 for 3.4 ounces),* and Water Wax Water Based Pomade 3 *($12.95 for 1.7 ounces);* **One 2 One by Redken**

One 2 One Smooth Anti-Frizz Creme *($12.50 for 3.4 ounces)*; **Robert Craig** Pomade *($8 for 2 ounces)*; **Rusk** Wired Internal Restructure Multiple Personality Styling Cream *($10.10 for 6 ounces)* and Str8 Anti-Frizz/Anti-Curl Lotion *($9.50 for 6 ounces)*; **Scruples** Total Accents Precision Creme *($9.95 for 5 ounces)*; **Collectives by Sebastian** Molding Mud Sculpting Bonder *($14.30 for 4 ounces)* and Grease Flexible Fixative *($8.10 for 1.5 ounces)*; **XTAH by Sebastian** XTAH Crude Clay Modeler *($17.50 for 4.4 ounces)*; **Terax** Luxcent Hair Pomade *($14 for 2.5 ounces)*; **Theorie** Smooth Styles Styling Creme for Definition and Smoothness *($6.17 for 5.5 ounces)*; **Blue by TIGI** Texturing Pomade with Essential Oils *($9.96 for 2 ounces)*, Hair Glaze *($9.95 for 1 ounce)*, and Thickening Cream with Essential Oils *($15.95 for 3.4 ounces)*; and **Trevor Sorbie** Glossaire *($9.49 for 2.6 ounces)* and Texturecreme Styler with Jojoba Oil *($9.99 for 5 ounces)*.

LIGHT TO MEDIUM HOLD: American Crew Fiber Pliable Molding Creme *($13.50 for 3.53 ounces)* and Thickening Lotion for Thicker Fuller Hair *($10.50 for 4.2 ounces)*; **Apple Pectin by Lamaur** Scentsates Apple Peach Styling Cream *($4.99 for 4 ounces)*; **Aveda** Self Control Hair Styling Stick *($18.60 for 2.5 ounces)*; **Pure-Fume by Aveda** Pure-Fume Brilliant Thermal Styling Creme *($14 for 8 ounces)*; **Back to Basics** Sunflower Sculpting Lotion *($3.95 for 4 ounces)*; **Basic Texture by Back to Basics** Be Thick Thickening Hair Creme *($9.95 for 6.8 ounces)*; **BioSilk** Molding Silk Designing Paste *($10 for 4 ounces)*; **Super Straight Hair by Freeman** Super Straight Hair Straightening Balm, Honeydew & Lilac *($3.69 for 5.3 ounces)*; **System Design by Hayashi** Texture Mud Design Adhesive *($13.90 for 3.5 ounces)*; **ISO** Bouncy Creme, Texture Energizer *($8 for 10.2 ounces)*; **I.C.E. by Joico** Forming I.C.E. Styling Creme *($12.80 for 4.2 ounces)* and Molder Texture Cream *($15 for 4.2 ounces)*; **Professional Prescription by Jheri Redding** Gelle Polish for Normal to Dry Hair *($4.49 for 8 ounces)*; **Ready to Wear by John Frieda** Shaping and Glossing Balm *($4.58 for 0.9 ounce)*; **KMS** Pomade Molding Gel *($14.50 for 4.06 ounces)* and Paste Molding Paste for All Hair Types *($12.50 for 3.5 ounces)*; **AMP: Amino-Magnesium-Panthenol by KMS** Volume Leave-in Thickening Cream for All Hair Types *($7.95 for 6 ounces)*; **Hair Play by KMS** Hair Play Defining Pomade *($10 for 4 ounces)*; **Hair Stay by KMS** Hair Stay Sculpting Lotion *($10.95 for 8.1 ounces)*; **Lange** Styling Creme with Marine Collagen *($9.49 for 8 ounces)*; **Bed Head by TIGI** A Hair Stick for Cool People *($17.96 for 2.7 ounces)*; **Tresemme** 4+4 Contour Hair Creme *($7.99 for 9 ounces)*; and **Vidal Sassoon** Hairline Essential Creme *($8.95 for 4 ounces)*.

MEDIUM TO FIRM HOLD: Kenra Molding Creme Firm Hold for Definition, Separation and Control 18 *($14.95 for 6.95 ounces)*; **Hair Play by KMS** Hair Play Molding Paste *($9 for 3.4 ounces)*; and **Paul Mitchell** Wax Works Control with Shine *($11.95 for 5 ounces)*.

The Best Hairsprays

When hairstyling is all done, hairspray is the classic way to make a hair design stay put. **General guidelines for use:** Apply in an even layer over hair for minimal hold or through the hair for overall hold. Aerosol hairsprays provide more of a light-weight mist, while pump hairsprays tend to concentrate the application. Generally both types are interchangeable and which one you chose just depends on personal preference.

<u>LIGHT HOLD:</u> **Alberto** Finishing Spritz, Firm Hold *($1.99 for 10 ounces)*, Hair Spray Hard to Hold *($2.99 for 8.5 ounces)*, Hair Spray Hard to Hold, Conditioning *($1.99 for 8.5 ounces)*, Hair Spray Hard to Hold, Extra Body *($1.99 for 8.5 ounces)*, Hair Spray Hard to Hold, Extra Body (Non-Aerosol) *($1.99 for 10 ounces)*, Hair Spray Hard to Hold, Unscented (Non-Aerosol) *($1.99 for 10 ounces)*, Hair Spray Hard to Hold, Silver *($1.99 for 8.5 ounces)*, Hair Spray Hard to Hold, Super *($1.99 for 8.5 ounces)*, and Hair Spray Hard to Hold, Unscented (Aerosol) *($1.99 for 8.5 ounces)*; **American Crew** Grooming Spray *($9 for 8.45 ounces)*; **Apple Pectin by Lamaur** Naturals Raspberry Leaves & Vitamin E Hair Spray *($4.49 for 11 ounces)*; **Aqua Net** 1 All-Purpose All Day All Over Hold, Fresh Fragrance and Unscented *($0.97 for 7 ounces)*; **Aussie** AirDo Flexible Hold Professional Styling Mist Aerosol *($2.97 for 7 ounces)*, AirDo Flexible Hold Professional Styling Mist Non-Aerosol (Unscented and Scented) *($2.97 for 8 ounces)*, Instant Freeze Aerosol *($2.83 for 7 ounces)*, Instant Freeze Non-Aerosol *($3.59 for 8 ounces)*, Mega Styling Spray, Aerosol *($2.78 for 14 ounces)*, Mega Styling Spray, Non-Aerosol *($2.83 for 12 ounces)*, Sprunch Spray Non-Aerosol (Scented and Unscented) *($3.59 for 12 ounces)*, and TwinFixx Spray Gel and Hairspray in One *($5.29 for 12 ounces)*; **Avon** Hair Care Techniques Tri-Nutriv Formula Finishing Hair Spray for Natural Hold and Control *($3.99 for 11 ounces)*, Hair Care Techniques Tri-Nutriv Formula Hair Spray for Extra Hold and All-Over Control Aerosol *($3.99 for 8 ounces)*, and Hair Care Techniques Tri-Nutriv Formula Mega Hold Styling Spritz *($3.99 for 7.6 ounces)*; **Back to Basics** Comfrey Natural Hold Finishing Spray *($6.95 for 8 ounces)*, Sunflower Firm Hold Hair Spray *($9.95 for 10 ounces)*, and Witch Hazel Firm Hold Hair Spray *($7.95 for 8 ounces)*, **BioSilk** Finishing Spray Natural Hold (Aerosol) *($10.80 for 10 ounces)* and Finishing Spray Firm Hold (Aerosol) *($10.80 for 10 ounces)*; **Bumble and Bumble** Hairspray *($9.20 for 8 ounces)*; **Conditions 3-in-1 by Clairol** Hairspray, Extra Hold (Aerosol—both Scented and Unscented) *($1.75 for 7 ounces)*, Hairspray, Extra Hold (Non-Aerosol—both Scented and Unscented) *($1.75 for 8 ounces)*, Hairspray, Natural Hold (Aerosol—both Scented and Unscented) *($1.75 for 7 ounces)*, and Sculpting Spritz *($1.75 for 8 ounces)*; **Finesse** Touchables Shaping Spray Dual Usage for Wet or Dry Hair *($2.08 for 7 ounces)*; **Salon Textures by Freeman** Salon Textures Shaping

Aire Hair Spray *($4.99 for 8 ounces)* and Salon Textures Zero Alcohol Aire Hair Spray *($4.99 for 8 ounces)*; **Garden Botanika** Hair Care Natural Finishing Spray *($8.50 for 12 ounces)*; **Jason Natural Cosmetics** Fresh Botanicals Hairspray Super Style Holding Natural Hold Alcohol Free (Non-Aerosol) *($4.66 for 8 ounces)*; **Jhirmack** Styling Spritz, Extra Hold Styling on Dry or Damp Hair *($2.99 for 8.4 ounces)*; **Puritives by KMS** Alcohol Free Hairspray Medium Hold *($10.25 for 8.45 ounces)*; **M.A.C.** Holding Spray *($7 for 8 ounces)*; **Mastey** Direction Shaper Spray *($5.90 for 5.1 ounces)*; **Logics by Matrix** Total Hold Spritz *($12.95 for 13.5 ounces)*; **Vital Nutrients by Matrix** BodyFusion Styling Spray *($9.86 for 10 ounces)*; **Phytotherathrie** Phytolaque Hair Spray for Sensitive Hair with Silk Proteins (Non Aerosol) *($15 for 3.3 ounces)*; **Salon Selectives** Perfect Curls Flexible Control Level 10 *($1.67 for 7 ounces)* **Salon Style by Lamaur** Protect 'N Shine Fixxer Hair Spray, Mega Hold with UVA Protectant *($2.22 for 10.5 ounces)*; **Collectives by Sebastian** Shpritz Light Finishing Spray *($8 for 10.2 ounces)*; **Laminates by Sebastian** Hair Spray (Aerosol) *($10.50 for 8.5 ounces)*; **Soft & Beautiful** Humidity Guard Holding Spray, Maximum Hold *($2.69 for 10.5 ounces)*; **Style by Lamaur** Hair Spray Maximum Control Mega Hold (Aerosol) *($1.29 for 7 ounces)*, Hair Spray Maximum Control Mega Hold (Non-Aerosol) *($1.29 for 7 ounces)*, Hair Spray Soft, Flexible Control Natural Hold (Aerosol) *($1.29 for 7 ounces)*, Hair Spray Long-Lasting Control Super Hold (Aerosol) Scented and Unscented *($1.29 for 7 ounces)*, and Hair Spray Long-Lasting Control Super Hold Scented and Unscented (Non-Aerosol) *($1.29 for 7 ounces)*; **Salon Formula by Suave** Hair Spray Extra Hold Aerosol *($0.78 for 7 ounces)* and Hair Spray Extra Hold Non-Aerosol *($0.78 for 7 ounces)*; **Herbal Care by Suave** Herbal Care Hairspray Non-Aerosol Flexible Hold Chamomile, Arnica & White Ginger *($1.39 for 8.5 ounces)* and Herbal Care Hairspray Aerosol Flexible Hold Chamomile, Arnica & White Ginger *($1.39 for 8.5 ounces)*; **TCB** Holding Spray, Jojoba & Chamomile, Exceptional Hold (Aerosol) *($3.29 for 11.9 ounces)*; **Terax** Aria Pura Volumizing Ecological Spray, Forte *($14 for 8.4 ounces)*, and Aria Pura Volumizing Ecological Spray *($14 for 8.4 ounces)*; **ThermaSilk** Heat Activated Shape & Hold Spray Firm Hold (Aerosol) *($2.99 for 7 ounces)*, Heat Activated Shape & Hold Spray Firm Hold (Non-Aerosol) *($2.99 for 10.5 ounces)*, Heat Activated Shape & Hold Spray Flexible Hold Aerosol *($2.99 for 7 ounces)*, and Heat Activated Shape & Hold Spray Flexible Hold Non-Aerosol *($2.99 for 10.5 ounces)*; **Tressa** Boost Spray Glaze with Bold Control *($7.99 for 8 ounces)*; **TRI** Aerogel (Non-Aerosol) *($10.99 for 8 ounces)*; **Victoria Jackson** Anti-Elements Holding Spray *($14.95, $9.95 for 8 ounces)*; **Collections by White Rain** Firm Hold Hair Spray Aerosol *($1.59 for 7 ounces)* and Extra Hold Hair Spray Aerosol Scented and Unscented *($1.59 for 7 ounces)*; and **Herbs & Blossoms by White Rain** Chamomile Hairspray Extra Hold *($1.07 for 7 ounces)*.

LIGHT TO MEDIUM HOLD: Adorn Hairspray for Long Lasting, Touchable Hold, Extra Hold (Aerosol) Scented and Unscented *($2.92 for 7.5 ounces)* and Hairspray for Long Lasting, Touchable Hold, Frequent Use No Build Up (Aerosol) *($2.92 for 7.5 ounces);* **All Ways Natural by African Pride** 911 Styling Spritz Extra Firm Hold *($2.71 for 8 ounces);* **Alberto Naturals** Non-Aerosol Hair Spray, Fruitsation (melon, wild berry, wheat germ extract), Super Hold *($1.99 for 10 ounces)* and Non-Aerosol Hair Spray, Vanilla Blossom (vanilla, honeysuckle, chamomile), Super Hold *($1.99 for 10 ounces);* **Aqua Net** 2 Super Hold All Day All Over Hold, Fresh Fragrance and Unscented *($0.97 for 7 ounces),* 3 Extra Super Hold All Day All Over Hold, Fresh Fragrance and Unscented *($0.97 for 7 ounces),* and 4 Ultimate Hold All Day All Over Hold, Fresh Fragrance and Unscented *($0.97 for 7 ounces);* **Texture Line by ARTec** Texture Freeze (Non-Aerosol) *($8.36 for 8 ounces)* and Texture Spray (Aerosol) *($9.76 for 10 ounces);* **Aubrey Organics** Natural Missst Hairspray *($6.35 for 4 ounces);* **Aussie** 12-Hour Humidity Spray *($2.83 for 12 ounces);* **Aveda** Air-O-Sol Witch Hazel Hair Spray (Aerosol) *($21 for 14.75 ounces);* **Back to Basics** Chamomile Sculpting and Volumizing Spray *($6.95 for 8 ounces);* **Beauty Without Cruelty** Natural Hold Hair Spray *($6.95 for 8.5 ounces);* **Bumble and Bumble** Holding Spray *($9.20 for 8 ounces);* **Citre Shine** Shaping Hair Spray *($3.42 for 8 ounces);* **Herbal Essences by Clairol** Hairspray, Extra Hold, for All-Over Control (Aerosol) *($3.48 for 8 ounces);* **Daily Defense by Clairol** Hairspray, Extra Hold for Lasting Control (Aerosol) *($3.18 for 8 ounces),* Non-Aerosol Hairspray, Extra Hold for Lasting Control *($3.18 for 8 ounces),* and Hairspray, Maximum Hold, for Lasting Control (Non-Aerosol) *($2.99 for 8.5 ounces);* **Conditions 3-in-1 by Clairol** Hairspray, Maximum Hold (Aerosol—both Scented and Unscented) *($1.75 for 7 ounces)* and Hairspray, Maximum Hold (Non-Aerosol—both Scented and Unscented) *($1.75 for 8 ounces);* **Clinique** Serious-Hold Hairspray Unscented *($10 for 6 ounces)* and Non-Aerosol Hairspray Unscented *($10 for 8 ounces);* **Dark & Lovely** Quik Freeze Super Shine Spritz *($3.49 for 8 ounces);* **Finesse** Touchables Hairspray Extra Hold, Aerosol (Scented and Unscented) *($2.08 for 7 ounces)* and Touchables Hair Spray Extra Hold, Non-Aerosol *($2.08 for 8.5 ounces);* **Focus 21 Changes** Flexible Hold Hair Spray (Non-Aerosol) *($3.49 for 12 ounces)* and Medium to Firm Hold Hair Spray (Non-Aerosol) *($3.19 for 8 ounces);* **Focus 21 Illusions** Design and Finishing Hair Spray, Medium Hold (Aerosol) *($4.51 for 10 ounces);* **Splash by Focus 21** Fashion Splash Design and Finishing Hair Spray, Extra Firm Hold (Aerosol) *($6.99 for 9.5 ounces),* Splash Finishing Spray *($2.97 for 12 ounces),* and Splash Flexible Hold Spray *($2.97 for 12 ounces);* **Framesi Biogenol** Color Care System Design Spray Strong Hold (Aerosol) *($9.90 for 10 ounces),* Color Care System Finishing Spray Firm Hold (Non-Aerosol) *($8.90 for 10 ounces),* Shine In Take Hold (Aerosol) *($8.49 for 10 ounces),* Hold 10 Extra Strong Hold *($9.99 for 10 ounces),* and Myste

Finishing Spray *($8.99 for 10 ounces)*; **Beautiful Hair by Freeman** Beautiful Hair Botanicals Hawaiian Ginger Conditioning Freeze Spritzer Maximum Hold *($3.49 for 8.5 ounces)* and Freeze Spritzer Mega Hold, Prescription for Maximum Hold, Honeysuckle, Marigold and Wild Chamomile *($2.48 for 8 ounces)*; **Papaya Provita by Freeman Papaya** Silk Miracle Control Ultra Spritzer with Ginseng Maximum Hold & Ultimate Control *($1.99 for 10.1 ounces)* and Papaya ProVita Sculpting Spritzer for Touchable Hold *($1.99 for 10.1 ounces)*; **Big Thick Hair by Freeman** Big Thick Hair Spritzer *($2.74 for 6 ounces)*; **Real Shiny Hair by Freeman** Real Shiny Hair Spritzer *($2.74 for 6 ounces)*; **Fudge** Hair Cement The Exceptional Finishing Spray *($9 for 10.01 ounces)*; **System 911 by Hayashi** Spray Plus Finishing Spray for Damaged Hair *($8.50 for 8.4 ounces)*, Freeze-It Working Spray *($7.90 for 8.4 ounces)*, and Quikk Fast Dry Working Spray (Aerosol) *($12.50 for 10.6 ounces)*; **System Hinoki by Hayashi** Finishing Spray Control and Shine for Fine and Thinning Hair *($7.90 for 8.4 ounces)*; **Infusium 23** Pro-Vitamin Hair Spray Extra Firm Hold Formula (Non-Aerosol) *($3.44 for 8 ounces)* and Pro-Vitamin Hair Spray Firm Hold Formula (Non-Aerosol) *($3.44 for 8 ounces)*; **ISO** Creative Hair Spray, Flexible Shaping Spray (Aerosol) *($8.49 for 10 ounces)* and Enduring Spritz Firm, Lasting Hold *($8.49 for 10 ounces)*; **Jheri Redding** Design Spritz, Super Hold (Non-Aerosol) Scented and Unscented *($2.24 for 14 ounces)*, Glossing Design Spritz, Super Hold (Aerosol) *($2.24 for 14 ounces)*, Flexible Hold Hair Spray (Aerosol) *($2.59 for 10.5 ounces)*, Flexible Hold Hair Spray (Non-Aerosol) Scented and Unscented *($2.24 for 12 ounces)*, and Shine Hair Spray, Super Hold (Aerosol) Scented and Unscented *($2.24 for 10 ounces)*; **Professional Prescription by Jheri Redding** Styling Spray for All Hair Types *($4.49 for 8 ounces)*; **Jhirmack** Extra Hold Hairspray Level 2 (Non-Aerosol) Scented and Unscented *($2.99 for 8.4 ounces)*, Silver Extra Hold Hairspray Level 2 (Aerosol) *($2.99 for 7 ounces)*, and Ultimate Hold Hairspray Level 3 (Non-Aerosol) *($2.99 for 8.4 ounces)*; **Frizz-Ease by John Frieda** Moisture Barrier Hair Spray (Aerosol) *($3.14 for 10 ounces)*; **Ready to Wear by John Frieda** Modeling Spray, Flexible Hold Spritz (Non-Aerosol) *($4.59 for 6.7 ounces)*; **Blue Line by Joico** Styling Spray Thermal Designing Spray *($8.65 for 8.45 ounces)*, Transformation Styling Spray *($8.95 for 8.45 ounces)*, JoiMist Firm Super-Hold Finishing Spray (Aerosol) *($8.95 for 10.5 ounces)*, and JoiMist Shaping Spray *($9.80 for 10.5 ounces)*; **ICE by Joico** Finisher Hair Spray Medium Impact (Aerosol) *($10 for 10.5 ounces)* and Fixer Hair Spray High Impact (Non-Aerosol) *($10 for 10 ounces)*; **Kenra** Capture Plus Spray Extra Firm Hold Finishing Formula 23 *($8.95 for 10.1 ounces)*; **KMS** HairHold Styling Spray, Medium Hold Spray for Finishing (Non-Aerosol) *($5 for 8 ounces)*, **ProliFixx** Finishing Spray, Medium Hold (Aerosol) *($9.95 for 9.5 ounces)*, ProliMaxx Finishing Spray, Maximum Hold (Aerosol) *($9.95 for 9.5 ounces)*, ProliForce Finishing Spray, Maximum Hold Spray for Finishing *($7.95 for 8 ounces)*, ProliFree

Alcohol-Free Hairspray, Medium Hold Spray for Finishing (Non-Aerosol) *($7.95 for 8 ounces)*, and **ProliMist** Pure Finishing Spray, Soft Hold Spray for Finishing *($9.95 for 12 ounces)*; **Flat Out by KMS** Stay Smooth Spray, Soft Hold, High Shine Finishing Spray *($8.95 for 7 ounces)*; **Hair Stay by KMS** Hair Stay Max Hold Spray (Non-Aerosol) *($12.95 for 8.5 ounces)*; **Hair Stay by KMS** Hair Stay Medium Hold Aerosol *($12.95 for 9.5 ounces)*; **L.A. Looks** Touchable Hold Finishing Spray (Level 2) (Aerosol) *($2.29 for 7.5 ounces)*, Touchable Hold Finishing Spray (Level 2) (Non-Aerosol) *($2.29 for 7.5 ounces)*, Finishing Spritz,. Extra Super Hold (Level 3) *($2.29 for 7.5 ounces)*, Finishing Spray (Level 2) (Aerosol), Style 'N Hold Shaping Spray, Mega Hold (Level 3) (Non-Aerosol) *($1.99 for 7 ounces)*, Style 'N Hold Shaping Spray, Ultimate Hold (Level 4) (Non-Aerosol) *($1.99 for 7 ounces)*, Ultimate Finishing Spray, Extra Super Hold (Level 3) (Aerosol) *($1.77 for 7 ounces)*, Ultimate Finishing Spray, Extra Super Hold (Level 3) (Non-Aerosol) *($2.29 for 7.5 ounces)*, and Ultimate Finishing Spray, Mega Hold (Level 4) (Aerosol) *($2.29 for 7.5 ounces)*; **Colors & Curls by L'anza** Finishing Freeze *($9.80 for 10.1 ounces)*; **Rebalance by L'anza** Special F/X, Light Styling Spray *($9.80 for 10.6 ounces)* and Styling Spritz, for Curling Iron Styling *($8.95 for 10.1 ounces)*; **Volume Formula by L'anza** Finishing Protector Dryspray *($9.96 for 8.5 ounces)*; **Studio Line by L'Oreal** Studio Line Mega Spritz Multi-Vitamin Formula Mega Hold *($2.99 for 8.5 ounces)*, Studio Line Mighty Mist Hair Spray Extra Hold *($2.99 for 8 ounces)*, and Studio Line Mighty Mist Hair Spray Mega Hold *($2.99 for 8 ounces)*; **Mastey** Fixe Firm Hold Finishing Hair Spray with Sunscreen *($5.90 for 5.1 ounces)*, Fixe Soft Hold Finishing Hair Spray with Sunscreen *($5.90 for 5.1 ounces)*, and Rigide Spritz for Maximum Hold with Sunscreen *($5.50 for 5.1 ounces)*; **Logics by Matrix** Thermal Fixative *($11.99 for 13.5 ounces)*; **Essentials by Matrix** Finishing Spray *($7.50 for 14 ounces)* and Proforma Hair Spray Aerosol *($12.95 for 12 ounces)*; **Biolage by Matrix** Complete Control Hair Spray Firm Hold *($13.50 for 10 ounces)*, Firm-Active Hair Spray Extra Firm *($14.25 for 8.5 ounces)*, Natural Finish Hair Spray *($8.50 for 10 ounces)*, and Finishing Spritz *($14.50 for 13.5 ounces)*; **Motions at Home** Light Hold Working Spritz for Curling and for Hold *($3.16 for 10 ounces)*; **Neutrogena** Hairspray for Permed or Color-Treated Hair, Natural Hold *($5.29 for 7 ounces)* and Hairspray for Permed or Color-Treated Hair, Super Hold *($5.29 for 7 ounces)*; **Nexxus** Headress Shaping Spray *($7.50 for 10.6 ounces)*, Hairspray Styling Versatility *($7.50 for 10.1 ounces)*, Maxximum Super Holding Hair Spray *($7.50 for 10.1 ounces)*, Sculpting and Finishing Spray Maxximum *($7.50 for 10.1 ounces)*, and Hair Spray Body Building Firm Hold *($7.50 for 10.1 ounces)*; **Pantene** Pro-Vitamin Hairspray Flexible Hold with Elastesse (Aerosol) *($2.79 for 8.25 ounces)*, Pro-Vitamin Hairspray Flexible Hold with Elastesse for Fine Hair (Aerosol) *($2.79 for 8.25 ounces)*, Pro-Vitamin Hairspray Flexible Hold with Elastesse Unscented (Non-Aerosol) *($2.79 for 10 ounces)*, and

Pro-Vitamin Wet or Dry Styling and Holding Spray, Extra Firm Hold (Non-Aerosol) *($2.79 for 8.5 ounces);* **Paul Mitchell** Fast Drying Sculpting Spray *($8 for 8 ounces);* **philosophy** hold that thought anti-frizz hair spray *($14 for 8 ounces);* **Phytotherathrie** Phytolaque Hair Spray for All Hair Types with Vegetal Lacquer Proteins (Non Aerosol) *($15 for 3.3 ounces)* and Phyto Style Holding Spray (Non-Aerosol) *($15 for 5 ounces);* **Professional** Brilliant Shine/Firm Hold Hairspray (Non-Aerosol) *($3.62 for 12 ounces),* Extra Hold Finishing Spray (Non-Aerosol) *($3.62 for 12 ounces),* Ultra-Shaping Hair Spray (Aerosol) *($4.34 for 10 ounces),* and Ultra-Shaping Hair Spray Plus (Aerosol) *($4.34 for 10 ounces);* **Rave** Sculpting Spritz Mega Hold *($1.99 for 14 ounces),* Hairspray 2-Super Hold Non-Aerosol *($1.49 for 7 ounces),* Hairspray 2 Super Hold Aerosol Scented or Unscented *($1.49 for 7 ounces),* Hairspray 3 Ultra Hold Aerosol Scented or Unscented *($1.99 for 14 ounces),* Hairspray 3 Ultra Hold Unscented Non-Aerosol *($0.89 for 7 ounces),* Hairspray Plus Conditioning Nutrients 3+ Ultra Hold *($1.49 for 7 ounces),* Microspray 3 Ultra Hold Micro Droplet Technology Aerosol *($1.59 for 3.5 ounces),* Microspray 4 Mega Hold Micro Droplet Technology Aerosol *($1.59 for 3.5 ounces),* and Hairspray 4 Mega Hold Aerosol Scented and Unscented *($1.50 for 14 ounces);* **Redken** Lift & Shine Finishing Spritz 15 *($7.50 for 8.5 ounces)* and Body & Bounce Sculpting Spray Gel 6 *($7.50 for 8.5 ounces);* **CAT by Redken** CAT Finishing Spritz *($7.75 for 10.1 ounces)* and Fat CAT Body Booster Plump Spray for Fine Hair *($10 for 11 ounces);* **Robert Craig** Spray Finishing 3-in-1 Formulation *($10 for 8 ounces);* **Salon Selectives** Finishing Spray Flexible Hold Level 10 Non-Aerosol *($1.67 for 7 ounces),* Finishing Spray Flexible Hold Level 10 Aerosol *($1.67 for 7 ounces),* Finishing Spray Maximum Hold Level 15 Non-Aerosol Scented and Unscented *($1.67 for 7 ounces),* Finishing Spray Maximum Hold Level 15 Aerosol *($1.67 for 7 ounces),* Spritz Fixx Ultra Hold Level 20 Non-Aerosol *($1.67 for 7 ounces),* Style Freeze Ultra Hold Level 20 Aerosol *($1.67 for 7 ounces),* Botanical Blends Finishing Spray Extra Hold Kiwi Jasmine Blend Aerosol Dual Usage *($1.67 for 7 ounces),* and Botanical Blends Finishing Spray Extra Hold Kiwi Jasmine Blend Non-Aerosol *($1.67 for 7 ounces);* **Salon Style by Lamaur** Design Elements Non-Aerosol Hair Spray Flexible Hold *($2.27 for 10 ounces)* and ProMist Quick Drying Hairspray, Mega Hold *($2.22 for 9.5 ounces);* **Silhouette Styling System by Schwarzkopf** Non-Aerosol Hairspray Natural Hold *($9.50 for 8.45 ounces)* and Non-Aerosol Hairspray Super Hold *($8.80 for 8.45 ounces);* **Scruples** V2 Double Volume for Hair *($9.95 for 8.5 ounces);* **Collectives by Sebastian** Shpritz Forte Extra Strength Finishing Spray *($8.50 for 10.2 ounces)* and Hold & Mold Spray Gel Styling and Finishing Spray *($10.30 for 10.2 ounces);* **Performance Active by Sebastian** Volumizer & Finishing Spray *($13 for 8.5 ounces);* **Sheenique** Silk Freez Spritz (Non-Aerosol) *($2.99 for 8 ounces)* and Super Hold Hair Spray (Aerosol) *($2.89 for 10 ounces);* **Optimum Care by Soft Sheen** Firm Holding Spritz *($3.59 for*

8 ounces) and Soft Holding Spritz *($2.99 for 8 ounces)*; **St. Ives** Swiss Formula Silk and Keratin, European Styling and Finishing Hairspray, Extra Hold *($1.78 for 10 ounces)* and Swiss Formula Silk and Keratin, European Styling and Finishing Hairspray, Ultimate Hold *($1.78 for 10 ounces)*; **Suave** Hairspray Extra Hold Aerosol *($0.78 for 7 ounces)*, Hairspray Extra Hold Non-Aerosol *($0.78 for 7 ounces)*, Hairspray Maximum Hold Aerosol *($0.78 for 7 ounces)*, and Hairspray Maximum Hold Non-Aerosol *($0.78 for 7 ounces)*; **Herbal Care by Suave** Herbal Care Hairspray Non-Aerosol Extra Hold Passion Flower, Goldenseal & Witch Hazel *($1.89 for 14 ounces)*; **Susan Lucci Collection** Pollution Shield Hairspray Healthy Hair Complex Advanced Formula *($12.75 for two 8-ounce containers)* and Collection Climate Control Hairspray Alcohol Free *($12.75 for two 8-ounce containers)*; **TCB** Designing Spritz, Chamomile, Almond Oil & Jojoba Oil, All Day Hold *($3.49 for 10 ounces)*; **Bone Strait by TCB** 12 Hour Holding Spritz, Lite Hold *($1.99 for 12 ounces)* and Spritz, Super Hold *($2.29 for 8 ounces)*; **Bed Head by TIGI** Hard Head Hard Hold Hairspray (Aerosol) *($11.95 for 10 ounces)*; **Blue by TIGI** Catwalk Medium Hold Working Hairspray *($11.95 for 8 ounces)*; **Trevor Sorbie** Affix Hair Spray for Extra Firm Hold *($8.55 for 10 ounces)*, Finishe Forme Energizing Hair Spray *($7.91 for 10 ounces)*, Spraye *($7.91 for 10 ounces)*, and Hot Shapes Thermo-Protective Spray for Heat Styling *($6.53 for 5 ounces)*; **TRI** Control and Finishing Mist *($6.99 for 8 ounces)*, Covert Control Holding Spray *($8.49 for 9 ounces)*, and Aerogel (Aerosol) *($8.99 for 6 ounces)*; **Vidal Sassoon** Finishing Hair Spray, Extra Hold (Aerosol) *($3.59 for 8.5 ounces)*, Non-Aerosol Finishing Hairspray Extra Hold Unscented *($2.99 for 10.2 ounces)*, and Styling Freeze, Maximum Hold (Non-Aerosol) *($2.24 for 8.5 ounces)*; **Collections by White Rain** Extra Hold Hair Spray For Extra Long Lasting Hold Non-Aerosol Scented and Unscented *($1.59 for 7 ounces)*, Extra Hold Hair Spray with Pro-Vitamin B5 Non-Aerosol *($0.86 for 8.75 ounces)*, Extra Hold Styling Spritz with Pro-Vitamin B5 *($0.99 for 7 ounces)*, Hair Spray Maximum Hold Aerosol *($1.59 for 7 ounces)*, and Maximum Hold Hair Spray with Chamomile & Rosemary Extracts Non-Aerosol *($0.99 for 7 ounces)*; **Willow Lake** White Lily and Jasmine Hair Spray, Extra Hold Aerosol *($3.76 for 8.5 ounces)*, Raspberry Leaf & Vitamin E Non-Aerosol Hair Spray, Extra Hold *($2.91 for 8 ounces)*, and Orange Blossom & Clove Spritz, Maximum Hold *($2.91 for 8 ounces)*.

    <u>MEDIUM TO FIRM HOLD:</u> **All Ways Natural by African Pride** 911 Super Spritz *($2.71 for 8 ounces)*; **Apple Pectin by Lamaur** Naturals Rose Hips & Lemon Grass Spritz *($3.99 for 8 ounces)* and Ultra Hold Spritz *($3.69 for 8 ounces)*; **Texture Line by ARTec** Texture Spray Firm (Aerosol) *($9.76 for 10 ounces)*; **Aura** Lavender Ultra-Firm Freezing Spray *($4.99 for 7 ounces)*, Witch Hazel Hair Spray (Non-Aerosol) *($4.69 for 8 ounces)*, and Witch Hazel Super Shaping Hair Spray (Aerosol) *($5.99 for 10 ounces)*; **Aveda** Firmata Firm Hold Hair Spray *($12.50 for 8.4 ounces)* and

Witch Hazel Medium Hold Hair Spray (Aerosol) *($9 for 8.45 ounces);* **Basic Texture by Back to Basics** Get Control Maximum Hold Hair Spray *($9.95 for 11.5 ounces);* **Bain de Terre** Finishing Mist *($6.95 for 13 ounces),* Finishing Spritz *($6.95 for 8 ounces),* Goldenseal Shaping Spray *($6.95 for 7.6 ounces),* and Mint Balm Spray Stylizer *($7.50 for 7.6 ounces);* **BioSilk** Spray Spritz Firm Hold Styling Spray (Non-Aerosol) *($8.80 for 10 ounces);* **Citre Shine** Mega-Hold Finishing Spray Styler, for Dry Application (Non-Aerosol) *($3.42 for 12 ounces)* and Mega-Hold Finishing Spray Styler, Professional Hair Spray (Aerosol) *($3.42 for 10 ounces);* **Herbal Essences by Clairol** Hairspray, Extra Hold for Lasting Control (Non-Aerosol) *($3.48 for 8.5 ounces),* Hairspray, Maximum Hold, for All-Over Control (Aerosol) *($3.11 for 8 ounces),* Hairspray, Maximum Hold for Lasting Control (Non-Aerosol) *($3.11 for 8.5 ounces),* and Styling Spritz, Maximum Hold, for Ultimate Control *($3.48 for 8.5 ounces);* **Final Net by Clairol** All-Day Hold Hairspray, Extra Hold, Light Scent *($2.59 for 12 ounces),* Hold that Moves Hairspray, Extra Hold, Scented and Unscented *($2.59 for 12 ounces),* Hold that Moves Hairspray, Regular Hold, Scented and Unscented *($2.59 for 12 ounces),* and Hold that Moves Hairspray, Ultimate Hold, Scented and Unscented *($2.59 for 12 ounces);* **Dep** Level 7 Finishing Hairspray Extra Super Hold *($3.19 for 8 ounces);* **Finesse** Touchables Hairspray Maximum Hold, Aerosol *($2.08 for 7 ounces)* and Touchables Hairspray Maximum Hold, Non-Aerosol *($2.08 for 8.5 ounces);* **BIO2 Tanicals by Focus 21** Flash Freeze Plus Design and Finishing Hair Spray, Extra Firm Hold (Aerosol) *($10.90 for 10 ounces)* and Flash Freeze Plus Shine Mango Design and Finishing Hair Spray, Extra Firm Hold (Non Aerosol) *($9.70 for 12 ounces);* **Salon Textures by Freeman** Salon Textures Easy Hold Aire Spritzer *($4.99 for 8 ounces);* **Exclusives by Goldwell** Exclusives Finishing Super Firm & Dry Spray *($9.50 for 8.5 ounces)* and Exclusives Finishing Super Firm Spray (Non-Aerosol) *($7.90 for 8 ounces);* **Bodacious by Graham Webb** Bodacious Finishing Hair Spray *($6.95 for 10 ounces);* **Classic Line by Graham Webb** Jet Stream *($7.95 for 8 ounces),* Finish Energy Lock Maximum Hold Hair Spray *($12.04 for 10 ounces),* and Finish Super Hold & Shine Firm Hold Hair Spray *($10.96 for 8.5 ounces);* **Intensives by Graham Webb** Intensives Total Control Silk Protein Finishing and Styling Hair Spray *($10.96 for 8 ounces),* Intensives Visible Control Silk Protein Finishing and Styling Hair Spray *($10 for 8 ounces),* and Intensives Vivid Color Hair Spray, Color Locking Protection with Firm Hold for Color Treated Hair *($12.72 for 10 ounces);* **Ion** Hydrolac Hair Spray Extra Firm Humidity-Proof Hold *($2.99 for 11 ounces),* Long-Lasting Hold Hair Spray with Electro Bond Proteins *($3.99 for 8 ounces),* Styling Spritz Super Hold for Freeze and Shine Styling, Wet or Dry *($3.99 for 8 ounces),* Flexible Hold Finishing Spray *($3.99 for 8 ounces),* Hard-to-Hold Hair Spray *($2.99 for 11 ounces),* Super Hold Spritz with Electro-Bond Proteins *($3.99 for 8 ounces),* Shaping Plus Styling Spray Super Hold for Hard to Control Styles *($4.99 for 10* *ounces)*, and Anti-Frizz Alcohol-Free Hair Spray *($3.99 for 8 ounces)*; **ISO** Ultimate Hold Shaping Spray, Firm Extra Hold (Aerosol) *($10.49 for 10 ounces)* and SportFinish Shaping Spray (Non-Aerosol) *($8.49 for 10.2 ounces)*; **Professional Prescription by Jheri Redding** Ultra Hold Hair Spray for All Hair Types *($2.69 for 11 ounces)*; **Jhirmack** Freeze Quick Drying Hairspray Level 4 (Aerosol) *($2.99 for 7 ounces)* and Freeze Quick Drying Hairspray Level 4 (Non-Aerosol) *($2.99 for 8.4 ounces)*; **I.C.E. by Joico** Mist Super-Hold Finishing Spray *($3.60 for 2 ounces)*; **Kenra** Artform Spray Firm Hold Styling and Finishing Spray 18 *($11.95 for 12 ounces)*, Endurance Fragrance-Free Long-Lasting Styling Spray 21 *($9.95 for 10.1 ounces)*, Volume Spray Super Hold Finishing Spray *($11 for 12 ounces)*, and Design Spray Light Hold Styling Spray 9 *($11.95 for 12 ounces)*; **Lange** Ultra-Hold Finishing Spray *($8.99 for 8 ounces)*; **Colors & Curls by L'anza** Dramatic F/X Super Hold Hairspray *($9.90 for 10.6 ounces)*; **Amplify Volumizing System by Matrix** Volumizing System Hair Spray *($13.75 for 10 ounces)*; **Icon for Men by Matrix** Controlling Spray (Aerosol) *($8.99 for 10 ounces)* and Natural Holding Spray *($8.99 for 8 ounces)*; **Logics by Matrix** Performance Spray *($10.94 for 10 ounces)*; **Essentials by Matrix** Vital Control Hair Spray *($12.95 for 14.8 ounces)* and Freeze Spray *($12.95 for 12 ounces)*; **Vavoom by Matrix** Freezing Spray *($12.25 for 14.8 ounces)*, Professional Styling Spray *($17.50 for 15 ounces)*, Shaping Spray (Aerosol) *($12.75 for 10 ounces)*, and Spritzing Spray Extra *($12.75 for 12 ounces)*; **Nexxus** Comb Thru Hair Spray *($7.50 for 10.6 ounces)* and Firmist Hair Spray *($7.50 for 10.6 ounces)*; **Nick Chavez Perfect Plus** Hairspray, Quick Drying, Super Hold *($10 for 8 ounces)*; **Pantene** Pro-Vitamin Hairspray Ultra Firm Hold (Aerosol) *($2.79 for 8.25 ounces)*, Pro-Vitamin Hairspray Ultra Firm Hold (Non-Aerosol) (Scented and Unscented) *($2.79 for 10.2 ounces)*, and Pro-Vitamin Fixation Spritz, Maximum Hold *($2.79 for 8.5 ounces)*; **Paul Mitchell** Super Clean Spray with Awapuhi *($9.50 for 10 ounces)*, Super Clean Extra Firm Holding Spray *($10 for 10 ounces)*, Freeze and Shine Super Spray *($9 for 8 ounces)*, and Soft Spray *($7 for 8 ounces)*; **Principal Secret** Super Control Hair Spray *($13, $9 for 10 ounces)*; **Professional** Sculpting Shaping Spray (Non-Aerosol) *($3.62 for 12 ounces)*; **Quantum** Finishing Spray for Firm, Flexible Hold *($4.99 for 11 ounces)* and Spritz for Firm Hold *($4.99 for 8 ounces)*; **Rave** Hairspray 4 Mega Hold Fresh Fragrance Non Aerosol *($0.89 for 7 ounces)*; **Redken Amino Pon** Hairspray Firm Hold 16 *($8 for 11 ounces)*; **Redken** Quick Dry Shaping Mist 18 *($9.90 for 11 ounces)*, Framework Designing Spray 20 *($10 for 11 ounces)*, Suspend Forming and Mending Spray Firm Control 16 *($7 for 5 ounces)*, and Direct Airosol Mist Ultra Hold 26S *($6.95 for 8.5 ounces)*; **Climatress by Redken** High Humidity Hairspray *($7.95 for 11 ounces)*; **One 2 One by Redken** Stay Firm Hold Treatment Spray *($9.50 for 5 ounces)*; **Rusk** Radical Hold *($9.95 for 8 ounces)*, Worx Atomizer Fixing/Finishing Spray *($12.50 for 10 ounces)*, Worx Working/Finishing Spray *($12.50 for 10 ounces)*, W8less Plus

Extra Hold Shaping and Control Myst *($11 for 10 ounces)*, W8less Shaping and Control Myst *($10 for 2 ounces)*, and Spray Bombe Working/Finishing Spray *($8 for 8 ounces)*; **Silhouette Styling System by Schwarzkopf** Hairspray Super Hold (Aerosol) *($15 for 13.6 ounces)*; **Scruples** Ultra Form Molding Spray *($6.95 for 8.5 ounces)*, High Definition Extra Dry Hair Spray *($4.95 for 1.5 ounces)*, Effects Fast Drying Styling Spray *($5.95 for 10.6 ounces)*, Effects Super Hold Finishing Spray *($5.95 for 10.6 ounces)*, Renewal Styling Spray for Colored Treated Hair *($6.50 for 8.5 ounces)*, Enforce Fast Drying Styling Spray *($7.50 for 8.5 ounces)*, and Enforce Plus Extra Firm Holding Spray *($7.50 for 8.5 ounces)*; **Senscience** Maximum Memory Firm Holding Spray *($8.99 for 6.5 ounces)*, Energy Spritz *($8.05 for 8 ounces)*, and Memory Mist Brushable Holding Spray *($7.99 for 6.5 ounces)*; **Shaper Slipline by Sebastian** Liquid Shaper Styling Gel and Fast Drying Hair Spray *($10.80 for 8.5 ounces)*, Liquid Shaper Plus, Extra Hold Hair Spray and Spray Gel *($9.95 for 8.5 ounces)*, Shaper Hair Spray Styling Mist for Hold and Control *($9.95 for 10 ounces)*, Shaper Plus Hair Spray Styling Mist for Super Hold and Extra Control *($18.30 for 18 ounces)*, and Shaper Zero g Weightless Hair Spray *($14.95 for 14.1 ounces)*; **Soft Sheen Alternatives** Firm Holding Spritz with MRC (Moisture Retention Complex) *($3.49 for 8 ounces)*; **Salon Formula by Suave** Spritz Ultimate Control *($0.78 for 7 ounces)*; **Sukesha** Freeze Frame Super Spray (Non-Aerosol) *($5.95 for 8 ounces)*, Styling Hair Spray, Working Spray with Firm Control (Non-Aerosol) *($5.95 for 8 ounces)*, Maximum Hold Hair Spray, Ultimate Hold Formula (Aerosol) *($6.95 for 10 ounces)*, and Shaping and Styling Hair Spray, Firm Design Formula (Aerosol) *($6.95 for 10 ounces)*; **TIGI** EnviroShape Firm Hold Hairspray *($11.50 for 10 ounces)*, Hold & Gloss Spray *($11.50 for 8 ounces)*, and Non-Aerosol Finishing Spray *($10.50 for 8 ounces)*; **Tressa** Sustain Design Spray, Maximum Hold for All Hair Types (Aerosol) *($9.99 for 10 ounces)*, Hair Spray Working and Finishing Spray (Aerosol) *($8.99 for 10 ounces)*, Sculpting Spray Flexible Holding Spray (Non-Aerosol) *($7.99 for 8 ounces)*, and Aliquis Design Spray, Firm Hold for All Hair Types *($8.99 for 8 ounces)*; **Vertu by Tressa** Air Form Finishing Mist *($15 for 14 ounces)*; **Tresemme** European Tres Hold Fixative Spray *($2.97 for 8.1 ounces)*, Two Extra Hold Working Hair Spray (Aerosol) *($2.97 for 13 ounces)*, Two Ultra Fine Mist Hair Spray *($2.97 for 11.2 ounces)*, European Tres Spray Styling Spritz, Super Hold *($3.69 for 10.5 ounces)*, 4+4 Extra Hold Brush Out Shaping Spray *($4.99 for 12.9 ounces)*, 4+4 Extra Hold Formula Hair Spray *($1.99 for 12.2 ounces)*, 4+4 Super Hold Styling Spritz *($3.99 for 12 ounces)*, and 4+4 Ultra Fine Mist Control Extra Hold Hair Spray *($1.99 for 12.2 ounces)*; **TRI** Prego Extra Extra Firm Hair Spray *($6.75 for 8 ounces)*; **Vidal Sassoon** Flexible Hold Hair Spray for Fine Hair with Formesilk (Aerosol) *($2.99 for 8.25 ounces)*, Flexible Hold Hair Spray for Fine Hair with Formesilk (Non-Aerosol) *($2.99 for 8.5* *ounces)*, Flexible Hold Hair Spray with Formesilk (Aerosol) *($2.99 for 8.25 ounces)*, Flexible Hold Hair Spray with Formesilk (Non-Aerosol) Scented and Unscented *($2.99 for 8.5 ounces)*, Ultra Firm Hold Hair Spray (Aerosol) *($2.99 for 8.25 ounces)*, and Ultra Firm Hold Hair Spray (Non-Aerosol) Scented and Unscented *($2.99 for 10.2 ounces)*; **Liquid Hair by Wella** Fast Finish Fixing Spritz *($8 for 6.8 ounces)* and Fast Finish Fixing Spritz *($8 for 6.8 ounces)*; **Herbs & Blossoms by White Rain** Angelica Hairspray Maximum Hold *($1.07 for 7 ounces)*.

Specialty Products

FAST DRY SHAMPOO AND CONDITIONER: **Active Express by Redken** Active Express Flash Wash Fast-Drying Shampoo *($7.50 for 10.1 ounces)*, Active Express Split Second Rinse-Out Conditioner *($7.95 for 8.5 ounces)*, and Active Express Quick Treat Treatment & Styler.

OIL-BASED SERUMS, SPRAYS, AND GELS: In many ways these are similar to silicone serums, sprays, and gels, though they do tend have a feel that is more "greasy" than silky. Their advantage for some hair types is that they can be more emollient and therefore in the long run more conditioning—but that's a fine line and one you may have to judge for yourself. As you may already have guessed, my preference is for the silicone versions earlier in this chapter. **General guidelines for use:** These are best used after shampooing and conditioning, on damp or dry hair. The serums and gels are best used before other styling products; the sprays can be used either before or after the hair is styled.

African Pride Miracle Sheen Oil Sheen & Conditioning Spray *($2.99 for 12.5 ounces)* and Wonder Weave Conditioning Sheen Spray *($3.49 for 2 ounces)*; **African Royale** BRX Braid & Extensions Spray On Shampoo *($3.99 for 12 ounces)*; **The Body Shop** Slick *($6.95 for 5.3 ounces)*; **Motions at Home** Oil Sheen and Conditioning Spray for Superb Sheen and Softness *($3.86 for 11.25 ounces)*; **Sheenique** Silk Oil Sheen Spray (Aerosol) *($3.19 for 10 ounces)*; **Soft Sheen** Oil Sheen Spray with MRC (Moisture Retention Complex) *($2.99 for 11.5 ounces)*; **Wanakee** Penetrating Nourishment for Braids *($21.95 for 8 ounces)*.

MOUSSES WITH DYE AGENTS: **Aubrey Organics** Chestnut Brown Natural Body Highlighter Mousse *($7.75 for 8 ounces)*, Golden Camomile Natural Body Highlighter Mousse *($7.75 for 8 ounces)*, and Soft Black Natural Body Highlighter Mousse *($7.75 for 8 ounces)*.

GELS WITH GLITTER: **Volume Formula by L'anza** Zero Weight Gel *($9.89 for 8.5 ounces)*.

CHAPTER ELEVEN

Problems? Solutions!

Holding on to Long Hair

If your hair hangs down to the middle of your back or longer, consider cutting it to just about shoulder length. I know you've probably read this recommendation elsewhere, but it is a good one. Those ends you keep thinking will get healthier if you just cut off an inch every now and then are not going to heal. The damage is more than just at the very ends. Hair becomes damaged just from being around a long time, especially if you've been dyeing it, styling it, or even just washing it frequently. Cutting off several inches will give you great volume and make your hair look incredibly healthy. It really will look like new.

No Time to Wash Your Hair

I've been so busy lately, there has been no time to do a thing with my hair, so I've been living in a ponytail, which is not my best look. To improve things, I take an extra few minutes to slick it back straight with some gel and hairspray, so it frames my face much better and looks rather elegant. I add a neutral-colored wrap around the cloth-covered rubber band I use to add a soft flair. But please, no big ribbons or banana clips—there's no other way than tacky to describe these accessories. This slicked-back look is a great way to get through a bad-hair day without looking like you're having one.

Battling with Fine, Limp Hair

Struggling with fine, limp hair isn't easy. It turns out that the less you do to fine hair, the better off it is. Anything that contains conditioners or styling agents just adds weight that drags things down. Consider a shorter cut and then color it. Hair color adds thickness to thin hair because it roughs up the cuticle, which creates artificially induced but natural-looking volume. Then all you have to do is use a gentle shampoo, period! Yes, less can mean more for this hair type when short is the style. The slight stiffness you get from not using a conditioner (instead of putting stiffness back in with a styling product) can also give you all the body you need. Give it a try. If you need to smooth things in place or reduce flyaways, take an anti-cling sheet from your dryer and rub it over your hair. You can also spray a tiny bit of hairspray on your fingertips and work them through the ends of your hair. This may be just what your hair is looking for.

Thick, Coarse Hair or Damaged Hair

If your hair is thick and coarse or chemically treated and damaged (which is really the same thing—chemically treated hair is always damaged), you may want to consider getting a bit more from your conditioner. Rather than investing in deep-conditioning products, take your regular conditioner and mix in a drop of M Professional Shine On Laminate, a pure silicone serum (yes, M Professional now has some hair products too), and a drop of safflower oil. Rub that into just the ends of your hair and not the roots—unless you have a dry scalp or very full hair you're trying to control, in which case the roots can take this treatment too—and let the mixture soak in for a while. Depending on your hair type, you can wash this mixture out or just rinse it off.

Growing Out a Perm

Perms can have such a, well, *permed* look, and the damage builds to almost complete hair degeneration with each successive perm you get. Sometimes the best and only option is to grow it out and never perm it again. When growing out a perm, you have a couple of choices. One is to cut it all off, a radical notion most women couldn't live with unless they are into a Demi Moore look. A better option is to cut off as much as you can stand and then follow the directions below for the tousled look.

Fast Fixes

No time to style? Try a tousled look. Use your fingers to separate your hair as you blow it dry. Lift at the roots and apply the heat there if you want more fullness. (I don't—my hair is plenty full on its own—so I slightly tug downward on my hair to make it lie a little flatter.) Add a slight amount of mousse when you're done to keep things neat and in place. It takes a while to get used to this look; at least it did for me. At first, I couldn't get over the fact that it looks messy and unstructured, but now it is my favorite hairstyle to use when I want to get out of the house fast.

A hairdresser friend gave me a great idea for when I look in the mirror and notice flyaways. Rather than applying hairspray or more mousse, which can make things sticky, she suggested that I take a tiny amount of moisturizer (which I always keep in my purse or briefcase for my hands), spread it all over my hands, and then use the little bit that doesn't get absorbed to coat the ends. She was right: voilà! No more frizzies!

Dry, Flaky Scalp

A dry or flaky scalp could be caused by a variety of things. Changes in weather can affect scalp moisture and cause flaking. Winter produces a dry climate in houses and offices, and the cold air outside can chap the skin, even on the scalp. Overwashing in the summer from swimming excursions can also cause a change in the scalp. Some medications, such as Accutane, can cause surface dryness too. Shampoos with strong detergent bases can dry out the scalp, as can some plant extracts such as peppermint or menthol.

The cause determines the course of action. If the products you're using are causing problems, stop! If you have to wash your hair frequently, don't lather more than once and try to massage the scalp as little as possible. If the environment in your house is a problem, put a humidifier in your bedroom, which can help the skin all over your body as well.

If you still are struggling with a dry scalp and dandruff isn't the culprit (dandruff would not be affected by any of the things suggested above), don't forget to massage a small amount of most any moisturizer such as Cetaphil Moisturizer, Lubriderm, or Eucerin Lite into your scalp at night when you plan to wash your hair the next morning.

If you scalp is constantly itchy and dandruff shampoos aren't helping, an over-the-counter cortisone cream such as Lanacort or Cortaid can be massaged into the scalp on nights when you plan to wash your hair the next morning.

By the way, the notion that drugstore dandruff shampoos are too harsh on the hair and salon brands are gentler is blatantly false. The active ingredients in salon brands are identical to those in Head & Shoulders, to mention just one line.

Styling Tricks of the Trade

Tension and heat are the keys to getting hair straight. The tighter you pull your hair and the better able you are to get heat on it, the straighter it will be. The reason stylists can get your hair so straight is because they are in the perfect position to get the necessary tension to make hair behave. Another trick that stylists use is to keep the blow-dryer moving instead of leaving it in one spot. Aiming the heat at the roots and making sure the roots are going in the direction you want—up for more fullness, down for straightening—is the best way to get control of your locks. Another styling essential is to move the blow-dryer down along the hair shaft instead of back and forth. Anything you can do to encourage the cuticle to lie flat will make your hair look smoother and shinier (that means no back-combing, which roughs up the cuticle, causing damage and dullness).

For coarse hair, the best styling help you can get is still hair serums, those pure silicone, oil-like products (like the one I mentioned above from M Professional) that add unbelievable shine and a silky feel to every strand. For thin or fine hair, the less you use the better. To help make normal or coarse hair behave, I find that the Studio Fix line from L'Oreal has a handful of gels and mousses that work great.

Static Electricity

Dry air means static electricity. A standard hairstylist trick for this problem is to spray a small amount of any hairspray on your hairbrush when you are done styling your hair and to brush it through from top to bottom. This one works for most of the day. No hairspray? Take your moisturizer, spread a very thin, imperceptible layer over your hands, and then gently smooth the tiny remaining amount over the flyaways. That will absolutely make them calm down.

Breakouts Along the Hairline

If you've been having problems with breakouts along your hairline, you need to be sure you're not having problems with your shampoo or conditioner. Change to a shampoo with no conditioning agents (such as protein, silicone, quaternium, or polyquaternium) or thickening agents (such as cetyl alcohol or stearyl alcohol), and use only the smallest amount of conditioner on the ends. Do this for a few days and see what happens. If the breakouts seem to be clearing up, you'll know you were using products that were too emollient for your scalp. Also, be sure the styling products you're using, especially hairsprays, gels, and mousses, aren't coming into contact with your skin. Styling products are a sure way to encourage breakouts, as the film-forming ingredients are great pore cloggers!

Hard Water

If you live in a hard water area, the use of a water softener can make a difference in how your hair and skin feel. What is hard water? The term "hardness" simply refers to the total concentration of calcium and magnesium ions present in the water. Why is hard water a problem? Hard water is an issue when it comes to any type of washing because it can take twice as much cleanser, shampoo, or laundry detergent to achieve the same level of cleanliness than it does for those using soft water. The other issue for hard water is that cleansing agents of any kind combine with the calcium and magnesium ions to form a film that doesn't easily rinse off, if at all. That film attaches to all kinds of surfaces including dishes, imperceptibly on clothes, bathtubs, and yes, skin and hair. In fact, the squeaky sound you may hear after washing your face or hair is due to the presence of calcium, not the effect of being clean. That means there really is no such thing as "squeaky clean." And yes, the film remains on your skin even after rinsing, which can clog pores and coat hair. According to several water-softening companies I called, the most economical way for you to soften household water is with an ion-exchange water softener. These types of units exchange the hard calcium and magnesium minerals with sodium, which has softening properties. This can be a far less costly process than trying to find hair-care products that make your hair feel softer and fuller. One word of warning: If you do choose to try a water softener in your home, when the "hard" minerals are removed, cleansers will no longer form a film and you won't get much of a "bathtub ring," but you may also experience a slippery feel on the skin and hair, almost too much "softness." That can take a while to get used to. It can also tend to make hair more flyaway, which would require different hair-care products than you would normally use when your hair was being rinsed with hard water.

CHAPTER TWELVE

Beauty that Respects Nature

Mankind's true moral test consists of its attitude toward those who are at its mercy: animals. And in this respect mankind has suffered a fundamental debacle, a debacle so fundamental that all others stem from it.

Milan Kundera, *The Unbearable Lightness of Being*

Animal Testing

The following is reprinted from my book Don't Go to the Cosmetics Counter Without Me, *4th Edition, because it accurately sums up my position on this very emotional, humane issue affecting any cosmetic you buy.*

I am proud to say that my cosmetics company, Paula's Choice and Paula's Select, does not test any aspect of its products on animals, and I donate a portion of its earnings to The Humane Society of the United States (HSUS) every year. Please check out HSUS's Web site at *www.hsus.org*. Its mailing address is The Humane Society of the United States, 2100 L Street N.W., Washington, D.C. 20037 (it can use your financial help as well).

HSUS's approach to the issue of animal rights and animal testing is one I agree with most strongly. The spring 1998 issue of *HSUS News* stated, "The HSUS shares with these scientists [the many who are opposed to or are uncomfortable with animal testing] the desire to eliminate the harmful use of animals in laboratories. In the meantime the HSUS is planning a campaign to urge the scientific community to adopt, as a priority goal, the elimination of all animal pain and distress in the laboratory. The HSUS believes that an emphasis on humane issues will lead to good science and will benefit, rather than harm, the advance of human knowledge."

For those of you unfamiliar with my full position on animal testing in cosmetics and in the medical research field, the following offers a discussion of the topic from my book *The Beauty Bible*.

Politically, I'm a moderate. I haven't always been. I grew up in the 1960s, and my politics have ranged from idealistic liberal to confused bipartisan. Now, as I stand on the cusp of the millennium, I can earnestly say I am convinced that few, if any, issues in life are black and white, or all or nothing. More and more often, I find that there is truth on both sides of the issues and the middle ground is often the only reasonable position. At least the middle ground is the only position that acknowledges the whole picture and not just one side. I vote both Republican and Democrat, depending on the individual and his or her voting record.

This middle position is also reflected in my perspective on animal testing as it pertains to cosmetics products and the health-care industry. While I unquestionably advocate the humane and ethical treatment of all life, especially unprotected and dependent life, I am not in favor of eliminating all forms of animal testing when it comes to health-care issues or human safety issues.

I feel terrible pain and anguish when I think of animals suffering in any way so I can put on mascara or clean my face. Many animal tests that are used to ascertain whether a cosmetic will hurt people are cruel and gratuitous. No one is ever going to eat 50 pounds of mascara. Forcing animals to do so in order to demonstrate how much mascara people can eat before they die makes me want to resign from the human race. How can anyone put an animal through such torture?

On the other hand, my older sister, who had breast cancer, my father, who had prostate cancer, my dearest friend's mother, who has Alzheimer's, my sister in-law who had melanoma, and my husband, who struggles with high blood pressure, all have undergone medical procedures and treatments that have prolonged and improved their quality of life—and all of these procedures and treatments have been proven effective and safe as a result of animal testing. I absolutely do not want to see even one animal die by being force-fed foundation or eyeshadow to prove it is a safe cosmetic formulation. And it would be my absolute preference in life that no animal suffer for any reason; yet if sacrificing an animal's life can help find the cure for Alzheimer's, prevent more cancers, or reduce the risks of high blood pressure and a host of other illnesses, I would and do support that research. Simultaneously, I actively donate money to animal-rights groups that are helping to encourage the creation of alternative testing methods so that eventually no animals will be needed for any kind of medical research.

Most of us are aware of the dramatic pictures distributed by animal-rights groups showing the terrible torment of animals in research laboratories. This is indeed a grotesque and painful exposé that all of us should be sickened by and do our best to change. But this narrow, shocking display does not address the results of animal research (the creation of safe products and medical treatments), nor does it represent the labs that treat animals humanely by caring for them and anesthetizing them.

Children who survive leukemia owe their lives to animal testing. Arthritis patients who can walk again owe their agility to animal testing. Successful excisions of brain tumors are due to animal testing—and on and on. Human health-care advancement and the use of animals to test various protocols and risks are inextricably linked and cannot be separated. This is the dilemma of animal testing.

There are many arguments from both points of view surrounding this issue. On one side are the animal-rights activists who claim there is no need or reason to ever use animal testing (or eat meat, use leather goods, or employ animals for any purpose other than as pets, and there are those who would say that even *that* is inappropriate). When it comes to animal testing, they point to alternative methods of research assessment that can be used. Spokespeople for People for the Ethical Treatment of Animals (PETA) and the National Anti-Vivisection Society (NAVS) claim that a preponderance of research proves that all animal testing is inconclusive and has no relation to what takes place in humans. Animal-rights activists insist that all animal testing is motivated by financial profit and stubborn old-fashioned doctors or "good old boys" who refuse to change. Their reasoning is that animal testing is big business, and no one wants to alter what they are doing and potentially lose money.

On the other side are a vast majority of physicians, medical research groups from most major universities, national medical organizations representing everything from cancer to heart disease, and pharmaceutical companies, all of which believe the use of animal models for research is essential to the evaluation of new and old medical treatments and procedures. These physicians and organizations often agree that in vitro (test tube–oriented) tests and computer model studies can replace some animal testing.

However, no one among these countless medical professionals would concede that all or even most animal testing is futile and immaterial. They can point to thousands of chemical substances and operations that were first determined to be safe and effective or dangerous and deleterious because of animal testing. Suggesting that these be stopped would halt most medical research, from AIDS to Alzheimer's to hair-growth products, and the development of any new drug.

The truth probably exists somewhere in the middle. Medical, pharmaceutical, and cosmetics industry experts freely admit that they were doing far more animal experiments than were needed to prove safety. Animal-rights activist campaigns inspired a vocal consumer base to force a major change in the number and type of animal tests being done. Many companies responded by reducing animal testing, changing to alternative methods whenever possible, and instituting humane treatment of their animals. Yet all or nothing is the goal of some animal-rights activists, and it may not be the goal of all consumers buying makeup, taking medicines, or considering medical procedures. Consumers should look at the whole issue and not just shocking pictures.

For example, according to an article in the January 1997 issue of *Drug and Cosmetic Industry* magazine, Gillette has been a boycott target of PETA since 1986. What PETA does not acknowledge is that, since its boycott, Gillette has reduced tests on animals by more than 90 percent, has contributed millions of dollars to alternative research, and has donated more than $100,000 to the Humane Society. You would think PETA would ease up on Gillette, but that isn't the case. It still lists Gillette among its companies to boycott. As long as a company does any animal testing, humane or otherwise, it is a target for PETA's condemnation. That is regrettable, because as a consumer you get only a limited perspective.

As a result of PETA's and NAVS's black-or-white position, you may be led to believe that The Body Shop is the greatest ally of animal rights since the inception of the concept. Yet, when faced with the publication of an article exposing The Body Shop's ambiguous animal-testing policy, owner Anita Roddick had her cabal of attorneys suppress the story from running in *Vanity Fair*. That only fueled the ire of reporter Jon Entine, who was then able to get his story published in *Business Ethics* and *Drug and Cosmetic Industry* magazines. It seems The Body Shop didn't want people to know its product development included use of ingredients that had been tested on animals; in fact, The Body Shop was banned from using the phrase "not tested on animals" on its products by West German courts in 1989. (The company subsequently began using the phrase "against animal testing.") According to a January 1997 article in *Drug and Cosmetic Industry* magazine, a research executive at The Body Shop in 1993 was quoted as saying that "the technology of alternative testing for raw materials has not yet sufficiently advanced to guarantee product safety." This story about The Body Shop was overlooked or completely ignored by both PETA and NAVS.

Most of us are against animal testing, but we also have the right to safe products and straight information about how that can best be accomplished. It would be wonderful if alternative, computer-based, and test-tube models were sufficient for establishing a cosmetic, drug, or medical procedure's safety, but that doesn't seem to be true, at least not now or in the near future. If alternatives become common practice, it will probably happen in the world of cosmetics first, mainly because cosmetics are not ingested, and alternative research methods for irritation studies are showing promise.

Frank Fairweather, head of clinical and pathological programs at the British Industrial Biological Research Association, is a frequent spokesperson in Europe on alternatives to animal testing of cosmetics. In a presentation Fairweather made at the Second World Congress on Alternatives to Animal Use in the Life Sciences, 1996, he said that "none of the alternative techniques could yet be reliably substantiated." He is hoping that research protocols can be quantified and then mimicked via in vitro methodology, but at this point, they don't exist, though he feels optimistic that in the next several years, tests will be developed that finally do away with the need for testing cosmetics on animals. I hope so too.

I will continue to earnestly support the humane and ethical treatment of animals, but I do not at this time support a complete ban on animal testing. I personally do not use animal testing, either directly or indirectly (meaning I don't hire third-party testing facilities to do my testing for me), for any of the cosmetic products I sell. I use only proven, long-established formulations and ingredients, as do many other companies that make claims about no animal testing. But because all of the cosmetics ingredients currently in use have at some point been tested on animals, especially sunscreens and other over-the-counter formulations such as skin lighteners, disinfectants, or chemical exfoliants and peels, no company can claim that the ingredients in its products involved no animal testing.

By creating products that are not tested on animals and by my support through financial contributions to such organizations as animal welfare groups and legal groups that fight for animal causes, I feel I am doing my part to help create a world in which fewer and fewer animals will be used for testing, and those that are will be treated humanely and ethically every step of the way.

I want my readers to know that I believe that their decisions and consumer activism in this area have been and continue to be vital. Cosmetics companies only started changing and looking for alternative methods because you, the consumer, brought pressure to bear and forced them to change. It is important to keep up this pressure. However, I feel it would be foolish to follow organizations like PETA and NAVS blindly unless you truly agree completely with their goal of abolishing all animal testing and creating a completely vegetarian society. **Instead, I encourage you to support organizations fighting for the welfare and safety of all animals, limited and humane animal testing, and continued research to find alternatives to animal testing in hopes that eventually someday no animal will have to be used in any research experiments.** This is completely in your power, because you, the consumer, have everything to say about what you buy and whom you buy it from, and that speaks loudly and clearly to all kinds of corporations and enterprises the world over.

Those of you who are very concerned about this issue may wonder why I include in my reviews product lines that test on animals. Although I personally support and donate money to the above-mentioned animal-rights group, I still feel strongly that it's my responsibility as a journalist to report on all types of cosmetics and hair-care products.

This is a consumer-oriented book about good and bad products, regardless of their research techniques. I cannot, in good conscience, avoid or ignore the companies that do animal testing. Women who disagree with my position on animal testing need consumer information too. But I can do my part by stating clearly which cosmetics companies do test on animals.

The following list is compiled from NAVS's 1999 booklet *Personal Care for People Who Care.* You can obtain your own free copy from The National Anti-Vivisection Society at 53 W. Jackson Street, Suite 1552, Chicago, IL 60604; phone (800) 888-NAVS; or visit its Web site at www.navs.org.

Animal Testing and Hair Care Products

Companies that do not test their finished products on animals:
Adorn
Almay
ARTec
Aubrey Organics
Aura
Aveda
Avon
Back to Basics
Bain de Terre
Beauty Without Cruelty
The Body Shop
Citre Shine
Clinique
Dark & Lovely
Dep
Focus 21
Framesi Biogenol
Freeman
Garden Botanika
Goldwell
Halsa
I.C.E.
Jason Natural
J. F. Lazartigue
Jheri Redding
John Frieda
Joico
Kenra
Kiehl's
KMS
L.A. Looks

L'Oreal
M.A.C.
Mastey
Neutrogena
Nexxus
Origins
Paul Mitchell
philosophy
Redken
Revlon
Schwarzkopf
Scruples
Sebastian
Soft & Beautiful
Thicker Fuller Hair
TIGI
TRI
Wash 'N Curl
Wella
White Rain
Zero Frizz

Companies that continue to test products on animals:
Alberto Culver
Aqua Net
Aussie
Clairol
Finesse
Head & Shoulders
Infusium 23
Jhirmack
Johnson & Johnson

Matrix
Motions at Home
Pantene
Pert
Prell
Quantum
Queen Helene
Rave
Salon Selectives
St. Ives
Style by Lamaur
Suave
TCB
ThermaSilk
Tresemme
Vibrance Organic Care
Vidal Sassoon

Companies with unknown animal-testing status:
African Pride
African Royale
AllWays Natural
American Crew
Apple Pectin by Lamaur
BioSilk
Bumble and Bumble
Denorex
Fudge
Graham Webb
Hayashi
Ion
ISO

Klorane
Lange
L'anza
M Professional
Nick Chavez
Nioxin
Ouidad
Phytotherathrie
Principal Secret
Professional
Progaine
Pro-Vitamin
Robert Craig
Rusk
Salon Style by Lamaur
Selsun Blue
Senscience
Sheenique
Soft Sheen
Sukesha
Sunglintz
Susan Lucci Collection
Tegren
Terax
Theorie
Tressa
Trevor Sorbie
Ultra Swim
Victoria Jackson
Wanakee
Willow Lake